A REFERENCE COMPANION TO THE HISTORY OF ABNORMAL PSYCHOLOGY

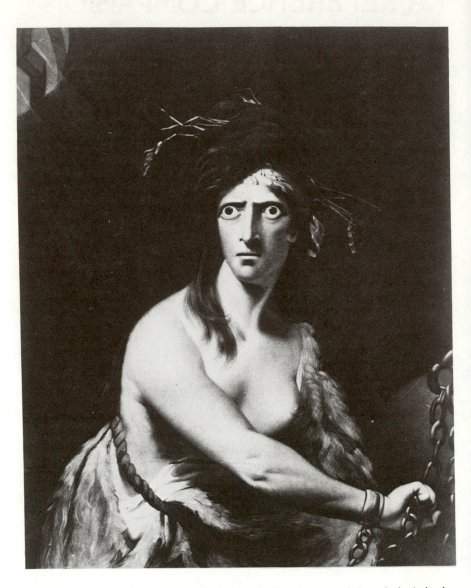

MADNESS. A dramatic representation of the breakdown of the mind: Agitation demands restraint by chains and ropes; the inappropriate clothing and the straw in the hair reflect disordered thought and the staring eyes suggest hallucination. Mezzotint by W. Dickson after R. E. Pine, 1775. By courtesy of the Wellcome Trustees, Wellcome Institute for the History of Medicine, London.

A REFERENCE COMPANION TO THE HISTORY OF ABNORMAL PSYCHOLOGY

John G. Howells
and
M. Livia Osborn

M — Z

GREENWOOD PRESS
Westport, Connecticut • London, England

Library of Congress Cataloging in Publication Data

Howells, John G.
  A reference companion to the history of abnormal
psychology.

  Includes index.
  1. Psychology, Pathological—Miscellanea.
2. Psychology, Pathological—Early works to 1900-
Miscellanea. I. Osborn, M. Livia, joint author.
II. Title.
RC454.4.H68   616.89   80-27163
ISBN 0-313-22183-9 (lib. bdg.)
ISBN 0-313-24261-5 (lib. bdg. : v. 1)
ISBN 0-313-24262-3 (lib. bdg. : v. 2)

Library of Congress Catalog Card Number: 80-27163
ISBN: 0-313-22183-9

First published in 1984

Greenwood Press
A division of Congressional Information Service, Inc.
88 Post Road West
Westport, Connecticut 06881

Printed in the United States of America

10 9 8 7 6 5 4 3 2 1

Contents

Illustrations

Acknowledgments

It gives us pleasure to record our grateful appreciation of help received from Miss Jessica Smith, Mrs. Patricia Smith, and the Department of Medical Illustration of the Ipswich Hospital.

Introduction

A Reference Companion to the History of Abnormal Psychology is a source book and a channel to the history of abnormal psychology. As it gleans from the pastures of the literature of abnormal psychology, it is also an analecta. As many of its entries were selected for their fascination, it is a delectus. As It hopes to be a ready servant to the reader, it is an ancilla. The book provides within its covers material of historical interest in the field of abnormal psychology that is not found in a single volume. By the term "abnormal" we mean the unusual as well as the frankly pathological. These two terms are taken in their historical context. For example, although conditions such as mental retardation and epilepsy are not now considered part of the field of abnormal psychology, they were in the past. Because they were not understood, the behavior they engendered was linked to psychiatric disorders.

The *Companion* paints on a broad canvas packed with holy springs, sacred plants, old superstitions, ancient fears, amulets, potions, strange beliefs, madhouses, scientific ideas, instruments of therapy, legal edicts, famous books, poets, painters, politicians, kings, queens, humble folk, popes, and debauchers, saints and sinners, healers and the healed, exploiters and the exploited, the wise and the foolish. A male soprano, FARINELLI, who, with his golden voice, cured Philip V of Spain of his melancholy, precedes an entry on FARMING, a method of therapy imposed on mental patients in eighteenth-century Scotland. MAHLER's emotional difficulties and the diagnosis of his condition by Freud give a new dimension to the understanding of his music. SPIRIT OF SKULL, as administered to Charles II of England, the SPINNING CHAIR, TOBACCO and its history, the strange symptoms of TARANTISM and the psychopathic activities of the THUGS are some of the entries that throw an unusual, intriguing, and often unexpected light on the history of abnormal behavior, its explanation and its treatment. Should the reader require brief biographical details and data on the major achievements of famous physicians of antiquity, psychiatrists, or psychologists and relatively modern workers in allied disciplines, especially in neurology, these will be found within the *Companion*, as well as entries on major hospitals of historical interest and material, which, although not abnormal or unusual, is relevant to the field. Again, the relevance of some entries is to be found in their historical context; a belief or a practice that today is considered commonplace, was once unusual, originated from a unexpected source, or was in advance of its time.

Whenever the opportunity presented, we have added a touch of human interest. We have deliberately paused on any unusual, intriguing, or humorous note; flesh has been added to bare bones, without deviating from the truth. Most entries have been completed with a bibliographical reference that the reader can consult for further information or use to begin the study of a particular subject.

The reasons for the selection of some entries are obvious, particularly in those entries concerning famous contributors to the field of abnormal behavior. There is, however, always some room for a difference of opinion, as each individual has a personal store of cherished particles of knowledge. Some of the material that is not directly a part of abnormal psychology leaves latitude for a personal element in selection. We hope our choice meets the requirements of most readers. The weight given to each entry called for considerable judgment. The key factor was its usefulness to the reader. Some material is readily available elsewhere, thus we have given it short space. Less accessible material that is likely to intrigue the reader is given more space. With a few exceptions, living people have been omitted.

The book is intended for those readers who have an interest in abnormal psychology in its broadest sense. The general reader will find not only pleasure but also information in the *Companion*. We believe the *Companion* will be equally at home on the shelves of professional and general libraries as on the private desk. As a reference work, it will, of course, have a particular appeal to the writer, researcher, teacher, and student in the field of abnormal psychology.

The foundation of the book rests on material gathered over the last twenty-five years. A still growing collection of books, articles, and notes accumulated for a quarter of a century seemed too precious to be left unused and its excitement unshared. Thus, over the last ten years, we set out to marshal the material in an easily retrievable form before offering to share it with others, who, like us, worship at the shrine of Clio.

Over 4200 entries are arranged in alphabetical order with frequent cross references. Structured reading is made possible by the category appendix. For example, a reader interested in the history of hypnosis will find categorized in the appendix those items referring to it. Another reader may wish to abstract items that would give him a collection of names of artists noted for their abnormal behavior. Yet another may wish to collect the names of saints invoked by the insane. All this and more is possible. Each reader can easily compile a bibliography for further reading in his field of interest by collecting the relevant references provided in each entry.

We have been particularly careful to assure the accuracy of our facts, but, like others before us, we have learned that sources sometimes disagree. Whenever posible, we have consulted original sources or those most likely to be exact. Nevertheless, we are bound to have made errors both of ommission and commission.

We found our material in the most unexpected places. We went from old texts to daily newspapers, from sacred books to profane manuals, from biographies to works of art, and all of them yielded a particle for inclusion. In the quest for relevant, useful, and intriguing material hundreds of books have been searched. Not unlike Burton's *Anatomy of Melancholy*, the *Companion* casts its net wide in time and place and harvests a multitude of facts, ranging from unusual objects and strange beliefs to brief biographies and little known anecdotal curiosities. We were fascinated, awed, amused, and, at times, depressed by what we found. It was impossible to record it all. Every reader will know of material he would like to see included; some— we hope most—he will find among our selection. Inevitably some material will not appear due to the limitations of our experience, or it may have been unavailable to us, or it may have been omitted to meet the constraints of space. Every reader, therefore, can find pleasure in adding to the items we make available.

Journal Abbreviations

Acta Paedopsychiat.
Acta Psychiatrica
  Scandinavica
Allg. Zeitschr. f. Psych.

Amer. Anthropologist
Am. Imago
Am. J. Clin. Hypn.

Am. J. Dis. Chil.

Am. J. of Medical Sciences

Am. J. Obstetr.
Am. J. Psychiat.
Am. J. Psychol.
Anatomischer Anzeiger
Ann. med. psychol.
Annals of Medical History
Archive de Psychologie
Archive für pathologische
  Anatomie und Physiologie
Archiv. für Psychiatrie
Arch. Gen. Psychiat.
Arch. Neur. Paris

Berliner Klinische Wchnschr.
Brain
Bristol Med.-Chir. J.
Brit. J. Dermatol.
Brit. J. Psychiat.

Acta Paedopsychiatrica
Acta Psychiatrica Scandinavica

Allgemeine Zeitschrift für
  Psychiatrie

American Anthropologist
American Imago
American Journal of Clinical
  Hypnosis
American Journal of Diseases
  of Childhood
American Journal of Medical
  Sciences
American Journal of Obstetrics
American Journal of Psychiatry
American Journal of Psychology
Anatomischer Anzeiger
Annales medico-psychologiques
Annals of Medical History
Archive de Psychologie
Archive für pathologische
  Anatomie und Physiologie
Archives für Psychiatrie
Archives of General Psychiatry
Archives of Neurology, Paris

Berliner Klinische Wochenschrift
Brain
Bristol Medico-Chirurgical Journal
British Journal of Dermatology
British Journal of Psychiatry

Bull. Hist. Med.	Bulletin of the History of Medicine
Bull. Menninger Clinic	Bulletin of the Menninger Clinic
Bull. Soc. d'anthrop. de Paris	Bulletin de la Societé d'anthropologie de Paris
Bull. Univer. de Lyon	Bulletin de l'Université de Lyon
Bulletins de la Societé de psychologie physiologiques	Bulletins de la Societé de psychologie physiologiques
Can. Med. Assn. J.	Canadian Medical Association Journal
Can. Psychiat. Ass. J.	Canadian Psychiatric Association Journal
Clin. Lect. Rep. London Hosp.	Clinical Lecture Report, London Hospital
Confinia Psychiat.	Confinia Psychiatrica
Developmental Medicine and Child Neurology	Developmental Medicine and Child Neurology
Encéphale	Encéphale
Epilepsia	Epilepsia
Episteme	Episteme
Essays in Applied Psychoanalysis	Essays in Applied Psychoanalysis
Hamdard	Hamdard
Hist. Med.	Histoire de la Médicine
Hist. Sci. Med.	History of Scientific Medicine
Indian Antiquary	Indian Antiquary
Indian J. Psychiat.	Indian Journal of Psychiatry
Int. J. Psychoanal.	International Journal of Psychoanalysis
Int. J. Psychoanal. Psychoth.	International Journal of Psychoanalytic Psychotherapy
Int. J. Soc. Psychiat.	International Journal of Social Psychiatry
Irrenfreund	Irrenfreund
Journal de Psichologie	Journal de Psichologie
J. Ethno-pharmacology	Journal of Ethno-pharmacology
J. Experimental Medicine	Journal of Experimental Medicine
J. Homosex.	Journal of Homosexuality
J. Ment. Sci.	Journal of Mental Sciences
J. Psychol. Med. Ment. Pathol.	Journal of Psychological Medicine and Mental Pathology

J. Psychol.	Journal of Psychology
J. Sex. Res.	Journal of Sexual Research
J. Hist. Behav. Sci.	Journal of the History of Behavioral Sciences
J. Hist. Med. & All. Sci.	Journal of the History of Medicine and Allied Sciences
J. Hist. Philosophy	Journal of the History of Philosophy
J. of the Polynesian Society	Journal of the Polynesian Society
Lancet	Lancet
Life Threatening Behavior	Life Threatening Behavior
Med. Hist.	Medical History
Med. J. Australia	Medical Journal of Australia
Med. Klin., Berlin	Medizine Klinik, Berlin
Medical Women's Federation J.	Medical Women's Federation Journal
Medico-Chirurgical Transactions	Medico-Chirurgical Transactions
Mem. Nat. Acad. Sci.	Memorandum of National Academy of Sciences
Milbank Memorial Fund Quarterly	Milbank Memorial Fund Quarterly
Minerva Medica	Minerva Medica
Mod. Lang. Rev.	Modern Language Review
Neurology	Neurology
New Zealand Med. J.	New Zealand Medical Journal
Practitioner	Practitioner
Proceedings of the Society of Psychical Research	Proceedings of the Society of Psychical Research
Proc. Roy. Soc. Med.	Proceedings of the Royal Society of Medicine
Psychiatric Annals	Psychiatric Annals
Psychiat. Neurol.	Psychiatria, Neurologia, Neurochirurgia
Psychiatric News	Psychiatric News
Psychiatry	Psychiatry
Psychoanal. Quart.	Psychoanalytic Quarterly
Psychol. Bull.	Psychological Bulletin
Psychol. Med.	Psychological Medicine
Psychological Rev.	Psychological Review
Review of English Studies	Review of English Studies
Revue Philosophique	Revue Philosophique
Rivista Sperimentale di Freniatria	Rivista Sperimentale di Freniatria

Soc. Psychiatry	Social Psychiatry
Spike Wave	Spike Wave
Trans. Stud. Coll. Physicians Phila.	Transactional Studies of the College of Physicians of Philadelphia
Transactions of the Amer. Ophthalmol. Soc.	Transactions of the American Ophthalmological Society
Trans. Ophthal. Soc. U.K.	Transactions of the Ophthalmological Society of the United Kingdom
Transcultural Psychiatric Research Review	Transcultural Psychiatric Research Review
World Medicine	World Medicine
World Psychiatric Assn. Bulletin	World Psychiatric Association Bulletin
Yale J. Biol. Med.	Yale Journal of Biology and Medicine
Zeitschrift für die gesamte Neurologie und Psychiatrie	Zeitschrift für die gesamte Neurologie und Psychiatrie

A REFERENCE COMPANION TO THE HISTORY OF ABNORMAL PSYCHOLOGY

M

MAB. In English folklore (q.v.) she was queen of the fairies. William Shakespeare (q.v.) described her in *Romeo and Juliet*, I, iv as the midwife of the fairies and said she helped at the birth of dreams (q.v.) in the brains of men.

MACBETH, LADY. The wife of Macbeth in the play *Macbeth* by William Shakespeare (q.v.). She is a psychopathic (*see* PSYCHOPATHY) character, unremorseful and unrestrained. After instigating dreadful deeds, she becomes unbalanced. Her symptoms include sleepwalking and ablutomania (q.v.). The doctor called to help her states that she is "troubled with thick-coming fancies that keep her from her rest" (*Macbeth*, 5.5), a diagnosis that provokes Macbeth's outburst, "Cure her of that!"

> Canst thou not minister to a mind diseased,
> Pluck from the memory a roothed sorrow,
> Raze out the written troubles of the brain
> And with some sweet oblivious antidote
> Cleanse the stuffed bosom of that perilous stuff
> which weights upon the heart?

[*Macbeth*, 5.5]

Bibliography: Shakespeare, W. *Macbeth*.

McCARTHY, JOSEPH RAYMOND (1909-1957). An American politician. He was notorious for his inquisitions and accusations of communism. President Harry S Truman (1884-1972) described him as a "pathological character assassin," thus underlining the unhealthy quality of his personality.
Bibliography: Griffin, R., and Theoharis, A. 1974. *The spectre: original essays on the Cold War and the origins of McCarthyism*.

MACDONALD, ARTHUR (1856-1936). An American anthropologist. He was a specialist in the criminology and education of psychopaths. His nu-

merous writings included books on suicide (q.v.) and insanity, hypnotism, psychoanalysis, alcoholism (qq.v.), and prisons. He also established standards for comparing normal and abnormal children.
Bibliography: MacDonald, A. 1905. *Man and abnormal man.*

McDOUGALL, WILLIAM (1871-1938). A British psychologist. Before turning to psychology he studied medicine to understand how the brain and the nervous system influence behavior. His biological approach to psychology was greatly influenced by the work of William James (q.v.). In 1920 McDougall emigrated to the United States, where he systematized and developed many of his views. A controversial figure, he supported eugenics (q.v.) and psychical research, which were unpopular causes at the time. He was a pioneer in physiological and social psychology and developed a system known as "hormic psychology," which asserted that all activity was not based solely on instinct but had a purpose and a goal as well. He wrote numerous books and papers, including *Physiological Psychology* (1905), *Social Psychology* (1908), and *Outline of Abnormal Psychology* (1926). McDougall's theories influenced Sigmund Freud (q.v.) when he formulated his group theories.
Bibliography: Boring, E. G. 1950. *A history of experimental psychology.*

MACH, ERNST (1838-1916). Austrian physicist and philosopher. He believed that all physical and psychological phenomena could be reduced to sensations, which were, therefore, the data of all sciences. His work established the basis of modern positivism (q.v.).
Bibliography: Boring, E. G. 1950. *A history of experimental psychology.*

MACHIAVELLI, NICCOLÒ (1469-1527). An Italian statesman and writer. He wrote the famous treatise, *Il Principe*, (*The Prince*) (1532) for Lorenzo de' Medici in which he asserted that political deceit and unethical methods are justified if they are used as means to a noble end. Political leaders should appear to have good qualities, even if they did not possess them. It is thought that Cesare Borgia was the model for the Prince. He considered man in relation to social and personal problems and dealt with psychological issues in a concrete manner that rejected the abstractions and theories of previous philosophers.
Bibliography: Fleischer, H. 1973. *Machiavelli and the nature of political thought.*

MACHINES. The advent of the use of machines in industry towards the end of the eighteenth century was also the advent of their use in psychiatry. Most of the contraptions introduced in the treatment of psychiatric patients were designed to revolve or swing the patient until he experienced vertigo, vomiting, and total exhaustion or loss of consciousness. The principle was to produce shock in the organism, which in turn, restored sanity. In practice,

these machines were used on patients who were considered uncooperative. Not surprisingly, it was reported that the machines had a salutary influence and treatment seldom had to be repeated. Erasmus Darwin, William S. Hallaran, and Benjamin Rush (qq.v.) were among the enthusiastic advocates of these devices. The machines were eventually abandoned, but not before a few fatal accidents had demonstrated how dangerous they were.
See also GYRATOR, ROTATORY MACHINE, SPINNING CHAIR, SWINGING CHAIR, TWIRL-ING STOOL, and WHIRLING CHAIR.
Bibliography: Kraepelin, E. 1962. *One hundred years of psychiatry.*

MACKLIN, CHARLES (c.1700-1797). An Irish actor and dramatist. He wrote and acted in *Love à la Mode* (1759) and *The Man of the World* (1781). His dignified and tragic portrayal of Shylock made him famous. He was an eccentric, arrogant, and quarrelsome man and an inveterate gambler. The death of his daughter is said to have caused his final mental breakdown. He became senile and was unable to remember his lines.
Bibliography: Winslow, L.S.F. 1898. *Mad humanity: its forms apparent and obscure.*

McLEAN ASYLUM. An American institution for the insane in Massachu-setts. It was opened in 1818 as part of a general hospital. Dr. Rufus Wyman was the first resident superintendent and the first medical man to hold such a position in America. He adopted the humane treatment advanced by Phi-lippe Pinel (q.v.) and William Tuke (q.v.). The first patient to be admitted was believed by his family to be possessed (*see* POSSESSION) by the devil and had been severely whipped by his father in an effort to exorcise (*see* EXORCISM) him. In the asylum (q.v.) his treatment was more clinical, and, on discharge, he became a prosperous pedlar. In 1821 the institution adopted the name McLean in gratitude to a Boston merchant, John McLean, who had given the asylum a large sum of money. At that time the hospital housed about two dozen patients. In 1826, Dr. Luther V. Bell (q.v.) became its physician and superintendent. Under Bell, many innovations were intro-duced, including a new heating system of circulating hot water that produced a warm current of air. In 1882, the first modern American training school for attendants was organized at McLean by Dr. Edward Cowles.
Bibliography: Fletcher Little, N. 1972. *Early years at the McLean Hospital.*

M'NAUGHTEN (or McNAUGHTON), DANIEL (?-1865). A British joiner born in Glasgow, Scotland. His name has been spelled sixteen different ways. He was illegitimate, and as a child he was said to be solitary and strange in his behavior. As an adult, he lived alone in lodgings, and, after he had been evicted, he slept in his workshop. He became paranoid (*see* PARANOIA), imagined that he was being followed by enemies with mur-derous intentions, and complained of violent headaches. After a short period in France, he returned to England completely convinced that the Tory party was against him. He planned to kill the prime minister, Sir Robert Peel (1788-1850) but shot his secretary, Edward Drummond, by mistake. His trial made history when he was acquitted on the grounds of insanity in 1843. The House of Lords, worried at the public outcry against the verdict, summoned the judges to explain how they had reached their decision. Their explanation resulted in the M'Naughten rules (q.v.). M'Naughten was admitted to Bethlem Royal Hospital (q.v.) where he spent the remaining twenty years of his life.

Bibliography: West, D. J., and Walk, A. 1977. *Daniel McNaughton: his trial and the aftermath.*

M'NAUGHTEN RULES. The legal rules introduced in the House of Lords in 1843 to clarify the law following the trial of Daniel M'Naughten (q.v.). The rules influenced the laws of Great Britain and the United States in their acceptance of insanity as a defence in criminal trials.

Bibliography: West, D. J., and Walk, A. 1977. *Daniel McNaughton: his trial and the aftermath.*

MADAME D. The designation given by Pierre Janet (q.v.) to one of his patients whom he investigated in depth at the Salpêtrière (q.v.). She was a thirty-four-year-old seamstress suffering from amnesia (q.v.). Janet treated her by hypnosis (*see* HYPNOTISM) and used her in his famous clinical demonstration of December 22, 1891. His concept of dynamic amnesia was based on observations made around this patient.

Bibliography: Charcot, J. M. 1893. *Clinique des maladies du système nerveux.*

MAD AS A HATTER *or* **THE MAD HATTER.** The expressions may be derived from episodes of organic psychosis (q.v.) in hat makers due to the toxic effect of mercuric nitrate, a chemical employed in the manufacture of felt hats. Robert Crab, a seventeenth-century haberdasher of hats, is believed to have been the original "mad hatter." After receiving a head injury in the Civil War of 1642, he developed religious mania (q.v.). He gave all his goods away and became a recluse and prophet. Another view bases the term on John Hatter (q.v.). The phrase, however, owes its popularity to the Mad Hatter in *Alice in Wonderland* (1865) by Lewis Carroll (q.v.). Carroll's Mad Hatter is thought to have been based on Theophilus Carter, a furniture dealer near Oxford who was known in his area as the Mad Hatter because he wore a top hat and was an eccentric.

Bibliography: Spalding, K. 1951. Poisoning from mercurous nitrate used in the making of felt hats. *Mod. Lang. Rev.* 46: 442.

MAD-DOCTOR. A term used in the eighteenth century to designate doctors dealing with insanity. Mad-business was the term then used for psychiatry (q.v.).

MADELINE (1853-1918). A patient of Pierre Janet (q.v.). She was admitted to Salpêtrière (q.v.) in 1896 with mystical delusions (q.v.), ecstasies (*see* ECSTASY), and signs of stigmata (q.v.). Janet met her when she was forty-two years old and remained in contact with her even after her discharge for approximately twenty-five years, which enabled him to compile a detailed case history. The theories he developed around Madeline were expounded by him in 1826 in a book entitled *De l'Angoisse à l'Extase*, that aroused violent controversy, especially among Catholics.
Bibliography: Ellenberger, H. F. 1970. *The discovery of the unconscious.*

MAD MAUDLIN. Also known as Bess O'Bedlam (q.v.). She was the companion of Tom O'Bedlam (q.v.) in the popular songs of the seventeenth century.
Bibliography: O'Donoghue, E. G. 1914. *The story of Bethlehem Hospital.*

MAD PARLIAMENT. The English Parliament assembled in Oxford in June 1258 to plan the reforms agreed upon by Henry III (1207-1272) and his barons. A contemporary chronicler named it *insigne parlamentum*, but the word *insigne* (famous) was read as *insanus* (mad), and the Parliament was erroneously named.
Bibliography: Steinberg, S. H., and Evans, I. H., eds. 1970. *Steinberg's dictionary of British history.*

MAD POET. The term by which Nathaniel Lee (q.v.) was known toward the end of his life.
Bibliography: 1964. *The Oxford companion to English literature.* ed. P. Harvey.

MAD-SHIRT. A garment used at the Pennsylvania Hospital (q.v.) to restrain patients. Thomas G. Morton, the historian of the hospital, described it as "a close-fitting cylindrical garment of ticking, canvas or other strong material without sleeves, which, drawn over the head, reached below the knees, and left the patient an impotent bundle of wrath, deprived of effective motion."
See also STRAIT-WAISTCOAT.
Bibliography: Morton, T. G. 1895. Reprint. 1973. *The history of the Pennsylvania Hospital, 1751-1895.*

MADWORT. The popular name for a species of the genus *Alyssum*. In antiquity it was used in the treatment of the insane to moderate violent and destructive behavior.
Bibliography: Law, D. 1969. *Herb growing for health.*

MAENADS. In Greek mythology (q.v.), women inspired by Dionysus (q.v.). It was believed that he endowed them with superhuman strength. They were not bound by any social convention and roamed the countryside

hunting wild animals. Because their rites led to frenzies, they became identified with madness.
Bibliography: Graves, R. 1960. *The Greek myths.*

MAGAZIN ZUR ERFAHRUNGSSEELENKUNDE. The first psychiatric journal ever published. It was begun in Berlin in 1783 by Karl Philipp Moritz (q.v.). Its full translated title was *Know Thyself, or Magazine for Empirical Psychology for Scholars and Laymen.* Three issues were published per year for ten years until the death of its founder. Its articles discussed a wide field, including psychoses (*see* PSYCHOSIS) and neurotic (*see* NEUROSIS) disorders. Special emphasis was given to childhood memories and to dreams (q.v.). The authors of the articles were usually physicians, teachers, clergymen, and lawyers. Moritz gave up his editorship for three years while he was in Italy but resumed control on his return having discovered that the new editor, C.F. Pockels had turned the journal into an instrument of attack against religion.
Bibliography: Eng, E. 1973. Karl Philipp Moritz's *Magazin Zur Erfahrungsseelenkunde* [Magazine for Empirical Psychology] 1783-1793. *J. Hist. Behav. Sci.* 9: 300-305.

MAGDALENE ASYLUMS. A term used for referring to institutions established for reclaiming prostitutes. The term was derived from Mary Magdalene, the woman who anointed Christ's feet and repented of her sins (Luke 7: 37).
Bibliography: 1978. *Brewer's dictionary of phrase and fable.*

MAGDALENE HOSPITAL. Originally, a charitable foundation in Bath, England. It was connected with the Priory Chapel of Saint Mary Magdalene. It originated in the seventeenth century as a hospital for lepers (*see* LEPROSY). When leprosy became less common, the hospital cared for idiots and insane paupers. It later was amalgamated with the municipal charities of Bath, but continued its care of mental defectives.
Bibliography: Kanner, L. 1964. *A history of the care and study of the mentally retarded.*

MAGENDIE, FRANÇOIS (1783-1855). A French physiologist. His family became impoverished during the French Revolution, and, as a youth, his frustration with a life of poverty made him depressed and apathetic. He speedily recovered when he was informed that he had inherited a large sum of money. Within a year he had spent his entire inheritance and was forced to return to his medical studies. He is now considered a founder of experimental physiology. Independently of Sir Charles Bell (q.v.), he discovered the function of the cerebrospinal nerve roots. His experiments advanced the study of the reflexes.

See also BELL-MAGENDIE LAW.

Bibliography: Haymaker, W., and Schiller, F. 1970. *The founders of neurology.* 2d. ed.

MAGGOT. In English folklore (q.v.) it was believed that moody or whimsical individuals had maggots in their brains.

Bibliography: 1978. *Brewer's dictionary of phrase and fable.*

MAGIC. Magico-religious practices have played a significant role in medicine, particularly psychiatry even from the earliest times. Primitive cultures have attributed supernatural forces to phenomena that they cannot understand and have tried to counteract their malevolent effects with magic rituals, amulets (q.v.), charms and by spoken words of special significance. Abnormal behavior has often been linked with magic practices. The powerful element of suggestion in all forms of magic has been an aetiological factor in mental disorders as well as a therapeutic tool. Religious beliefs and an increasing understanding of the laws of nature have caused the persecution of magicians and witches (*see* WITCHCRAFT) at various times but their observations and experimentations have often pointed the way to truth.

Bibliography: Sperber, P. A. 1973. *Drugs, demons, doctors, and disease.*

MAGIC MOUNTAIN, THE. A novel by Thomas Mann (q.v.) written in German in 1924. It describes the patients in a tuberculosis (q.v.) sanatorium in the Swiss Alps and their interaction. Psychoanalysis (q.v.), hypnotism (q.v.), and other forms of psychiatric treatment are discussed. The book portrays the mood swings often connected with tubercular patients and reflects the emotional turmoil felt by many Europeans during that period. The theme of the novel was suggested to Mann by visits to a sanatorium at Davas, Switzerland, where his wife was a patient.

Bibliography: Mann, T. 1970. *The magic mountain,* trans. H.D.L. Porter.

MAGIC SHOT. A foreign body, which in primitive medicine is believed to be a spirit that enters the victim's body and causes illness. The foreign body can be a splinter of wood or bone. The term lingers in the German word *Hexenschuss,* or lumbago, which literally means "witch-shot." The fear of injections in primitive people is explained by this belief.

Bibliography: Pollack, K. 1968. *The healers,* trans. E. A. Underwood.

MAGNAN, VALENTIN (1835-1916). A French physician. He began his career by investigating the brain changes occurring in general paralysis of the insane (q.v.). His first paper was published in 1864, and discussed the toxic effect of absinthe (q.v.). He later studied the neurological and mental changes brought about by alcoholism (q.v.) and, because alcoholism was particularly prevalent in France at that time, advocated the establishment of special hospitals for alcoholics. He also organized a special laboratory for the study of alcoholism and drug addiction. He lectured widely, and his theory of hereditary mental degeneration was accepted both in France and abroad. Eugen Bleuler (q.v.) studied under him and was influenced by him. Magnan was against the physical restraint (q.v.) of mental patients and promoted its abolition. His theories were popularized in many novels, including those by Émile Zola (q.v.).

Bibliography: Zilboorg, G. 1941. *A history of medical psychology.*

MAGNET. A lodestone. The magnet's property of attracting iron and steel has been known since the time of Thales of Miletus in the sixth century B.C. The name may have been derived from the Greek shepherd, Magnet, who discovered its properties or from the city of Magnesia in Asia Minor, where it was first found. It was used in medicine from ancient times to draw out poisons and humors (q.v.). Avicenna (q.v.) advised it as an antidote for iron in the organism, which he considered poisonous. Dioscorides (q.v.) wrote that the magnet could draw out humors and differentiate between chaste and adulterous women; when placed in the bed of the chaste woman, he believed that she would reach for her husband, while in the bed of the adulterous woman, it would cause her to have bad dreams (q.v.) and to fall out of bed. Aetius of Amida (q.v.) used it in the treatment of mental disorders, and Paracelsus (q.v.) believed in a "universal fluid" that acted on the body like a magnet. Ambroise Paré (q.v.) used magnets in poultices in the treatment of hernias, and the entire concept of magnetism (q.v.) as a cosmic fluid was the base of the doctrine developed by Franz Mesmer (q.v.). Even toward the end of nineteenth century, Cesare Lombroso (q.v.) was using "correctly orientated" magnets in the treatment of certain nervous disorders.

MAGNETISM. Although the concept took its name from the magnet (q.v.), it had nothing to do with it. Franz Mesmer (q.v.), while treating patients with magnets, discovered that it was not their effect, but some other force, which he compared to a magnetic force, that brought about cures. He came to believe that a special "fluid" emanating from himself affected the patients. He discarded magnets and relied solely on what he called "animal magnetism" (q.v.) absorbed from the magnetic fluid that he thought filled the universe. An imbalance of this fluid, according to him, would result in illness. Mesmer and his followers developed various contraptions and techniques, and magnetism became a popular and expensive form of treatment. Patients, singly or in groups, were magnetized by the establishment of a flow of "fluid" from the therapist. They then would experience a therapeutic "crisis" that consisted of convulsions and attacks of crying or laughing.

Many cures were reported, and the popular imagination was stimulated by literary works concerned with it. In 1784 the Académie des Sciences (q.v.) appointed a committee to investigate it and its findings condemned it. Philippe Pinel (q.v.) was among those who refused to take the new vogue seriously and jokingly said that he would not mind prescribing "to the ladies the charming manoeuvre of magnetism," but he would hastily send the men to the drug store. Although magnetism eventually fell into disrepute and was ridiculed in plays and satirical cartoons, it helped the understanding of phenomena that later formed the basis for the dynamic approach in psychiatry. *See also* HYPNOTISM and MESMERISM.

Bibliography: Buranelli, V. 1975. *The Wizard from Vienna: Franz Anton Mesmer and the origins of hypnotism.*

MAGNUS MORBUS. A Latin term meaning "the great disease." It was another of the many terms for epilepsy (q.v.).

MAGNUS, RUDOLF (1873-1927). A German physiologist. With Sir Charles Sherrington (q.v.), he undertook research on the reflex mechanism of the central nervous system. Working with other scientists at the University of Utrecht, he contributed a vast amount of literature to the field of neurology (q.v.).

Bibliography: Haymaker, W., and Schiller, F. 1970. *The founders of neurology.* 2d. ed.

MAHLER, GUSTAV (1860-1911). A Czech-Austrian composer. He was one of twelve children in a Jewish family. His parents did not love each other or their children. Five of the children died of diphtheria, one committed suicide, one died of a brain tumor, and another was killed in an accident. Of those left, Aloys was unstable, and Gustav was oversensitive, lonely, and anguished. His mother, a sickly woman, spent most of her time in bed. He married when he was forty-one years old, a woman twenty years his junior, who had little in common with him, and he neglected her to the point of cruelty. After finding a love letter addressed to her his emotional difficulties and his mood swings worsened. He became impotent and eventually agreed to see Sigmund Freud (q.v.), who, during a walking consultation in Leyden, Holland, diagnosed a mother-fixation. Mahler was said to have been cured and to have found a new attachment to his wife, but nine months later he died of a streptococcal infection. The manuscript of his tenth symphony, which was composed during a time of emotional stress, is marked with scrawled phrases, one of which reads, "the devil dances with me; madness takes hold of me. Cursed one, destroy me that I may forget

that I am. . . ." His wife, Alma Mahler Werfel, lived to the age of 85; she died in New York in 1964, after a life full of lovers and husbands.
Bibliography: Mitchell, D. 1958. *Gustav Mahler*.

MAIMAKTERION. A period of the year in ancient Greece corresponding approximately to November and December. The storms and strong winds occurring at that time were said to cause raging madness, and propitiatory offerings were made to Zeus (q.v.) as a preventive measure.
Bibliography: Vaughan, A. C. 1719. *Madness in Greek thought and customs*.

MAIMONIDES, ABRAHAM (1186-1237). A physician, son of Moses Maimonides (q.v.). He followed the humoral theory (q.v.) of Galen (q.v.) and believed that the brain must be kept dry to function properly. According to him, overeating could affect the brain adversely. He claimed passions interfered with reason, and, therefore, rage, hatred, and vindictiveness, as well as overindulgence in eating or sexual pleasure, were to be avoided. In moderation these activities were considered beneficial by him, for "celibacy often drives those who are unused to such sexual abnegation to melancholy and insanity."
Bibliography: Rosenblat, S. 1927. *The high ways to perfection of Abraham Maimonides*.

MAIMONIDES, MOSES (1135-1204). A Spanish philosopher and physician, born in Córdoba. His father was a rabbi, and his intellectual pursuits greatly influenced Maimonides' development. After Córdoba was captured by the Almohads, his family led a fugitive life and eventually settled in Cairo. There, he studied medicine, and the knowledge of his skills reached Saladin (1138-1193), sultan of Egypt, who appointed him court physician. Maimonides combined Greek and Jewish thought in a rational system of psychology, that emphasized the psychosomatic nature of many disorders and stressed the importance of emotional factors in therapy. In *Hygiene of the Soul* Maimonides wrote, "The physician should notice that every sick person is not cheerful, and he should, therefore, remove the mental effects which cause that depression, for in this way is the health maintained." His influence in medicine and Christian philosophy lasted throughout the Middle Ages (q.v.).
Bibliography: Rosner, F., and Muntner, S., eds. 1970-1971. *The medical aphorisms of Moses Maimonides*. 2 vols.

MAINE DE BIRAN, FRANÇOIS PIERRE (1766-1824). A French philosopher, son of a physician. His real name was Marie François Pierre Gonthier de Biran. He spent his life studying psychology. He believed that voluntary effort was the basic working principle of the mind, which was raised by consciousness from sensation to perception. According to him, emotions, instincts, and habit fell below the conscious level and were re-

vealed in somnambulism (q.v.) and in dreams (q.v.). His writings influenced many nineteenth-century psychiatrists, including Pierre Janet (q.v.).
Bibliography: Cresson, A. 1950. *Maine de Biran: sa vie, son oeuvre.*

MAIN PUTERI. A healing ceremony performed in West Malaysia. If the patient is suffering from mental disorders, he is interviewed by the healer, who falls into a trance to the accompaniment of music and chants as the patient acts out his difficulties. Exorcism (q.v.) may be attempted. The ceremony lasts all night, and in the morning, the healer and his helpers leave after advising the patient and his family.
Bibliography: Kramer, B. H. 1970. Psychotherapeutic implications of a traditional healing ceremony: the Malaysian Main Puteri. *Transcultural Psychiatric Research Review.*7:149-51.

MAISON BELHOMME. A private institution owned by Dr. J.E. Belhomme (q.v.) in Paris at the time of the French Revolution. It was one of many *maisons de santé* that accepted wealthy patients who were suffering from venereal disease and mental disorders. Philippe Pinel (q.v.) often visited this institution to observe mental patients.
Bibliography: Galdston, I. 1967. *Historic derivations of modern psychiatry.*

MAJOR, HERMAN WEDEL (1814-1854). A Norwegian physician and reformer in the field of mental health. At the request of the Norwegian government he drafted Norway's first mental health legislation, which was passed in 1848. He advocated a national mental health service that included provisions for chronic and acute patients and the establishment of new mental hospitals.
Bibliography: Retterstøl, N. 1975. Scandinavia and Finland. In *World history of psychiatry*, ed. J. G. Howells.

MAKARENKO, ANTON SEMENOVICH (1888-1939). A Russian physician who has had considerable influence on child-rearing practices in the USSR. He emphasized the need for cooperation between parents in raising children, recommended caution in administering punishment, and especially noted the importance of the father. Makarenko's pedagogic system has been regarded as the basis for a model psychotherapeutic community.
Bibliography: Issacs, B. n.d. *Makarenko: his life and work.*

MALABAR. An area on the southwest coast of India. It was customary among sick people there to dedicate themselves to their idols in return for a cure. Once well, they would fatten themselves for several months and then cut off their own heads on the appropriate feast day in honor of the god who had saved them from death.
Bibliography: Fedden, H. R. 1938. *Suicide.*

MALACARNE, M. VINCENZO (1744-1816). An Italian anatomist, physician, and professor at the universities of Pavia and Padua. He wrote on

cretinism (q.v.) and goiter and was well known for his anatomical studies. He introduced the term "enteroid processes" (q.v.) to describe the convolutions of the brain, thus stressing their similarity to the intestines.
Bibliography: Clarke, E., and Dewhurst, K. 1972. *Illustrated history of brain function.*

MALAGRIDA, GABRIEL (1689-1761). An Italian Jesuit missionary to Portugal. His mystic practices were carried to extremes and his writings were full of absurdities. Despite his obvious derangement, he occupied an important position in the order. When his involvement in a plot to assassinate the king of Portugal was discovered, he was brought to trial as a heretic and burnt at the stake.
Bibliography: Ireland, W. W. 1889. *Through the ivory gate.*

MALARIA THERAPY. In the fourth century B.C. Hippocrates (q.v.) observed that physical illnesses often relieve mental illnesses; in the beginning of the eighteenth century Georg Stahl (q.v.) believed that a fever during madness was an indication that the "soul" was fighting the disorder. At the end of the nineteenth century, Julius Wagner von Jauregg (q.v.) suggested that malaria could be used as a form of therapy for general paralysis of the insane (q.v.). Wagner von Jauregg put his theories into practice in 1917. Compared to other forms of therapy, malaria proved successful and was adopted. In the United States it was first used in Saint Elizabeth's Hospital (q.v.) in Washington, D.C., and the hospital staff published the first paper in English on the results of its use in treatment.
Bibliography: Lewis, N.D.C.; Hubbard, L. D., and Dyar, E. G. 1924. Malaria treatment of paretic neuro-syphilis. *Amer. J. Psychiat.* 4:175.

MAL DES ARDENS. The name given to the episodes of mass hysteria (q.v.) that swept Holland and the province of the Rhine in 1373. Those affected ran about aimlessly singing and dancing, carrying flowers in their hands, and wearing garlands on their heads. It was said that their abdomens were greatly distended, which suggests that a physical illness, possibly linked with toxemia, may have caused the epidemics.
Bibliography: Hecker, J.F.C. 1844. *Epidemics in the Middle Ages,* trans. B. G. Babington.

MAL D'HERCULE. A term used by Aretaeus of Cappadocia (q.v.) for epilepsy (q.v.). The term was derived from Heracles (q.v.) who was believed to suffer from fits of madness, which were confused with epilepsy.
Bibliography: Esquirol, J.E.D. 1845. Reprint. 1965. *Mental maladies: a treatise on insanity.*

MAL D'ORIENT. Another term for homosexuality (q.v.). The term was derived from the belief that homosexuality had spread to European countries only after the crusades. The returning men were said to have learned the practice from the East, hence "oriental evil."

MAL DU SIÈCLE. The strange melancholy (*see* MELANCHOLIA) fashionable in the early nineteenth century. It oscillated between gentle lassitude and violent despair. Waves of discontent and moodiness added to the morbid brooding that found expression in the artistic output of the time.

MALEBRANCHE, NICHOLAS (1638-1715). A French philosopher. He abandoned the study of theology and turned to philosophy after reading the works of Réne Descartes (q.v.). His major book, entitled *De la Recherche de la Verité* and published in 1674, combined mysticism and psychological approach in the search for the causes of error.
Bibliography: Gouhier, H. 1926. *La philosophie de Malebranche.*

MALINOWSKI, BRONISLAW KASPER (1884-1942). A Polish anthropologist, greatly influenced by Sir James Frazer's (q.v.) *The Golden Bough* (q.v.). Malinowski applied psychological principles to the investigation of anthropological phenomena and used psychoanalytical theory to describe and explain his findings. He studied primitive mechanisms for dealing with sex and death, the significance of the family among Australian aborigines, magic (q.v.), culture, and religion. Among his works are *Myth in Primitive Psychology* (1926) and *The Dynamics of Culture Change* (1945).
Bibliography: Firth, R., ed. 1957. *Man and culture: an evolution of the work of Bronislaw Malinowski.*

MALLEUS MALEFICARUM (THE WITCHES' HAMMER). The title of a book written by two German Dominican brothers, Johann Jacob Sprenger (q.v.) and Heinrich Kraemer (q.v.). It became a textbook for the Inquisition (q.v.). It was approved by Pope Innocent VIII (q.v.) in 1484, backed by Maximilian I (1459-1519), Holy Roman emperor-designate, in 1486, and finally, in 1487, it received permission for publication from the faculty of theology at the University of Cologne, which had resisted it for as long as possible. The book was divided into three parts: the first asserted the existence of devils and witches (*see* WITCHCRAFT); the second described methods of detecting witchcraft; and the third established procedures for trials in civil courts and listed the punishments for offenders. It was a fanatical work, but accepted by State and Church, and was aimed at the detection and punishment of heretics. Although it clearly stated that a physician was to be consulted if there were any reason to believe that the accused was sick in body or mind, it attributed to the devil any disease that could not be explained or cured by drugs (q.v.). Delusions (q.v.) and hallucinations (q.v.) were regarded as reflections of evil thoughts and, therefore, condemned. Inexplicable forms of abnormal behavior were similarly condemned, and a number of mentally ill men, women, and children became enmeshed in the working of the Inquisition, although the *Malleus Maleficarum* was not deliberately intended to be used against them. It was translated into English

in 1928, by the Reverend Montague Summers (1880-1948), who regarded it as being "among the most important, weightiest and wisest books of the world."
Bibliography: Zilboorg, G. 1969. *The medical man and the witch during the Renaissance.*

MALOPTERURUS ELECTRICUS. The Nile electric catfish. It is still used by some African tribes for shock therapy. The practice was originally learned from Greek and Roman invaders.
See also ELECTROICHTHYOLOGY.
Bibliography: Kellaway, P. 1946. The part played by electric fish in the early history of bioelectricity and electrotherapy. *Bull. Hist. Med.* 20: 112-37.

MANAGE. A village in the district of Hainault, Belgium. In 1892 a group of Brothers of Charity founded in the village the first Belgian asylum for idiots.
Bibliography: Barr, M. W. 1904. *Mental defectives.*

MANCHESTER LUNATIC HOSPITAL. An institution founded in Manchester, England, in 1766. It was attached to the infirmary, or general hospital, which was known as the Manchester Royal Infirmary, and contained twenty-two cells for wealthy private mental patients. Its "Anti-maniac" therapy was carried out under the supervision of Dr. John Ferriar (q.v.) who introduced many innovations. In 1848, the asylum was moved to Cheadle and became known as the Cheadle Royal Hospital (q.v.). Henry Maudsley (q.v.) was appointed as its medical superintendent in 1859. He instituted many reforms, including the introduction of occupational therapy (q.v.), and reorganized the management of patients.
Bibliography: Brockbank, E. M. 1934. *A short history of Cheadle Royal from its foundation in 1766 for the humane treatment of mental diseases.*

MANDALA. A Sanskrit term meaning "magic circle." It implies a highly complex mental picture of the world and an awareness of the spiritual truth that is at its center. As a religious symbol, it is used in rituals to aid contemplation. In the Middle Ages (q.v.) Christian mandalas showed Christ in the center and the four evangelists at the cardinal points. Carl G. Jung (q.v.) became particularly interested in the mandala symbolism when he found that it often occurred in the dreams (q.v.) and hallucinations (q.v.) of patients.
Bibliography: Hannah, B. 1976. *Jung: his life and work.*

MANDEVILLE, BERNARD (1670-1733). An English satirist and physician, born in Holland. He settled in London but never had a successful practice. In 1711 he wrote a work entitled *A Treatise of the Hypochondriack and Hysterick Passions*, which discussed neurotic (*see* NEUROSIS) disorders in the light of his personal experiences during his own illness. In his book,

The Fable of the Bees, published in 1714, he asserted that "private vices are public benefits." Its contents were considered offensive, and in 1723 the Grand Jury of Middlesex condemned the book. The subsequent publicity and controversy caused it to go into nine editions.
Bibliography: Mandeville, B. 1711. Reprint. 1976. *A treatise of the hypochondriack and hysterick passions.*

MANDI-MINJAK-MENDIDI. A Chinese ceremony performed in some parts of Indonesia. The term literally means "bathing in boiling oil." A statue of a god is brought out of a temple and taken through the streets in a procession. The devotees, encouraged by the priests and the suggestive atmosphere, go into a state of trance, during which they perform dangerous acts without hurting themselves. They have been known to walk on fire and even immerse their hands in boiling oil.
Bibliography: Kline, N. S. 1963. Psychiatry in Indonesia. *Am. J. Psychiat.* 119: 809-15.

MANDRAGORA, *or* **MANDRAKE.** A plant of the nightshade family, important in the pharmacopoeia of many cultures. It grows, among other places, in India, China (q.v.), Spain, Italy, and Palestine. Its forked root vaguely resembles a human form, hence its name, which means "dragon resembling man." Magic (q.v.) properties have been attributed to it, and in earlier times, its price made it worthwhile for the unscrupulous to manufacture imitations from the roots of other plants. For a long time it was regarded as the best remedy for anxiety, madness, and pain. It was also thought to be an aid to fertility, an antidote against all poisons, and an aphrodisiac, known as the "love-apple." Hippocrates (q.v.) believed it to be beneficial in the treatment of depression, and Avicenna (q.v.) used it to dull the senses of patients undergoing operations. Later physicians recommended it for insomnia. It was considered to be most efficacious if it had grown under gallows and had been watered by human blood. Elaborate ceremonials surrounded its collection because it was said to emit a horrid shriek that could drive men mad when it was pulled from the ground. To prevent this, it was uprooted by a dog who was tied to it and then called from a safe distance.
Bibliography: Scott, J. 1946. *The mandrake root.*

MANES. The ghosts of the dead. According to ancient Roman beliefs, they would not rest until their wishes had been fulfilled by those still alive.
Bibliography: 1978 *Brewer's dictionary of phrase and fable.*

MANIA. A word used in the past to indicate insanity. According to Jean Esquirol (q.v.), the term was derived from the Greek *mene*, meaning "moon" (q.v.), as the moon was believed to cause mental disorders and maniacs were

said to be "moon-struck." In the early classifications of mental disorders, the term was reserved for states of abnormal excitement. Some Latin authors, however, Cicero (q.v.) among them, preferred the term "furor" (q.v.). In the humoral theory (q.v.), mania was attributed to an excess of yellow bile (q.v.).
Bibliography: Zilboorg, G. 1941. *A history of medical psychology.*

MANIA, CAESAR. A term derived from the concept of the absolute power of the Caesars. It is seldom used. Eugen Bleuler (q.v.) defined it as "a feeling of being absolute master of life and death among savages."

MANIA SINE DELIRIO. Insane without delirium (q.v.). Jean Esquirol (q.v.) recognized that an individual could be insane, or maniacal, without being in a state of delirium, or confusion of mind. He first used the term.
Bibliography: Esquirol, J.E.D. 1845. Reprint 1965. *Mental maladies: a treatise on insanity.*

MANIAS PARTICULARES. One of the first books dealing with psychiatric disorders to be printed in the New World. It appeared in Lima, Peru, in 1791; its author was Father Francisco Gonzales Laguna.
Bibliography: Leon, C. A., and Rosselli, H. 1975. Latin America. In *World history of psychiatry*, ed. J. G. Howells.

MANIC-DEPRESSIVE PSYCHOSES. The first mention of this group of diseases as such occurred in the 1899 edition of the *Textbook of Psychiatry* written by Emil Kraepelin (q.v.). The observation that the symptoms of certain disorders are alternating states of abnormal exhilaration and depression is much older; for example, Aretaeus of Cappadocia (q.v.) described a disease that expressed itself in these two states in the first or second century A.D.
Bibliography: Kraepelin, E. 1899. *Lehrbuch der Psychiatrie.*

MANICHAEUS (or MANI) (216?-?276). The Persian founder of Manichaeism, a synthesis of Gnosticism, Zoroasterism, other Persian religions, and Christianity. It was based on the belief of the coeternal existence of God and Satan. Its adherents advocated voluntary death and suicide (q.v.). Manichaeus was accused of heresy and crucified.
Bibliography: Rosen, G. 1971. History in the study of suicide. *Psychol. Med.* 1: 267-85.

MANN, HORACE (1796-1859). An American educator and reformer. Following his plea for better provisions for the insane whom he regarded as wards of the state, the Massachusetts legislature appointed a committee to investigate their conditions. It was found that many of the mentally ill still were kept in prisons or workhouses, were treated cruelly, or, at best, neglected. Following the passage of legislation, the Worcester County Lunatic Asylum was erected in 1833 to remedy the situation. On Mann's advice, the first patients were drawn primarily from the prisons. Mann was an advocate of "moral treatment" and a firm believer that mental illness was curable. He introduced many educational innovations and revolutionized the public school system.

Bibliography: Deutsch, A. 1949. *The mentally ill in America.*

MANN, THOMAS (1876-1955). A German novelist. His mother was half Portuguese West Indian, temperamental and artistic; he settled with her in Munich to study at the university but he never completed the course and left to live with his brother in Italy, where he wrote his first masterpiece *Buddenbrooks* (1901). It was the story of four generations of a family similar to his own. This and his subsequent novels demonstrate his deep concern for mankind and the influence of Arthur Schopenhauer (q.v.), Friedrich Nietzsche (q.v.) and the romantic poets. His novels, which often reflected his own personal conflicts, are psychological studies of individuals torn between the realm of the imagination and reality. The themes of the seductive aspects of death frequently occur in such works as *The Magic Mountain* (q.v.) and *Death In Venice* (1912). His short story, entitled *Disillusionment*, describes how an arid environment can influence affective development. Mann regarded Freudian psychoanalytic concepts as a translation of Schopenhauer's metaphysical ideas. On the eightieth birthday of Sigmund Freud (q.v.), Mann read an address in his honor. In 1933, to demonstrate his opposition to the Nazi regime, he left Germany for Switzerland and eventually moved to the United States.

Bibliography: Thomas, R. H. 1956. *T. Mann: the mediation of art.*

MANNHEIM, KARL (1893-1947). A Hungarian sociologist. He taught in Germany and London and was deeply interested in the relationship between education and society. He believed that the democratization of the intelligentsia as well as the upsurge of the workers was at the center of the crisis experienced by society in the twentieth century. Mannheim dedicated himself to the problem of establishing a balance that would reassert the role of reason. He believed that planning could be achieved through applied psychology and sociology, or social education. His works include *Diagnosis of Our Time* (1943) and the posthumously published *Essays on Sociology and Social Psychology* (1953).

Bibliography: Raison, T., ed. 1969. *The founding fathers of social science.*

MAN OF FEELING, THE. A novel by the Scottish author Henry Mackenzie (1745-1831), called the historian of feeling by Sir Walter Scott. It contains a graphic and poignant description of a visit to Bethlem Royal

Hospital (q.v.) that ends with a moving scene in which the sad plight of a young woman who has lost her reason following the death of her lover reduces the visitors to tears.
Bibliography: Mackenzie, H. 1967. *The Man of Feeling*, ed. B. Vickers.

MANON LESCAUT. The heroine of a famous eighteenth century romance by the Abbé Prévost (real name, Antoine François Prévost d'Exiles [1697-1763]). She represents a type of woman whose actions are dictated by a complete lack of morality. Her treatment of others and her disregard of conventions is amoral rather than immoral. In 1893 Giacomo Puccini (q.v.) composed an opera of the same name based on the novel.
Bibliography: Prévost, A. F. 1949. *Manon Lescaut*, trans. by L. W. Tancock.

MANTEGAZZA, PAOLO (1831-1910). An Italian physician, anthropologist, and medical writer. He worked in Italy, Latin America, and the United States and wrote many literary and scientific works. His views were materialistic; he regarded love as a physiological process that could be attributed solely to glandular secretions. In his book, *Il Secolo Neurotico* (*The Neurotic Century*) published in 1887, he asserted that all the manifestations of superior intelligence in the eighteenth century were the product of neurosis (q.v.). According to him, neuroticism was born in 1789 from the philosophy of liberty, equality and fraternity and had produced neurotic literature, politics, and philosophy.
Bibliography: Rosselli, H. 1968. *Historia de la psiquiatria en Colombia*.

MAPOTHER, EDWARD (1881-1940). A British psychiatrist. He worked in both the clinical and academic fields as a physician and as a teacher. He wrote on schizophrenia (q.v.), alcoholic morbidity, and the mental symptoms associated with head injury. He played a constructive part in the development of the Maudsley Hospital (q.v.) in London. Among his works is the notable *The Schizophrenic Paranoid Series*, published in four volumes between 1929 and 1939.
Bibliography: Slater, E. 1972. The psychiatrist in search of a science. I: early thinkers at the Maudsley. *Brit. J. Psychiat.* 121:591-98.

MAQLÛ. The main psychiatric textbook of Babylonian medicine (q.v.). It dealt with mental disorders caused by witchcraft (q.v.) performed on images. It described the burning and slow melting of images representing persons believed to persecute patients suffering from delusions.
Bibliography: Moss, G. C. 1967. Mental diseases in ancient Mesopotamia. In *Diseases in antiquity*, ed. D. Bramwell and A. T. Sandison.

MARASCOS. A Greek poet mentioned by Aristotle (q.v.) as an example of an individual who functioned better when mentally ill than when sane.

He was said to write beautiful verses during attacks of mania (q.v.) but only mediocre ones during periods of sanity.
Bibliography: Zilboorg, G. 1941. *A history of medical psychology.*

MARAT, JEAN PAUL (1743-1793). A French revolutionary. The only time he remembered rebelling as a child was when he was unjustly punished and shut in his room; he was so indignant that he threw himself out of the window. He was extremely ambitious. At the age of five he wanted to be a school teacher, at fifteen a professor, at eighteen an author, and at twenty a creative genius (q.v.). He studied medicine and practiced for some time in London in Soho Square. The University of St. Andrew's in Scotland gave him an honorary degree, and he became well known as a physician. In 1789 he turned his interests to politics and was imprisoned several times for his revolutionary beliefs. While hiding in the sewers of Paris, he contracted a skin disease which he retained for the rest of his life. He became one of the most bloodthirsty leaders of the French Revolution (q.v.); he demanded the death of the king, and coldly calculated that an efficient organization could put to death 260,000 men in a single day. Many thought that he was insane. He had to spend much of his time immersed in water to relieve the pain of his skin disease. He was stabbed to death in his bath by Charlotte Corday (1768-1793) in the belief that she was freeing France from its worst enemy.
Bibliography: Gottschalk, L. R. 1942. *J. P. Marat: a study in radicalism.*

MARBE, KARL (1869-1953). German psychologist and philosopher, born in Paris but raised and educated in Germany. He was a pupil of Wilhelm Wundt (q.v.). In 1896 he was appointed lecturer at the University of Würzburg, which then was developing a school of psychology under Oswald Külpe (q.v.) whom he later succeeded. Marbe's study on judgment undertaken in 1901 was one of the school's first important contributions to psychology. He found that the rational conclusions arrived at by the mind are the result of introspection, rather than a conscious psychological process. His work on the psychology of thinking was based on systematic experimentation. Marbe also was interested in animal psychology, the psychology of advertising, and in many aspects of industrial psychology, including the link between personality and accidents.
Bibliography: Murchison, C., ed. 1936. *A history of psychology in autobiography.* Vol. 3.

MARC, CHARLES CHRETIEN HENRI (1771-1840). A Dutch psychiatrist. He studied in Germany before moving to Paris in 1795. As a youth he had suffered from such severe depression that he had considered suicide (q.v.). This personal experience became the source of his interest in suicide and led to a wider field that encompassed all the basic issues of judicial psychiatry. His major work, which was published in 1840, dealt with legal

psychiatry (q.v.) and was entitled *De la Folie Considérée dans ses Rapports avec les Questions Medico-Judiciaires*. He was held in such high regard that he became first physician to the king and was elected president of the Academy of Medicine.
Bibliography: Mora, G. 1971. Anniversaries. *Am. J. Psychiat.* 128:729.

MARCÉ, L.W. (1828-1864). A French physician. He and Jules Falret (q.v.) described four clinical varieties of general paralysis of the insane (q.v.): paralytic, congestive, expansive, and melancholic. Valentin Magnan (q.v.) worked under him at the Bicêtre (q.v.).
Bibliography: Marcé, L. W. 1862. *Traité pratique des maladies mentales.*

MARCELLE (1871-?). A patient of Pierre Janet (q.v.) at the Salpêtrière (q.v.) in 1891. She was twenty years old and had been admitted with disorders of memory (q.v.) and thought, as well as difficulty in moving her legs. Janet carefully investigated her history, which had included several traumatic events. Following them Marcelle had retreated into a dreamlike world. He treated her through hypnosis (*see* HYPNOTISM) and automatic writing. His experiences with this patient convinced him of the therapeutic value of psychological analysis and helped him to formulate the principles on which his work was based.
Bibliography: Janet, P. 1903. *Névroses et idées fixes.*

MARCHI, VITTORIO (1851-1908). An Italian physician. After teaching anatomy at the University of Modena, he worked at the Mental Hospital of San Lazzaro in Reggio Emilia and later became assistant to Camillo Golgi (q.v.). When he failed to be appointed to the chair of histology at the University of Palermo, he dedicated himself to clinical practice and became chief of the Hospital of Jesi. There he instituted a neurological clinic and a histological laboratory. He died of meningitis, following an ear infection. He had diagnosed his illness himself and accurately predicted the time of his death. His contributions to neuroanatomy include a method of staining histological preparations that was widely used and allowed the study of the distribution of degenerative nerves.
Bibliography: Haymaker, W., and Schiller, F. 1970. *The founders of neurology.* 2d. ed.

MARCHIAFAVA, ETTORE (1847-1935). An Italian physician. He conducted important research on infectious and degenerative diseases of the nervous system. Marchiafava became the first to describe syphilitic cerebral arteritis. His study of malaria still has not been surpassed and remains a

classic in the field. He was personal physician to the Italian royal family and to three popes.
Bibliography: Haymaker, W., and Schiller, F. 1970. *The founders of neurology.* 2d. ed.

MARCUS AURELIUS ANTONINUS (A.D. 121-180). A Roman emperor. He was a Stoic (*see* STOICISM) and a pacifist notwithstanding the constant wars of his reign. Although he was often lonely and sad, he never allowed bitterness to govern his actions. His principal work *Meditationes*, discussed suicide (q.v.) as a duty. After his death, he was worshipped by his subjects, who believed that he would appear to them in dreams (q.v.).
Bibliography: Birley, A. 1966. *Marcus Aurelius.*

MĂRCUTA ASYLUM. The first secular psychiatric hospital in Rumania. In 1846 patients were transferred to it from the hermitage of Balamuci, which had treated patients gathered from various monasteries since 1838. The Mărcuta Asylum was located on the grounds of a former monastery near Bucharest. Dr. Protici, a psychiatrist and one of its first superintendents, introduced enlightened treatment of patients and initiated occupational therapy (q.v.). The hospital remained active until 1923 when it was replaced by the Central Hospital for Mental and Nervous Diseases, now known as the G. Marinescu Hospital.
Bibliography: Predescu, V., and Christodorescu, D. 1975. Rumania. In *World history of psychiatry*, ed. J. G. Howells.

MARE. An abbreviation for nightmare (q.v.) or incubus (q.v.). A mare was a female hag (q.v.) or demon that caused nightmares.
Bibliography: 1978. *Brewer's dictionary of phrase and fable.*

MARGARET (1240-1275). Eldest daughter of Henry III (1207-1272) of England. At the age of eleven she married Alexander III (1241-1286) of Scotland, who was a year her junior. In 1255 her parents sent a physician, Reginald of Bath (q.v.) to investigate reports of her illness. He found her melancholy (*see* MELANCHOLIA) and pale but ready to discuss her troubles with him. The many restrictions and poor living conditions imposed upon her by the Scottish nobles were the cause of her melancholy, which was further exacerbated by the fact that she had never been allowed to sleep with her husband. Parental intervention improved matters, and her depression disappeared.
Bibliography: Talbot, C. H., and Hammond, E. A. 1965. *Medical practitioners in medieval England.*

MARÍA. A novel by the Colombian poet Jorge Isaacs (1837-1895), published in 1867. María, the heroine, is said to have been based upon Ester

Isaacs, a cousin of the author. She suffered from the psychiatric disorders vividly described in the novel. The physician in the novel, Dr. Mayn, was Dr. Mayne, an English physician living in Colombia, who treated Ester Isaacs.
Bibliography: Rosselli, H. 1968. *Historia de la psiquiatria en Colombia.*

MARIA I (1734-1816). A queen of Portugal. She married her uncle, Pedro III (1717-1786). Both of them were weak and mentally unstable. After the death of her husband in 1786 and her eldest son in 1788, she became deeply depressed. Reputedly the anxiety produced by the French Revolution increased her instability and in 1792, her son John VI assumed power because she was considered to be deranged.
Bibliography: Beirão, C. 1944. *Maria I.*

MARIABERG. The first government-sponsored institution in Germany for the care of mentally retarded children. It was founded in 1847 and based on Abendberg Institution (q.v.). It was housed in a former convent that had been built by Count Hugo von Montfort as a promise to the Virgin Mary whom he had petitioned when his children disappeared. Although they were found dead, the count kept his promise. The building had been abandoned by the nuns before Dr. Heinrich Karl Rösch (q.v.) was asked by Wilhelm I (1781-1869) of Württemberg to organize an institution for mentally retarded children and to use the convent and its grounds for that purpose. The institution's patroness was Queen Olga, and Wilhelm Griesinger (q.v.) was among its advisors.
Bibliography: Kanner, L. 1964. *A history of the care and the study of the mentally retarded.*

MARIAMNE THE HASMONAEAN (c.60-29 B.C.). The second of the ten wives of Herod the Great (q.v.). Her husband suffered from paranoid jealousy (q.v.), which combined with the machinations of Mariamne's vile mother, destroyed the marriage. Herod ordered her to be killed if he died before her. When she discovered the arrangement, she denied him her love and sent her portrait to Mark Antony in defiance. Her husband killed her and ordered the death of her sons, mother, brother, and grandfather. She was a predictable subject for murder.
Bibliography: Perowne, S. H. 1956. *The life and times of Herod the Great.*

MARIA PADILLA. An opera by Gaetano Donizetti (q.v.) in which Don Ruiz, the father of the heroine, is driven mad by his daughter's shameful liaison with the king. When the king has him lashed, the torture precipitates the old man's breakdown.
Bibliography: Ashbrook, W. 1965. *Donizetti.*

MARIAZELL. An Austrian shrine at Zell. In the seventeenth century, individuals made pilgrimages to it to be cured of their illnesses. Christoph

Haizmann (q.v.) went there to be freed from the devil by exorcism (q.v.). During his first visit in 1677, he was cured temporarily after three days and three nights of continuous exorcism. He believed, however, that the devil and the symptoms of possession (q.v.) had returned and the following year again asked the monks of the shrine for ceremonies and prayers. After these ceremonies he apparently was cured.

Bibliography: Hunter, R., and Macalpine, I. 1956. *Schizophrenia 1677.*

MARIE. A patient of Pierre Janet (q.v.). She was considered insane and brought to the hospital of Le Havre at the age of nineteen. Her symptoms, which included blindness in one eye, manifestations of terror, delirium (q.v.), and body contortions, appeared monthly after menstruation. Using hypnotism (q.v.), Janet.was able to uncover the various traumatic events in her life that had given rise to the disorders. Her cure was brought about by catharsis (q.v.). He used her case history to demonstrate "the importance of fixed subconscious ideas and the role they play in certain physical illnesses, as well as in emotional illnesses."

Bibliography: Janet, P. 1889. *L'automatisme psychologique.*

MARIE, PIERRE (1853-1940). A French neurologist. After studying law, he turned to medicine and worked at the Salpêtrière (q.v.) under Jean Martin Charcot (q.v.). He described several new clinical conditions of the nervous system and collaborated with Charcot on some of them. Progressive muscular atrophy, acromegaly—a term he coined—and cerebellar heredoataxia were among the disorders he named. His work on aphasia stimulated many subsequent studies. He succeeded Charcot in the chair of neurology (q.v.).

Bibliography: Marie, P. 1928. *Traveaux et mémoires.*

MARIJUANA (*or* MARIHUANA). The term by which Americans and Mexicans refer to the drug derived from *Cannabis sativa* (q.v.). Although it decreases sexual ability, it is usually taken in cigarettes as a stimulant of sexual fantasies.

MARINESCU, GEORGES (1864-1938). A Rumanian neurologist and pupil of Jean Martin Charcot (q.v.). His studies and research covered a wide range of subjects and greatly contributed to the advancement of Rumanian and international neurology (q.v.). He described new aspects of brain pathology and studied normal brain cells and the etiopathogenesis of hysteria (q.v.). The primary Rumanian mental hospital in Bucharest is now known as the G. Marinescu Hospital (formerly the Central Hospital for Nervous and Mental Diseases).

Bibliography: Haymaker, W., and Schiller, F. 1970. *The founders of neurology.* 2d. ed.

MARJORAM. *Origanum vulgare,* an aromatic herb usually found on hilly slopes. Marjoram means "joy of the mountain." Herbalists believed it to

have medical properties and used it in the treatment of depression, anxiety, sleep disorders, and enuresis (q.v.).
Bibliography: de Baìracli Levy, J. 1974. *The illustrated herbal handbook.*

MARKUS FAMILY. The fictitious name given by the Swiss psychiatrist J. Jörger to a family of vagrants. In 1918 he studied members of the group and found that twenty percent of them were imbeciles (q.v.), thus demonstrating the hereditary nature of mental deficiency. He also discovered that this family and the Zero family (q.v.) had a common ancestor.
See also EUGENICS.
Bibliography: Jörger, J. 1918. Die familie Markus. *Z. ges. Neurol. Psychiat.* 43:76-116.

MARLBOROUGH, (JOHN CHURCHILL), DUKE OF (1650-1722). An English nobleman, soldier, and politician. In 1716 he suffered a stroke, after which senile dementia reduced him to a state of imbecility (*see* IMBECILE). For an additional fee, his servants would exhibit him to visitors who were viewing the treasures of his palace, Blenheim.
Bibliography: Hayward, A. 1864. *Diaries of a lady of quality.*

MARRIAGE. In the eighteenth and nineteenth centuries, marriage was often used as a form of therapy for nervous disorders in women. The rationale behind this treatment was the assumption that hysteria (q.v.), traditionally connected with the uterus (q.v.), was essentially a sexual disorder. The results of marriage therapy were almost always disastrous.

MARSHALL, ANDREW (1742-1813). A Scottish surgeon and anatomist. After studying arts and divinity at the University of Edinburgh, he turned to medicine and emigrated to London. Although he was not on the staff of Bethlem Royal Hospital (q.v.), he was allowed to observe patients there. He believed that mental disorders were due to brain pathology and quarreled with John Hunter (q.v.), who did not share his views. In 1815 he published a book entitled *The Morbid Anatomy of the Brain in Mania and Hydrophobia.* He may have been instrumental in persuading his nephew James Murray (q.v.) to leave funds in his will for the erection of Murray Royal Hospital (q.v.).
Bibliography: Hunter, R., and Macalpine, I. 1963. *Three hundred years of psychiatry.*

MARSHMALLOW. *Althea officenalis,* a small plant, found mostly in Europe near the sea. It is also known as hollyhock. It was used in antiquity in the treatment of epilepsy (q.v.). Pliny the Elder (q.v.) was among those who advocated it as a safe remedy.
Bibliography: Morton, J. F. 1977. *Major medicinal plants.*

MARSTON, WILLIAM MOULTON (1893-1947). An American psychologist. In 1934 he developed a test for deception that was based upon

variations in the systolic blood pressure. The test became popularly known as the "lie detector."
Bibliography: Marston, W. M. 1938. *The lie detector test.*

MARTIN, EVERETT DEAN (1880-1941). An American sociologist. For twenty years (from 1918 to 1938) he was director of the Cooper Union Forum, the most important center in the United States for free discussions on subjects of educational and political importance. His investigations included studies on the formation and behavior of crowds, a field in which he became an authority.
Bibliography: Martin, D. D. 1920. *The behaviour of crowds.*

MARTIN, JOHN (1789-1854). An English painter, brother of Jonathan Martin (q.v.). His early life was dominated by his mother's forceful personality. As a child, he was afraid of the dark and imagined ghosts and goblins in every corner. He acted as an interpreter for his brother who could not speak, and some of his paintings seem to be a continuation of this role. Their subjects parallel Jonathan's religious ravings in their use of large, apocalyptic, visionary landscapes with disordered time-scales, scenes of destruction, and burning cities.
Bibliography: Feaver, W. 1975. *The art of John Martin.*

MARTIN, JONATHAN (1782-1838). An English tanner, the son of an unstable father and a neurotic (*see* NEUROSIS), eccentric mother. She claimed she possessed visionary powers and reared five of her thirteen children to fear the Lord and the terrors of hell. As a child, Martin was extremely lonely; he was tongue-tied from birth until the age of six, when the frenulum was cut. He suffered from nightmares (q.v.) and frightening fantasies. Although he did not go to school, he taught himself to read and write. When he was twenty-two years old, he was press-ganged into the navy and spent six years at sea. He became fanatically religious, accused the clergy of immorality, and threatened the life of the bishop of Oxford. He was brought to court, found insane, and ordered to an asylum (q.v.) from which he escaped several times. His religious fanaticism, fanned by dreams (q.v.) and visions, led him to intensify his campaign against the clergy whom he called "blind hypocrites, serpents and vipers of hell, wine bibbers and beef eaters." To punish them, he decided to set fire to York Minster. He was again tried but, having been found insane, was committed to Bethlem Royal Hospital (q.v.) for the remainder of his life. His only son was probably schizophrenic (*see* SCHIZOPHRENIA) and committed suicide (q.v.) shortly after his father's death.
Bibliography: Balston, T. 1945. *The life of Jonathan Martin.*

MARTIN, LILLIEN JANE (1851-1943). An American psychologist, pupil of Georg E. Müller (q.v.). She was the founder and director of the Old Age

Counseling Center in San Francisco, California. Among other topics, she wrote on mental hygiene, old age, the mental training of young children, and personality as revealed by the content of images.
Bibliography: Martin, L. J. 1927. *Round the world with a psychologist.*

MARULÍC, MARKO (MARCUS MARULUS) (1450-1524). A Yugoslavian writer and poet born at Split, on the Dalmation coast. In 1765 his biographer, a learned Jesuit, Daniel Farlati, while listing Marulíc's works included a volume entitled *Psychologia de Ratione Animae Humanae (Psychology: on the Human Soul).* This work seems to indicate that Marulíc wrote what may have been the first book on psychology in the world, although he did not necessarily coin the term "psychology."
Bibliography: Brozĕk, J. 1973. Psychologia de Marcus Marulus. *Episteme* 7: 125-31.

MARX, KARL (1818-1883). A German social philosopher and founder of modern communism. Although his father was a Jew, Marx grew to dislike Jews. He married a descendent of an aristocratic German family and led a life strictly controlled by middle-class values. After he was expelled from Paris and Brussels because of his political activities, he settled in London. The family experienced extreme poverty but tried to retain their middle-class standards, even to the point of redeeming their watches from a pawnbroker before a holiday. He loved his children, who regarded him as a kind of god, and was deeply affected by the death of two sons and a daughter. Marx suffered from a large number of disorders, including migraine (q.v.) and some nervous complaints. His youngest daughter, Eleanor, suffered from depression and psychosomatic disorders, possibly resulting from the strain of conforming to the rules of middle-class behavior so important to her family. She committed suicide (q.v.). Marx's doctrines became clear in the famous *Communist Manifesto* written with Friedrich Engels (q.v.) in 1848. His major work, *Das Kapital (Capital* [q.v.]) appeared in 1867.
Bibliography: Payne, R. 1968. *Marx.*

MARY I (1516-1558). A queen of England, daughter of Henry VIII (1491-1547) and Catherine of Aragon (1485-1536). Her father was very fond of her, but was forced to declare her illegitimate after he married Anne Boleyn in 1533. Mary, like her mother, was rigid and overreligious, but also intelligent and accomplished. Following her adolescence, which was made difficult by her father's rejection and her stepmother's jealousy, Mary became depressed and suffered from insomnia, headaches, attacks of anxiety, and psychosomatic symptoms related to the digestive and genital systems. In 1554, she married Philip II (q.v.) of Spain, nine years her junior. Her much publicized pregnancy, which was accompanied by lavish preparations for the baby, turned out to be false (pseudocyesis [q.v.]), and after ten months

she had to recognize that she was not pregnant. A further period of deep depression culminated in a second episode of pseudocyesis from which she emerged despairing, humiliated, and even more rejected by her unloving husband. She died in willful isolation, some say of grief, having lost all appetite for life.
Bibliography: Erickson, C. 1978. *Bloody Mary.*

MARYLAND HOSPITAL. A hospital founded in the United States in Spring Grove, Maryland, in 1797 by an act "to encourage the establishing of a hospital for the relief of indigent sick persons and for the reception and care of lunatics." In 1808 the hospital, which was having financial problems, was taken over as a private enterprise by two physicians, James Smythe and Colin Mackenzie. Shortly after their deaths, public opinion pressed for the return of the hospital to public control, which was achieved in 1828. Five years later the hospital became an institution exclusively dedicated to the care and treatment of the insane.
Bibliography: Deutsch, A. 1949. *The mentally ill in America.*

MASADA. A hill fortress on the Dead Sea and a Jewish stronghold against the Romans in the first century A.D. After three years of siege, the 960 surviving defenders committed mass suicide (q.v.) rather than surrender to the Romans.
Bibliography: Yadin, Y. 1966. *Masada.*

MASOCHISM. A term related to the idea that pain gives pleasure. It was coined by Richard von Krafft-Ebing (q.v.) who derived it from Leopold von Sacher-Masoch (q.v.), an eighteenth-century German novelist whose heroes derived sexual pleasure from cruel treatment.
Bibliography: Krafft-Ebing, R. von. 1886. *Psychopathia sexualis.*

MASON'S MADHOUSE. A private asylum orginally established in Stapleton, England in 1738 by Joseph Mason. In 1760, the establishment was transferred to Fishponds, near Bristol, and in 1788 Joseph Mason Cox (q.v.) took charge of it. He advertised his enterprise, emphasizing that it was dedicated exclusively to "cases of insanity, hypochondriasis, and other chronic nervous affections." In 1844 following complaints against its management, the asylum, then called Fishponds Private Lunatic Asylum, was the subject of a public inquiry. Its affairs, as described by the inquiry, were printed in a volume of 800 pages. The asylum remained in the hands of the same family until 1852. In 1859 it was finally closed down and the premises were sold. Another Fishponds asylum (now Glenside Hospital) was opened nearby in

1860; it was a public mental hospital and it had no connection with Mason's Madhouse.
Bibliography: Hunter, R., and Macalpine, I. 1963. *Three hundred years of psychiatry.*

MASSACHUSETTS SCHOOL FOR IDIOTIC AND FEEBLE-MINDED CHILDREN. An American institution for mentally retarded children in Waltham, Massachusetts. It was opened in 1848 as a wing of the Perkins Institution for the Blind. It was the first school for mentally retarded children in America and owed its inception to the efforts of Dr. Samuel Gridley Howe (q.v.). After functioning successfully for three years, it was granted its own premises in South Boston. Edouard O. Seguin (q.v.) spent a brief period helping at the school. The school moved to Waltham where it became known as the Walter E. Fernald State School, after one of its superintendents.
Bibliography: Kanner, L. 1964. *A history of the care and study of the mentally retarded.*

MASS HYSTERIA. Hysteria (q.v.) involving several individuals. The phenomenon has been observed since antiquity. Early examples can be found, for example, in the cult of Dionysus (q.v.). During the Middle Ages (q.v.), epidemics of delirium (q.v.) with ecstasies (*see* ECSTASY) were frequent, especially among religious communities. Johann Weyer (q.v.) was one of the few who recognized that the epidemics were caused by the influence of one sick individual upon others. In the nineteenth century Prosper Despine (q.v.) wrote about these phenomena, which he attributed to "moral contagion." Other famous examples include Aix-en-Provence, the Loudun nuns, the Shakers, and mal des Ardens (qq.v.).
Bibliography: Sirois, F. 1974. *Epidemic hysteria.*

MASTER IN LUNACY. During the Middle Ages (q.v.), the title given to the master of the courts. In English law, the master in lunacy regulated the administration of lands belonging to lunatics.
Bibliography: Steinberg, S. H., and Evans, I. H. 1970. *Steinberg's dictionary of British history.*

MASTURBATION. In the nineteenth century, masturbation was regarded as a cause of insanity. Jean Esquirol (q.v.) in his book, *Mental Maladies: A Treatise on Insanity,* wrote: "Masturbation, that scourge of human kind, is more frequently than is supposed, the cause of insanity, especially among the rich." In some cultures, for example, the Tarascan of Latin America, masturbation is performed openly, while in others it is strongly opposed.

Bibliography: Ellis, A., and Abarbanel, A., eds. 1961. *The encyclopaedia of sexual behaviour*.

MATHARI MENTAL HOSPITAL. A mental hospital opened in Nairobi, Kenya in 1910. It provided accommodation for two European and eight African mental patients.
Bibliography: Carman, J. A. 1976. *A medical history of the colony and protectorate of Kenya*.

MATHURIN, DE LARCHANT, SAINT. A French saint. In the fourteenth century, the clergy of the Hôtel-Dieu (q.v.) sent insane patients to the shrine of this saint. Those wishing to pray on behalf of an insane patient also were sent there.
Bibliography: Rosen, G. 1968. *Madness in society*.

MATILDA OF COLOGNE. Probably a murderess. The chronicles of the life of Saint Thomas à Becket (1118?-1170) record her as insane. She is described as shouting, using foul language, and striking whoever wanted to restrain her. According to the chronicles, she was tightly bound with ropes, and, after raving for some hours, she came to, declaring that she had seen Saint Thomas in a dream (q.v.). Three stained glass windows in the Trinity Chapel at Canterbury Cathedral (q.v.), England, depict her story.
Bibliography: Rackham, B. 1957. *The stained glass windows of Canterbury Cathedral*.

MATIRUKU. A form of hypomania found among the Fijians. The term literally means "low tide in the morning." It is used as a figurative expression to describe someone who is periodically insane.
Bibliography: Price, J., and Karim, I. 1978. Matiruku, a Fijian madness: an initial assessment. *Brit. J. Psychiat.* 133: 228-30.

MATSUMOTO, MATATARO (1865-1943). A Japanese psychologist. He trained at Yale University under Edward W. Scripture (q.v.). After his training, he traveled throughout America and Europe inspecting psychological laboratories. On his return to Japan, he designed a psychological laboratory (q.v.) for Tokyo University; it was the first such laboratory in Japan. In 1906 he became professor of psychology at Kyoto University and founded a second laboratory there. His research and writings were primarily in the field of applied psychology. He also wrote on the psychology of intelligence, the psychology of art and the psychology of old age.
Bibliography: Misiak, H., and Sexton, V. S. 1966. *History of psychology*.

MATTHEWS, JAMES TILLEY (?-1814). A London tea broker. In 1798 he became insane and was admitted to Bethlem Royal Hospital (q.v.). John

Haslam (q.v.), the hospital apothecary, wrote a book describing his symptoms and the patient himself illustrated it with representations of the weird instruments of torture that appeared in his hallucinations (q.v.). The book was the first single psychiatric history to be published. Matthews died in a private asylum to which he had been transferred for a change of air.
Bibliography: Haslam, J. 1810. *Illustrations of madness.*

MAUDSLEY, HENRY (1835-1918). An English psychiatrist and founder of the Maudsley Hospital (q.v.) in London. Born on a Yorkshire farm, he led a cheerless childhood, especially after his mother's death, which caused his father to become withdrawn and uncommunicative. His paternal uncle and maternal aunt provided him with some of the affection that he was missing. When he was fourteen years old, his aunt sent him as a private pupil to the house of the Reverend Alfred Neuth at Oundle. In 1850, Maudsley went to University College Hospital and was apprenticed for five years to Clover the resident medical officer. His first post was as assistant medical officer at the Wakefield Asylum (q.v.), and after a brief spell in Brentwood Asylum, he became medical superintendent of the Cheadle Royal Hospital (q.v.) when he was twenty-three years old. He remained there for three years, during which he effected many improvements. In his first paper, *Correlation of Mental and Physical Forces, or, Man, a Part of Nature* (1859), he theorized that man's consciousness, moral nature, and all his other psychological attributes were closely dependent on the physical structure of his brain. *Physiology and Pathology of Mind*, published in 1867, was his first important publication; it was soon translated into German, Italian, French, and Japanese and made him well known throughout the world. He was greatly concerned with the problems of the will in disease and crime and urged the need for early and voluntary treatment of the mentally ill. He also recognized the importance of training physicians in this field. In 1908 Maudsley's plans for a university psychiatric clinic devoted to early treatment, research, and post-graduate training were accepted by the London County Council. Although it was some time before the plans were put into practice, the building finally was completed in 1915. Maudsley regarded insanity as "the result and evidence of a discord between the man and his surroundings," yet he also believed in an organic pathological aetiology. This dual explanation of mental disorders influenced the development of psychiatry in British mental hospitals. Maudsley's wife was the daughter of John Conolly (q.v.).
Bibliography: Allderidge, P. H. 1976. Historical notes on the Bethlem Royal Hospital and the Maudsley Hospital. In *Essays and notes on the history of medicine*, ed. P. H. Allderidge.

MAUDSLEY HOSPITAL. A psychiatric hospital in London. It was founded by Henry Maudsley (q.v.). In 1909 Maudsley contributed a large sum of money and a bequest toward its establishment, and it came under the control of the London County Council. It was created to provide a small hospital for acute mental disorders which would be separated from the large asylums. It had a large staff and facilities for research as well as teaching. The building was completed in 1915, but it was not fully functioning until 1923. It was the first of such institutions to be termed a "mental hospital." Under special legislation it became the first mental institution controlled by a public authority to accept voluntary patients. In 1946 it amalgamated with Bethlem Royal Hospital (q.v.).

Bibliography: Allderidge, P. H. 1976. Historical notes on the Bethlem Royal Hospital and the Maudsley Hospital." In *Essays and notes on the history of medicine*, ed. P. H. Allderidge.

MAUGHAM, WILLIAM SOMERSET (1874-1965). An English novelist and playwright. He was born, spent part of his life, and died in France. His childhood was unhappy and lonely. His mother died when he was eight years old, and his father's death followed within two years. He was brought up by an uncle who was a rigid, childless, and unsympathetic clergyman. Maugham's wretched school years were the prelude to hard medical study at Saint Thomas Hospital in London. Although he qualified, he never practiced. His success as a writer, and later as a dramatist, did not change his melancholic (*see* MELANCHOLIA) outlook on life, and he remained tormented by childhood griefs and indignities and oversensitive about his height and appalling stammer. He was a homosexual (*see* HOMOSEXUALITY), a fact that he was afraid to admit even to himself. When his mistress, Syrie Wellcome, became pregnant, he married her but left her within a year for Gerald Haxton who remained his companion for the next twenty-five years. As Haxton was banned from England, they settled in France. Maugham once said that he had "never enjoyed living"; his real world was the one that he created in his writings. His novel *Of Human Bondage* (1915) was partially autobiographical, and, although he wrote it to regain his peace of mind, it only served to sharpen his feelings; and he could not read certain passages without breaking into tears.

Bibliography: Morgan, T. 1980. *Somerset Maugham*.

MAULÉVRIER, FRANÇOIS ÉDUARD COLBERT, MARQUIS DE (1675-1706). A French brigadier in the king's army. His intelligence and valor did not disguise his ambitious scheming and lack of self-control. He fell in love with the dauphine, Marie Adelaide of Savoy (1685-1712), and for over a year he pretended to have lost his voice in order to be able to whisper to her. Eventually, rage over the princess' rejection and paranoid jealousy unbalanced his mind. He was confined to his house and watched by his wife and devoted friends. One morning, however, he managed to

elude them, and threw himself out of an upper window. He died on the cobblestones below.
Bibliography: Norton, L. 1978. *First lady of Versailles*.

MAUPASSANT, GUY DE (1850-1893). A French writer. His mother is said to have been a neurotic, hysterical woman, who was overly possessive of her children. He was influenced and encouraged by the novelist Gustave Flaubert (q.v.), a close friend of his mother. Maupassant was an eccentric and a womanizer, who boasted of his sexual prowess and claimed that he could attain twenty physical climaxes in succession; he enjoyed proving his potency visually to his friends. In his early thirties he became addicted to ether (q.v.) inhalations, which he had tried in an effort to relieve his excruciating headaches. The feeling of unreality and levitation caused by the ether pleased him, and he continued to use it for the rest of his life. In the last decade of his life, he suffered from physical and mental illness. He was depressed and weary and developed strange ideas that culminated in such a feeling of depersonalization that he could not recognize himself in the mirror. Syphilitic (*see* SYPHILIS) infection led to paralysis, partial blindness, and madness. In 1892 he tried to commit suicide (q.v.) by cutting his throat and was admitted to Dr. Blanche's asylum at Passy. His delusions (q.v.) included the belief that he was the younger son of the Virgin Mary and that the little branches he stuck into the ground would grow into "little Maupassants." During delirium (q.v.) he often believed that his thoughts had escaped from his head; he would search for them and rejoice when he thought he had found them, describing them as shaped like brightly colored butterflies. After a year in the asylum he died. The first of the approximately three hundred short stories he wrote was *Boule de Suif*, which was immediately recognized as a masterpiece. Among his most famous novels are *Une Vie* (1883), *Bel-Ami* (1885), and *Pierre et Jean* (1888). All his writings reflect a sombre, morbid, often macabre, mood, as well as an interest in the bizarre and the abnormal, as shown in *Le Horla* (1887), the story of a hunted man that is probably based on Maupassant's own hallucinatory experiences.
Bibliography: Lanoux, A. 1967. *Maupassant, le bel-ami*.

MAUTHE DOG. The ghost of a black spaniel that was believed to haunt Peel Castle on the Isle of Man. Its nightly visits to the guardroom forced the soldiers to refrain from profanity in its presence and to have a companion during their rounds. According to legend, a drunken soldier once elected to do the rounds alone; he later was found speechless with terror and died within three days. In 1871 when the skeleton of Simon, bishop of Sodor and Man in the thirteenth century, was uncovered, the bones of a dog were found in the same grave.
Bibliography: 1978. *Brewer's dictionary of phrase and fable*.

MAXWELL, WILLIAM (1581-1641). An English medical author. In 1689 he wrote a book entitled *De Medicina Magnetica* in which he discussed a

"universal fluid." He believed that the fluid was responsible for the influence exerted by man on fellow men and matter. Franz Mesmer (q.v.) presumably borrowed the concept of magnetism (q.v.) from Maxwell.
Bibliography: Cope, Z. 1957. *Sidelights on the history of medicine.*

MAYA (*or* **MAHAMAYA**) (?-c.563 B.C.). The mother of Buddha (q.v.). She provides an example of psychosomatic death brought about by an acute emotion. Before conceiving she dreamed that a little white elephant had entered her womb; when her son was born she died of joy.
Bibliography: Brewster, E. W. 1956. *The life of Gotama the Buddha.*

MAYAKOVSKY, VLADIMIR VLADIMIROVICH (1894-1930). A Russian poet and playwright. His comfortable childhood ended with the death of his father, which plunged the family into poverty. As an adult, his love affairs and friendships brought him sorrow and disillusionment. Although he enthusiastically greeted Marxism and was ready to applaud the changes that were occurring, the death of Nikolai Lenin (q.v.), which he celebrated in a poem full of sadness, left him uncertain of the future and isolated. His works, previously full of propaganda, became critical of the new regime, which turned against him. His physical health was poor, frustration and depression haunted him, and he shot himself, leaving a suicide (q.v.) note in which he said that his love boat had been smashed against the rock of everyday trivialities.
Bibliography: Charters, A., and Charters, S. 1979. *I Love.*

MAYERNE, THEODORE TURQUET DE (1573-1655). A Swiss-born physician. In 1603 he settled in England, where he was regarded as the authority on mental diseases. He was physician to several kings in England and on the continent. He was a follower of the humoral theory (q.v.), but his treatment was more elaborate than that of his contemporaries. Herbs, bleeding (q.v.), purging (q.v.), emetics, blistering, and anointing were used by him. One of his prescriptions contained twenty-seven items alone. He was accused by his enemies of introducing iatrogenic illness by over-prescribing mercury (q.v.) and antimony (q.v.). Twenty-three volumes of his case notes are in the British Museum, and among them are interesting comments on James I of England and VI of Scotland (q.v.), one of his royal patients. There is a monument to him in St. Martin-in-the-Fields in London.
Bibliography: Tuke, D. H. 1882. *History of the insane in the British Isles.*

MAYO, THOMAS (1790-1871). A British physician. As a young man he was interested in psychiatric disorders and coauthored with his father a book entitled *Remarks on Insanity* (1817). In it they presented a plan of therapy that included physical and psychic measures, which reflected their belief in the importance of somatic elements in mental disorders. Mayo later modified

his views and became interested in mental pathology, particularly in its relationship to crime. He wrote several books on the legal aspects of crimes committed by persons presumed insane and encouraged investigations into the problems of double personalities. His *Medical Testimony and Evidence in Cases of Lunacy* appeared in 1854. He also was interested in mesmerism (q.v.) and believed that it could help to ascertain the events that lead to attacks of insanity.
Bibliography: Hunter, R., and Macalpine, I. 1963. *Three hundred years of psychiatry.*

MAZDEJESNAN (fl. c. 500 B.C.). A Persian physician. He was known as the "victor of sickness." He treated his patients by touching them with magic wands, but they had such faith in him that cures by suggestion were numerous.
Bibliography: Cesbron, H. 1909. *Histoire critique de l'hystérie.*

MAZE. One of the best known of the performance tests used in animal psychology. It was introduced in 1901 by William S. Small (q.v.), who designed it for the study of intelligence in laboratory animals. The test was modeled on the maze at Hampton Court (q.v.) in England.
Bibliography: Boring, E. G. 1950. *A history of experimental psychology.*

MAZEPPA. An opera by Peter Tchaikovsky (q.v.). The heroine, Maria, is forcibly married to Mazeppa, who murders her father and her lover. She ends her days in madness.
Bibliography: Rosenthal, H., and Warrack, J. 1964. *Concise Oxford dictionary of opera.*

MAZORRA. A mental hospital in La Habana, Cuba, originally called Hospital San Dionisio. It was founded in 1828. One of its early directors was José Joaquin Munoz, a pioneer in Cuban psychiatry and a follower of the doctrines promulgated by Jean Esquirol (q.v.) and Jules Baillarger (q.v.).
Bibliography: Leon, C. A., and Rosselli, H. 1975. Latin America. In *World history of psychiatry*, ed. J. G. Howells.

MEAD, GEORGE HERBERT (1863-1931). An American social psychologist. He tried to formulate a scientific basis for social psychology (q.v.). In his book *Mind, Self and Society* (1934), he emphasized that the mind of the individual cannot be studied in isolation but rather must be related to society. He developed a pragmatic social behaviorism.
Bibliography: Mead, G. H. 1956. *The social philosophy of George Herbert Mead.*

MEAD, MARGARET (1901-1978). An American anthropologist. She was a student and collaborator of Ruth Benedict (q.v.). Mead's work, influenced

by Karl Abraham (q.v.) and Sigmund Freud (q.v.), covered a wide field. She studied many primitive societies, focusing her attention on the links between culture and personality. She also wrote on child nurturing practices and the cultural aspects of adolescence. Among her best known books are *Coming of Age in Samoa* (1928), *Sex and Temperament in Three Primitive Societies* (1935), *Male and Female* (1949), and *American Women* (1966).
Bibliography: Mead, M. 1972. *Blackberry winter*.

MEAD, RICHARD (1673-1754). An English physician. He believed that mental disorders were incompatible with physical illness, especially tuberculosis (q.v.). He observed that extreme emotional experiences can disturb mental balance, irrespective of the type of emotion aroused. He was a physician at the Bethlem Royal Hospital (q.v.), where he tried to care for the insane by using medications and lessening the stresses playing on their minds, rather than by coercion and physical restraint (q.v.).
Bibliography: Hunter, R., and Macalpine, I. 1963. *Three hundred years of psychiatry*.

MEADOW PARSNIP. A herb growing in most European countries. Herbalists recommend an infusion made from it in the treatment of all nervous complaints, including hysteria, hypochondriasis, epilepsy, and Saint Vitus dance (qq.v.).
Bibliography: Leyel, C. F. 1949. *Heart-ease*.

MECHANISTIC THEORIES. Theories that attempt to explain mental phenomena in terms of mechanical responses. One of the first philosopher/physicians to offer a mechanical explanation for sensation and perception was Democritus (q.v.). In the seventeenth century, René Descartes (q.v.) subscribed to a mechanistic concept of natural phenomena, but he distinguished between phenomena appertaining to the body and those of the mind. The phrenologists (*see* PHRENOLOGY) also held views consistent with a mechanistic theory of behavior. Additional examples can be found in modern schools of psychology.
Bibliography: Watson, R. I. 1963. *The great psychologists*.

MEDEA. A sorceress in Greek mythology (q.v.). In the legends of Jason and Medea, she murders Jason's intended bride and is driven by unbearable conflict to kill her own children. In psychiatry the term "Medea complex" is used to describe those mothers who have death wishes toward their off-

spring. Usually the death wish is motivated by a desire for revenge against the father. The term was first used by F. Wittels, in 1944.
Bibliography: Stern, E. S. 1948. The Medea complex: mother's homicidal wishes to her child. *J. Ment. Sci.* 94:321.

MEDICAL INQUIRIES AND OBSERVATIONS UPON THE DISEASES OF THE MIND. The first American book on psychiatry. It was written by Benjamin Rush (q.v.) in 1812.
Bibliography: Dain, N. 1964. *Concepts of insanity in the United States, 1789-1865.*

MEDICI. Among the Arabs and in the Middle Ages (q.v.) the *medici* were those practitioners of medicine who investigated with their senses. The *physici* used logical arguments to reach their conclusions and were regarded as superior to the medici.
Bibliography: Talbot, C. H. 1967. *Medicine in medieval England.*

MEDICINA GYMNASTICA. A book written by Francis Fuller (1670-1706) and first published in 1705 in London. In it the author recounted his own experiences with a cutaneous infection that did not respond to ointments, bleeding (q.v.), or hydrotherapy; it so worried him that he became a hypochondriac (*see* HYPOCHONDRIASIS). By chance he discovered that his hypochondriasis responded to horseback riding (q.v.), and he was soon cured. This caused him to advise exercise, especially horseback riding, for hypochondria and hysterical (*see* HYSTERIA) disorders. According to him, it was important that rider and horse should suit each other's temperament. The book was such a success that by 1777 it was in its ninth edition.
Bibliography: Hunter, R., and Macalpine, I. 1963. *Three hundred years of psychiatry.*

MEDICINAL DAYS. In Hippocratic (*see* HIPPOCRATES) doctrine, the days when crises were likely to occur, and the days when it was safe to administer medicines (medical days). Number lore can be found in the early systems of medicine in many cultures. It may be based upon the observation of periodicity of some pathological phenomena.
See also ANNIVERSARY REACTION and MENSIS MEDICALIS.
Bibliography: Garrison, F. H. 1929. *An introduction to the history of medicine.*

MEDICINA MUSICA. The first English book on music therapy (q.v.). It was written by an apothecary named Richard Browne and first published in 1727 under a longer title. The second edition in 1729 bore the title *Medicina Musica.* He recommended music not only for diseases of the body but especially for diseases of the mind. He went on to stress its power

to "sooth the turbulent affections" and calm "maniacal" patients who had not responded to physical remedies.
Bibliography: Hunter, R., and Macalpine, I. 1963. *Three hundred years of psychiatry.*

MEDICO-PSYCHOLOGICAL ASSOCIATION OF GREAT BRITAIN AND IRELAND. *See* ASSOCIATION OF MEDICAL OFFICERS OF ASYLUMS AND HOSPITALS FOR THE INSANE.

MEDIUM. A person claiming to be able to mediate between the living and the dead by communicating with the dead while in a state of trance. The ancient Greeks and Romans practiced the art of mediumship. In the middle of the nineteenth century there was an upsurge of interest in psychical phenomena, and some mediums became famous. Seances became socially acceptable and fashionable. The credulity of the believers was matched by the ingenuity of the charlatans: illusions and hallucinations (q.v.) were easily provoked in an atmosphere charged with suggestion and tension. In London, crystal balls were the rage of the time, Queen Victoria and Prince Albert practiced "table-turning" and in Florence so-called guaranteed turning tables were sold for high prices. Mediums and their seances quickly lost their popularity when, toward the end of the century, they were subjected to scientific investigation.
Bibliography: Pearsall, R. 1972. *The table rappers.*

MEDIUM, THE. An opera by Gian-Carlo Menotti (1911-). It describes the tragedy of a woman caught between the world of reality and the world of the supernatural. The composer was inspired to use this theme after he had attended a séance with some friends and was struck by their pathetic anxiety to believe that they could communicate with their dead daughter.
Bibliography: Harewood, ed. 1969. *Kobbe's complete opera book.*

MEDUNA, LADISLAS JOSEPH VON (1896-1964). A Hungarian psychiatrist who emigrated to the United States in 1939. On the basis of his comparison of the brains of schizophrenic (*see* SCHIZOPHRENIA) and epileptic (*see* EPILEPSY) patients, he concluded that the two diseases were incompatible. Thus, in 1935, he introduced Metrazol therapy (q.v.) for schizophrenia. In 1946, he originated carbon dioxide therapy (q.v.) for neurotic (*see* NEUROSIS) disorders. Rejecting psychodynamic theories and psychoanalysis (q.v.), he believed in the efficacy of psychopharmacology.

He founded the Society of Medical Psychiatry and helped to establish the *Journal of Neuropsychiatry*.
Bibliography: Wortis, J., ed. 1966. *Recent advances in biological psychiatry*. Vol. 8.

MEERENBERG HOSPITAL. A mental hospital in the Netherlands. Founded in 1849, it was the first Dutch hospital to introduce the nonrestraint system.
Bibliography: Gerdes, E. 1876. Reprint. 1971. *Meerenberg en de Kranzinnigen*.

MEGARIS. A part of ancient Greece. Its inhabitants were proverbial for their stupidity, yet Euclid (fl. 300 B.C.) was a Megarian and founded a school of philosophy there.
Bibliography: 1978. *Brewer's dictionary of phrase and fable*.

MEGRIMS. A term originating from a corruption of hemicrania, which, in Greek, meant half the skull. The term "migraine" (q.v.) is derived from it. It was used also to indicate silly whims and fantasies.
Bibliography: 1978. *Brewer's dictionary of phrase and fable*.

MEINONG, ALEXIUS (1853-1920). An Austrian philosopher and psychologist. He was a pupil of Franz Brentano (q.v.) in Vienna. After taking a degree in philosophy, he remained in Vienna as a professor. Although he was not an experimentalist and his work was in the field of theoretical psychology and the theory of knowledge, in 1894 he founded the first Austrian psychological laboratory (q.v.) located in Graz. He established a general theory of value that was based on psychological assumptions and expressed in a new terminology.
Bibliography: Boring, E. G. 1950. *A history of experimental psychology*.

MEJIA, EPIFANIO (1838-1913). A Colombian poet. To support his family of twelve children, he engaged in commerce and agriculture. In 1869 he became deranged, possibly schizophrenic (*see* SCHIZOPHRENIA). He spent more than thirty years in a mental hospital and died without regaining his reason. During his insanity he was happy and tranquil, believing that he lived in an ideal world. His best known poems are *Can del Antioqueno* and *Historia de una Tortola*.
Bibliography: Rosselli, H. 1968. *Historia de la psiquiatria en Colombia*.

MELAMPOD. Another term for hellebore (q.v.). It is derived from Melampus (q.v.).
Bibliography: 1978. *Brewer's dictionary of phrase and fable*.

MELAMPUS. In Greek mythology (q.v.), the son of Amythaon. The early Greeks believed him to be the first mortal to receive prophetic power and to practice medicine. According to legend, he rescued and reared some young serpents whose parents had been killed, and, in gratitude, they licked his ears, thus giving him the ability to predict the future and to understand the language of the birds. Serpents have remained a symbol of the healing art since that time. Melampus was said to have obtained a share of the kingdom of Argos by using hellebore (q.v.) to cure its women who had fallen victims to an epidemic of lycanthropy (q.v.) and roamed about imagining that they were cows.

Bibliography: Virgil. *Eclogues—Georgics*, trans. H. R. Fairclough.

MELANCHOLIA. A term derived from the Greek, meaning "black bile" (q.v.). An excess of this humor (q.v.) was believed to be responsible for depression. The term came to be used for both the humor and the disorder. Among the earliest writings on melancholy are those of Hippocrates (q.v.). In his classification of mental disorders, he used the term "melancholia" to indicate states of abnormal depression. Climatic (*see* CLIMATE) conditions, astral influences, incorrect diets (q.v.), and constitutional mental characteristics were among the aetiological factors of melancholia. Greco-Roman physicians, represented by Aretaus of Cappadocia (q.v.), attributed "amorous melancholy" to the tribulations of love. Galen (q.v.) thought that melancholy was due to *succus melancholicus*, or melancholic humor, which affected the sensual soul and made the patient depressed. Avicenna (q.v.) believed that the seat of melancholy could be found in the stomach (q.v.), the spleen (q.v.) and the liver (q.v.). In the Middle Ages (q.v.), it sometimes was attributed to the devil. Later, more sophisticated workers modified this belief by attributing melancholy to guilt about sin. Timothy Bright (q.v.) and Robert Burton (q.v.) were among the many authors who wrote about melancholy in the sixteenth and seventeenth centuries. Jacques Ferrand (q.v.) was particularly interested in what he called "erotic melancholy," or erotomania (q.v.). The term often covered reactive depression and psychotic (*see* PSYCHOSIS) depression and confused the symptoms of the two. As reactive depression is a common symptom in neurosis (q.v.) the term often embraced this condition also. Historically, melancholy has been fashionable in two periods. The first spans the latter part of the sixteenth century and the first part of the seventeenth, and the second occurred in the nineteenth century, when it was regarded as "interesting" and the sign of a cultured person. In that century, poets and society ladies cultivated it. Daniel H. Tuke (q.v.) devoted a number of pages to melancholia in his *Dictionary of Psychological Medicine* (1892) and subdivided it into more than fifty different forms, from *active melancholia*, characterized by agitation, to *melancholia zoanthropia*, characterized by the patient's belief that he has been transformed into an animal.

Bibliography: Zilboorg, G. 1941. *A history of medical psychology.*

MELANCHOLIA, DE. A treatise by Constantine the African (q.v.) written in the eleventh century. Mental disorders are discussed in it, and their aetiology is attributed to humoral imbalance. He considered the brain or the stomach (q.v.) to be the seat of melancholia (q.v.). Other psychiatric symptoms, such as guilt, withdrawal, and delusions (q.v.), and their causes are also described.

MELANCHOLIA ANGLICA. A term coined by François Sauvages (q.v.) to indicate depression with suicidal (*see* SUICIDE) thoughts. He believed it to be endemic in England.
See also ENGLISH MALADY.

MELANCHOLY JACQUES. An expression derived from William Shakespeare's (q.v.) *As You Like It.* Jean Jacques Rousseau (q.v.) was often referred to as "Melancholy Jacques" because of his constant gloomy expression and his morbid sensibility.
Bibliography: 1978. *Brewer's dictionary of phrase and fable.*

MELANCHTHON, PHILIP (1497-1560). A German scholar and religious reformer. His real name was Schwarzerd, which he hellenized into Melanchthon. He was a friend and associate of Martin Luther (q.v.). He believed that "the variety of melancholic diseases proceeds from the stars." He is credited with coining the term "psychology" meaning the study of the soul. In spite of his enlightened, humanistic views, he regarded the burning of heretics as just and proper.
Bibliography: Manschrek, C. 1958. *Melanchthon, the quiet reformer.*

MELANCOLICO, EL. A Spanish play written in 1611 by Tirso de Molina (1584?-1648). The character of Rogerio, the moody hero, is believed to have been based on Philip II (q.v.).
Bibliography: Bushee, A. H. 1939. *Three centuries of Tirso de Molina.*

MELESTA. A small island among the Hebrides in Scotland. It was believed that all its inhabitants were either born insane or became so before death.
Bibliography: Tuke, D. H. 1882. *History of the insane in the British Isles.*

MELILOT. A term literally meaning "honey lotus." It is used to designate a herb similar to clover. Herbalists believe it to be efficacious in the treatment of nervous disorders, especially those involving the eyes.
Bibliography: Law, D. 1969. *Herb growing for health.*

MELUN. A term from the Middle Ages (q.v.) indicating a chalet for the insane.
Bibliography: Foucault, M. 1967. *Madness and civilization.*

MELVILLE, HERMAN (1819-1891). An American novelist. He began his working life at the age of fifteen as a bank clerk, but in 1839 he left New York and went off in search of adventure on the sea. This period provided the inspiration for many of his works, especially his masterpiece *Moby Dick* (1851). Both his father and his brother had suffered from mental disorders, and he too was often depressed to the point of despair. His personality and emotional problems are reflected in his story *Bartleby the Scrivener* (q.v.).
Bibliography: Mumford, L. 1962. *Herman Melville: a study of his life and vision.*

MEMORIAS DE LA CASA DE ORATES. The title of the first psychiatric book in Chile. It was written by the Argentinian psychiatrist Ramon Elquero, physician in charge of the Casa de Orates, or House for the Insane in Santiago during the 1860s.
Bibliography: Leon, C. A., and Rosselli, H. 1975. Latin America. In *World history of psychiatry*, ed. J. G. Howells.

MEMORY. Early philosophers were greatly concerned with problems of memory. In the fourth century B.C. Aristotle (q.v.) wrote a treatise on *Memory and Forgetting*. In the seventeenth century, Francis Bacon (q.v.), in his analysis of psychological attributes, classified memory, understanding, and imagination as the three faculties of the soul. His analysis influenced the study of psychology for a long time. Juan Vives (q.v.) devoted a third of his work *De Anima et Vita* (1538) to phenomena related to the memory, as well as other things, in terms of association. In the nineteenth century, the work of Hermann Ebbinghaus (q.v.) initiated experimental studies on memory and its measurement, which resulted in more research in the field of psychology and education. Georg E. Müller (q.v.) was among the pioneers in this area of study.
Bibliography: Brett, G. S. 1912. *A history of psychology.*

MEMPHIS. An Egyptian city. A temple of healing was established there in honor of Imhotep (q.v.), and the city later became famous for its hospital and for its school of medicine.
Bibliography: Hurry, J. B. 1928. *Imhotep.*

MENDEL, GREGOR JOHANN (1822-1884). An Austrian biologist and abbot in the Order of St. Augustine. In the garden of the monastery at Brünn he experimented with peas and discovered their dominant and recessive characteristics. From this he developed theories of heredity that were

later rediscovered and on which the science of modern genetics is based. His work has considerably influenced psychiatric genetics.
Bibliography: Wilson, J. 1929. *A manual of Mendelism.*

MENECRATES OF SYRACUSE. A physician who, according to the Greek scholar Athenaeus in the second century A.D. 1, suffered from the delusion (q.v.) that he was Zeus.
Bibliography: Moss, C. G. 1967. Mental Disorders in Antiquity. In *Diseases in antiquity*, ed. D. Brothwell and A. T. Sandison.

MENIPPUS. A Greek Cynic (*see* CYNICS) philosopher of the third century B.C. He was a pupil of Diogenes (q.v.). A bitter man, he used satire even against his fellow philosophers. On losing his fortune, he hanged himself.
Bibliography: Diogenes Laertius. *Lives of Eminent Philosophers.* Vol. 2, trans. R. D. Hicks.

MENNINGER FOUNDATION. A nonprofit American psychiatric organization chartered in 1941. It developed from the Menninger Clinic, which was founded in Topeka, Kansas, in 1919, by Dr. Charles F. Menninger (1862-1953) and his eldest son, Karl Menninger (q.v.). Charles Menninger's youngest son, William, later joined them. Begun as a group practice, in 1925 the clinic expanded into a sanatorium and was housed in a converted farmhouse. Within ten years the clinic was one of the best private mental hospitals in the United States. Needing financial support for education and research, the Menninger Foundation was established on April 23, 1941 as a nonprofit corporation. In addition to clinical services, it provides a training program, facilities for research, and preventive activities. Its practice is based largely on psychoanalysis. It employs a staff of over 1,000 people.
Bibliography: Menninger Foundation. 1961. *Interdisciplinary research on work and mental health; a point of view and a method.*

MENNINGER, KARL AUGUSTUS (1893-   ). An American psychiatrist. In 1919, he joined his father in establishing the Menninger Clinic in Topeka, Kansas, for the practice of general medicine and psychiatry. In 1941 the Menninger Foundation (q.v.) was developed from the clinic. He has contributed to research in psychosomatic medicine (q.v.), criminology, suicide (q.v.), industrial and military psychology and classification. Among his many books are *The Human Mind* (1930), *Man Against Himself* (1938), and *The Vital Balance* (1963).

MENSIS MEDICALIS. A medical month, based on the Galenic tradition of a lunar month of twenty-six days. These days were regarded as particularly favorable for diagnosis or therapy, which was linked to astrology (q.v.).
See also MEDICINAL DAYS.
Bibliography: Zilboorg, G. 1941. *A history of medical psychology.*

MENTAL AFTER-CARE ASSOCIATION. An association founded in England in 1879 by the Reverend Henry Hawkins (q.v.), the chaplain for

Colney Hatch Asylum (q.v.). Its objective was to provide convalescent homes for those patients recently discharged from mental hospitals. Its first president was Lord Anthony Shaftesbury (q.v.), and its membership included the leading psychiatrists of the time.

Bibliography: Hunter, R., and Macalpine, I. 1974. *Psychiatry for the poor.*

MENTAL DEFECTIVE SCHOOLS. Nineteenth-century schools for the mentally retarded. They reflected the humanitarian attitude of the century. In the first three decades of the nineteenth century in France, Guillaume Ferrus (q.v.) at Bicêtre (q.v.) and L. Falret at the Salpêtrière (q.v.) were pioneers in the establishment of an instructional program for mental defectives. In 1837 Edouard Seguin (q.v.) established a private school that was based in part on the ideas of Jean Itard (q.v.). In Switzerland, Jakob Guggenbuhl (q.v.) founded the Abendberg Institution (q.v.) for cretins (*see* CRETINISM) in 1842, and in Germany, C. W. Saegert was the founder of an establishment in Berlin termed "Institution for the Care and Education of Idiots." In England, due primarily to the efforts of John Conolly (q.v.) institutions were opened at Bath, Colchester, and Earlswood, as well as other places. In the United States the first public provisions for the training of mental defectives were inaugurated in 1857 at the Ohio State Lunatic Asylum. These were followed by the establishment of similar schools in other states.

Bibliography: Kanner, L. 1964. *A history of the care and study of the mentally retarded.*

MENTAL HYGIENE. The term was first used in the United States in 1843 by Dr. William C. Sweetser (q.v.), the author of a book entitled *Mental Hygiene or an Examination of the Intellect and Passions Designed to Illustrate their Influence on Health and Duration of Life.* This volume was followed in 1863 by a work written by Isaac Ray (q.v.) and entitled *Mental Hygiene.*

Bibliography: Zilboorg G. 1964. *A history of medical psychology.*

MENTAL HYGIENE MOVEMENT. A movement initiated in 1909 in the United States after the publication of *The Mind that Found Itself* by Clifford Beers (q.v.). In the same year, a group of prominent psychiatrists and psychologists including Adolf Meyer (q.v.) and William James (q.v.) founded the National Committee for Mental Hygiene, which later became known as the National Committee for Mental Health. In England a similar organization, known as the National Council for Mental Hygiene, came into existence. It merged later with other voluntary organizations and founded the National Association for Mental Health (q.v.).

Bibliography: Deutsch, A. 1949. *The mentally ill in America.*

MEPHISTOPHELES. A name derived from the Greek, meaning "not loving light," hence "lord of darkness" and "spirit of destruction." He appears

in both Christian and pagan medieval legends. In the play *Faust*, Johann Wolfgang von Goethe (q.v.) endows him with supernatural power as the tempter of Faust with whom he makes a pact entailing the exchange of Faust's soul for the chance of comprehending all experience, including personal feeling, culture, politics, and history.
Bibliography: 1978. *Brewer's dictionary of phrase and fable*.

MERCIER, DÉSIRÉ JOSEPH (1851-1926). A Belgian cardinal. He was a theologian and a pioneer of neoscholastic psychology, which reintroduced the doctrines of Aristotle (q.v.). In 1891 he established a psychology laboratory (q.v.) at the University of Louvain. His book on the history of psychology, entitled *The Origins of Contemporary Psychology*, was published in London in 1918.
Bibliography: Gade, J. A. 1934. *The life of Cardinal Mercier*.

MERCURIALE, GERONIMO (MERCURIALIS, HIERONYMUS) (1530-1606). An Italian physician. He wrote essays on melancholia (q.v.) and mania (q.v.) and described several types of each. He pointed out that melancholic people often suffered from digestive disorders and affections of the heart, which made them anxious and fearful. Melancholia, according to him, was due to a life of pleasure and luxury. He distinguished three types of mania: sanguineous, bilious, and melancholic. For the first he prescribed bleeding (q.v.) for the second cholagogues, and for the third purges (*see* PURGING) and cauterization (q.v.). He was also the author of works on skin diseases, pediatrics, and an illustrated treatise on medical gymnastics.
Bibliography: Castiglioni, A. 1946. *A history of medicine*, ed. and trans. E. B. Krumbhaar.

MERCURY. A metallic chemical element. In the Middle Ages (q.v.), it was used in the treatment of skin diseases including those of syphilitic (*see* SYPHILIS) origin. Later it became a form of therapy for unspecified mental disorders, because it was believed that the increase in salivation produced by it would help the body to reject morbid juices. Benjamin Rush (q.v.) was an enthusiastic advocate of its use.
Bibliography: Rush, B. 1812. *Medical inquiries and observations upon the diseases of the mind*.

MERLIN. A prophet, magician, and poet in Welsh tradition. He was said to be the son of a maiden and a demon or an incubus (q.v). Although he was redeemed by baptism, he retained his father's gifts of divination. During the battle of Arthured in A.D. 573, he became insane.
Bibliography: Jarman, A. O. H. 1960. *The legend of Merlin*.

MERXHAUSEN. A cloister in Germany belonging to the monks of St. Augustine. In 1553 it was adapted to function as a mental hospital.

MÉRYON, CHARLES (1821-1868). A French etcher. He was the illegitimate son of an English physician and a French dancer. His father provided financially for his education but gave him little emotional support. Méryon appears to have brooded over his illegitimacy, which he regarded as a great social handicap. When his wish to become a painter was frustrated by his discovery that he was color blind, he became an etcher. His behavior began to show signs of paranoia (q.v.), and he began to express delusions (q.v.) and feelings of unfounded guilt. At the age of thirty-six, he was arrested and taken to the asylum of Charenton-Saint-Maurice, where he was said to suffer from melancholic (*see* MELANCHOLIA) madness. His symptoms occasionally were mild enough to permit some artistic output, but it was usually bizarre, although technically good. One of his delusional works was an illustrated legislative plan, *The Lunar Law*, which, among other things, suggested that all people should be forced to sleep in an upright position. Almost continually hallucinated (*see* HALLUCINATION) he believed himself to be Christ. Toward the end of his life, he refused food and eventually died of malnutrition.
Bibliography: Fama, P.G. 1973. Charles Méryon: a biographical and psychiatric reassessment. *New Zealand Med. J.* 28: 448-55.

MERZBACHER, LUDWIG (1875-?). A German physician practicing in Argentina. In 1908 he described a familial hereditary condition in which the cerebral white matter of the brain degenerates. He described its symptomatology, which includes lack of coordination, speech disorders, and mental retardation, and called it "aplasia axialis extracorticalis congenita." A German neurologist, Friedrich Pelizaeus (q.v.) had previously reported the condition in 1885. It has since become known as Pelizaeus-Merzbacher disease. Merzbacher also demonstrated that some forms of mental deficiency are associated with structural anomalies in the brain.
Bibliography: Merzbacher, L. 1908. Weitere Mitteilungen über eine eigenartiage hereditär-familiäre Erkrankung des Zentral-nervensystems. *Med. Klin., Berlin* 4: 1952-95.

MESCALINE. The active principle of the peyote (q.v.).

MESMER, FRANZ ANTON (1734-1815). An Austrian physician, born in Switzerland. He studied Paracelsus' (q.v.) theories of mental illness and the methods of treatment used by Jan Van Helmont (q.v.) from whom he derived his doctrine of magnetic fluid or celestial force, which he believed could be applied by the use of magnetic rods. He described his belief in his book *De Planetarum Influxu* (1776). He later abandoned the rods, when he became convinced that he had discovered "animal magnetism" (q.v.), a personal fluid that could pass from the therapist to the patient. In 1779 he described his new ideas in his work *Mémoire sur la Decouverte du Mag-*

netisme Animal. He applied his doctrines to individuals and groups, which he gathered round his famous baquet (q.v.). His success was, of course, due to suggestion as the royal commission appointed in 1784 by the French government to investigate his practices realized. They found that imagination (q.v.) rather than magnetism was the basis of his cures, and he was discredited. He died in obscurity, but, for a time, he had achieved immense popularity, especially in France. His seances were attended by many famous people, including Philippe Pinel (q.v.). Although he has often been represented as a charlatan, he focused attention on hypnotic phenomena, and there is evidence that he was a cultured and fashionable man, a patron and friend of composers. Wolfgang Amadeus Mozart's (1756-1791) early opera *Bastien und Bastienne* was given its premiere in the garden of Mesmer's beautiful house in Vienna.

Bibliography: Walmsley, D. M. 1967. *Anton Mesmer*.

MESMERISM. The name given to Franz Mesmer's (q.v.) process, which often produced dramatic hypnotic (*see* HYPNOTISM) phenomena. Mesmer first used it in Austria but met with such hostility there that he moved to Paris. From there mesmerism spread to other countries, where it was put to various uses. In England, John Elliotson (q.v.) enthusiastically advocated it; in London, James Esdaile (q.v.) applied it to produce anaesthesia, and in the United States it was propagated by the public demonstrations of Charles Poyen, a French magnetizer. Mesmerism helped to redress the balance between physical and emotional phenomena and led to the development of psychotherapy (q.v.).

See also MAGNETISM.

Bibliography: Thornton, E. M. 1976. *Hypnotism, hysteria and epilepsy: an historical synthesis*.

MESOPOTAMIAN PSYCHIATRY. Medicine in ancient Mesopotamia was based on magic (q.v.) and religion. Whatever the illness, the patient's life history was taken into account in the diagnosis and treatment of it. Disease was regarded as punishment for sin, and mental disorders were attributed to demoniac possession (q.v.). Magic, astrology (q.v.), and divination were employed by the priest-physicians. Dream (q.v.) interpretations played an important part.

Bibliography: Alexander, F. G., and Selesnick, S. T. 1966. *The history of psychiatry*.

MESSALINA, VALERIA (?-48 A.D.). The third wife of the Emperor Claudius. Her lust and cruelty made her name a byword for vice. She was executed by order of her husband.

Bibliography: Seutonious. *The twelve Caesars*, trans. R. Graves.

MESSER, AUGUST (1867-1937). A German psychologist and philosopher. He was influenced by the work of Oswald Külpe (q.v.) under whom he

studied at Würzburg. Messer used introspection to explore thought processes and by means of free and constrained associations came to the conclusion that mental content was linked to psychic processes. From this he developed a system that combined content psychology with act psychology (q.v.). His studies in Würzburg resulted in his book *Experimentelle-psychologische Untersuchungen über das Denken*, which was published in 1906.
Bibliography: Boring, E. G. 1950. *A history of experimental psychology.*

MESSERSCHMIDT, FRANZ XAVER (1736-1784). A German sculptor. He rose from poverty to fame and became assistant professor of sculpture at the Academy of Vienna. He expected to become full professor on the death of the head of the department, but there were objections to his appointment. Count Wenzel Kauniz (1711-1794), the prime minister, wrote to Empress Maria Thérèsa (1717-1780) that Messerschmidt had "shown signs of some confusion" in "a perfectly healthy imagination." He added that Messerschmidt also suffered from what amounted to persecution mania (q.v.) and could not be trusted with pupils. Disappointed at not receiving the professorship, Messerschmidt retired to Bratislava. He lived in isolation and remained bitter, persecuted, and too proud to accept favors from would-be benefactors. His sculptures, usually busts or heads, were studies of human physiognomy that often showed considerable passion. In many sculptures he was his own model and worked from a mirror into which his grimacing image was projected and then endlessly reproduced in marble. He believed that demons, jealous of his skill, tormented him.
Bibliography: Kris, E. 1952. *Psychoanalytic explorations in art.*

METALLIC TRACTORS. Rods made of iron and brass that were devised and patented by Dr. Elisha Perkins (q.v.) an American physician. They were brought to England by his son toward the end of the eighteenth century. The rods were supposed to effect cures by the transference of "animal electricity." They were successfully marketed in various parts of the country until 1799 when Dr. John Haygarth of Bath, England, demonstrated that wooden rods, painted to resemble iron, had the same effect and concluded that the cures were due to the "patient's imagination."
Bibliography: Hunter, R., and Macalpine, I. 1963. *Three hundred years of psychiatry.*

METAPSYCHOLOGY. Sigmund Freud (q.v.) coined this term by analogy with the metaphysics of Aristotle (q.v.). It expresses the concept of a doctrine that goes beyond psychology.
Bibliography: Watson, R. I. 1963. *The great psychologists.*

METEORS. Shooting stars. They were believed to be "the excrements of the stars" that brought catastrophes to earth and caused physical and mental disease in men. This belief was held by Saint Hildegard of Bingen (q.v.) and Paracelsus (q.v.) among others.

METHODISM. A nonconformist Christian sect founded in England by John Wesley (q.v.). Its impact on the workers and its influence on the poor was regarded with suspicion by the middle classes. Its doctrines were accused of causing "religious mania," and Jules Falret (q.v.) went so far as to link Methodism with the frequency of suicide (q.v.) in England.
Bibliography: Leigh, D. 1961. *The historical development of British psychiatry.*

METLINGER, BARTHOLOMAEUS (?-1492). A German pediatrician. The first known reference to microcephaly occurs in his book *Ein Regiment der jungen Kinder*, which was published in Augsburg, Germany, in 1473. It was the first handbook on the care of children written in German and, therefore, understandable to those who had no knowledge of Latin.
Bibliography: Still, G. F. 1965. *The history of paediatrics.*

METOPOSCOPY. The practice of predicting the future and reading the past from the lines on the forehead. It was known and practiced in antiquity. In the sixteenth century, Girolamo Cardano (q.v.) was the greatest exponent of metoposcopy, although he admitted that it was a fallible art. According to the rules that he devised, seven horizontal lines on the forehead corresponded to seven planets, each linked with personal characteristics. Other minor lines and marks were also considered before compiling a forecast of future events for an individual. Cardano wrote a book on the subject entitled *Metoposcopie.*
Bibliography: Wykes, A. 1969. *Doctor Cardano physician extraordinary.*

METRAZOL THERAPY. Intravenous injections of metrazol were introduced as a form of shock therapy by Ladislas Meduna (q.v.) in 1935. He used this drug to produce convulsions in schizophrenic (*see* SCHIZOPHRENIA) patients on the rationale that epileptic (*see* EPILEPSY) seizures had been observed to reduce the symptoms of psychosis (q.v.).
Bibliography: Goldenson, R. M. 1970. *The encyclopedia of human behavior.*

METZ. A French city. The town's records show that the mentally ill were cared for in the two monasteries founded there by Sigibaldus (q.v.) in A.D. 850. Guardians and hospital attendants for the insane had to swear an oath that they would conscientiously fulfil their duties. One of the earliest asylums exclusively for the mentally ill existed in Metz in 1100.
Bibliography: Walsh, J. J. 1970. *Medieval medicine.*

MEUMANN, ERNST (1862-1915). A German educational psychologist and pupil of Wilhelm Wundt (q.v.). His *Oekonomie und Technik des Ler-*

nens (1903) deals with various aspects of learning. With Wundt he conducted experiments on the time sense and devised special apparatus for this type of research. In his later years he wrote on esthetics. In 1903 he founded the *Archiv für die gesamte Psychologie*.
Bibliography: Boring, E. G. 1950. *A history of experimental psychology.*

MEYER, ADOLF (1866-1950). An American psychiatrist and neurologist, born in Switzerland. In 1892, after qualifying in Zürich, he emigrated to the United States. In 1910, after various clinical and academic appointments, he became professor of psychiatry at the Johns Hopkins Hospital in Baltimore, Maryland, and director of the Henry Phipps Psychiatric Clinic (q.v.) in 1913. He rejected investigations based on autopsies and preferred to observe living patients. He introduced the term "psychobiology," (q.v.) meaning the study of mental life and behavior in relation to other biological processes, and this approach and his understanding of the patient's total personality and reactions greatly influenced American psychiatric education. He forged an affective link between European and American psychiatry and brought new concepts to both. He recognized the importance of considering the patient's background in developing a treatment program and the need to educate the public about mental health in order to prevent certain mental disorders. He was active in the mental hygiene movement (q.v.) and actually suggested the term "mental hygiene."
Bibliography: Winters, E. E., ed. 1950-1952. *The collected papers of Adolf Meyer.* 4 vols.

MEYER, CONRAD FERDINAND (1825-1898). A Swiss poet and novelist, born near Zürich. His family included an adopted child who was mentally defective. His mother was a fanatic Calvinist, who suffered from severe headaches and depression. She had a nervous breakdown soon after his birth. Throughout her life, she would not allow her children to kiss her, yet she was extremely possessive. In 1856, when Meyer was thirty-one years old, she committed suicide (q.v.), and it was only then that he felt himself free. He was an introverted, insecure, depressed man who suffered from a physical deformity: a bone disorder caused him to have an enormous head, while his body was exceptionally thin. His beard did not grow until he was forty years old because of an endocrine imbalance. He was seen so seldom that people sometimes thought that he had died. Brief periods of happiness produced such anxiety in him that he would burst into tears. Meyer was admitted to a mental hospital for the first time when he was twenty-seven. He suffered from delusions (q.v.), depression, and suicidal impulses. It was only after he was forty that he began to write and developed a more normal personality. Intricate psychological situations and complex personality de-

scriptions characterize his work. He wrote epic poems and historical novels of which *Der Heilige* (1880) is one of the best remembered.
Bibliography: Hohenstein, L. 1957. *Conrad Ferdinand Meyer.*

MEYER, MARY (*née* **POTTER BROOKS**). Wife of Adolf Meyer (q.v.). She helped her husband in his work by visiting female patients to learn about their backgrounds and social histories. She is regarded as the first American social worker.
Bibliography: Alexander, F. G. and Selesnick, S. T. 1966. *The history of psychiatry.*

MEYNERT, THEODOR HERMANN (1833-1892). A German neurologist and psychiatrist. He came from a rather Bohemian family. His father was a writer, and his mother was an opera singer. He anticipated many developments in both neurology and psychiatry. His histological studies of the nervous system gave him a sound basis for understanding the function and structure of the cortex. He is credited with the first description of "association neurones" in 1868. Paranoia (q.v.), which he called *amentia*, was described by him. His concepts were dynamic, but his approach to mental disease was purely anatomical. He even objected to the term "psychiatry" because he advocated minimal restraint (q.v.) in asylums (q.v.). Auguste Forel (q.v.) spent several months with Meynert but was disconcerted by the disorder and dirt of the department at the asylum and by Meynert's aloofness. Sigmund Freud (q.v.) studied under him at the medical school in Vienna and obtained his first knowledge of clinical psychiatry there.
Bibliography: Haymaker, W., and Schiller, F. 1970. *The founders of neurology.* 2d. ed.

MICAWBER. A byword for an incurable optimist. It is derived from Wilkins Micawber, a character in *David Copperfield* by Charles Dickens (q.v.). Dickens based the character on his father. Micawber never doubted that all his ill founded schemes would lead to fortune, despite the fact that they each ended in grief.
Bibliography: Dickens, C. 1849-1850. *David Copperfield.*

MICHELANGELO BUONARROTI (1475-1564). An Italian sculptor, painter, and poet. His genius (q.v.) was marked by his stubbornness and his hypersensitivity. He was passionately loyal to his friends but could not be polite to those he disliked. He was generous and avaricious, suspicious and jealous. His extravagances puzzled those around him, and his violence was often frightening. Many of his works were never completed, possibly because he was tormented by doubts and self-criticism. His contemporaries called him "the divine madman," and he himself wrote that "there is no better way of keeping sane and free from anxiety than being mad." It is

possible that he was never in love with a woman. Even Vittoria Colonna (1490-1547), who entered his later years, probably represented an intellectual rather than intimate relationship. Although his letters and love poems to men have been interpreted as displaying a tendency to homosexuality (q.v.), in the context of the period they were not sensual and probably no more than expressions of platonic friendship.
Bibliography: Murray, L. 1980. *Michelangelo.*

MICHON, PIERRE, ABBÉ BOURDELOT (1610-1685). A French physician. He was interested in the correlation between handwriting and character traits. The term "graphology" (q.v.) was coined by him.
Bibliography: Rand, H. A. 1962. *Graphology.*

MICHOTTE, ALBERT EDOUARD (1881-1965). A Belgian psychologist. Working at the laboratory of Louvain University, he conducted experimental work in and research on the processes involved in choice. He also studied problems of perception, movement, and learning and devised new investigation techniques for them. In the latter part of his life he turned his attention to the perceptual phenomena of causality.
Bibliography: Michotte, A. et al. 1962. *Causalité, permanence et réalité phénoménales.*

MICRONOMANIA. A term coined by Benjamin Rush (q.v.) to describe what was later called moral insanity. It is presently referred to as psychopathy (q.v.). Rush called the total absence of this quality "anomia" (q.v.).
See also INSANITY, MORAL.
Bibliography: Rush, B. 1786. Reprint 1972. *Two essays on the mind,* intro. E. T. Carlson.

MICROSCOPE. Although this instrument in a rudimentary form was probably invented as early as the thirteenth century by Roger Bacon (q.v.) and was employed in medicine as early as the seventeenth century, it was not used to study brain pathology until the nineteenth century, when histopathological changes in the brains of patients suffering from general paralysis of the insane (q.v.) were observed under its lenses.
Bibliography: Zilboorg, G. 1941. *A history of medical psychology.*

MIDDLE AGES. A period in Western European history marked by more than usual sadness and pessimism. Plague, disease, and death were constant sources of anxiety and depression. Superstition was rampant. The belief that disease was sent by God as a form of retribution for sin led to feelings of guilt and practices aimed at the expiation of guilt and the postponement of impending doom. Witchcraft (q.v.) was alternatively blamed for all ills and used as a protection against them. The concept of the "whole man," which was held by medieval medicine, meant that diseases of body and soul were

recognized and attributed respectively to physical agents or less tangible causes. Treatment consisted of herbal remedies, adjustments in diet (q.v.), bleeding (q.v.), and exorcism (q.v.), which at times included beating the patient to drive the devil out of him. To this period belong such mass phenomena as flagellants (q.v.) and dancing mania (q.v.), which can now be attributed to group hysteria (q.v.) or ergot poisoning (q.v.) and other toxic states. No special provisions for the care of the insane existed. They were admitted into the hospitals of monasteries and religious organizations as part of the Christian duty of caring for the sick.
Bibliography: Huizinga, J. 1954. *The waning of the Middle Ages.*

MIDDLESEX HOUSE. A private nursing home for mental patients. Situated near London, it operated from 1791 until 1811 and was typical of the so-called free house (q.v.), an establishment in which the supervision of treatment remained with the patient's doctor. Among its amenities it boasted of comfortable apartments and "an excellent shower bath," all for "moderate terms."
Bibliography: Hunter, R., and Macalpine, I. 1963. *Three hundred years of psychiatry.*

MIDSUMMER MADNESS. Because excessive heat and the moon (q.v.) were believed to be two causes of madness, the time of full moon in midsummer was considered particularly dangerous.
Bibliography: 1978. *Brewer's dictionary of phrase and fable.*

MIGNONETTE. *Reseda lutea,* a plant found in both wild and cultivated states. *Reseda* means "calm" and indicates its narcotic properties. In France, peasants used pillows stuffed with it to promote sleep.
Bibliography: de Bairacli Levy, J. 1974. *The illustrated herbal handbook.*

MIGRAINE. Paroxysmal attacks of headache with visual and gastric disorders. In antiquity it was believed that the gods inflicted migraines on mortals who had offended them. Many primitive cultures have attributed migraine to evil spirits that can be released from the head by trepanation (q.v.). Incantations (q.v.) for its treatment existed in Mesopotamia about four thousand years before Christ, and Hippocrates (q.v.) wrote a treatise on migraine. The term is derived from "hemicrania," a word first used by Galen (q.v.) to describe the condition. He believed that it was caused by ascending vapors that were excessively hot or cold. Among the medieval superstitions connected with migraine, was the belief that if birds used discarded hair to build their nests, the head that had lost the hair would experience pain. Witches (*see* WITCHCRAFT) were believed to burn hair stolen from those they wished to harm. Ancient herbals recommend many remedies for it that are connected with astrology (q.v.). Magical (*see* MAGIC) rituals, prayers, holy water, and exorcism (q.v.) have been used to drive out the

devils causing migraine. Saint Hildegard of Bingen (q.v.) was probably a sufferer, but she believed her symptoms to be miraculous visions. In more recent times, Thomas Jefferson, Friedrich Nietzche (q.v.), Sigmund Freud (q.v.) and Charles Darwin (q.v.) have been among the famous people tormented by migraine.
Bibliography: Friedman, A. P. 1973. *Headache.*

MIHARA. A volcano on the Japanese island of O-shima. Following the suicide (q.v.) in 1933 of a nineteen-year-old girl, Kiyoko Matsumoto (1914-1933), who traveled there from Tokyo with the express aim of jumping into the crater, it became famous for the number of people who threw themselves into its crater. In 1933, 143 people died there, and, in 1934, 167 people committed suicide. The volcano became a center of attraction for the curious, as well as suicidal, and a tourist industry prospered on the island. The government intervened, guards were placed round the crater, and it became a criminal offence to purchase a one-way ticket to O-shima.
Bibliography: Fedden, H. R. 1938. *Suicide.*

MILESIAN MAIDENS. The maidens of Miletus, an ancient seaport of Western Asia Minor, once conceived a desire to hang themselves, which resulted in an epidemic of suicide (q.v.). The Milesians passed a law stating that all maidens hanging themselves should be dragged naked to their grave by the rope that had hanged them; such shame was too great, and the epidemic stopped.
Bibliography: Plutarch. *Moralia*, vol 3, trans. F. C. Babbitt.

MILL, JAMES (1773-1836). A Scottish historian, philosopher, and psychologist, one of the chief representatives of associationism (q.v.). The son of a shoemaker, he was originally destined for the church. He went to London where he supported himself, his wife, and their nine children through his work in journalism. In addition, he helped his father, his brother, and his sisters. His fortunes improved when his *History of India*, begun in 1806, was published finally in 1817. While this work was dictated by financial needs, his psychological efforts were the result of personal interest in the field and culminated in the publication of *Analysis of the Phenomena of the Human Mind* in 1829. It was an exposition of mechanistic associationism that reduced all mental functioning to a mechanical law and rejected the belief that the mind had purpose and activity. Mill recognized eight sensations: vision, hearing, smell, taste, touch, and muscular sensation, disorganization sensation, and alimentary tract sensations. He explained the mind and its contents by a combination of simple elements.
Bibliography: Boring, E. G. 1950. *A history of experimental psychology.*

MILL, JOHN STUART (1806-1873). A British philosopher and economist. He was a child prodigy with an estimated I.Q. of 190. He was educated by his father, James Mill (q.v.). By the age of three he was learning Greek; by the time he was eight years old, he had read most of the classic Greek works and was accomplished in philosophy, Latin, algebra and history. His father entrusted him with the education of his younger brothers and sisters. Although he had no childhood in the accepted sense, he did not realize what he was missing because the isolation in which the family lived did not offer him the opportunity for comparison. He grew up like an intellectual machine, showing no emotions. He described his home in his memoirs as a miserable place that was devoid of any lighter element. In his later life he dedicated himself to fighting exploitation and promoting freedom of thought. After beginning as a clerk in the East India Company, he rose to head of the examiner's office. In 1836, Mill became seriously ill with what was described as "an obstinate derangement of the brain," which was attributed to excessive intellectual strain. His relationship with his father was such that he did not dare to disagree with him, however, seven years after the death of James Mill, he published his first major work *System of Logic* (1843) in which he used a concept of association that was different from his father's. He believed in what was termed the "chemistry of the mind" whereby simple ideas combined, like elements in a chemical process, to generate complex ideas that did not necessarily resemble the original sources. This concept was widely accepted and greatly influenced the development of psychology. In 1851 he married Harriet Taylor (?-1858). He described her as "in part the author" of his best works. Her death deeply affected him and every year he spent six months at Avignon in France to be near her grave. In addition to books on politics and economics, his other major works of interest to psychology are *Examination of Sir William Hamilton's Philosophy* (1865) and an annotated edition of his father's *Analysis of the Phenomena of the Human Mind* (1869). Shortly before his death, he published an *Autobiography* (1873), which included an account of his painful education by his father.

Bibliography: Ryan, A. 1970. *John Stuart Mill.*

MILLER, MISS FRANK. The pseudonym of a young American woman who sent notes about her day-dreaming and hypnagogic experiences to Théodore Flournoy (q.v.) with whom she had studied for six months in Geneva. She was an easy subject for suggestion and autosuggestion (q.v.) and could imagine hearing verses, long poems, and even dramas. She tried to trace the sources of these fantasies by examining her past life and the material she had read. Flournoy originally published her notes in French, and Carl G. Jung (q.v.) discussed them in detail in his study of myths and their link with daydreams and fantasies.

Bibliography: Miss Frank Miller. 1967. Some instances of subconscious creative imagination. In *The collected works of Carl Jung. Vol. 5*, ed. and trans. by R. F. C. Hull.

MILLER, WILLIAM (1782-1849). An American farmer and founder of the Second Adventists or Millerites, in 1831. He predicted that the world would end in 1843, and the millennium would commence. He estimated his followers to be as many as 100,000. Presumably they were among the most unstable members of the community, as a number of them became deeply depressed by his predictions and some went so far as to commit suicide (q.v.). *See* MILLERISM.

Bibliography: Nichol, F. D. 1944. *The midnight cry.*

MILLERISM. The popular term for the doctrines of William Miller (q.v.). Many mental derangements were attributed to millerism. Jean Esquirol (q.v.) strongly condemned the movement and described it as an "epidemic monomania." The Millerites prepared for the end of the world in 1843 by giving up property and work. When the world did not end in 1843, a date was set for it in 1844. On October 22, 1844, they assembled, chanting prayers and dressed in white garments; some of them climbed trees in an effort to be among the first to meet the Lord, when he descended from the sky. When nothing happened, the leaders claimed that a mistake had been made and that the year should have been 1844 of the Jewish calendar. Followers went home and continued in their delusion (q.v.). "Miller maniacs," wrote Esquirol in *Mental Maladies: A Treatise on Insanity*, "were almost daily brought to the doors of Mad Houses, worn out and exhausted by the ceaseless orgies of this devoted sect."

Bibliography: Nichol, F. D. 1944. *The midnight cry.*

MILL-REECK. A term used in Scotland to indicate a form of organic psychosis (q.v.) in miners caused by lead poisoning (q.v.).

MILLS, CHARLES KARSNER (1845-1931). An American neurologist. He is remembered for his medico-legal work and for his description in 1900 of unilateral ascending paralysis (Mills disease), which was followed in 1906 by his description of unilateral descending paralysis. He was the author of *A Treatise of the Nervous System and Its Diseases*, which was published in 1898.

Bibliography: Haymaker, W., and Schiller, F. 1970. *The founders of neurology.* 2d. ed.

MILLS, HANNAH (?-1790). An English Quaker (q.v.) girl who was a patient in the York Lunatic Asylum (q.v.). Her family was refused permission to visit her, and she died under mysterious circumstances in the asylum. The events prompted the Society of Friends to suggest the establishment of an institution for their own members. This led to the foundation of the York Retreat (q.v.).

Bibliography: Tuke, S. 1813. Reprint. 1964. *Description of the retreat.*

MILTON, JOHN (1608-1674). An English poet. His first poem was written on the occasion of the death of his sister's child. His years of formal education at Cambridge were not altogether as loftily moral as some of his verses. His involvement in religious controversy and politics often made it necessary for him to go into hiding. His personal life also caused him distress. His first wife, an adolescent girl whom he married in 1643 when he was thirty-three years old, left him after a few months of marriage and refused to return until 1645. This event prompted him to begin a series of four pamphlets on divorce, written between 1643 and 1645. He maintained that the most important reason for divorce should be incompatibility and that a forced continuation of a loveless union was a crime against human dignity. When she did return, she was accompanied by her whole family of ten, made refugees in the Civil War. After his wife's death in 1652, he remarried. He married for a third time in 1663. His restlessness is reflected in his continuous changing of houses. He lived in no less than eleven houses in London alone. Of all his works, *Samson Agonistes* (1671) best projects his own emotional state. It is full of questioning and despair, exalting the public cause and vituperating women. Like Samson, Milton was blind, having lost his sight in 1652. According to John Aubrey (q.v.), he managed to remain cheerful and found solace in music. His verses about a troubled dream have been said to be a description of the workings of the insane mind:

All we affirm or what deny and call
Our knowledge or opinion; then retires,
Into her private cell, when nature rests
Oft in her obscure mimic fancy wakes,
To imitate her; but misjoining shapes,
Wild work produces oft, and most in dreams,
Till matching words and deeds long past or late.
Bibliography: Hanford, J. H. 1949. *John Milton, Englishman.*

MIND, GOTTFRIED (1768-1814). A Swiss painter. He came from a family of cretins (*see* CRETINISM) and was himself of low intelligence. A dwarf with a large goitre and rachitic legs, he was deaf and possessed a limited vocabulary. From his childhood on he drew pictures of cats, thousands of them in all forms and guises, in sorrow, in anger, in joy, and in all the moods usually attributed to humans. He became known as the "Raphael of Cats." Bibliography: Winslow, L.S.F. 1898. *Mad humanity: its forms apparent and obscure.*

MIND. The first British psychological journal. It was founded in 1876 by Alexander Bain (q.v.). Groom Robertson, a pupil of Bain and a professor of the philosophy of mind and logic, was appointed editor by Bain, who supported the journal financially until 1892, when Robertson died. Its contents were predominantly philosophical. Bibliography: Boring, E. G. 1950. *A history of experimental psychology.*

MINERAL WATERS. A fashionable form of treatment for mental disorders in the nineteenth century. Some of the most famous springs were at Bath

and Tunbridge Wells in England; Doberan, Toplitz, Baden-Baden, and Pyrmont in Germany; Vichy in France; and Spa in Belgium. It was from the last resort that the term "spa" came to be applied to resorts with similar facilities.
Bibliography: Searle, M. 1977. *Spas and watering places.*

MINGAZZINI, GIOVANNI (1859-1929). An Italian neurologist. He contributed to a better understanding of the mechanisms of motor aphasia and established the syndrome of striatal hemiplegia, also known as Mingazzini's lenticular hemiplegia. He was reputed to be parsimonious, known to be emotional, and vented his irritation with loud and hearty oaths. He vigorously opposed fascism, but despite his liberal views he was able to continue his work in Rome. In Rome the popular saying "go to Mingazzini" was synonymous with "you are mad."
Bibliography: Haymaker, W., and Schiller, F. 1970. *The founders of neurology.* 2d. ed.

MINNIE BRANDON. The title of a psychological novel, published in 1899, by the French writer Leon Hennique. It is the story of a young woman with a double personality: Minnie, charming and virtuous, and Brandon, a vicious shrew. It had considerable success in a period when people were becoming more aware of the unconscious (q.v.).
Bibliography: Hennique, L. 1899. *Minnie Brandon.*

MIRABEAU, HONORÉ GABRIEL RIQUETI COMTE DE (1749-1791). A French statesman. His father hated his mother and hated him to the point of physical repugnance, all the more because he resembled his paternal grandfather. As a child, Mirabeau was constantly reminded of how ugly he was and how base. He was compared to a vile worm and constantly punished. His tutors were deliberately chosen for their cruelty and encouraged to beat him. His docility infuriated his father, who made him use his mother's name, sent him to the strictest schools, and wanted to have him placed in a reformatory. He did have Mirabeau imprisoned for an adolescent love affair and nearly succeeded in having him sent to a penal settlement. Mirabeau grew up to be sullen and, at times, vicious. He married but then eloped with another woman. During a public quarrel with his father, he overplayed his hand, libeled him, and was imprisoned for three years. When he was released he dedicated himself to politics, hoping to establish a strong constitutional monarchy. His views were sound and he had a large following but never gained the complete trust of either the royalists or Jacobins.
Bibliography: Vallentin, A. 1949. *Mirabeau: voice of the revolution.*

MIRACLE WATER. A remedy for nervous disorders, epilepsy (q.v.), and hysteria (q.v.) in Russian folk medicine. To produce the miracle water, a woman had to wear around her neck a small bottle filled with water during a number of acts of sexual intercourse; the bottle had to touch the bodies of both partners who had to experience a climax simultaneously. If these conditions were fulfilled, the water was said to have the necessary curative powers. Another type of miracle water was obtained from certain springs; it had to be collected during moonless nights, and the folk healer carrying it had to pass through a cemetery. It was believed that the water had to be associated with strong emotions, either fear or love, to be effective.

See also FEAR WATER.

Bibliography: Kourennoff, P. M., and St. George, G. 1970. *Russian folk medicine.*

MIRAGLIA, BIAGIO (1814-1885). An Italian physician, patriot, and man of letters. He was a follower of phrenology (q.v.). In 1843 he became physician of a mental hospital in Aversa (q.v.) in southern Italy. He abolished restraint (q.v.) and instituted many beneficial innovations, such as a system of ventilation for the wards and the presentation of dramas by the patients. Alexandre Dumas Pére (q.v.) was among those who attended and admired these performances. Miraglia also compiled a classification of mental disorders, wrote on phrenology, planned a model asylum (q.v.), and founded the Società Frenopatica Italiana (q.v.), as well as two psychiatric journals and the chair of psychiatry at the University of Naples.

Bibliography: Mora, G. 1958. Biagio Miraglia and the development of psychiatry in Naples in the eighteenth and nineteenth centuries. *J. Hist. Med. allied Sci.* 13:504-23.

MIROIR ROTATIF (ROTATING MIRROR). A device consisting of two mirrors rotating in opposite directions. It was used by Jules Luys (q.v.) to hypnotize (*see* HYPNOTISM) patients. Frequently he hypnotized several of them at the same time. Patients gazed at the mirror, while the voice of the hypnotist droned on suggesting sleep.

Bibliography: Vincent, R. H. 1897. *The elements of hypnotism.*

MIRROR WRITING. A way of writing in reverse from the right to the left. Individuals with certain brain disorders and some left-handed people occasionally write in this fashion. The most famous mirror-writer of all was Leonardo da Vinci (q.v.).

Bibliography: Critchley, M. 1928. *Mirror-writing.*

MISALA. An acute disorder usually found among young African males and characterized by excitement leading to frenzy and acts of aggression. It resembles amok (q.v.), but it is less violent and of shorter duration.

Bibliography: Goldenson, R. M. 1970. *Encyclopedia of human behavior.*

MISES, DR. Pseudonym of Gustav Theodor Fechner (q.v.). In his earlier years he wrote a number of satirical papers under the pseudonym, Dr. Mises.

In them he derided materialistic interpretations of the functions of the mind. Among these early papers are *Proof that the Man is made of Iodine* and *Comparative Anatomy of the Angels*.

Bibliography: Flugel, J. C. 1945. *A hundred years of psychology.*

MISHIMA, YUKIO (1925-1970). A Japanese writer. His original family name was Hiraoka. His grandmother was the dominant personality of the family and took him away from his mother when he was a few weeks old. She brought him up in her own house, overprotecting him and treating him as if he were a girl. He was an adolescent when she died and he was forced to face adjustment to a boys' world at school. His wish to hide his acquired feminine manners made him overcompensate, and concentrate on building up his body and acting the part of a strong, aggressive male. This resulted in the need to act all the time and concentrate on himself. He was constantly depressed and dwelt on thoughts of a heroic death before reaching old age. Narcissism (q.v.), homosexual (*see* HOMOSEXUALITY) tendencies, and mistrust permeate all his works, especially the autobiographical *Confession of a Mask* (1949). He loved to be photographed naked in sadomasochistic poses that depicted hara-kiri (q.v.), accidents, or executions. Notwithstanding his bisexuality, his marriage was reasonably happy. Admiring the samurai of old Japan and wanting his country to return to the ways of that era, he formed a private army of intellectual young men, garbed in a special uniform of brown, gold, and green. Their aim was to protect the emperor and restore the sacred tradition of the country. With a few of his followers he stormed the army barracks in Tokyo, delivered an impassioned speech from the balcony, and then turned away and impaled himself on a Samurai sword. His friend Morita cut off his head before going through the same ritual, being decapitated by another member of their group. The official reports of the event stated that Mishima must have been insane. He left behind some 100 books that mirror his own narcissistic needs and morbid eroticism.

Bibliography: Nathan, J. 1975. *Mishima: a biography.*

MISTLETOE. A semiparasitic plant linked with many ancient myths and legends. When found on oak trees, it was selected as a remedy against epilepsy (q.v.) because the oak was believed to be a strong tree that was not easily felled. Pliny the Elder (q.v.) described various elaborate rituals for its gathering in his *Historia Naturalis*. It was also a favorite remedy of Galen (q.v.). The Druids regarded it as a holy plant and a panacea for many ills. Special ceremonies for its harvest were observed, and it was cut only when they were told in a vision to do so. The priests dressed in white vestments,

white bulls were sacrificed, and a golden sickle was used to cut it. By the eighteenth century, however, Richard Mead (q.v.) claimed that it was useless.
Bibliography: Leyel, C. F. 1949. *Hearts-ease.*

MITCHELL, SILAS WEIR (1829-1914). An American neurologist and psychiatrist. He is considered one of the founders of neurology (q.v.) in the United States and the instigator of many innovations and experiments. He was "contract surgeon" to a hospital in Philadelphia during the Civil War, and his experiences there formed the basis of his *Gunshot Wounds and Other Injuries of Nerves,* which was published in 1864. This volume was followed by other works on the neurological aspects of wounds. His interest in neurology was responsible for his tendency to concentrate on the somatic aspects of mental and emotional disorders. He believed that attending college could cause women to have nervous breakdowns and thought that the "railroad age" was responsible for many nervous disorders. He devised a rest cure (q.v.) that became a standard form of therapy for functional neuroses (*see* NEUROSIS). At times Mitchell's approach was unorthodox; on one occasion he set fire to the bed of an hysterical (*see* HYSTERIA) woman, to prove that she could walk if she so wished. He was also known as a poet and a novelist.
Bibliography: Walter, R. D. 1970. *S. Weir Mitchell, M.D.—neurologist: a medical biography.*

MITFORD, JOHN (1782-1831). An English writer and poet. He spent some time in the navy, before becoming a journalist in London. In 1811 he was certified insane and sent to a private asylum (q.v.) for two years. Twelve years later, in 1825, he published two pamphlets relating his experiences as a patient. He gave lurid descriptions of how sane persons were imprisoned in madhouses by their relatives and how some criminals escaped punishment by feigning madness. The pamphlets appealed to the general public because of their sensational details, which were usually of sexual character. Toward the end of his life he became an alcoholic (*see* ALCOHOLISM) and was sent to a workhouse where he died.
Bibliography: Parry-Jones, W. Ll. 1972. *The trade in lunacy: a study of private madhouses in England in the eighteenth and nineteenth century.*

MITHRIDATE. An ancient panacea made up of a large number of substances, including opium (q.v.). Its name derives from Mithridates VI (c. 132-63 B.C.), known as Mithridates the Great, who was king of Pontus and Bithynia (a part of modern Turkey on the Black Sea). He was said to have lived in fear of being poisoned and to have made himself immune by taking small doses of poisonous substances regularly. Mithridate was still in use at

the time of Felix Plater (q.v.). It was listed for the last time in the fifth London Pharmacopoeia in 1746.
Bibliography: 1978. *Brewer's dictionary of phrase and fable*.

MNEMONICS. A device to assist the recall of related data. The term is derived from the Greek. Mnemosyne, in Greek mythology (q.v.) was the daughter of heaven and earth, the mother of the nine Muses, and the goddess of memory (q.v.).
Bibliography: Graves, R. 1960. *The Greek myths*.

MNEMOSYNE. *See* MNEMONICS.

MODIGLIANI, AMEDEO (1884-1920). An Italian-Jewish painter and sculptor. He left Italy in 1906 and lived in Paris. He was an alcoholic (*see* ALCOHOLISM) and a drug addict. The long limbs and excessively elongated necks of his figures may have been the result of visual distortion caused by his addiction to hashish (q.v.), which he ate spread on bread and butter or mixed with sugar. His widow killed herself and their unborn child by jumping out of a window a few days after his death from tuberculosis (q.v.) at the age of thirty-five.
Bibliography: Mann, C. 1980. *Modigliani*.

MODIOLUS. A hand trephine devised by the Italian anatomist and surgeon Fabricius ab Aquapendente (1537-1619) to gain access to the cranium. In a modified form, it is still used by neurosurgeons for leucotomy and hypophysieal stalk section.

MOEBIUS, PAUL JULIUS (1853-1907). A German psychiatrist who was particularly interested in the correlation between psychopathology and artistic and cultural activity. He wrote pathographies of a number of great men, such as Jean Jacques Rousseau, Arthur Schopenhauer, and Johann Wolfgang von Goethe (qq.v.). According to him, hysteria (q.v.) was a psychological disorder that produced physical symptoms. In his book *On the Physiological Imbecility of Women* (1901), he theorized that women in general were feebleminded but remarked that this was fortunate because as such they were not dangerous. His classification of mental disorders into endogenous and exogenous groups was accepted by Emil Kraepelin (q.v.). Moebius' imaginative work and literary ability contributed to the influence he exercised over his contemporaries. Psychoanalysts imitated his pathographies and applied their concepts to life histories and childhood memories. Periodic ophthalmoplegic migraine (Moebius' disease) was first described by him in 1884.
Bibliography: Zilboorg, G. 1941. *A history of medical psychology*.

MOHAMMED (*or* MAHOMET) (570-632). An Arabian prophet, born in Mecca. His father, a poor merchant, died when he was an infant, and his mother died when he was still a child. He was raised by his uncle. When he was twenty-four years old, he married a wealthy widow, who was fifteen years older than he. At the age of forty, he experienced his first revelation during a period of meditation, which he spent alone in a cave for several days. After seeing the angel Gabriel and hearing voices, he returned home shaking and worried that his mind had become deranged. According to tradition he was so worried that he contemplated throwing himself over a precipice. From contemporary accounts it has been surmised that he was subject to epileptic (*see* EPILEPSY) fits and at times fell into a coma. He was treated by cupping on the back of the head. His hallucinations (q.v.) of sight and hearing reflected his mystical preoccupations. At the time of his death he had nine wives. The religion he preached, Islam, became a strong uniting force in the Arab world.

Bibliography: Rodinson, M. 1973. *Mohammed*, trans. A. Carter.

MOHAMMED TUGHLAK (c.1290-1351). An Indian sultan, king of Delhi. He came to the throne after arranging the death of his father. He was skilled in physics, logic, astronomy, and mathematics. It was said that if one of his subjects suffered from an intriguing disease, he would treat him personally. He was as famous for his generosity as for his cruelty. His own life was rigid, and he condemned intemperate pleasures in others. His schemes, however, were irrational to an extreme degree. Once, to punish the inhabitants of Delhi, he ordered all of them to leave the city, which then remained empty and desolate. During one march he lost a tooth and ordered it to be buried with great ceremony and a monument erected over it. He was a mixture of incredible cruelty, generosity, intelligence, egotism and lack of judgment. Reports of his behavior led William W. Ireland (q.v.) to assert that he was insane.

Bibliography: Ireland, W. W. 1885. *The blot upon the brain: studies in history and psychology.*

MOIRAE. In Greek mythology (q.v.) the three divinities of fate, or destiny, which even the gods could not escape. They corresponded to the Latin concept of the Parcae.

Bibliography: Graves, R. 1960. *The Greek myths.*

MOLIÈRE (1622-1672). A French playwright and actor. His real name was Jean Baptiste Poquelin. He was educated by the Jesuits. After an unhappy marriage, he poured his bitterness in his comedies. He mercilessly ridiculed women, courtiers, physicians, and clergymen. His psychological portraits were powerful; but some of his disgruntled victims successfully pressed for the suppression of some of his plays. He dealt openly with madness, upheld good sense, and denounced pretensions and false values. The clergy of the time never forgave him for his treatment of them and on his death denied

him a church burial. *Le Malade Imaginaire* contains a masterful portrait of an hypochondriac (*see* HYPOCHONDRIA).
Bibliography: Lewis, D.B.W. 1959. *Molière*.

MOLINOS, MIGUEL DE (1628-?1697). A Spanish priest. He was sentenced by the Inquisition (q.v.) to life imprisonment for his contemplative doctrine known as quietism (q.v.). He was said to practice sexual aberrations and to encourage his followers in the same acts, which he regarded as devoid of sin and purifying. Toward the end of his life he reversed his opinions. His *Spiritual Guide* was published in Rome in 1675.
Bibliography: Dudon, P. 1921. *Le quietiste espagnol Michel Molinos*.

MOLL, ALBERT (1862-1939). A German psychiatrist. He studied sexual psychopathology and emphasized that corporal punishment of children might lead to unhealthy stimulation in the child, in the individual administering the punishment, and in the onlookers. He was the first to use the term "libido" (q.v.) to indicate evolutionary sexual instinct. In 1926 he organized an international congress on sexual research in Berlin. He was interested in hypnotism (q.v.) and wrote and lectured on it; he also introduced hypnotic psychotherapy (q.v.) into Germany.
Bibliography: Moll, A. 1936. *Ein leben als arzt der seele-erinnerungen*.

MOLLES. Supernatural beings. They were said to cause insomnia and nightmares (q.v.). Caelius Aurelianus (q.v.) discussed them in his writings.
Bibliography: Semelaigne, A. 1889. *Études historiques sur l'aliénation mentale dans l'antiquité*.

MOLL FLANDERS. A novel written by Daniel Defoe (q.v.) in 1721. He described the book on the title page as containing "The Fortunes and Misfortunes of the famous Moll Flanders, &c, who was born in Newgate, and during a life of continued variety, for threescore years, besides her childhood, was twelve years a Whore, five times a Wife (whereof once to her own brother), twelve years a thief, eight years a transported Felon in Virginia, at last grew rich, lived honest, and died a Penitent." The book offers a vivid picture of the social conditions of the time and also contains a good description of Newgate Prison (q.v.), which was known to Defoe.
Bibliography: Defoe, D. 1721. Reprint. 1971. *The fortunes and misfortunes of Moll Flanders*, ed. G. A. Starr.

MOLOCH (MOLECH). A Canaanite idol mentioned in the Bible (q.v.). Children were burnt in sacrifice to it. In *Paradise Lost*, John Milton (q.v.) presented Moloch as a leader of the fallen angels. The name is often used in relation to unnatural sacrifices of a horrid nature.
Bibliography: 1932. *The Oxford companion to English literature*, ed. P. Harvey.

MONAKOW, CONSTANTIN VON (1853-1930). A Russian neurologist who became naturalized Swiss. As an adolescent, he was such an indolent student that his father told him to leave home. Against his father's wishes, he chose a career in medicine and became interested in neurology (q.v.) early in his studies. Monakow became physician in a Swiss asylum and began the experiments on the thalamus that stimulated much of his subsequent work. He also wrote on problems of philosophy and morality and their impact on everyday life. He was a picturesque and unusual individual; the poetess Maria Waser wrote a biographical novel about him, *Begegnung am Abend*, published in 1933.

Bibliography: Haymaker, W., and Schiller, F. 1970. *The founders of neurology*. 2d. ed.

MONASTERIES. During the Middle Ages (q.v.) in Western Europe, medical science was preserved by the work of members of religious communities. Saint Benedict of Nursia (q.v.) had emphasized literary work, usually copying ancient manuscripts for the monastic libraries, in his *Regula Monochorum*, and a knowledge of medicine had been imparted to his monks at the monastery of Monte Cassino in Italy by Flavius Cassiodorus (q.v.) during his years of refuge there. Hence, the monasteries became repositories of theoretical knowledge in a world that was temporarily rejecting cultural pursuits. At the same time they were centers of healing because of the Christian tradition of caring for the sick of body and mind. Bethlem Royal Hospital (q.v.) is one religious foundation that in time became dedicated solely to the mentally ill. Not surprisingly, treatment was colored by religious practices, and therefore exorcism (q.v.), application of sacred objects, prayers, visits to holy places, and, when all else failed, whippings to expel the devils were common.

Bibliography: Poynter, F.N.L., ed. 1964. *The evolution of hospitals in Britain*.

MONDRIAN, PIET (1872-1944). A Dutch abstract painter. He was a deeply religious man who was influenced by the ideas of the theosophists. As his art developed, he became less concerned with depicting reality. The subject and content of his work became symbolic images of any experience, which he called the equivalence of opposite, or neo-plastic art. His straight lines and the exclusive use of three primary colors and black and white have been interpreted as a projection of his obsessive compulsive personality.

Bibliography: Elgar, F. 1968. *Mondrian*, trans. T. Watton.

MONGOLISM. A term used in 1866 by Dr. John Langdon Down (q.v.) to describe a genetic condition leading to defective development. Those affected have a superficial facial resemblance to individuals of the Mongolian race. In Down's time the evolutionary stage of the Caucasian race was regarded as more advanced than that of other races, and therefore mentally defective people were believed to be "throw backs" to an earlier stage. The

condition is now termed Down's syndrome, or autosomal trisomy of group G.
Bibliography: Down, J.L.H. 1866. Observations on an ethnic classification of idiots. *Clin. Lect. Rep. London Hosp.* 3: 259-62.

MONIZ, ANTONIO CAETANO DE ABREU FREIRE EGAS (1874-1955). A Portuguese physician. His godfather added Egas Moniz, the name of the Portuguese hero to his names at his christening. He later used it as a pen name and finally wholly adopted it. He became a world famous neurologist later in his life, after he ceased his political involvement. Moniz devised a method of diagnosing brain tumors, and in 1935 he became the first to employ leucotomy to relieve psychosis (q.v.). He shared a Nobel Prize in physiology and medicine for this procedure in 1949. In 1944 he renounced his position of professor of neurology at the University of Lisbon and became involved in publishing various works on politics and art, as well as an autobiography entitled *Confideñcias de un investigador científico* (1949).
Bibliography: Haymaker, W., and Schiller, F. 1970. *The founders of neurology.* 2d. ed.

MONKEYS. The expression "to get one's monkey up," meaning to be irritable or enraged, is derived from the belief that monkeys are easily roused to anger.
Bibliography: 1978. *Brewer's dictionary of phrase and fable.*

MONKHOUSE HILL. A poem by Thomas Bakewell (q.v.). It was published anonymously in 1807 and described the plight of the insane in a parish workhouse:

> There see the idiot's vacant stare,
> And th' wild maniac's frantic glare.
> Where tho' strong chains the body bind,
> No fetters can restrain the mind.

Bibliography: Bakewell, T. 1807. *The Moorland bard.*

MONKS. Most religious fraternities in the Middle Ages (q.v.) made provisions for those monks who became sick because of the oppressive closeness and rigid rules of the monasteries. Sleep disorders, headaches, and other psychosomatic symptoms were understood to have a psychic aetiology, and the patients were treated by periods of rest in sister houses in the country.
Bibliography: Poynter, F.N.L., ed. 1964. *The evolution of hospitals in Britain.*

MONOMANIA. A term suggested by Jean Esquirol (q.v.) for a "form of insanity, in which delirium is partial, permanent, gay or sad." The word was admitted into the dictionary of the French Academy in 1835.
Bibliography: Esquirol, J.E.D. 1845. Reprint. 1965. *Mental maladies: a treatise on insanity.*

MONOMANIE INCENDIAIRE. "Arson insanity," a term used by the French physician Ulysses Trelat (q.v.) to defend psychotic (*see* PSYCHOSIS) patients found guilty of arson. By claiming that they could not be held responsible for their actions in that particular area of behavior, he was able to shield them from punishment.

Bibliography: Zilboorg, G. 1941. *A history of medical psychology.*

MONRO. The surname of a British family that served Bethlem Royal Hospital (q.v.) for four generations and practiced psychiatry for five. JAMES MONRO, (1680-1752) became physician to Bethlem Royal Hospital (q.v.) in 1728 and remained there until his death. His son JOHN (1715-1791), after ten years of traveling in Europe and a period in Edinburgh studying insanity, became joint physician with his father at Bethlem Royal Hospital and continued in the post after his father's death. He is particularly remembered for his *Remarks on Dr. Battie's Treatise on Madness* (1758). It was an attack on the work of Dr. William Battie (q.v.) and gave rise to a bitter and much publicized controversy. It was the first psychiatric book written by a physician from Bethlem Hospital. Monro believed that madness could not be understood properly and that no treatment would cure it. He also owned a private asylum known as Brooke House (q.v.), which remained in the family for many years. His son THOMAS (1759-1833) held several offices in the College of Physicians and in 1792 succeeded him at Bethlem. In 1816, however, he and John Haslam (q.v.) were dismissed after an investigation of the case of William Norris (q.v.). He was well known to his contemporaries for his interest in art and his patronage of young artists, including Joseph Turner (q.v.) and John Linnell (1792-1882). His son EDWARD THOMAS (1790-1856) took his place at Bethlem, and he too appears to have been unsatisfactory as the commissioners in lunacy (q.v.) investigated his affairs in 1852. He refused to resign, and, as a compromise, he was appointed consultant physician, which he remained until his death. The last of the Monros to dedicate his work to the mentally ill, was HENRY (1817-1891). He held no appointment at Bethlem but was physician at Saint Luke's Hospital for Lunatics (q.v.) and treated private patients at Brooke House. In 1864 he became president of the Medico-Psychological Association (q.v.). He was a philanthropist and an artist in his own right. His book *Remarks on Insanity* was published between 1850 and 1851 and advocated a theory of insanity based on neurological pathology.

Bibliography: Leigh, D. 1961. *The historical development of British psychiatry.*

MONRO, ALEXANDER (1733-1817). A Scottish anatomist, the son of Alexander Monro (1697-1767), a noted anatomist. In 1783 Monro described the connection between the lateral ventricles of the brain that is now known as *foramen of Monro.* He also was interested in "animal electricity" and conducted experiments on the nervous system with opium (q.v.) and metallic substances to determine the nature of the electrical discharges of the brain. He was the author of *Observations on the Structure and Functions of the*

Nervous System, which was published in 1783. His son Alexander (1773-1859) wrote on anatomy and held a joint professorship with him. The three Alexander Monros were distinguished by the appellation primus, secundus and tertius.

Bibliography: Wright-St. Clair, R. E. 1964. *Doctors Monro.*

MONROE, MARILYN (1926-1962). The assumed name of Norma Jean Mortenson, an American film actress. She had a depriving childhood and emerged in adolescence as a sex symbol. After divorcing Joe Di Maggio (1914-   ) she married the playwright Arthur Miller (1915-   ). She was a helpless, sensitive person, who longed to be accepted as a serious actress. Hysteria (q.v.), drugs (q.v.), and bouts of deep depression eventually led to her suicide (q.v.). She occasionally wrote poetry and once wrote:

> Help Help
> Help I feel life coming closer
> When all I want is to die.

Bibliography: Robinson, D., and Kobal, J. 1974. *Marilyn Monroe.*

MONROSE, CLAUDE LOUIS (1783-1843). A French actor. After a brilliant career, he became insane. His symptoms included loss of personality and the belief that he was the characters he had impersonated. He was placed in an asylum and released only to act the role of Figaro in a performance organized for his benefit. He performed perfectly until he had to say the words "Il est fou" ["he is mad"]. At this point he broke down and had to retire from the stage. He returned to the asylum and remained there for the rest of his life.

Bibliography: Winslow, L.S.F. 1898. *Mad humanity: its forms, apparent and obscure.*

MONSIEUR. The name of a black poodle, constant companion of Agrippa (q.v.). Many people who regarded Agrippa's enlightened views as heretic were fully convinced that the little dog was an incarnation of the devil.

Bibliography: Morley, H.1856. *The life of Henry Cornelius Agrippa von Nettesheim.*

MONTAIGNE, MICHEL EYQUEM DE (1533-1592). A French essayist. He was inclined toward a realistic interpretation of psychological phenomena. Interested in human feelings and behavior, he came to believe that emotions could be powerful enough to cause psychic and physical disorders, or even death. According to him, imagination (q.v.) could produce strange phenomena, which then were attributed to evil spirits. Montaigne was the first to refer to the English tendency for suicide (q.v.), which he attributed

to the climate (q.v.). He, himself, believed that unendurable pain or an unacceptable form of death justified suicide.
Bibliography: Frame, D. M. 1965. *Montaigne, a biography.*

MONTANUS. The leader of an heretical movement of the second century A.D. known as montanism. It originated in Phrygia and lasted for about fifty years, except for a few remnants in isolated areas. He maintained that the end of the world was near and that no forgiveness was possible for Christians who had fallen from grace. With his women companions, Prisca and Maximilla, he delivered divine revelations to his followers in whom he induced such guilt that they often became hallucinated (*see* HALLUCINATION).
Bibliography: Labriole, P. de. 1913. *La crise montaniste.*

MONTANUS, GIOVANNI BATTISTA (1493-1552). A prominent Italian physician. He believed that clinical practice should be based on observation. He is considered the founder of the method of bedside teaching of medicine. He refuted the idea that the devil could cause mental illness and treated melancholia (q.v.) with frequent baths (q.v.) and bleeding (q.v.).
Bibliography: Castiglioni, A. 1946. *A history of medicine,* ed. and trans. E. B. Krumbhaar.

MONTESQUIEU, CHARLES LOUIS DE SECONDAT BARON DE LA BRÈDE (1689-1755). A French political philosopher. Although he admired the English people, he believed that the foggy atmosphere of England was the principal cause of its great number of suicides (q.v.). In his *Lettres Persanes* (1721) he defended the practice of suicide.
Bibliography: Shackleton, R. 1961. *Montesquieu: a critical biography.*

MONTESSORI, MARIA (1870-1952). An Italian physician and pioneer in education. She was the first Italian woman ever to obtain a medical degree. Her position as assistant physician at the psychiatric clinic of the University of Rome led to her interest in mentally retarded children. In 1898, after studying psychiatry and pedagogy, she founded a school for feebleminded and defective children in which she successfully practiced the teachings of Edouard Séguin (q.v.). She later developed her own methods for the education of normal children. In 1907, she opened a *casa dei bambini* (children's home) for the slum children of Rome. It was the first of the many Montessori schools that flourished in several European countries. Her methods were based on the belief that children should be guided but not coerced and that freedom to experiment and use their own initiative together with training of the senses is more conducive to healthy development than formal teaching. She designed special materials for children, including child-sized furniture. She lectured widely, and her books have been translated in fourteen lan-

guages. The first of them appeared in English in 1912 under the title of *The Montessori Method*.
Bibliography: Standing, E. M. 1958. *Maria Montessori*.

MONTEZ, LOLA. *See* GILBERT, MARIA DELORES ELIZA ROSANNA.

MONTROSE ROYAL MENTAL HOSPITAL. A mental hospital in Scotland founded by Susan Carnegie (q.v.) in 1781. The funds for it were collected primarily from members of her own family. Originally the patients were under the care of a general practitioner in Montrose, but in 1834 William A. F. Browne (q.v.) was appointed physician superintendent.
See also ROYAL ASYLUMS.
Bibliography: Henderson, D. K. 1964. *The evolution of psychiatry in Scotland*.

MONUMENT, THE. A Doric column 67 meters high, designed by Sir Christopher Wren (q.v.) and erected in London between 1671 and 1677 to commemorate the Great Fire of London. It became popular as a place for suicide (q.v.) after a Miss Elizabeth Moyes threw herself from it in 1839. The reason given for her suicide was the need to support herself, following the reduced circumstances of her father, a baker.
Bibliography: Winslow, L.S.F. 1898. *Mad humanity: its forms, apparent and obscure.*

MONUMENT OF SYMPATHY. The name of a piece of sculpture in Thailand (q.v.). It stands outside the male section of Dhonburi Mental Hospital and represents a nurse with two patients. It was erected by a local merchant in gratitude for the care given to his mentally ill son.
Bibliography: Sangsingkeo, P. 1975. Thailand. In *World history of psychiatry*, ed. J. G. Howells.

MONYHULL HALL. A hospital for mental defectives, organized on the colony system and established in 1908 in Birmingham, England. Until its establishment, mentally retarded persons needing institutional care had been kept in workhouses. The Monyhull colony was an innovative idea that provided valuable experience for similar institutions in Britain and elsewhere.
Bibliography: 1958. *Birmingham Regional Hospital Board: Monyhull Hall.*

MOON. The belief that the moon has a special influence on the mind and on human affairs has been prevalent from ancient times. Many religious beliefs have been woven around the moon, which, at various times, has been personified as a goddess. She was Ishtar to the Babylonians, Asthoreth to the Phoenicians, and to the Greeks, Artemis, the chaste huntress who cruelly punished those who failed to worship her. The Romans called her Diana (q.v.) and greatly honored her. Even the term "lunacy" (*see* LUNATIC) reflects the early beliefs in the moon's influence, as it is derived from the

Latin word *luna*, meaning moon. Plutarch, Pliny the Elder, Hippocrates, and the Bible (qq.v.) have all asserted its noxious influence on the mind and attributed nightmares (q.v.) as well as madness to it. Julius Caesar (q.v.) used the German tribes' fear of the evil effect of the moon to conquer them. Aretaeus of Cappadocia (q.v.) and Rhazes (q.v.) wrote that epileptic (*see* EPILEPSY) seizures were governed by the moon. In the Middle Ages (q.v.) it was believed that insanity, idiocy (*see* IDIOT), and epilepsy were caused by the moon. Saint Hildegard of Bingen (q.v.) wrote that "a male born on the 17th day of the moon will be an idiot," and added that other defects were also related to certain phases of the moon. Leech books (q.v.) and herbals considered the phases of the moon to be crucial in prescribing treatment, especially bleeding (q.v.), and in indicating the days during which curative herbs were to be collected. In *Diseases that Deprive Man of His Reason* (1567), Paracelsus (q.v.) wrote that lunatics were those mad persons affected by the power of attraction of the moon "which tears reason out of man's head by depriving him of humors and cerebral virtues." The same belief persisted in the time of William Shakespeare (q.v.) whose plays are rich in references to the moon as the "sovereign mistress of true melancholy"; in 'Othello' we find:

> It is the very error of the moon,
> She comes more near the earth than she was wont
> And makes men mad.

In 1791 the French psychiatrist Joseph Daquin (q.v.) wrote in his *Philosophie de la Folie*, "it is a well established fact that insanity is a disease of the mind upon which the moon exercises an unquestionable influence." Jean Esquirol (q.v.) concluded that the moon affected the insane through its light, which excited some and frightened others. In Italy, Cesare Lombroso (q.v.) also firmly believed in the effects of the moon on mental disorders. In eighteenth-century England, William Blackstone (q.v.), a great jurist, writing on English law, defined a lunatic as one who has lost his reason but enjoys lucid intervals "depending upon the changes of the moon," and in Bethlem Royal Hospital (q.v.), until 1808, patients were chained and flogged at certain phases of the moon as a preventive against violence. In England the Lunacy Act of 1842 stated that a lunatic was a person "afflicted with a period of fatuity in the period following after the full moon." Although in the twentieth century it is difficult to find firm statements about the influence of the moon, many studies have considered the phases of the moon in relation to mental hospital admissions, suicide (q.v.), murder, pyromania, destructive urges, anxiety, migraine (q.v.), childbirth, and marriage problems. Man's landing on the moon has not abated many superstitions.

Bibliography: Oliven, J. F. 1943. Moonlight and nervous disorders: a historical study, *Am. J. Psychiat.* 99:579-84.

MOONBEAMS. The title of a patient's magazine begun in 1904 in the Midlothian and Peebles District Asylum, now known as the Rosslynlee Hospital, in Scotland. In view of the aetiological significance given to the moon (q.v.) in mental disorders, the title is not without humor.

See also JOURNALS BY PATIENTS.

Bibliography: 1971. *Rosslynlee Hospital,* Roslin, Midlothian.

MOONEY, JAMES (1861-1921). An American ethnologist. The Bureau of American Ethnology sent him to the West of the Mississippi to study the ghost-dance religion (q.v.) of the Indian tribes. He also studied Irish customs and the ways in which people react to prolonged stress under poverty and oppression.

Bibliography: Mooney, J. 1965. *The ghost-dance religion and the Sioux outbreak of 1890,* cd. A.F.C. Wallace.

MOONRAKERS. The people of Wiltshire, England. The nickname was derived from the story that when they were caught raking a pond to recover kegs of smuggled brandy on a moonlit night they pretended stupidity and claimed to be trying to rake the reflection of the moon (q.v.) from the water.

Bibliography: 1978. *Brewer's dictionary of phrase and fable.*

MOORE, JOSEPH WALDRON (1879-1957). An American physician. With Hideyo Noguchi (q.v.) he demonstrated that the spirochete found in the brain tissue of patients dying from general paralysis of the insane (q.v.) was *Treponema pallidum,* the same spirochete that causes syphilis (q.v.). Following this laboratory demonstration, general paretics were treated with arsenicals and other drugs used for syphilitic disorders but without marked success.

Bibliography: Noguchi, H., and Moore, J. W. 1913. A demonstration of treponema pallidum in the brain in cases of general paralysis. *J. Experimental Medicine.* 17: 232-38.

MORA. A seventeenth-century town in Sweden. In 1669 a large number of people in the town were tried for witchcraft (q.v.). The mass hysteria (q.v.) was begun by children who claimed to have been carried away by witches. Eighty-five of the accused were burnt.

Bibliography: Russell, J. B. 1980. *A history of witchcraft.*

MORAL INSANITY. *See* INSANITY, MORAL.

MORAL MEDICINE. A term employed in the nineteenth century to denote a form of psychiatric treatment addressed to the emotions, rather than to physical remedies. It consisted of a total regime directed toward changing the attitude of the patient, and it included what now we would call psychotherapy (q.v.). Jean Esquirol (q.v.) in his *Mental Maladies: A Treatise on Insanity* (1845) wrote "moral medicine, which seeks in the heart for the cause of the evil, which sympathizes and weeps, which consoles, and divides with the unfortunate their sufferings, and which revives hope in their breast, is often preferable to all other." William A. F. Browne (q.v.), writing in 1844, gave the following definition: "Much of what is designated moral treatment consists in the conferences and controversies of the officers with the patients in the attempt to disentangle the intricacies and confusions of thought; to substitute precise for vague conceptions, hopes for fears, reason for impulse, to convince of error." Charles Dickens (q.v.) also was impressed by the approach and wrote about what he had seen of its application in America in *American Notes for General Circulation* (1842).

Bibliography: Bockoven, J. S. 1963. *Moral treatment in American psychiatry.*

MORE, SIR THOMAS (1478-1535). An English humanist and lord chancellor of England at the time of Henry VIII (1491-1547). He was famous for his scholarship and rectitude. More was the author of many works, one of which, *Utopia* (1515), his greatest, describes an ideal social system. For some time (c. 1516-1523), he lived at Crosby Place, Bishopsgate, across the street from Bethlem Royal Hospital (q.v.). In a sermon entitled *Four Last Things* (c.1523) he discussed the madness of sin and mentioned Bethlem: "Think not that everything is pleasant that men for madness laugh at. For thou shalt in Bedlam see one laughing at the knocking of his head against a post, and yet there is little pleasure therein." In his *Apology* (1533) he gave another example of his observations gathered at Bethlem Royal Hospital and mentioned a man who had been "put into Bedlam, and afterwards by beating and correction gathered his remembrances to come again to himself." Such methods as these were accepted as correct in the treatment of the insane, and no cruelty was implied. More fell from grace in consequence of his unbending honesty, which did not allow him to agree with Henry VIII's devious manoeuvres; he was tried for treason, imprisoned, and beheaded in the Tower of London.

Bibliography: Chambers, R. W. 1935. *Sir Thomas More.*

MOREAU DE TOURS, JACQUES JOSEPH (1804-1884). A French psychiatrist and pupil of Jean Esquirol (q.v.). He believed that dreams (q.v.)

provided material for understanding emotional disorders and psychotic symptoms. Although he did not use the term "dynamic," the concept of evolution and regression in psychiatric illness began with him. Janet (q.v.) was greatly influenced by him. His book, *Du Hachisch et de l'Aliénation Mentale: Études Psychologiques'* (1845), described from his personal experiences the effects of hashish or cannabis indica (qq.v.). He claimed that self-restraint and the awareness of events was not altogether lost during periods of intoxication and that it was possible to remember actions and feelings brought about by the drug on recovery. He also encouraged many of his pupils and friends, including Théophil Gautier (q.v.)., to experiment with cannabis. Moreau de Tours was the first to produce "artificial psychoses" for research purposes by administering certain drugs. La Société Moreau-de-tours, dedicated to his memory, was founded in France in 1959 for the advancement of psychopharmacology.

Bibliography: Baruk, H. La vie et l'oeuvre de Moreau de Tours. *Ann. méd. Psychol.* 2: 27-32.

MOREL, BENEDICT AUGUSTIN (1809-1873). A French psychiatrist, born in Vienna and educated in Paris. For a time he was secretary to Jules P. Falret (q.v.) at the Salpêtrière (q.v.). He was an excellent clinician and diagnostician. Although early in his career he emphasized the importance of emotional pathology, he later developed a classification of mental disorder that centered on heredity. He believed that mental disease was the result of physical, intellectual, and moral degeneration (q.v.), which, in turn, was derived from hereditary weaknesses. A congenitally deformed external ear, now referred to as "Morel's ear," was regarded as one of the stigmata of degeneration. Morel predicted the onset of madness in Ludwig II of Bavaria (q.v.) by the look in the patient's eyes. The term "dementia praecox" (q.v.), which was later utilized by Emil Kraepelin (q.v.), was first used by Morel to denote a rapid mental impairment. He is credited also with using the term "obsession" (q.v.) for the first time in its present-day sense, and he described a form of neurosis (q.v.) that he called "emotional delusion." Morel wrote on forensic psychiatry and contributed to the history of mental diseases with a historical review of psychiatry in Belgium, Germany, Italy, Switzerland, Great Britain, and the United States that covered the years 1844 to 1850. Among his writings are *Traité des Dégénérescences, Physiques, Intellectuelles et Morales de l'Espèce Humaine* (1857), and *Traité de Maladies Mentales* (1860).

Bibliography: Zilboorg, G. 1941. *A history of medical psychology.*

MOREL, FERDINAND (1888-1957). A Swiss psychiatrist, unrelated to Benedict A. Morel (q.v.). After attending the course on neuropathology given by Jean Charcot (q.v.) at Salpêtrière (q.v.), he acquired clinical experience at Saint Anne's Hospital (q.v.) in Paris, under André

Thomas and Gaétan de Clerambault (q.v.). In 1938 he became professor of psychiatry and director of the Bel Air Psychiatric Hospital. Morel is best known for his neurologically orientated psychiatric theories, which opposed those of Sigmund Freud (q.v.). He objected to leucotomies and had reservations about shock therapies. His name is connected with the Steward-Morel-Morgani syndrome, which is also known as metabolic cranipathy. His best known work, *Introduction a la Psychiatrie Neurologique*, was published in 1947.

Bibliography: Wildi, E. Ferdinand Morel. 1957. *Psychiat. Neurol.* 134: 346-49.

MORENO, JACOB LEVY (1892-1974). A psychiatrist, born in Bucharest, Rumania, in a Spanish-Jewish family. He was educated in Vienna, where, toward the end of World War I, he launched a journal of existential literature entitled *Daimon*. In 1921 he founded in Vienna the Theater of Spontaneity, from which psychodrama (q.v.) developed. Eleven years later, in 1932, he introduced the term "group psychotherapy" (q.v.), which he had developed from using drama in the treatment of disturbed children. His work in the United States led to the foundation of the Moreno Institute and Theatre of Psychodrama. Moreno's methods were imitated widely and further developed in group work with psychiatric patients.

Bibliography: Moreno, J. L. 1953. *Who shall survive? foundations of sociometry, group psychotherapy and sociodrama.*

MORGAGNI, GIOVANNI BATTISTA (1682-1771). An Italian physician and founder of pathological anatomy. His father died when he was seven years old and his mother dedicated her life to his education. When he was fifteen years old, he was sent to Bologna to study medicine and philosophy. Eventually he became professor of medicine at the University of Bologna and taught anatomy at the University of Padua. He believed that diseases were related to particular organs and that autopsies could reveal the cause of the patient's symptoms. He was particularly interested in the pathology of the brain. He correlated the clinical data and anatomical findings he had collected in his last and greatest book, *De Sedibus et Causis Morborum per Anatomen Indagatis*, which was published in 1761, when he was seventy-nine years old. The book was written in the form of letters, and the first parts contain chapters on phrenitis (q.v.), madness, and melancholia (q.v.). In 1769 it was translated into English with the title *The Seats and Causes of Diseases Investigated by Anatomy*. Morgagni also wrote on Latin classics and archaeology. He continued to teach to the last year of his life.

Bibliography: Cameron, G. R. 1952. The life and times of Gianbattista Morgagni, F.R.S. *Notes and records of the Royal Society of London.* Vol.9.

MORGAN, CONWAY LLOYD (1852-1936). A British psychologist, professor of psychology at the University of Bristol. He was a pioneer in the field of comparative psychology. Recognizing the dangers of relying excessively on animal psychology, he formulated a law, referred to as "Lloyd Morgan's canon," that stated: "In no case may we interpret an action as the outcome of the exercise of a higher psychical faculty, if it can be interpreted as the outcome of the exercise of one which stands lower in the psychological scale." In a book entitled *Animal Life and Intelligence* and first published in 1890, he opposed the theories put forward by George Romanes (q.v.). In 1895, he wrote more about his experiences in the field of animal behavior in *Introduction to Comparative Psychology* (1895).

Bibliography: Watson, R. I. 1963. *The great psychologists.*

MORGANNWG HOSPITAL. A mental hospital in Wales in the county of Glamorgan. It opened as the Glamorgan County Asylum in 1864 with Dr. David Yellowless (q.v.) as its first medical superintendent. It was one of the first large mental hospitals in Wales, where, until the early part of the nineteenth century, psychiatric patients had been cared for at home, or in workhouses or jails.

Bibliography: Annear, M.W.A. 1968. *Morgannwg Hospital, 1864-1964.*

MORIA. A term used by John Mason Good (q.v.) to designate fatuity, a subdivision of the class Neurotica in his classification of mental disorders. *See also* ALUSIA, APHLEXIA, ECPHRONIA, EMPATHENIA, and LAGNEIA FUROR.

MORISON, ALEXANDER (1779-1866). A Scottish psychiatrist. As a postgraduate student, he trained in Paris under Philippe Pinel (q.v.) and Jean Esquirol (q.v.) and was influenced greatly by Esquirol. He traveled widely and at times thought of settling in Russia or the West Indies but eventually took up residence in London to practice medicine, despite the fact that he was more interested in agriculture. His interest in psychiatry was confirmed when he was appointed visiting physician to the private lunatic houses of Surrey in 1809. For a while he tried unsuccessfully to establish a professorship of mental disease, financed by Mrs. Coutts the wife of a wealthy banker to whom he was private physician. Further support for his effort had come from the royal family because of the illness of George III (q.v.), but the project was opposed by professors at the university. He then gave private lectures in Edinburgh and London in which he covered many aspects of the diagnosis, course, prognosis, and treatment of mental disorders. He became physician to the Bethlem Royal Hospital (q.v.). Morison was one of the original members of the Association of Medical Officers of Asylums and Hospitals for the Insane (q.v.) and the founder, with Anthony Ashley Cooper, the earl of Shaftesbury (q.v.) of the Society for Improving the Conditions of the Insane (q.v.).

Bibliography: Morison, A. 1848. *Lectures on the nature, causes and treatment of insanity.*

MORITA, SHOMA (1874-1938). A Japanese psychiatrist. He was a severe critic of psychoanalysis. He evolved his own theory of neurosis (q.v.) which, like the therapy he suggested, was based on Zen Buddhism (q.v.) and was particularly suitable for Japanese patients. Morita therapy assumes that the patient has become unduly self-conscious because of his illness and is overly preoccupied with his physical and mental health. Using a directive approach, it attempts to develop realistic attitudes toward life through bed rest, work, and strict discipline.

Bibliography: Ikeda, K. 1968. Morita's theory of neurosis and its application in Japanese psychotherapy. In *Modern perspectives in world psychiatry*, ed. J. G. Howells.

MORITZ, KARL PHILIPP (1757-1793). A German writer of novels and travel books. He also wrote on psychology. In 1783 he published the *Magazin zur Erfahrungsseelenkunde* (q.v.), the first psychiatric journal in the world. His autobiography, written in the form of a novel and entitled *Anton Reiser* (q.v.), contains remarkable insightful descriptions of psychological development.

Bibliography: Henning, H. 1908. *K. P. Moritz.*

MORLAND, GEORGE (1763-1804). An English painter. His childhood was marred by the extreme rigidity of his father who was also a painter and to whom he was apprenticed. Morland compensated for the rigidity of his childhood in late adolescence and adulthood by turning to excessive drinking and every kind of debauchery, which left him broken in health and spirits. His inability to settle his debts and his recurring seizures due to alcoholism (q.v.) necessitated his institutionalization in a London sponge-house, a place of preliminary imprisonment, where he died of what his contemporaries called "brain-fever."

Bibliography: Williamson, G. C. 1904. *Morland.*

MORNING GLORY. The popular name for a tropical climbing plant in the Convolvulaceae family. Its seeds have hallucinogenic properties. The Aztecs regarded it as sacred and employed its black seeds in their magic (q.v.) rites of divination (q.v.). In Hawaii it is called "wood rose," and the seeds are used by the poorer natives to obtain a feeling of euphoria, which is followed by the more unpleasant symptoms of a hangover. The psychoactive properties of morning glory are due to amides of lysergic acid. It

has enjoyed a certain popularity among young people, especially in the United States.
Bibliography: Emboden, W. 1972. *Narcotic plants.*

MORON. A term derived from the Greek and used to indicate a class of mentally retarded people. It was introduced by Henry H. Goddard (q.v.) in 1910, when he devised a new classification of mental deficiency.
Bibliography: Kanner, L. 1964. *A history of the care and study of the mentally retarded.*

MOROTA, YUJIRO (1858-1912). A Japanese psychologist, trained in the United States. He became the first professor of psychology at the University of Tokyo. In collaboration with Granville Stanley Hall (q.v.), he conducted research on dermal sensitivity. He introduced the theories of Zen Buddhism (q.v.) to the West in 1905 in a paper presented by him at the Fifth International Congress of Psychology in Rome. He deplored the limitations of Western laboratory investigations into psychological problems and favored the study of human activities in the wider context of society.
Bibliography: Misiak, H., and Sexton, V. S. 1966. *History of psychology.*

MOROTROPHIUM. A Latin term meaning "house for lunatics." There is no record of special hospitals for the insane in the Roman empire, but an institution existing in Byzantium (q.v.) in the fourth century A.D. was described by this term and may have been one of the earliest such hospitals.
Bibliography: Zilboorg, G. 1941. *A history of medical psychology.*

MORPHEUS. In Greek mythology (q.v.), he was the god of dreams and son of Hypnos (q.v.) the god of sleep. His name means "fashioner" or "molder," because he gave shape to dreams. Morphine (q.v.) is named after him.
Bibliography: Graves, R. 1960. *The Greek myths.*

MORPHINE. The principal alkaloid of opium (q.v.). In 1803 Charles Derosne, a French apothecary, isolated it as "salt of opium." Friedrich Wilhelm Sertürner, a German apothecary, followed the same process in 1804 and is usually credited with its discovery. He named it after the god of dreams, Morpheus (q.v.). Morphine became better known after 1817, when Louis Gay-Lussac, a French chemist, stressed its importance.
Bibliography: Morton, J.F. 1977. *Major medicinal plants.*

MORPHINISM. A term introduced in 1873 by Carl Fiedler (1835-1921), a German physician, to describe the effects of morphine (q.v.) addiction.
Bibliography: Zilboorg, G. 1941. *A history of medical psychology.*

MORPHY, PAUL CHARLES (1837-1884). An American chess player. He had demonstrated his exceptional skill from childhood. He could defeat the best players even blindfolded. His memory (q.v.) was extraordinary and hours after a game was over, he could remember every move he had made even while playing several people simultaneously. He was a calm, imaginative, and unflappable player, chivalrous and unwilling to obtain any financial gain from chess. Finding no one who would challenge him and sickened by the allegations against him, he retired from playing in his early twenties. His attitude toward chess turned to revulsion, and he took up law but became increasingly solitary and introverted. He finally became paranoid and believed he was being poisoned and that his clothes had been stolen from him. He died of apoplexy at forty-seven.

Bibliography: Jones, E. 1951. The problem of Paul Morphy. In *Essays in applied psychoanalysis*.

MORSELLI, ENRICO (1852-1929). An Italian psychiatrist and neurologist. He was professor of psychiatry in Turin and wrote on anthropology and mental disease. His laboratory of experimental psychology (q.v.), which may have been one of the first to be founded, produced valuable studies on the personality of the insane. He was particularly interested in problems of multiple personality and published a detailed case history of one of his patients, Elena F. (q.v.), in 1930. He believed in the clinical usefulness of hypnotism (q.v.), attended hypnotic demonstrations, and was himself hypnotized by the magnetizer Alfred d'Hont (q.v.), who figured prominently in his writings.

Bibliography: Morselli, E. 1886. *Il magnetismo animale*.

MORTALITY IN THE INSANE. Mortality rates among the insane held in the large and overcrowded asylums (q.v.) of the nineteenth century were high. Jean Esquirol (q.v.) summarized the situation as follows:

The tables of mortality, published by the physicians of London and York, are the more favourable, because they receive at those hospitals those individuals only, who offer the most favourable indications for a cure, and consequently, most widely removed from mortality: whilst at the Salpêtrière, Bicêtre, and Charenton, more than one third of the insane admitted, come to terminate their existence at these hospitals. We must also take notice of the accidental circumstances which modify the mortality. Thus we have observed at the Hôtel-Dieu of Paris, that when the smallpox was epidemic, a greater number of the insane died.

Bibliography: Esquirol, J.E.D. 1845. Reprint. 1965. *Mental maladies: a treatise on insanity*.

MORZINE. A French town in Savoy. In the late 1850s a group of children in the town became hysterical (*see* HYSTERIA) and were believed to be possessed (*see* POSSESSION) by demons. The hysteria spread to the adults, and many people became convinced that they were bewitched and their souls would go to hell. Services of exorcism (q.v.) were conducted by the clergy

to no avail, and the town was torn by episodes of mass hysteria for about five years. Life returned to normal only after the intervention of physicians who treated those affected.
Bibliography: Sirois, F. 1974. *Epidemic hysteria.*

MOSES. A biblical prophet and lawgiver to the people of Israel in the thirteenth century B.C. According to tradition, he was hidden by his mother in a basket placed in the bulrushes to escape the pharaoh's decree that all male infants should be killed. Found and raised by the pharaoh's daughter, he became the leader of his people. He killed, cursed, and commanded, but the Bible (q.v.) refers to him as meekest of all men (Num. 12: 13). Michelangelo's (q.v.) statue of Moses provoked the only piece of art criticism written by Sigmund Freud (q.v.), "The Moses of Michelangelo," published anonymously in 1914. Freud was said to have projected into the article his own feelings. The last of Freud's books to be published in his life time was also about Moses. Entitled *Moses and Monotheism*, it again reflects his fascination with the prophet. The work, published in 1939, was considered extremely controversial because of Freud's suggestion that Moses was an Egyptian who had been killed by the Hebrews.
Bibliography: Freud, S. 1939. *Moses and monotheism: three essays.*

MOSSO, ANGELO (1846-1910). An Italian psychologist. He is known for his studies on fatigue and his introduction of psychological measurements into physiology. He also wrote on fear.
Bibliography: Mosso, A. 1891. *Fatigue.*

MOTHER-SICK. An old expression meaning "hysterical." Because hysteria (q.v.) was believed to be connected with the womb, the term "the mother" became synonymous with hysteria.
Bibliography: 1978. *Brewer's dictionary of phrase and fable.*

MOTHERWORT. Popular name given to two herbs, *Chenopodium* and *Leonurus*, that are indigenous to Europe and some parts of Asia. The name "motherwort" was given to them in England, where they were used in the treatment of hysteria (q.v.) ("fits of the mother"). They were also popular in the treatment of depression. Nicholas Culpeper (q.v.), referring to Chenopodium, which he called *Arrach*, wrote "there is no better herb to drive melancholy vapours from the heart, to strengthen it, and make the mind cheerful, blithe and merry." The same author advised the rich to keep it for their poor neighbors as well as for their own household. John Gerard (q.v.) regarded Leonurus with the same respect, and modern herbalists still believe it is useful for various complaints, including irritability and hysteria.
Bibliography: le Strange, R. 1977. *A history of herbal plants.*

MOTT, FREDERICK WALKER, SIR (1859-1926). A British neurologist. Under his leadership, the pathological laboratory of the London county asylums at Claybury, England, became an important center of neuropathological research. He also conducted valuable investigations into the pathology of mental disorders at Maudsley Hospital (q.v.), which he helped to found. In 1899 he founded and edited a journal entitled *Archives of Neurology*. Mott wrote with great energy on practically every aspect of neuropathology.

Bibliography: Meyer, A. 1973. Frederick Mott, founder of the Maudsley laboratories. *Brit. J. Psychiat.* 122: 497-516.

MOUNT HOPE RETREAT. An institution in Baltimore, Maryland, founded by a Roman Catholic Order. In 1842 it was organized as an asylum for the insane and was supported by private charitable funds.

Bibliography: Tuke, D. H. 1892. *A dictionary of psychological medicine.*

MOUSSORGSKY (*or* MUSORGSKI), MODEST PETROVICH (1839-1881). A Russian composer. He abandoned his military career because of a nervous disorder and became a composer of many successful songs, before becoming famous for his opera *Boris Gudunov*. Other works remained unfinished as he became an alcoholic (*see* ALCOHOLISM) and was unable to concentrate for long periods. He eventually died of alcoholism. Many of his compositions were completed by his friend Nicolai Rimsky-Korsakov (q.v.).

Bibliography: Calvocoressi, M. D. 1974. *Mussorgsky*, ed. G. Abraham.

MOXA. Small combustible cones produced by a plant grown in the East and introduced into Europe by Prosper Alpinus (q.v.). They were placed on the body and ignited to cauterize (*see* CAUTERIZATION) the skin, a treatment for insanity still in use in the nineteenth century.

MUGGLETON, LODOWICKE (1609-1698). An English heresiarch, apprenticed to a tailor. With his cousin John Reeve (1608-1658), Muggleton claimed to be a witness of *Revelation* 11. Both men were puritanical and their fanatical approach to religious matters gained some followers but led to clashes with the Quakers (q.v.). Muggleton denied the Trinity and believed that the Devil had become incarnate in Eve. His preoccupation with guilt and its expiation was expressed in numerous writings, which eventually led to his imprisonment for blasphemy. Some of his doctrines anticipated Emanuel Swedenborg (q.v.). The sect he founded, the Muggletonions, lasted into the early twentieth century.

Bibliography: Williamson, G. C. 1919. *Lodowick Muggleton.*

MUGWORT. *Artemisia vulgaris*, one of the many species of the daisy family. In antiquity the plant was considered sacred and believed to ward off "devil sickness" and demoniac possession (q.v.). It was recommended

for this purpose in the herbal of Apuleius Platonicus, which dates from the fifth century B.C. John Gerard (q.v.) recommended it in the treatment of epilepsy (q.v.).
Bibliography: le Strange, R. 1977. *A history of herbal plants.*

MÜLLER, ANTON (1755-1827). A German physician and one of the first to devote himself to the care of the mentally ill. He worked in a hospital for the insane and attempted to abolish harsh treatment and brutal restraint (q.v.). He wished to humanize the management of patients.
Bibliography: Zilboorg, G. 1941. *A history of medical psychology.*

MULLER, CATHARINE. A medium (q.v.), better known by her pseudonym of Helene Smith. In 1894 she met Théodore Flournoy (q.v.) at a seance. He became interested in her abilities and began a five-year investigation of her activities. She claimed that in previous lives she had been an Indian princess, Marie Antoinette, and a Martian; she spoke an unknown language. Flournoy published a book about her psychopathology that caused violent controversy, and the medium would have nothing more to do with him after it appeared. She inherited a fortune from an American woman who wished her to stop working as a saleswoman and devote herself completely to spiritualism, which she did. She lived in isolation in a world of fantasy. Her paintings, executed during periods of somnambulism (q.v.), were exhibited in France and Switzerland after her death.
Bibliography: Flournoy, T. 1900. *From India to the planet Mars: a study of a case of somnambulism with glossolalia.*

MÜLLER, GEORG ELIAS (1850-1934). A German physiologist and philosopher with interests in psychology. As a young man he studied philosophy and history, but later devoted himself to natural science. He was a pupil of Rudolph Lotze (q.v.) who greatly influenced him. In 1873 he published his doctoral thesis, a dissertation on sensory attention, which was widely quoted for many years. He then turned to psychophysics and studied phenomena of vision and memory (q.v.). He became professor at Gottingen, where he established a well known laboratory of experimental psychology (q.v.). His *Abriss der Psychologie*, published in 1924, encompassed the whole field of psychology.
Bibliography: Watson, R. I. 1963. *The great psychologists.*

MÜLLER, JOHANNES PETER (1801-1858). A German physiologist, the fifth child of a shoemaker. His studies covered a wide field and greatly contributed to advances in neurology and in psychology. His famous *Handbook of Physiology* was published in 1838. Notwithstanding his brilliant intellect and the recognition of his achievements, Müller was prone to depression and would take large doses of opium (q.v.), especially in his last years.

He was found dead in his bed. His great work, a textbook of physiology (1833-1840), is comprised of more than three quarters of a million German words.
Bibliography: Watson, R. I. 1963. *The great psychologists.*

MUNCH, EDVARD (1863-1944). A Norwegian painter. Tuberculosis (q.v.) and insanity were prevalent in his family. His mother died when he was five years old; his sister died when he was thirteen; another sister and his grandfather died in an asylum. These events left him with a morbid anxiety about physical and mental illness. He was further handicapped by his home atmosphere of petty restrictions and piety. While in Paris, he met Paul Gauguin, Vincent Van Gogh, and Henri de Toulouse-Lautrec (qq.v.) and was greatly influenced by them. He went through periods of severe depression and mental agitation with a pathological interest in death and destructive love, which were reflected in many of his gloomy works. His series of paintings, *The Frieze of Life*, took over ten years to execute and revolved around the theme of fear, anguish, and obsessional love. His work attracted much attention in spite of its disturbing symbolism. Denying that art had anything to do with pleasure, he once wrote that "painting is for me like being ill or intoxicated: an illness of which I do not want to be cured. . . . " Writing about his famous work, *The Scream* (1893), he stated, "I hear the scream of nature."
Bibliography: Hodin, J. P. 1972. *Edward Munch.*

MÜNCHHAUSEN, KARL FRIEDRICH HIERONYMUS, BARON VON (1720-1797). A German cavalry officer descendant of an old aristocratic family. He became proverbial for the exaggerated stories of his exploits which he narrated with great gusto and self-satisfaction. The earliest version of his tales was written in English in 1785 by Rudolph Erich Raspe (1737-1794). One of Münchhausen's tales refers to the Royal College of Physicians of London whose residence he claimed he had lifted with a balloon to revenge himself on doctors. Clergy, undertakers, sextons, and grave-diggers then found themselves short of work because the death rate fell sharply when the doctors were suspended in mid-air for three months. The term "Münchhausen syndrome" was first used by R. Asher in 1951 to describe a condition in which some individuals pretend dramatic signs of acute illness and invent stories of previous attacks in order to gain admission to hospitals and, often, undergo repeated surgical operations.
Bibliography: Raspe, R. E. et al. 1948. *Singular travels, campaigns, and adventures of Baron Münchhausen*, ed. J. Carswell.

MUNK, HERMANN (1839-1912). A German physiologist. His discoveries concerning the role of the brain in vision, hearing, and somato-sensory functions contributed to neurology (q.v.). He established an understanding of cortical blindness and mind blindness. Munk's contributions often have been underestimated.

Bibliography: Haymaker, W., and Schiller, F. 1970. *The founders of neurology*. 2d. ed.

MÜNSTERBERG, HUGO (1863-1916). An American psychologist who pioneered in applied psychology. He was a pupil of Wilhelm Wundt (q.v.) and taught in several German universities before becoming a professor of psychology at Harvard University in 1892. In 1905 he became director of the psychological laboratory (q.v.) there. He proposed an action theory of consciousness (q.v.) that advanced the understanding of psychological processes. Legal and industrial psychology and psychic research were among his main interests. He was a pioneer also in the field of social psychology and advocated a wider use of psychological tests in schools and industry, as well as in assessing the reliability of witnesses in court cases. Münsterberg popularized psychology in his many books. He died during World War I, deeply disappointed at the hostilities between the United States and Germany.

Bibliography: Münsterberg, M. 1922. *Hugo Münsterberg: his life and work*.

MUNTHE, AXEL (1857-1949). A Swedish doctor and writer. He began his medical studies in Upsala in 1874 but eventually qualified in Paris in 1880 after a period of study at the University of Montpellier. As a student he met Jean Martin Charcot (q.v.) at the Salpêtrière (q.v.), and it may have been this experience that influenced his subsequent interest in psychological medicine and neurology rather than gynecology in which he had specialized. He settled in Paris where his fluency in several languages attracted a cosmopolitan clientele, mostly of rich women, suffering from neurotic disorders, real or imagined. However, he did not hesitate to rush to Naples, Italy, in 1884, when the city was stricken with cholera. From there he wrote *Letters from a Mourning City*, a series of articles, later published in one volume. He returned to Italy and established himself as a fashionable practitioner in Rome. Eventually he reached Capri, the island he had first fallen in love with in 1876, during a brief visit whilst convalescing from pulmonary tuberculosis. In Capri he built his dream house, Villa San Michele. Munthe is best remembered for the book which describes this house; mostly autobiographical, he dictated *The story of San Michele* in English to his Russian secretary Natascina Khalutine, because by then he was nearly blind. Restless and excitable, he was a sufferer from insomnia and often used morphine (q.v.) to obtain sleep. Munthe is remembered as a generous but extremely reserved man, who had a particular fascination for women. Queen Victoria of Sweden, who made him her personal physician, had a villa built in Capri to be near him. He died when he was ninety-one years old at the Court of

Stockholm, where he had been a guest of the royal family for the last six years of his life.
Bibliography: Munthe, G., and Uexkull, G. 1953. *The story of Axel Munthe*.

MURASAKI SHIKIBU (c.978-1031). A Japanese novelist and court figure. She wrote a famous diary (1007-1010) and a novel, *Genji Monagatari* (*The Tale of Genji*), which is the oldest full novel in the world and one of the greatest works in Japanese literature. It contains a sensitive awareness of human emotions.
Bibliography: *Lady Murasaki. The tale of Genji*. 1935. trans. A. Waley.

MURATORI, LUDOVICO ANTONIO (1672-1750). An Italian antiquary and historian, librarian to the Duke of Modena. His book on the power of human imagination (q.v.), *Della Forza della Fantasia Umana*, (1740) reveals him to be an early psychologist. In it he discussed in detail how fantasy influenced dreams (q.v.) during which the individual could fulfil his secret wishes. Muratori believed that pathological humors (q.v.) could cause disturbing dreams. He also gave his views on visions and delusions (q.v.) and asserted that strong passions influence the imagination.
Bibliography: Mora, G. 1975. Italy. In *World history of psychiatry*, ed. J. G. Howells.

MURRAY, GEORGE REDMAYNE (1865-1939). An English physician. In 1891 he became the first to employ hypodermic injections of thyroid extracts in the treatment of cretinism (q.v.). The improvement shown by patients so treated gave impetus to research on the link between endocrine glands and certain mental disorders.
Bibliography: Alexander, F. G., and Selesnick, S. T. 1966. *The history of psychiatry*.

MURRAY, JAMES (1781-1814). A Scottish philanthropist. He was a bachelor who inherited the wealth that had been left to his father by his half brother, William Hope. Murray stipulated in his will that two-thirds of his estate should be used to found a hospital for "lunatic persons," which led to the establishment of Murray Royal Hospital (q.v.) in 1826. Murray's uncle was the physician Andrew Marshall (q.v.) and may have inspired him to use some of his wealth for a mental hospital.
Bibliography: Henderson, D. K. 1964. *The evolution of psychiatry in Scotland*.

MURRAY ROYAL HOSPITAL. A mental hospital in Perth, Scotland. It was founded in 1826 with funds left in the will of James Murray (q.v.) whose family retained a connection with the administration of the hospital for many years. It was granted a royal charter of incorporation by George IV (1762-1830) in 1827. Even the first official report of the hospital in 1828 mentions that no patient was confined to his room and that all efforts had been made to avoid a gloomy appearance in the building. Occupational therapy (q.v.)

included gardening, reading, music, and games. From its original eighty patients, it grew rapidly. The hospital produced a magazine, the *Excelsior* (q.v.) founded in 1857, and from 1854 on, had its own Mechanics Institute, which provided educational classes and talks given by visiting lecturers. The first physician of the asylum was Dr. William Malcom. He was appointed even before building was begun and gave help and suggestions in its establishment. The hospital is now known as Perth Royal Mental Hospital. *See also* ROYAL ASYLUMS.

Bibliography: Chambers, W. D. 1927. Murray Royal Hospital, Perth. *Report of the Physician-Superintendent for the Year Ending 31st March 1927.*

MURUT. A mountain people of central Borneo, almost unknown until World War II. Their classification of mental illness comprises several categories. They distinguish between psychosis (q.v.), which they attribute to the influence of spirits residing in wells or trees, and neurosis (q.v.), which they call "worry of the mind" and attribute to human ill-wishers using poisonous charms and witchcraft (q.v.). Treatment consists of attempts by professional healers to placate the spirits and thus drive them out of the patient. Incantations, special lotions, fumigation (q.v.), and fasting (q.v.) are among the methods used.

Bibliography: Schmidt, K. E. 1967-1968. Some concepts of mental illness in the Murut. *Int. J. Soc. Psychiatr.* 14: 24-31.

MUSIC THERAPY. The therapeutic effects of music have been known and exploited throughout the world since antiquity. In Greek mythology (q.v.), Apollo (q.v.) is both god of music and of medicine. Aesculapius (q.v.) was said to cure diseases of the mind by using song and music, and music therapy was used even in ancient Egyptian temples. Plato (q.v.) believed that music not only temporarily affected the emotions but could even influence the character of an individual. Aristotle (q.v.) thought that music affects the soul. Celsus (q.v.) advocated the sound of cymbals and running water for the treatment of mental disorders, and the Bible (q.v.) contains many examples of music used to induce hallucinations (q.v.) and ecstasy (q.v.) as well as to cure mental disorders (see Plate 9). David played his harp to relieve the melancholy of Saul (Samuel: I, 16). In the Middle Ages (q.v.) music was used to exhaust whole crowds of people suffering from mass hysteria (q.v.) and was recommended specifically for the treatment of mental disorders by Bartholomaeus Anglicus (q.v.). The Turks appointed singers and musicians to play to the insane, believing that pleasant sounds would strengthen their spirits and reduce the bile (q.v.). Timothy Bright, Robert Burton, and William Shakespeare (qq.v.) all believed in the healing power of music and Shakespeare made many references to it in his plays (The Tempest; Henry IV, Part II, the Merchant of Venice, etc.). In the eighteenth century music was believed to be helpful in soothing the "passions of the soul," and

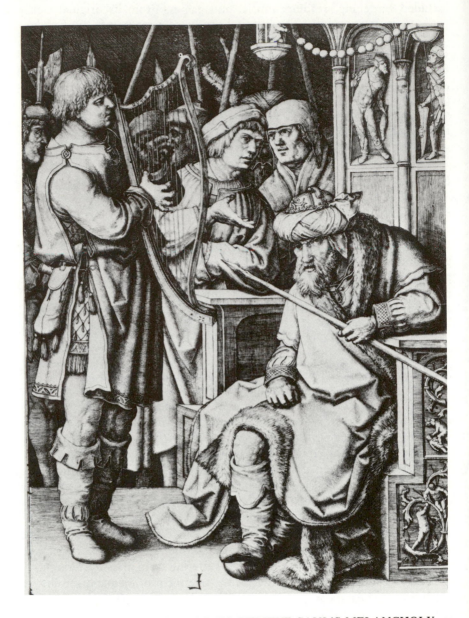

9. DAVID PLAYING THE HARP TO RELIEVE SAUL'S MELANCHOLY, as shown in a 1508 engraving by Lucas van Leiden. By courtesy of the Wellcome Trustees, Wellcome Institute for the History of Medicine, London.

Medicina Musica (q.v.) was dedicated to this form of therapy. Philip V (q.v.) could be cured of his depression only by the songs of Carlo Farinelli (q.v.). Nineteenth-century medical literature makes frequent references to music therapy, and most mental hospitals promoted concerts, dances, and brass bands (q.v.) for their patients. Jean Esquirol (q.v.) often employed music in treatment but with little success and came to believe that the ancients had exaggerated its effect. He found it to be more beneficial in the treatment of melancholia (q.v.) than in any other form of mental disorder. George III (q.v.) was offered music to relieve his symptoms during the last period of his illness.

Bibliography: Critchley, M., and Henson, R. A., eds. 1977. *Music and the brain.*

MUSK. A substance secreted by the preputial gland of the musk deer. In the *Great Herbal* of the sixteenth century, the strong smell of musk is recommended for "weakness of the brain."

Bibliography: Rohde, E. S. 1972. *Old English herbals.*

MUTISM. Psychopathological mutism sometimes was attributed to demoniac possession (q.v.). In the sixteenth century, Pierre Leloyer (q.v.) was among those who held this belief.

Bibliography: Zilboorg, G. 1941. *A history of medical psychology.*

MYERS, CHARLES SAMUEL (1873-1946). A British psychologist and leader in the field of experimental psychology. As a young man, he was interested in racial anthropology and conducted an investigation of ancient skulls found in Suffolk, England. He also joined an expedition to the Torres Straits and Sarawak, where he conducted research on the native population. In 1899, he became house physician to Saint Bartholomew's Hospital (q.v.) in London. Poor health forced him to seek a better climate, and he went to Egypt for a year. On his return he eventually settled in Cambridge and became director of the university's psychological laboratory (q.v.) until 1921, when he became director of the National Institute of Industrial Psychology. His research on the senses, industrial psychology, and shell shock greatly influenced British psychology. Shell shock he observed at first hand during his war service in France. He was the cofounder and first president of the British Psychological Society (q.v.) and the cofounder and editor of the *British Journal of Psychology* (q.v.). Most of his later work was devoted to applied psychology, especially in industry. He was the author of several books, including *A Textbook of Experimental Psychology* (1909).

Bibliography: Murchison, C., ed. 1936. *A history of psychology in autobiography.* Vol. 3.

MYERS, FREDERICK WILLIAM HENRY (1843-1901). An English poet and writer. He was particularly interested in the question of life after death.

His research led him into the field of parapsychology and investigations of hypnotism (q.v.), hysterical (*see* HYSTERIA) states, and personality. He believed that men possessed superior and inferior functions. Superior functions included the possibility of communication with spirits. He systematized the idea of an unconscious (q.v.) mind and attributed to it the weaving of fantasies, a function which he called "mythopoetic." In 1882 he founded with others the Society of Psychical Research. His most comprehensive work, *Human Personality and its Survival of Bodily Death*, was published posthumously in 1903.
Bibliography: Ellenberger, H. F. 1970. *The discovery of the unconscious.*

MYREPSOS, NICHOLAS. A thirteenth-century Byzantine physician born in Alexandria. For his book of pharmaceutical recipes he collected antidotes derived from the Arabs and the school of Salerno. His *Antidotarium*, comprised of some 2,656 recipes, gave impetus to the use of pharmacological remedies in the treatment of physical and mental disorders.
Bibliography: Zilboorg, G. 1941. *A history of medical psychology.*

MYRTLE. An evergreen shrub. Its leaves are used in Eastern medicine for the treatment of cerebral afflictions, especially epilepsy (q.v.). In the Middle Ages (q.v.) brushes made from twigs of myrtle were used to sprinkle holy water in exorcism (q.v.) ceremonies, and infusions of myrtle leaves were prescribed for hysteria (q.v.).
Bibliography: le Strange, R. 1977. *A history of herbal plants.*

MYTHOLOGY. The traditions preserved in mythological narratives reflect the beliefs of the people to whom they belong. They often represent efforts to explain natural phenomena, behavior that is not readily understood, and emotional reactions to stressful situations. The psychoanalytic school of psychiatry gave new impetus to the study of myths, as the interpretation of dreams (q.v.) often is based on them. Both Sigmund Freud (q.v.) and Carl G. Jung (q.v.) engaged in the study of mythology, and many of their followers imitated them.
See also NORSE MYTHOLOGY.
Bibliography: Robinson, H. P. and Wilson, K. 1962. *The encyclopaedia of myths and legends of all nations.*

N

NÄCKE, PAUL (?-?). A German sex pathologist. He wrote on homosexuality (q.v.), and, in translating Havelock Ellis' (q.v.) term "Narcissus-like," introduced the term *narcismus* into German in 1899. He used it to describe a form of sexual deviation in which the individual is in love with himself. He was an admirer of Sigmund Freud (q.v.) with whom he shared some concepts of sexuality.
Bibliography: Sulloway, F. J. 1979. *Freud: biologist of the mind.*

NADIA. A patient of Pierre Janet (q.v.). She was obsessed (*see* OBSESSION) with the fear of becoming fat and refused food, although she ate greedily in secret. Janet recognized that the symptoms were not those of ordinary anorexia nervosa (q.v.) and concluded that Nadia had an obsession about her body and its functions that was related to her anxiety about being despised and rejected.
Bibliography: Janet, P. 1903. *Les obsessions et la psychasthénie.*

NAGEL, WILIBALD A. (1870-1910). A German physiologist. He was particularly interested in the psychophysiology of sensation and published papers reporting the results of his research on vision, taste, smell, and touch. In 1905 he edited the *Handbuch der Physiologie* to which he contributed papers on the senses and the specific energies of nerves.
Bibliography: Boring, E. G. 1950. *A history of experimental psychology.*

NAGEOTTE, JEAN (1866-1948). A French physician. He worked at Bicêtre (q.v.) and then at the Salpêtrière (q.v.). He promoted a better understanding of the pathological changes occuring in the nervous system of tabetics.

Bibliography: Haymaker, W., and Schiller, F. 1970. *The founders of neurology*. 2d. ed.

NAGOYA. A town in Japan. The first Japanese institution for the feeble-minded was built there, following an earthquake in 1890. At that time, R. Ishii established a private orphanage for children who had lost their parents in the disaster and among them was an imbecile child, who gave him the idea of opening a special department for the mentally retarded. The institution was a development of this department and housed twenty retarded children.

Bibliography: Barr, M. W. 1904. *Mental defectives*.

NAJAB UD DIN UNHAMMAD. An Arab physician who lived between the eighth and ninth centuries. His original writings have been lost, but their contents were recorded in later medical commentaries. In his treatise he described and classified many mental disorders, including acute delirium (q.v.), bizarre behavior, agitation, depression, phobia, paranoia (q.v.) and psychopathic (*see* PSYCHOPATHY) personality. He believed that heat ascending to the brain could cause its degeneration, which in turn would give rise to mental symptoms. He ascribed neurotic (*see* NEUROSIS) disorders to excessive study and depression to impure or exaggerated love. Like other Arab physicians, he believed that treatment should consist of a good diet (q.v.), baths (q.v.), diversion, including music, and occasionally bleeding (q.v.).

Bibliography: Zilboorg, G. 1941. *A history of medical psychology*.

NAM. The fictitious name given to a family by Arthur H. Estabrook and Charles B. Davenport (q.v.) in their genetic study of feeblemindedness. The family lived in the mountains of western Massachusetts. At the end of their study, the two workers concluded that its members had a preponderance of alcoholics (*see* ALCOHOLISM) and demonstrated a remarkable lack of ambition.

See also EUGENICS.

Bibliography: Estabrook, A. H., and Davenport, C. B. 1912. *The Nam family: a study in cacogenics*.

NANCY SCHOOL. A loosely connected international group of physicians interested in mental disorders. They met in Nancy, France, under the inspiration of Ambroise-August Liébeault (q.v.). Their approach to hypnotism (q.v.) was different from that of Jean Martin Charcot (q.v.) at the Salpêtrière (q.v.) in that they believed hypnotic phenomena were the result of suggestion, which their method of treatment depended upon, and not pathology.

The school, begun in 1866, gave a new orientation to psychiatry, shifting its attention from psychosis (q.v.) toward the recognition of emotional disorders. The term psychotherapy (q.v.) was popularized by the Nancy school toward the end of the nineteenth century.

Bibliography: Chertok, L., and de Saussure, R. 1979. *The therapeutic revolution: from Mesmer to Freud.*

NANSEN, FRIDTJHOF (1861-1930). A Norwegian polar explorer and anatomist. He was a pupil of Camillo Golgi (q.v.). Nansen collected a large number of animal specimens, ranging from simple organisms to small mammals, and used them for detailed histological studies, especially of the central nervous system. His original observations have been associated with the neuron theory developed by Wilhelm His (q.v.) and August Forel (q.v.).

Bibliography: Hoyer, L. N. 1957. *Nansen: a family portrait.*

NAPOLEON I (NAPOLEON BONAPARTE) (1769-1821). Emperor of the French, born in Corsica. His mother subjected him to the dangers of war even before he was born, as she followed her husband in battle despite her pregnancy. As a child he was unruly, and his outbursts of rage terrified everybody. He completely dominated his elder brother, Joseph (1768-1844). Only his mother could manage him and he loved her. As an adolescent, he was undersized, poorly nourished, moody, awkward, taciturn, often lost in a fantasy world, and completely self-centered. Later in life he suffered from nervous indigestion, migraine (q.v.), and psychogenic dermatitis. He was prone to seizures that may have been due to epilepsy (q.v.). Charles Maurice de Talleyrand (1754-1838), in his memoirs, described how one evening Napoleon had fallen to the ground, groaning and shaken by convulsions suggestive of an epileptic fit. His attitude toward women was curious: those he used, he despised, and those he admired, he idealized unrealistically. He deeply loved his first wife, Josephine Beauharnais (1763-1814), despite her selfishness and many infidelities, but he divorced her when it became obvious that she was sterile. His intellectual processes were exceptionally quick. He could dictate simultaneously to four secretaries on four different subjects, and his memory (q.v.) also was extraordinary. In middle age, and declining health, his irascibility became explosive and he often gave vent to roaring rages. His attitude toward suicide (q.v.) was uncompromising. Fearing an epidemic when two of his soldiers committed suicide, he issued an order of the day that stated a soldier should know how to overcome the grief and melancholy of his passions and should bear his mental afflictions manfully. Yet, Charles-Tristan de Mantholon, (1783-1853), his faithful follower and biographer, wrote that in a period of depression he had tried to commit suicide by drinking a preparation of opium (q.v.), but he was persuaded to take an antidote. Under stress, he would often collapse in

tears. Georges Lefebvre (1874-1959), the great historian of the French Revolution, wrote that "Napoleon was more than anything else a temperament."
Bibliography: Cronin, V. 1973. *Napoleon.*

NAPOLEON III (CHARLES LOUIS NAPOLEON BONAPARTE) (1808-1873). President of the French Republic and later emperor of the French. Although he underwent many struggles for power and survived many intrigues and revolts, he was considered an irresolute man. He was often in poor health, depressed, and, at times, under the influence of opiates. After a bloodless revolution in Paris in 1870, he was exiled to England, where he died. His psychological make-up has intrigued many historians because of its contradictions. The unsettled political climate around him and the political meddling of his wife were probably contributory factors to the aetiology of his depression.
Bibliography: Williams, R. L. 1971. *The mortal Napoleon III.*

NARCISSISM. The term, derived from Narcissus (q.v.), is believed to have been used in psychological literature for the first time by Alfred Binet (q.v.) in 1887. Binet compared those fetishists who take themselves as the preferred sexual object to the legend of Narcissus. Havelock Ellis (q.v.) used the term "Narcissus-like" in 1898 in a paper on normal sexual activity. Paul Näcke (q.v.) translated Ellis' concept into German and applied it to a sexual perversion. Around 1910 Sigmund Freud (q.v.) adopted the term in the second edition of his *Three Essays on the Theory of Sexuality* and dwelt on the concept at some length in 1914 in his *On Narcissism: An Introduction.*
Bibliography: Sulloway, F. J. 1979. *Freud: biologist of the mind.*

NARCISSUS. In Greek mythology, (q.v.) the beautiful son of a river god and a nymph. He had never experienced love until he saw his own reflection in a pool of water and fell in love with it. One myth claims that he thought the reflection was a beautiful nymph, dived into the pool to reach her, and drowned, but another story claims he pined away because he could not approach the object of his love. His boy was transformed into the flower narcissus. Plutarch (q.v.) thought that the term derived from the Greek word *narke*, meaning "numbness", and that the narcissus was used to produce narcosis.
Bibliography: Graves, R. 1960. *The Greek myths.*

NARCOSYNTHESIS. A technique developed by Roy Grinker (1900-   ) and J. P. Spiegel during World War II. It attempts to bring back lost memories by means of narcotic drugs, such as sodium pentothal.
Bibliography: Grinker, R. R., and Spiegel, J. P. 1945. *War neuroses.*

NARDUS ROOT. *Nardostachys jatamansi*, a plant that grows at 13,000 to 15,000 feet on the Alpine Himalayas. The use of its root in Indian medicine can be traced as far back as 1000 to 800 B.C. It was used to induce sleep in cases of insomnia and in those cases of mental disorder in which the patients became overly excited.

Bibliography: Siddiqui, S. 1969. Need for research in plant drugs. *Hamdard* 12: 422.

NARRENSCHIFF (SHIP OF FOOLS). A literary work by the satirical poet and humanist, Sebastian Brant (1457?-1521). It was written in German dialect and first published in 1494. It deals with the shipping of fools from their native place to the Land of Fools. The fools, each representing a fashionable foible, are divided according to their type of folly and are reproved for their behavior. They represented officials and courtiers whom Brant condemned for their corrupted way of life. The work became world famous and was translated into several languages. An English adaptation by Alexander Barclay was published in 1509. The theme inspired *The Ship of Fools* (q.v.) painted by Hieronymous Bosch (q.v.).

Bibliography: Brant, S. 1494. Reprint 1971. *The ship of fools*, trans. W. Gillis.

NARRENTURM. A circular building for the confinement of the insane erected in Vienna, Austria, in 1784 by order of Emperor Joseph II (1741-1790). Its name means "tower of the mad," and it housed as many as 250 patients on its five floors. Because it was the first large hospital in Europe built exclusively for the insane, it was regarded as a show piece, and public visiting was allowed on payment of a fee. The inside of the tower was hollow with a square building in the center that was joined to the circle at each corner. The medical staff and the keepers were housed in the square building, and the insane were kept in the circular part. Some fifty years after its inauguration, conditions badly deteriorated, and it became the object of much criticism by visitors. In 1853, after a new hospital was built outside Vienna, the Narrenturm cared only for chronic and dangerous patients. It ceased to be a hospital in 1869 and became a storage place and museum.

Bibliography: Kraepelin, E. 1962. *One hundred years of psychiatry.*

NASSE, CHRISTIAN FRIEDRICH (1778-1851). A German psychiatrist and proponent of scientific psychiatry. After searching for a sound theory of mental disorders, he decided that neurological changes were responsible not only for psychosis (q.v.) but also for neurotic (*see* NEUROSIS) disorders. He despaired of the classification used at the time and wrote: "Those who talk to us about lunacy, insanity, and diseases of the mind should first be asked what they mean by those expressions; it is only luck if a mutual understanding can be reached. . . ." In 1838 he founded a journal, *Zeitschrift für die Beurteilung and Heilung der Seelenzustände* to provide a forum for discussion. He advocated that all physicians should be instructed in psychiatry and that general hospitals should have clinical wards for mental patients, who would be drawn from neighboring

asylums and be replaced every two or three months. Despite these views he still thought that harmless lunatics should be cared for by the clergy.
Bibliography: Kraepelin, E. 1962. *One hundred years of psychiatry.*

NATHUSIUS, MARIA (1817-1857). A German writer of pious stories. She campaigned vigorously for the establishment of special institutions for mentally retarded children. Because of her efforts, two such institutions—one for boys and one for girls—were established in the Harz region.
Bibliography: Kanner, L. 1964. *A history of the care and study of the mentally retarded.*

NATIONAL ASSOCIATION FOR MENTAL HEALTH. *See* MENTAL HYGIENE MOVEMENT.

NATIONAL ASSOCIATION FOR THE PROTECTION OF THE INSANE AND THE PREVENTION OF INSANITY. An American organization founded in 1880 in Cleveland, Ohio, during the annual meeting of the National Conference of Social Work. Its members were primarily psychiatrists, neurologists, and social workers, but it also included a number of interested laymen. From 1883 to 1884 it published its own journal, *The American Psychological Journal*, but the association ceased to exist after four years. Its disintegration was due in part to powerful opposition from the Association of Medical Superintendents of American Institutions for the Insane, now known as the American Psychiatric Association (q.v.).
Bibliography: Deutsch, A. 1949. *The mentally ill in America.*

NATIONAL HOSPITAL FOR NERVOUS DISEASES. The first neurological center in the world. It was founded in Queen Square, London, in 1859 for the Relief of Paralysis, Epilepsy, and Allied Disorders.
Bibliography: Holmes, G. 1954. *The National Hospital, Queen Square 1860-1948.*

NATIONAL INSTITUTE OF MENTAL HEALTH (NIMH). The National Mental Health Act (q.v.) passed by the United States Congress in 1946 authorized the Public Health Service to establish a national institute of mental health, now located in Bethesda, Maryland. The institute began functioning in 1949. Through grants to states and institutions it supports all aspects of mental health work.

NATIONAL MENTAL HEALTH ACT. An act passed by the United States Congress in 1946. It was of great importance to American psychiatry because it emphasized that the primary need was no longer in the field of custodial care of the insane, but in providing a wider program of prevention

and treatment within the community, which embraced family, school, and industrial problems, as well as delinquency in various fields.
Bibliography: Rosen, G. 1968. *Madness in society.*

NAWNKOTE. A village in the Punjab, India. As late as the second half of the nineteenth century, hysterical (*see* HYSTERIA) girls were believed to be possessed (*see* POSSESSION) by the devil. They were strung up by their feet on the village ancient banyan tree and swung about to the sound of drums to exorcise (*see* EXORCISM) the demons.
Bibliography: Mehta, Ved. 1972. *Daddyji.*

NAZARETH. An ancient town in Palestine, which the Jews regarded as proverbial for the stupidity of its inhabitants.
Bibliography: 1978. *Brewer's dictionary of phrase and fable.*

NEBUCHADNEZZAR (c.600-561 B.C.). A king of Babylon. According to the book of Daniel in the Bible (q.v.) he was emotionally unstable and suffered from insomnia and bad dreams (q.v.). During attacks of fury he ordered all the wise men of Babylon to be destroyed and ordered others to be thrown into a furnace. He later fell into an unkempt state for a period of seven years. His appearance resembled that of a wild animal, thus offering an early example of lycanthropy (q.v.). He recovered and lived to be eighty-three years old. The opera *Nabucco* by Giuseppe Verdi (1813-1901) is based on events surrounding his life and vividly describes him. William Blake (q.v.) depicted him crawling on all fours like a beast.
Bibliography: Wiseman, D. J. 1956. *Chronicles of Chaldaean kings.*

NECROMANCY. The practice of black magic (q.v.) and occult power. Necromancers were supposed to be able to converse with the spirits of the dead and to know the future. In the Bible the Witch of Endor called up Samuel (I. Sam. xxviii, 7ff.).

NEI CHING. A Chinese canon of medicine, dating from c. 249 B.C. It claimed that the brain was composed of the same material as the marrow of the bones and that the skull served as the main reservoir. Abundant marrow corresponded with good health. The doctrine of the pulse is also discussed in this canon. In insanity, a "deep" and "quick" pulse was considered a bad prognosis.
Bibliography: Morse, W. R. 1938. *Chinese medicine.*

NEILL, ALEXANDER SUTHERLAND (1884-1973). A British educationalist born in Scotland. In 1921, to practice his revolutionary ideas on child education, he founded an international school in Dresden, Germany. Political events forced him and his handful of pupils to move to Vienna and

then to England, where he finally settled in Leiston, Suffolk in 1924. Summerhill School was thus founded. Neill advocated personal freedom for his pupils, who were allowed to attend classes when they wanted. The pupils ran the school by a voting system and called their teachers by their first names—to them the founder was simply "Neill." He wrote several books on education and an autobiography.
Bibliography: Neill, A. S. 1972. *"Neill! Neill! Orange Peel!".*

NEMESIUS. A fourth-century Christian philosopher and bishop of Emesa, Syria. In his book, *On the Nature of Man* he allocated cogitation and reason to the middle ventricle of the brain, sensation to the anterior ventricle, and memory (q.v.) to the posterior ventricle. He vividly demonstrated how reason can be affected, while sensation and motion remain intact by asking a crowd outside his window which vessels brought in by a man should be thrown out. Nemesius threw out the indicated vessels and then asked if a workman in the room should also be thrown out. The crowd, thinking this a joke, said "yes," whereupon he threw the workman out. A follower of the theories of Galen (q.v.), he believed that the seat of grief is in the opening of the stomach (q.v.).
Bibliography: 1959. *Symposium: The history and philosophy of the brain and its functions.*

NEMINSKY, VLADIMIR PRAVDICH (1879-1952). A Russian physiologist. He was one of the pioneers of electroencephalography in Russia.
Bibliography: Brazier, M.A.B. 1971. Vladimir Pravdich Neminsky. *Spike Wave* 1: 17-22.

NENEK. A state of possesssion (q.v.) recognized by the Jale people of the Central Mountains of West Guinea. Those affected are usually young males. They are seized by tremor, run about erratically, and are incapable of rational communication. Treatment consists of sprinkling water on the patients and, if the patients are overly aggressive, physically restraining them.
Bibliography: Koch, K. F. 1968. On possession behavior in New Guinea. *J. of the Polinesian Society* 77: 135-48.

NEO-FREUDIANS. A term used to designate those psychopathologists who broke away from Freudian theories and stressed the importance of social influences. They were closer in their beliefs to the tenets of Alfred Adler (q.v.) than Sigmund Freud (q.v.).
Bibliography: Watson, R. I. 1963. *The great psychologists.*

NEPENTHES. An Egyptian drug mentioned in the *Odyssey* (q.v.). Helen of Troy added it to the wine given at a feast to relieve her guests of the sorrowful thoughts oppressing them. She was said to have learned the use of nepenthes from an Egyptian woman, Polydamma. The drug has been identified with opium (q.v.), although some people think it may have been cannabis indica (q.v.). The word is derived from Greek and means "no pain."

Bibliography: Simon, B., and Ducey, C. 1975. Ancient Greece and Rome. In *World history of psychiatry*, ed. J. G. Howells.

NERO CLAUDIUS CAESAR (A.D. 37-68). A Roman emperor. He was born feet first, which was considered a bad omen in Roman superstition. Both his mother, Agrippina the Younger (q.v.) and his father, Domitius, came from disturbed families in which insanity may have existed. The Roman historian Seutonius (fl. A.D. 119) reported that his father, when congratulated on the birth of a son, said, "Nothing can spring from Agrippina and myself but what is detestable, and an evil to the public." His father died when he was two years old, and he was adopted by the Emperor Claudius, whom he succeeded when Claudius was poisoned by Agrippina. She in turn was murdered by Nero's orders. As an adolescent he had been sensitive, cultured, and affectionate, but as an adult he was extremely cruel, extravagant, and vain. He was said to suffer attacks of epilepsy (q.v.). His behavior was dissipated and his mood oscillated between depression and mania (q.v.). He murdered Octavia, his first wife, and in a fit of temper he kicked to death his second wife Poppaea, who was pregnant at the time. A pyromaniac, he is said to have set Rome on fire and watched its destruction while reciting verses about the burning of Troy. He brought about the death of many people in his entourage, including Lucius Annaeus Seneca (q.v.). On hearing the news of an uprising against himself, he committed suicide (q.v.) on June 9, A.D. 68, the anniversary of his murder of Octavia, his first wife.

Bibliography: Grant, M. 1973. *Nero*.

NERVAL, GÉRARD DE (1808-1855). The pseudonym of the French writer and poet Gérard Labrunie. As an orphan, he spent most of his unhappy childhood with an uncle. He achieved early fame with his translation of Johann Wolfgang von Goethe's (q.v.) *Faust*. An inheritance allowed him to travel, but it only increased his restlessness. He became notorious for his dissipation and eccentricities, which included a tame lobster that he exercised in the streets. His many love affairs were superficial and disappointing. Increasing anxiety necessitated medical attention and finally admission to an asylum run by Dr. Etienne Blanche. Following Dr. Blanche's suggestion that he should write about his illness, he produced *Aurélia* (1855). One winter night he hanged himself from a lamppost, "asking as he went away: Why did I come?" In his delusion (q.v.) he thought that the apron string

with which he hanged himself, was the girdle of Madame de Maintenon
(1635-1719).
Bibliography: Rinsler, N. 1973. *Gérard de Nerval.*

NERVOUS SLEEP. A term used by James Braid (q.v.) to describe mes-
meric (*see* MESMERISM) trances.
Bibliography: Boring, E. G. 1950. *A history of experimental psychology.*

NESTORIANS. Followers of Nestorius (?-c.451), patriarch of Constan-
tinople (q.v.), and founder of a religious sect declared heretical in 451.
Following the declaration, Nestorius and his followers were persecuted.
Many of them dedicated themselves to the sick and became physicians of
great repute. Their knowledge of Greek brought the works of Hippocrates,
Aristotle, and Galen (qq.v.) to the Arabs and influenced the approach to
physical and mental disorders in Persia and Arabia (*see* ARABS).
Bibliography: Baker, B. 1908. *Nestorius and his teaching.*

NETTLES TREATMENT. Whipping with green nettles. It was prescribed
as a remedy for hysterical (*see* HYSTERIA) fits in women. Dr. Robert Waring
Darwin (1766-1848), the father of Charles Darwin (q.v.), was a firm believer
in this form of treatment.

NEUMANN, HEINRICH WILHELM (1814-1884). A German psychiatrist. He belonged to a school known as "romantic psychiatry," which
emphasized the psychogenesis of mental disorders, the symbolism of symptoms, and the usefulness of psychotherapy (q.v.). His approach to mental
illness was based on the principle that the patient and not the disorder needs
treatment. Neumann regarded classification as superfluous and believed that
the personality as a whole should be considered in diagnosis and treatment.
He asserted that anxiety resulted from frustrated drives and hysteria (q.v.)
from frustrated sexuality (q.v.). He believed life was a constant process of
destruction and reconstruction and that although the physician should treat
body and mind together, mental illnesses would be best treated by psychic
means. His work was not recognized immediately, but his views were revived with the advent of "moral medicine" (q.v.) and probably inspired
some of the theories of Sigmund Freud (q.v.).
Bibliography: Neumann, H. W. 1859. *Lehrbuch der Psychiatrie.*

NEURASTHENIA. A term and concept coined in 1869 by George M.
Beard (q.v.). The term described a syndrome that included pathological
fatigue and nervous exhaustion. It was discussed in a paper entitled "Neurasthenia or Nervous Exhaustion," which appeared in the *Boston Medical
and Surgical Journal.* According to Beard, neurasthenia was more prevalent
in America than anywhere else. Sigmund Freud (q.v.) became preoccupied

with neurasthenia, which he regarded as a sexual neurosis (q.v.) caused by masturbation (q.v.) and inhibited in men by seduction by women at an early age.
Bibliography: Chertok, L., and de Saussure, R. 1979. *The therapeutic revolution: from Mesmer to Freud.*

NEUROLOGY. The study of the nervous system. The term was coined in the seventeenth century by Thomas Willis (q.v.). In modern times, neurology has made its greatest advances during wars because of the opportunity they have provided for the study of gunshot wounds. In the United States, for example, neurology as a profession came into existence during the Civil War. The National Hospital for Nervous Diseases (q.v.), founded in London in 1859 with the name of National Hospital for the Relief of Paralysis, Epilepsy, and Allied Disorders was the first neurological center in the world.
Bibliography: Riese, W. 1959. *A history of neurology.*

NEUROPATHOLOGY. The study of pathological aspects of the nervous system. Neuropathology became established as an important branch of medicine in the eighteenth century through the work of William Cullen (q.v.).
Bibliography: Goldston, I. ed. 1967. *Historic derivations of modern psychiatry.*

NEUROPHYSIOLOGY. The study of the physiology of the nervous system. As a branch of medicine, it originated in the seventeenth century with the work of Francis Glisson (q.v.).
Bibliography: Zilboorg, G. 1941. *A history of medical psychology.*

NEUROSIS. A term derived from the Greek, meaning "disorder of neuron." It was first used by William Cullen (q.v.) in 1776 in his *Synopsis Nosologiae Methodical.* Under the title "neuroses" he proposed to include those diseases of the nervous system that had a somatic basis. Henry Maudsley (q.v.) used the term "neurosis" to indicate an altered nerve function that was linked to an altered mental function. Sigmund Freud (q.v.) used the term *Angstneurose,* or anxiety neurosis, which according to him, was a physiological disorder derived from physical sexual causes. The term now is used confusingly to indicate dysfunction of the psyche. Past terms used to cover more or less the same group of disorders include melancholia, hypochondria, hysteria, neurasthenia, and psychoneurosis (qq.v.).
Bibliography: Cope, Z. ed. 1957. *Sidelights on the history of medicine.*

NEURYPNOLOGY. A term invented by James Braid (q.v.) in 1842 to replace the term "mesmerism" (q.v.) from which he wished to disassociate himself. The prefix "neuro" was later dropped, leaving "hypnology," and its derivatives.

Bibliography: Chertok, L., and de Saussure, R. 1979. *The therapeutic revolution: from Mesmer to Freud.*

NÉVROSES DE L'HISTOIRE, LES. The title of a book by Lucien Nass published in Paris in 1908. It considers those personal neuroses which have had an impact on the course of world history.

Bibliography: Nass, L. 1908. *Les névroses de l'histoire.*

NEWCASTLE, AUSTRALIA. The first institute for idiots in Australia was established in Newcastle in 1878. It was housed in a former barracks.

Bibliography: Barr, M. W. 1904. *Mental defectives.*

NEWCASTLE LUNATIC ASYLUM. A mental hospital in Newcastle upon Tyne, England. It was first established in 1764 and could accommodate nineteen patients. In 1767 a new and larger building was provided for it, and it became known as the Pauper Hospital for Lunaticks for Newcastle, Northumberland, and Durham. It was said to be spacious and offer humane treatment. Its first physician in charge was Dr. John Hall (q.v.). By 1824 conditions had badly deteriorated, and extensive reforms and alterations were undertaken. The asylum then was renamed Bath Lane Asylum because it was in the same street as the public baths. It remained in use until 1856.

Bibliography: Le Gassicke, J. 1972. Early history of psychiatry in Newcastle-upon-Tyne. *Brit. J. Psychiat.* 120: 419-22.

NEW ENGLAND COLONIES LEGISLATION. The General Laws and Liberties of the Massachusetts Colony stated in 1641 that "Children, Idiots, Distracted Persons, and all that are strangers or new comers to our Plantation, shall have such allowances and dispensations in any case, whether Criminal or others, as Religion and Reason require."

Bibliography: 1648. Reprint. 1929. *The laws and liberties of Massachusetts.*

NEW ENGLAND SYSTEM. A custom originating in the northeastern United States in the seventeeth century. It consisted of auctioning the town's paupers to people who undertook to care for them at the lowest fee. As the town paid the fee for their care to the purchasers, the purchaser offering the lowest fee was successful. Paupers of both sexes and of all ages, even those physically or mentally ill, were publicly presented for auction. In some cases the town's authorities stipulated a certain standard of care, but often the successful purchaser was free to do what he liked with the paupers, who, in effect, were his slaves.

Bibliography: Deutsch, A. 1949. *The mentally ill in America.*

NEWGATE PRISON. A notorious prison in London. It was already in existence in the twelfth century. The worst criminals were sent there, but

it also held paupers and the insane. The appalling conditions there inspired Elizabeth Fry's (q.v.) efforts for prison reform. Overcrowding and lack of air and water often caused epidemics. Public executions were conducted at Newgate Prison and attracted a large public until 1868. Daniel Defoe (q.v.) was among its many famous prisoners. It was demolished in 1903.
Bibliography: Babington, A. 1971. *English Bastille: Newgate Gaol.*

NEW MOON, THE. The first British monthly periodical written and edited by mental patients. It was also one of the first journals to be published in an asylum. With the encouragement of the progressive Dr. William A. F. Browne (q.v.), it was begun in 1844 at the Crichton Royal Hospital (q.v.) in Dumfries, Scotland.
See also JOURNALS BY PATIENTS.

NEWNESS. A movement in New England in the second half of the nineteenth century. Its adherents were followers of an eccentric, a Mr. Alcott, a self-educated man. He was a vegetarian who further restricted his diet by eating only those vegetables that grew upward, for example, potatoes or radishes were banned because they grew down. He regarded daylight and clothing as damaging, so he exercised in the night, garbed in a single white vestment that caused him to be mistaken for a ghost. A cold winter brought about his conversion to a more traditional way of dress, and his followers disbanded.
Bibliography: Tuke, D. H. 1892. *A dictionary of psychological medicine.*

NEWTON, SIR ISAAC (1642-1727). An English mathematician and natural philosopher. He had an unsettled childhood; his father died before he was born, and his adored mother remarried and placed him in the care of his grandmother whom he disliked intensely. At the age of fourteen, after the death of his stepfather, he returned to live with his mother, whom he loved to the exclusion of all other women. He was an anxious and distrustful individual with a tendency to belittle himself and an abnormal dread of controversy. Various theories, including a fire in his house that destroyed most of his notes, rumors that his advancement was due to a beautiful and fond niece, exhaustion, and mercury (q.v.) poisoning, have been advanced to explain the serious mental illness he suffered in 1693. It was diagnosed as phrenitis (q.v.) and the symptoms included insomnia, loss of memory and paranoid delusions (q.v.) that led him to accuse his friends, John Locke (q.v.) and Samuel Pepys (q.v.) among them, of plotting against him. Newton influenced psychological thinking with a model of visual perception in which he stated colors were "sensations" related to elements of the psyche, rather than qualities of matter. He was one of the founding members of the Royal Society (q.v.) and later became its president. George Cheyne (q.v.) related that whenever Newton wished to stretch his mental faculties to the maximum, he would reduce his diet to a small quantity of bread and sack (wine) and water. The force of gravity, which he discovered, was believed by Franz Mesmer (q.v.) and his followers to be responsible for recurring diseases and epidemics.

Bibliography: Manuel, F. E. 1968. A portrait of Isaac Newton.

NEWTON, JAMES. A seventeenth-century London quack. Around 1674, he advertised (see ADVERTISING) himself as an "expert in madness and melancholy." He owned a private madhouse on Wood's Close, Clerkenwell Green, in the parish of St. James and promised to cure even the most obdurate cases of insanity. His establishment was taken over from the Newton family by William Battie (q.v.) in 1754 and in 1776 by John Monro (q.v.), who passed it to his son. It continued to be used as a private asylum until 1803.

Bibliography: Hunter, R., and Macalpine, I. 1963 *Three hundred years of psychiatry.*

NEW YORK CITY HALL. The residence of New York city administration. In 1971 archeologists digging in its grounds found fragments that confirmed the same site had been occupied by a lunatic asylum and house for vagrants in the eighteenth century. New York passed through a difficult phase in its civic life and the archeologists in writing of these findings to the mayor added, "If you sometimes feel that presiding over the city is like being broke and locked up in a madhouse, you are right."

Bibliography: *Daily Telegraph*, April 7, 1971.

NEW YORK EARLY ASYLUMS. The first record of an asylum in New York dates back to 1677 and refers to a one-man asylum (q.v.) built for a lunatic by the name of Peter Paull. The first institution built specifically for the insane came into existence in 1736. It was also used as a workhouse and a house of correction. The inmates were kept busy spinning, knitting, and sewing, unless they were so unruly that they required incarceration in special cells. In 1826 separate wards, known as insane pavilions, were reserved for mental patients at Bellevue Hospital, and in 1839 a city asylum was opened in Blackwell's Island in the East River. Charles Dickens (q.v.) inspected it during his visit to America in 1842 and reported unfavorably on the conditions he saw there.

Bibliography: Deutsch, A. 1949. *The mentally ill in America.*

NEW YORK STATE PSYCHIATRIC INSTITUTE AND HOSPITAL. A mental hospital in New York equipped with therapeutic, research, and teaching facilities. Legislation authorizing the city of New York to acquire land for the foundation of a psychopathic hospital dated back to 1904 when Dr. Adolf Meyer (q.v.) had been one of its promoters; but plans were shelved until 1929. The first director of the New York State Psychiatric Institute

and Hospital was Dr. George H. Kirby (1875-1935). The twenty-story building, overlooking the Hudson River, is one of the finest hospitals in the world.
Bibliography: Deutsch, A. 1949. *The Mentally Ill in America.*

NICHOLAS, SAINT (?-c.350). Patron saint of Russia, scholars, travelers, merchants, and children. As Saint Nicholas, or Santa Claus, he became associated with Christmas, first in Germany and later in other countries. Little is known of his life, but traditionally he has been identified with the bishop of Myra in Lycia, Asia Minor. He is said to have cared for the idiot (q.v.) and the imbecile (q.v.).
Bibliography: Meisen, K. 1931. *Nikolauskult und Nikolausbrauch in Abendland.*

NICHOLLS, FRANK (1699-1778). An English physician and anatomist, physician to George II (q.v.). In 1750 his Lumleian Lecture of 1748 was published under the title *De Anima Medica.* He believed that the state of mind of a feverish patient was linked to psychological forces.
Bibliography: Nicholls, F. 1750. *De anima medica*

NICHOLSON, MARGARET (c.1750-1828). An English domestic servant. In 1786 she attempted to stab George III (q.v.) with a blunt dessert knife. She suffered from the delusion (q.v.) that the Crown of England owed her property and asserted that she had no intention of killing the king, but merely was trying to attract attention to her cause. The king was unharmed, and his assailant was declared insane by Dr. Thomas Monro (q.v.). She was confined to Bethlem Royal Hospital (q.v.) for George III emphatically declared that she should not be punished.
Bibliography: Fisk, J. 1786. *The life and transactions of Margaret Nicholson.*

NICOLETTE. The heroine of *Aucassin and Nicolette,* an early thirteenth-century French romance in prose and verse. It contains a remarkable example of psychological healing in the episode of the sick pilgrim who lay near death but recovered when Nicolette approached his bed and lifted her gown and smock to bare her lovely body to his sight.
Bibliography: MacKinney, L. 1965. *Medical illustrations in medieval manuscripts.*

NIDER, JOHANNES (c.1380-1440). A German Dominican prior and professor of theology. He did not believe that witches (*see* WITCHCRAFT) could change themselves into animals and thought that visions were merely dreams (q.v.). In his book *Formicarius* (q.v.) he discussed theological, philosophical, and social issues, including superstitious practices and witchcraft.
Bibliography: Robbins, R. H. 1959. *The encyclopedia of witchcraft and demonology.*

NIETZSCHE, FRIEDRICH WILHELM (1844-1900). A German philosopher and writer. Following the death of his father, a Protestant minister, he was brought up in a household of women who overprotected and dominated him. He was an odd and solitary child. By the age of ten he had written over fifty poems and had given evidence of his genius (q.v.). In his youth he dramatically abandoned the Christian faith, shunned society, and went to live in solitude in the Swiss mountains. At the age of twenty-five he was appointed professor of classical philology at Basel, but increasing ill health forced him to resign after ten years. He suffered from severe insomnia and migraine (q.v.) and is said to have had as many as 118 attacks of migraine in a single year. In 1889, he was struck by general paralysis of the insane (q.v.). For the remainder of his life his sister cared for him in her house at Weimar. Much of his work is obscure and may have been the product of distorted thinking, caused by his mental illness. His most famous book, *Thus Spake Zarathustra* (1883-1891) is the story of a prophet, a projection of the author, and his utterances are expressions of his nihilistic doctrine, according to which "nothing is true" and science is "inimical to life and destructive." He wrote on resentment, repression, and sublimation and advocated the development of a superman who would be capable of realizing man's potentials to the full by disregarding morals. Nietzsche became a legend in his own lifetime, and his work has influenced many individuals; it was particularly exploited by nazism.

Bibliography: Hayman, R. 1980. *Nietzsche: a critical life.*

NIGHT ATTENDANT SERVICE. The night watch of patients who are mechanically restrained (*see* RESTRAINT). In the formalized institutional care of the mentally ill, there was no provision for supervision during the night until 1929. The patients were simply locked up in their cells and strapped in bed. In 1829 a patient's death at Lincoln Asylum (q.v.) during the night was caused by the harness that restrained him. This event led to the rule that night attendants should supervise patients who were mechanically restrained.

Bibliography: Deutsch, A. 1949. *The mentally ill in America.*

NIGHTINGALE, FLORENCE (1820-1910). A British philanthropist and reformer, born in Florence, Italy, and named by her mother after the place of her birth. She was the younger of two children of a wealthy family. Despite social conventions against her vocation, she trained as a nurse in Germany and Paris, and then returned to London where she was appointed superintendent of a nursing home. She felt that she had a mission in life, but was so shy and sensitive that her ambition was not to be noticed, despite her elegant and distinguished appearance. Nursing and medical practice in hospitals and on the battlefields were reformed by her reorganization and by providing professional training for nurses. In 1860 she founded the first training school for nurses at Saint Thomas' Hospital in London. Contrary to popular belief, she had a practical approach to her work and wrote "a woman who takes a sentimental view of Nursing (which she calls 'ministering,' as if she were an angel) is of course, worse than useless . . . ." She was also quick to realize the emotional influence of a nurse on her patients. She was a victim of poor health and for more than fifty years was confined to her room, communicating with people mostly by letters, even when the recipients were in the same house. She would consent to see no more than three or four persons a day, one at a time and for only a few minutes each. Her final years were increasingly stressful; she deteriorated mentally, was nearly blind, and expected death every day.

Bibliography: Woodham-Smith, C. 1950. *Florence Nightingale.*

NIGHTMARE. A horrible dream (q.v.), a night terror. In the Middle Ages (q.v.) it was believed that an incubus (q.v.) or succubus (q.v.) actually sat on the sleeper and caused him to have frightening dreams (see Plate 10). John Gerard (q.v.), in his herbal, published in 1597, recommended the seeds of peony (q.v.) against "the disease called the Night Mare, which is as though a heavy burthen were laid upon them and they oppressed therewith, as if they were overcome with their enemies or overprest with some great weight or burthen, . . ."

Bibliography: Oswald, I. 1968. Sleeping and dreaming. In *Modern perspectives in world psychiatry,* ed. J. G. Howells.

NIJINSKY, VASLAV (1890-1950). A Russian ballet dancer and choreographer. His talent was recognized throughout the world, but his style and nonclassical approach to ballet was controversial. Before marrying an Hungarian dancer, Romola de Pulszky, he had been closely associated with Sergei Diaghilev (1872-1929). At the beginning of World War I, as a Russian, he was interned in Hungary with orders to reside at the house of his parents-in-law with his wife and baby daughter. His in-laws were so antagonistic to him that he tried unsuccessfully to be transferred to a prisoner of war camp. Even the nurse engaged to breast-feed the baby disliked the couple and starved the baby. Nijinsky sent her away and assumed responsibility for the baby, bottle-feeding her and spending most of his time in her company. Eventually he was allowed to join the Russian Ballet company in the United States, but Diaghilev's old feelings for Nijinsky caused strife. Nijinsky and his family then found peace in Switzerland but for only a brief period that ended when he was found diagnosed as schizophrenic (*see* SCHIZOPHRENIA) by Eugen Bleuler (q.v.). Among those who were consulted about his state were Julius Wagner von Jauregg, Emil Kraepelin, Sandor Ferenczi, Sigmund Freud, and Carl G. Jung (qq.v.), as well as faith healers and fakirs (q.v.). When Diaghilev came to see him and asked him to dance

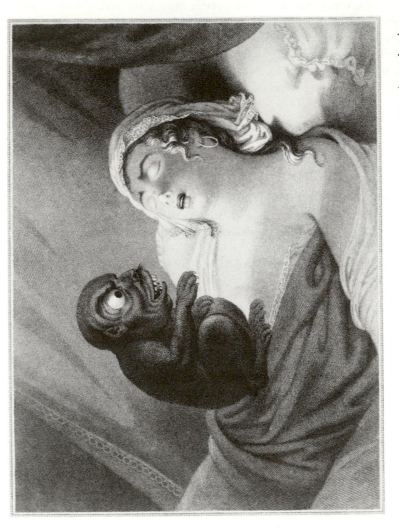

10. NIGHTMARE. An 1810 engraving by J. P. Simon showing a monster oppressing a sleeping woman and thus causing her to have terrible dreams. By courtesy of the Wellcome Trustees, Wellcome Institute for the History of Medicine, London.

again, he answered "I cannot, I am mad." He remained insane until his death.
Bibliography: Nijinsky, R. 1933. *Nijinsky.*

NILE ELECTRIC CATFISH. *See* MALOPTERURUS ELECTRICUS.

NIOBE. A legendary figure in Greek mythology (q.v.). She was said to be the wife of Amphion, king of Thebes. She had seven sons and seven daughters and boasted of her superiority to Leto, the goddess mother of Apollo (q.v.) and Artemis. To punish her, Leto sent her two children to destroy all Niobe's sons and daughters. Amphion committed suicide (q.v.) and Niobe, crying inconsolably, was turned into a weeping stone by Zeus (q.v.). She symbolizes grief.
Bibliography: Graves, R. 1960. *The Greek myths.*

NIOPO. The native name for snuff made from the seeds of the *Anadenanthera peregrina* tree. It is used by Indian tribes in Latin America to produce intoxication and hallucinations (q.v.). The snuff is made by roasting and powdering the seeds. Tribesmen going on a hunt use it to sharpen their senses and produce above normal alertness.
Bibliography: Emboden, W. 1972. *Narcotic plants.*

NIRVANA. A Buddhist concept. A state of mind devoid of passions and tranquil. Individuality is extinct, and the mind is absorbed in contemplation of God.
Bibliography: Stcherbatsky, T. 1927. *The conception of Buddhist nirvana.*

NISSL, FRANZ (1860-1919). A German neurologist. By introducing new methods of staining histiological preparations, he advanced the knowledge of the constituents of nerve cells. He devised a new classification of normal cells, and his work on pathological modifications greatly contributed to the understanding of some mental diseases, especially general paralysis of the insane (q.v.). He was a devoted worker, both in laboratory research and clinical practice but always retained his sense of humor and liking for practical jokes, as for example, pretending to be drunk to Kraepelin (q.v.), his chief, who was a strong antagonist of alcoholism.
Bibliography: Haymaker, W., and Schiller, F. 1970. *The founders of neurology.* 2d. ed.

N'JAYEI SOCIETY. An African secret tribal society of the Mende tribe in Sierra Leone. Like similar societies, it engages in ritualistic medicine that

functions through communal practices. It specializes in the treatment of mental disorders.
Bibliography: Lambo, T. A. 1975. Mid and West Africa. In *World history of psychiatry*, ed. J. G. Howells.

NOBEL, ALFRED BERNHARD (1833-1896). A Swedish philanthropist and the inventor of dynamite and other items. As a child he was often sick and suffered frequent seizures and violent spasms of vomiting. His mother, who slept in his room to look after him, encouraged his dependence on her. The intense relationship with his mother led to sexual difficulties for him in later life. Normal physical relationships with women were repugnant to him, and he never married. His brother once said that if the doctor who had attended his brother's birth had known how miserable his life was going to be, he would have mercifully killed him at his first breath. Nobel hated his own appearance and became a philanthropist as a compensation for the love he needed.
Bibliography: Halarz, N. 1959. *Nobel*.

NODDY. A term used to denote a person of poor intelligence. It may be derived from the verb "to nod," referring to the continuous head nodding of some idiots.
Bibliography: 1978. *Brewer's dictionary of phrase and fable*.

NOEGENETIC LAWS. Three qualitative laws, according to which the mind creates new mental content, enunciated by Charles E. Spearman (q.v.). The three laws relate to "apprehension of experience," "education of relations," and "education of correlates."
Bibliography: Spearman, C. 1923. *The nature of intelligence and the principles of cognition*.

NOGUCHI, HIDEYO (1876-1928). A Japanese bacteriologist. In 1913, with Joseph W. Moore (q.v.), he obtained a pure culture of the spirochete *Treponema pallidum* from the brain tissues of patients suffering from general paralysis of the insane (q.v.) and thus proved the link between this mental disorder and syphilis (q.v.).
Bibliography: Noguchi, H., and Moore, J. W. 1913. A demonstration of the treponema pallidum in the brain in cases of general paralysis. *J. Experimental Medicine* 17: 232-38.

NOIZET, F. J. (1792-1885). A French general and magnetist (*see* MAGNETISM). He emphasized the need for trust between the magnetist and his subject and believed that the effect of animal magnetism (q.v.) was a result of the action of the magnetist's vital fluid, impelled by his will, on the magnetized individual.

Bibliography: Noizet, F. J. 1854. *Mémoire sur le somnambulism et le magnétisme animal.*

NOLLEKENS, JOSEPH (1737-1823). An English sculptor. After studying in Rome, he returned to England and became the most fashionable sculptor of his day. His income was increased further by stock exchange speculations and the buying and selling of antiques. Despite his prosperity, he and his wife were incredibly miserly and devised numerous ways to minimize their household expenditures. They skimped on fuel, candles, and soap. Their house was cold and gloomy; daylight entered through broken panes of glass mended with putty; and their table crockery and cutlery consisted of a few odd items. Nollekens' clothes were little better than rags. On his death, he left a fortune in money, property, and paintings.

Bibliography: Smith, J. T. 1949. *Nollekens and his times.*

NOLLET, JEAN ANTOINE (1700-1770). A French abbé and physicist. In his work *Essai Sur l'Electricité des Corps,* published in Paris in 1765, he described the application of the lodestone in magnetic treatment and admonished that more research was needed to understand how magnetic electricity worked.

Bibliography: Tinterow, M. M. 1970. *Foundations of hypnosis: From Mesmer to Freud.*

NONINJURIOUS TORTURE. The term used by Johann C. Reil (q.v.) to describe a method of treatment for psychiatric disorders. It involved frightening and angering patients through realistic theatrical representations of cruel, morbid, and, in general, disturbing events. Sudden loud noises and unexpected plunges in water were also included in his psychological techniques. It was rationalized that the treatment acted on the patient's senses, which were either too dulled or overexcited. Reil published a description of these methods in 1803.

Bibliography: Reil, J. C. 1803. *Rhapsodien über die Anwendung der psychischen Curmethode auf Geisteszerrüttungen.*

NONNE, MAX (1861-1939). A German neurologist. In 1902 he wrote *Syphilis und Nervensystem* in which he stated his belief that progressive paralysis was not a specific syphilitic (*see* SYPHILIS) disease of the brain but played an important role in its production.

Bibliography: Haymaker, W., and Schiller, F. 1970. *The founders of neurology.* 2d. ed.

NONRESTRAINT MOVEMENT. The movement for the abolition of mechanical means of restraint (q.v.) in mental hospital. It spread throughout

Europe and the United States during the first half of the nineteenth century. The term was introduced by John Conolly (q.v.), one of the most enthusiastic exponents of nonrestraint; other medical men with the same aims were Vincenzo Chiarugi, Philippe Pinel, Jean Esquirol, William Tuke, and Robert Gardiner Hill (qq.v). Before becoming a generally accepted practice, nonrestraint generated a great deal of controversy. Isaac Ray (q.v.), for example, was among those who did not accept its doctrines. Its implementation was slow, and often leather implements or solitary confinement were merely substituted for chains and irons. Eventually moral medicine (q.v.) brought about a more humane approach to the management of the mentally ill.
Bibliography: Zilboorg, G. 1941. *A history of medical psychology.*

NONSENSE SYLLABLE. A syllable that conveys as little meaning as possible. The nonsense syllable, for example, zov or ciz, was invented in 1885 by Hermann Ebbinghaus (q.v.). He found that ordinary words were not suitable for his experiments on learning and memory (q.v.). Thus, he made a list of meaningless syllables that would not be familiar to his subjects, and would not evoke special associations.
Bibliography: Ebbinghaus, H. 1885. *Ueber das Geolächtnis.*

NORFOLK COUNTY ASYLUM. A mental hospital situated in Thorpe near Norwich in England. It is now known as Saint Andrew's Hospital. It is the oldest English county asylum (q.v.) still surviving. When it was first opened in 1814, it was managed by a lay "master."

NORRIS, WILLIAM (c.1760-1815). An insane American patient at Bethlem Royal Hospital (q.v.). In 1814, he was discovered incarcerated in a small, dark, and damp cell at Bethlem Hospital. He had been kept chained to the wall by iron rings to his hand, foot, and neck for at least ten years as punishment for threatening the apothecary and striking a keeper. He was freed but died shortly after his release. The case roused public feelings and led to an inquiry demanding the dismissal of Thomas Monro (q.v.) and John Haslam (q.v.).
Bibliography: Masters, A. 1977. *Bedlam.*

NORSE MYTHOLOGY. The old Icelandic sagas (*Åsatroen*) contain many examples of abnormal behavior, including anxiety and depression leading to suicide (q.v.), anger developing into uncontrollable rage necessitating physical restraint (q.v.), and disorders attributed to possession (q.v.). The term "berserk" (q.v.), literally meaning "clothed in bearskin," is derived from an old Norse term referring to warriors who were so carried away in the heat of the battle that they did not feel pain. Insanity and its symptoms and treatment are also mentioned in the sagas.

See also MYTHOLOGY.

Bibliography: Retterstøl, N. 1975. Scandinavia. In *World history of psychiatry*, ed. J. G. Howells.

NORTHAMPTON GENERAL LUNATIC ASYLUM. A mental hospital in England. It was opened in 1838 and was the first English hospital to practice nonrestraint from its inception. Its first medical superintendent was Thomas O. Prichard (q.v.). The poet John Clare (q.v.) was a patient there after his escape from Dr. Matthew Allen's (q.v.) private asylum.

NORTHCLIFFE, VISCOUNT. See HARMSWORTH, ALFRED .

NOSOGRAPHIE PHILOSOPHIQUE. A monumental work in three volumes by Philippe Pinel (q.v.). It was published in 1798. In it he classified mental disorders into mania (q.v.), melancholia (q.v.), dementia, and idiocy (*see* IDIOT).

Bibliography: Pinel, P. 1798. *Nosographie philosophique.*

NOSTALGIA. A term coined by Johannes Hofer in 1678 to describe an extreme longing for one's country. In the eighteenth and early nineteenth centuries, it was regarded as a mental disorder that could lead to melancholia (q.v.) and insanity. The British army recognized nostalgia as a disease and regarded it as serious enough to post home a soldier suffering from it. Robert Hamilton (1749-1830), an army doctor, described the symptoms in a young recruit in a paper entitled *History of a Remarkable Case of Nostalgia Affecting a Native of Wales, and Occuring in Britain.* Karl Jaspers (q.v.), writing in 1910, listed eighty-six references to nostalgia.

Bibliography: Editorial. 1976. Nostalgia: a vanished disease. *Brit. med. J.* 2: 857-58.

NOSTRADAMUS (or **MICHEL DE NOTREDAME,** or **NOSTRE-DAME) (1503-1566).** A French astrologer (*see* ASTROLOGY) and physician. He was believed to be able to predict the future, and his horoscopes were accepted as true. Catherine de Medici (1519-1589) invited him to her court, where he correctly prophesized the manner of death of her husband, Henry II (1519-1559) of France. Charles IX (1550-1611) appointed him physician-in-ordinary. His controversial book of prophecies, *Centuries*, published in 1555, was finally condemned by the pope in 1781.

Bibliography: Laver, J. 1942. *Nostradamus.*

NOUS. A Greek term used by Aristotle (q.v.) to indicate the highest element in man. It has been translated as "mind" or "intellect," but, more finely

defined, it would correspond to the capacity for actualizing pure form—the concept, rather than the particular object that can be perceived through the senses. According to Aristotle, *nous* survives the body and is immortal. The term is used colloquially to indicate possession of intellect.
Bibliography: Downey, G. 1965. *Aristotle.*

NUMBERS. Because medicine frequently was linked with astrology (q.v.), special attention was often paid to dates, lunar phases, months, and days of the week. Hippocrates (q.v.) devised a theory of crisis in sickness related to number. Galen (q.v.) contradicted this doctrine, which later was revived enthusiastically by Girolamo Cardano (q.v.), who strongly believed in the medical significance of numbers.
See also MEDICAL DAYS and MENSIS MEDICALIS.
Bibliography: Garrison, F. H. 1929. *An introduction to the history of medicine.*

NURSES. In the Middle Ages (q.v.) the care of the mentally ill usually was entrusted to religious orders. Although some orders specialized in this work, no special training was offered. The first training program for mental nurses was provided in France by Madame Louise de Marillac le Gras (q.v.) in her petites maisons (q.v.), institutions for the insane. Philippe Pinel (q.v.) also tried to organize a body of women known as the *Filles de service*, to look after discharged patients, but the venture lasted for only a few years. In England, William A. F. Browne (q.v.) organized formal lectures for nurses at the Crichton Royal Hospital (q.v.) in 1854. The first permanent training school for mental nurses in the United States was organized by Dr. Edward Cowles in 1882 at the McLean Asylum (q.v.). Dr. Cowles was also the first to use women nurses in male wards. The first official certificate in mental nursing was instituted in England in 1897 by the Medico-Psychological Association (q.v.).
Bibliography: Walk, A. 1961. The history of mental nursing. *J. Ment. Sci.* 107: 1-
17.

NUT. A slang expression for the head. It is also used to denote someone who is crazy or demented. Hence mental asylums (q.v.) were often referred to as "nut houses."
Bibliography: 1979. *Brewer's dictionary of phrase and fable.*

NUTMEG. *Myristica fragrans*, an evergreen aromatic tree. It is indigenous to the East, where its fruit is employed in the treatment of delirium tremens (q.v.) and insomnia. Arab physicians prescribed it as early as the seventh century A.D. Its hallucinogenic properties and the stupor it induces have been known since the Middle Ages (q.v.), but the first description of its effects written by a scientist occurred in 1576 in a work entitled *Plantarum*

seu Stiripium Historia by Matthias de l'Obel (c.1538-1616), botanist and physician to James I (q.v.).
Bibliography: Emboden, W. 1972. *Narcotic plants.*

NYMPHOMANIA. The exaggerated desire in women for sexual gratification. It was regarded as a sign of mental disorder. In the eighteenth century, M.D.T. de Bienville (q.v.) gave it the status of a syndrome, which served to emphasize the belief that female sexuality (q.v.) was abnormal. His book, entitled *La Nymphomanie ou Traité de la Fureur Utérine*, was published in 1771, and the term "uterine furor" took its place in the nosology of mental disorders.

NYMPHS. Semidivine maidens in Greek mythology (q.v.). They were believed to be able to possess (*see* POSSESSION) people and drive them mad. Those so affected were called *nympholeptos.*
Bibliography: Nilsson, M. P. 1940. *Greek folk religion.*

O

OAF. A term derived from the word "elf." Its meaning of "lout" or "idiot" (q.v.) is a reference to the old belief that a retarded child was a changeling (q.v.) who had been left in place of the baby stolen by the elves.
Bibliography: 1978. *Brewer's dictionary of phrase and fable.*

OATES, TITUS (1649-1705). A psychopathic (*see* PSYCHOPATHY) impostter, the son of an English Anabaptist pastor who had been accused of murder when a woman drowned while being baptized by him. Oates was an epileptic (*see* EPILEPSY) and was so repulsive looking that his mother thought he was an idiot (q.v.) and his father could not bear to have him near. He was expelled from his school and Cambridge University. Oates became notorious for his impostures and frauds. He invented the Popish Plot of 1678 and caused the deaths of many innocent Roman Catholics. Eventually his perjury was discovered, and in 1685 he was flogged and imprisoned. He regained his liberty and received a pension when William III (1650-1702) came to the throne in 1688.
Bibliography: Lane, J. 1949. *Titus Oates.*

OAT STRAW BATHS. An old Russian remedy for "calming the nerves." A pound of dry straw was boiled for twenty minutes, and the strained liquid added to a tub of water in which the patient bathed.
Bibliography: Kourennoff, P. M., and St. George, G. 1970. *Russian folk medicine.*

OBEAH. A West African term for a practice employed in witchcraft (q.v.) in which an object is put into the ground in the belief that it will bring ill luck, sickness, or even death to those for whom it was intended.
Bibliography: 1978. *Brewer's dictionary of phrase and fable.*

OBERSTEINER, HEINRICH (1847-1922). An Austrian neurologist. He was particularly interested in psychological research, experimentally induced epilepsy (q.v.) and psychosomatic disorders. He wrote extensively on the morphology of the nervous system and described his findings from personal observation. The Institute of Neurology at the University of Vienna was founded by him in 1882.

Bibliography: Haymaker, W., and Schiller, F. 1970. *The founders of neurology.* 2d. ed.

OBLIGING DREAMS. A term coined by Sigmund Freud (q.v.) in 1920. He used it in his paper *The Psychogenesis of a Case of Female Homosexuality.* According to him the content of such dreams (q.v.) represent the patient's infantile wish to please her father, and her adult wish to fool him, and displace her affection from father to therapist. In the dream the patient acts as if she were cured.

Bibliography: Freud, S. 1974. The psychogenesis of a case of female homosexuality (1920). *Standard edition.* Vol. 18. ed. J. Strachey.

OBLOMOVSHTCHINA. A Russian word describing a state of severe abulia (q.v.). It is derived from the name of Oblomov, the principal character in the novel *Oblomov* (1858) by the Russian writer Ivan Goncharov (q.v.). Complete idleness and passivity was not uncommon in the wealthy landowners of czarist Russia; an extreme example was the Wolf Man (q.v.).

Bibliography: Goncharov, I. 1858. *Oblomov.*

OBREGIA, ALEXANDRU (1860-1937). A Rumanian psychiatrist. He originally specialized in histology and spent ten years as a professor of histology before becoming a professor of psychiatry. He was an organizer, teacher, and founder of institutions, among which the most important was the Bucharest Central Hospital for Mental and Nervous Disorders (q.v.). His research focused on alcoholism (q.v.) and periodical manic-depressive psychoses (q.v.) for which he coined the term "cyclophrenia" (q.v.). He was the first to use suboccipital puncture for the analysis of the cerebrospinal fluid.

Bibliography: Predescu, V., and Christodorescu, D. 1975. Rumania. In *World history of psychiatry*, ed. J. G. Howells.

OBSESSION. An uncontrollable desire to dwell on a thought or perform a particular act. The term, in this sense, was first used by Benedict Augustin Morel (q.v.) in 1861.

Bibliography: Laughlin, H. P. 1967. *The neuroses.*

OCCLEVE or HOCCLEVE, THOMAS (c.1368-?1437). A minor English poet. His works contain descriptions of madness and melancholia (q.v.) expressed in terms of the medical knowledge of the time and the religious attitudes toward mental disorders. His portraits of madmen, melancholics, and diseased sinners are so vivid and detailed that it has been assumed that he was describing his own symptomatology. A *Complaint* (c. 1421) and a *Dialogue to a Friend* (c. 1422) appear to be autobiographical descriptions of his nervous breakdown. Biographical material is also found in the long preface to his *De Regimen Principum* (*On the Government of Princes*). (c.1411-12).

Bibliography: Doob, P.B.R. 1974. *Nebuchadnezzar's children: conventions of madness in Middle English literature.*

OCCUPATIONAL THERAPY. The clinical prescription of activities to keep the patient occupied in body and mind. References to occupational therapy can be found as far back as the Ebers papyrus (q.v.), which mentions that treatment in the asylums for the mentally ill in the Egyptian temples of Saturn (q.v.) included various forms of recreation and occupation. The Greeks and the Romans also recognized the usefulness of occupying the mind in cases of depression. Both Avicenna (q.v.) and Rhazes (q.v.) recommended occupational therapy, and, at later periods, Constantine the African (q.v.) and Bartholomaeus Anglicus (q.v.), among many other early medical writers, urged some form of activity. Organized occupational therapy began in the early nineteenth century following a course parallel with the development of moral medicine (q.v.). Philippe Pinel (q.v.) noted in his *Treatise on Insanity* (1801) that the patients at Bicêtre (q.v.) "were supplied by the tradesmen of Paris with employments which fixed their attention." Jean Esquirol (q.v.) firmly believed in keeping mental patients busy and implemented occupational therapy at the Salpêtrière (q.v.). Another famous early example of organized occupational therapy is the regime instituted by the mental hospital of Aversa (q.v.) near Naples, Italy. In the 1820s the patients there were employed in farming (q.v.), cloth manufacturing, printing, and translating. In the twentieth century occupational therapy has been systematized and recognized as a profession.

OD (or ODYLIC FORCE). A force alleged to permeate the universe. It is said to manifest itself as colored rays or marked changes in temperature, but only very sensitive people are said to be able to discern these manifestations.

Bibliography: Drewer, J. 1952. *A dictionary of psychology.*

ODOR OF THE INSANE. George Man Burrows (q.v.) believed that mania (q.v.) was characterized by a peculiar odor, which, once recognized, could be regarded as a sure sign of the disease, even if there were no other proof of it. He compared it to the scent of henbane (q.v.) in a state of fermentation but added that he knew of nothing that resembles it.

Bibliography: Burrows, G. M. 1828. *Commentaries on insanity.*

ODYSSEY. An epic poem by Homer (q.v.) probably written in the eighth century B.C. Covering ten years in the life of Odysseus, it describes many psychological situations. Emotional disorders are understood to be caused by adverse emotional stimuli, and dreams (q.v.) are given special significance. Nepenthes (q.v.), an herbal drug, is mentioned as a pain reliever, but most often counseling and prayers are employed to alleviate mental anguish. Those medical practitioners mentioned in the *Odyssey* are judged successful by the fame that has preceeded them and the memory that has followed their visits, both powerful psychological elements.

Bibliography: *The Odyssey*, trans. A. Cook.

OEDIPUS. According to the Greek myth, the son of Laius, king of Thebes, and his wife Jocasta (q.v.). An oracle (q.v.) had predicted that Laius would be killed by his son. To avoid the prophecy coming true, Laius ordered that his son should be exposed on a mountain. But the shepherd who took Oedipus to the mountain pitied the baby and gave him to the childless Polybus, king of Corinth. In adolescence, Oedipus was told also by the oracle that he would kill his father and marry his mother. Horrified, he left Polybus whom he believed to be his father. As he journeyed toward Thebes, he met his real father on the way, slew him in a quarrel, and, as a prize for solving the Sphinx's riddle, was given Jocasta as a wife. Guilt stricken when he realized the truth, he blinded himself, and Jocasta committed suicide (q.v.). From this legend Sigmund Freud (q.v.) derived the expression "Oedipus complex," in which children in late infancy are said to form a sexual attachment to the parent of the opposite sex — usually the love of a son for his mother. The essential difference between legend and Freud's concept is the fact that Oedipus had no knowledge of the identity of his parents, while the manifestations of infantile sexuality are supposed to occur in children who are aware of their relationships with their parents.

See also ELECTRA.

Bibliography: Freud, S. 1930. *Three contributions to the theory of sex*, trans. A. A. Brill.

O FACTOR. A factor put forward by Charles E. Spearman (q.v.). He suggested that each individual manifests an "oscillation" of ability from one moment to another. Although this oscillation varies from person to person, it is present in most activities.

See also G FACTOR, P FACTOR, and W FACTOR.

Bibliography: Spearman, C. E. 1927. *Abilities of man, their nature and measurement*.

OFHUYS, GASPAR (1456-1523). A Flemish monk. As well as being an *infirmarius* who cared for sick brethren, he was also the chronicler of his monastery, the Roode Clooster. In his writings he mentioned the case of Hugo van der Goes (q.v.), who was taken ill with frenzy of the brain and

recovered after he had repented of his sins. The description of the illness provides an account of fifteenth-century ideas about mental disorders.
Bibliography: Rosen, G. 1968, *Madness in society*.

OHIO HOSPITAL FOR EPILEPTICS. The first American institution dedicated exclusively to epileptics (*see* EPILEPSY). It was opened in 1893 at Gallipolis, Ohio. It was planned on the cottage system (q.v.) and originally was known as the Asylum for Epileptics and Epileptics Insane.
Bibliography: Deutsch, A. 1949. *The mentally ill in America*.

OHIO STATE ASYLUM FOR THE INSANE. An American institution, established in 1835 at Columbus. It was built entirely with funds provided by the state, and its administration was also in the hands of the state. Its first superintendent was William M. Awl (q.v.), who had provided the impetus for its foundation.
Bibliography: Deutsch, A. 1949. *The mentally ill in America*.

OKEY, ELIZABETH AND JANE. Two epileptic (*see* EPILEPSY) sisters. They were patients of John Elliotson (q.v.), who used them in public demonstrations of magnetism (q.v.). They claimed they were able to predict the outcome of disease and approaching death and believed that their clairvoyance (q.v.) allowed them to prescribe for their own ailments. Elliotson allowed Elizabeth to be tested by Thomas Wakley (1795-1862), the founder and editor of *The Lancet*. Wakley decided that the "magnetization" claimed by Elliotson was self-suggestion.
Bibliography: Thornton, E. M. 1976. *Hypnotism, hysteria, and epilepsy: an historical synthesis*.

OKNOS. The personification of delay and hesitancy appearing in Greek legend. He was said to be continuously occupied in making a straw rope, but the labor was made futile by an ass eating the rope as fast as he could twine it. Sometimes he was pictured as busily loading the ass with sticks that continuously fell off the animal's back.
Bibliography: Harvey, P. 1959. *The Oxford companion to classical literature*.

OLDENBURG, HENRY (c.1617-1677). A German philosopher. His first interest was in theology and the classics, but he later turned to science and medicine through travel and contact with famous contemporary men in those fields. He was a great admirer of Baruch Spinoza (q.v.). He became the secretary of the Royal Society (q.v.) of London and edited twelve volumes of its *Philosophical Transactions* (1664-1666). To disseminate knowledge

among those of similar interest, he evolved the scientific article. Until then, information had been disseminated in the form of letters.
Bibliography: 1900. *The dictionary of national biography.* 2nd ed.

OLD NORTHAMPTON MANOR HOUSE. A building in London, in the Clerkenwell area, once belonging to the earls of Northampton. In the latter part of the seventeenth century it was used as a private madhouse by Dr. James Newton (q.v.), a self-proclaimed expert in madness and melancholia (q.v.). It remained in his family until 1754, when it was taken over by Dr. William Battie (q.v.). On the death of Battie it was bought by John Monro (q.v.). His son Thomas Monro (q.v.) was the last to use it as a madhouse. It closed in 1803, and the building was converted into a boarding school.
Bibliography: Storer, J., Storer, H. S., and Cromwell, T. 1828. *History and description of the parish of Clerkenwell.*

OLEUM CEPHALICUM. An ointment prepared by a London quack, Thomas Fallowes (q.v.). It was used in the treatment of lunacy. The patient's head was shaved, and the ointment, a vesicant, was rubbed into the scalp until blisters appeared. The blisters were said to allow the noxious black vapors responsible for madness to escape.
Bibliography: Hunter, R., and Macalpine, I. 1963. *Three hundred years of psychiatry.*

OLIVER, CHARLES AUGUSTUS (1853-1911). An American ophthalmologist. He discovered the ocular symptoms of mongolism (q.v.), and described them in 1891. He also wrote *The Correlation Theory of Color Perception* and *Ophthalmic Methods in Recognition of Nerve Disease.*
Bibliography: Oliver, C. A. 1891. A clinical study of the ocular symptoms found in the so-called Mongolian type of idiocy. *Transactions of the Amer. Ophthalmol. Soc.* 6: 140-48.

OLOLIUQUI. Small seeds obtained from the snake vine used by the Aztecs to produce hallucinations (q.v.). In the sixteenth century, the Spanish conquistadors became concerned about ololiuqui, for they believed that those who used them were communicating with the devil. Their efforts to eradicate the practice met with little success, and the Aztec priests continued to use them in their ceremonies. To this day Mexican folk healers practicing curanderismo (q.v.) prepare a concoction from the seeds to obtain hallucinations that will reveal the nature of ailments and give them clairvoyant powers. Ololiuqui have been found to contain lysergic acid diethylamide (q.v.).
Bibliography: Emboden, W. 1972. *Narcotic plants.*

ONANISM. A term derived from the Bible (q.v.). It is used incorrectly as a synonym for masturbation (q.v.). Correctly used it refers to *coitus inter-*

ruptus: "And Onan knew that the seed should not be his; and it came to pass, when he went in unto his brother's wife, that he spilled it on the ground, lest that he should give seed to his brother" (Gen. 38: 9).

O'NEILL, EUGENE GLADSTONE (1888-1953). An American playwright, the son of a famous Irish-American actor; the family was continuously on the move and his birth occurred in a New York hotel. After spending a year at Princeton University, he roamed the world, gold hunting, working as a sailor, and spending time around the docks of New York. At twenty he married his first wife, but he never lived with her and did not meet his son until the boy was twelve years old. At twenty-three he tried to commit suicide (q.v.). In 1912 he contracted tuberculosis (q.v.), and it was in a sanatorium that he began to write plays. After his release, he spent a year at Harvard University studying with George Pierce Baker (1866-1935). Despair, illness, and alcohol coupled with his first-hand experience of low life gave a particular poignancy and realism to his plays. He remarried, had two children, was divorced, and married for a third time. His writing became a compulsion, and his plays became so long that it was impossible to produce them; *Mourning Becomes Electra* had thirteen acts. At thirty-seven, after being treated for alcoholism by a New York psychoanalyst, Dr. Gilbert V. Hamilton, O'Neill gave up drinking completely. He remained restless, superstitious, and unhappy. His brother died of alcoholism, his first son became an alcoholic and committed suicide, his second son became a drug addict, and his only daughter, Oona, married Charlie Chaplin (1889-1977) against his wishes. She was never reconciled with her father. The tremor that began to afflict him in adolescence advanced to the point when he could write no longer. The disorder was never properly diagnosed during his life, but an autopsy revealed that it was due to a cerebellar degeneration. O'Neill died of pneumonia, in Boston; his death, like his birth, occurred in the anonymity of an hotel room. His finest play *Long Day's Journey Into Night*, produced posthumously in 1956, is biographical and depicts the stormy life of his family.
Bibliography: Gelb, A., and Gelb, B. 1960. *O'Neill.*

ONYX. A gem. In the Middle Ages (q.v.) it was believed to bring sorrow and bad dreams (q.v.). Those who wore it were said to become irritable and quarrelsome.
See also PRECIOUS STONES.
Bibliography: Evans, J. 1922. *Magical jewels.*

OPAL, THE. An American periodical paper by and for mental patients. It was founded in 1850 at Utica state hospital (q.v.). It was written, edited, and printed in the institution and obtained wide recognition. It ceased publication in 1861, after most of the patients involved in its production were discharged.

See also JOURNALS BY PATIENTS.

Bibliography: Deutsch, A. 1949. *The mentally ill in America.*

OPERA. In a number of operas a character, usually a woman, loses her reason. Gaetano Donizetti (q.v.), who died insane, explored insanity in many of his operas: there are "mad scenes" in *Maria Padilla, Lucia di Lammermoor, Anna Bolena, Linda di Chamounix,* and *Torquato Tasso* (qq.v.). Vincenzo Bellini (1802-1835) introduced madness in *I Puritani* and *Il Pirata* (qq.v.). Some other instances are *Hamlet* by Ambroise Thomas (1811-1896), *Elektra* by Richard Strauss (1864-1949), *La Gioconda* (q.v.) Amilcare Ponchielli (1834-1886), *The Rake's Progress* by Igor Stravinsky (1882-1971), *Ruddigore* (q.v.) by Arthur Sullivan (1842-1900), *Mazeppa* (q.v.) by Peter Tchaikovsky (q.v.), and *Erwartung* (q.v.) by Arnold Schoenberg (1874-1951).

Bibliography: Rosenthal, H., and Warrack, J. 1964. *Concise Oxford dictionary of opera.*

OPERATIONISM. Linked with the ideas of Ernst Mach (q.v.). Operationism took its source from physics and philosophy and emerged in the 1930s. In 1944 the *Psychological Review* (q.v.) conducted a symposium on operationism; one of the six participants, Burrhus F. Skinner (1904–), defined it "as the practice of talking about (1) one's observations; (2) the manipulative and calculational processes involved in making them; (3) the logical and mathematical steps which intervene between earlier and later statements; and (4) nothing else."

Bibliography: Skinner, B. F. 1945. Symposium on operationism, 1944. *Psychological Rev.* 52: 241-94.

OPICINUS DE CANISTRIS (fl.1296-1350). An Italian cleric with a talent for drawing and some knowledge of medicine. When he became ill during a period of emotional stress, he began to record dreams (q.v.), visions, and obsessional (*see* OBSESSION) thoughts in a series of drawings that amount to a pictorial autobiography. These drawings show his obsession with creating a system of the universe. They are overcrowded with minute and disorderly details. The religious community in which he lived tolerated his derangement; Opicinus, himself, believed he was a victim of divine possession and never mentioned insanity in his notes.

Bibliography: Kris, E. 1953. *Psychoanalytic explorations in art.*

OPIUM. A white sticky juice exuded by the seedpods of the opium poppy as soon as the petals fall. If it is not collected within ten days, this complex chemical is broken down by the plant's own chemistry. Early references to

the plant of joy, the opium poppy, can be found in Summarian tablets more than 4000 years old. The Assyrians and the Babylonians considered opium an aphrodisiac. From the early Egyptians, until the end of the nineteenth century, it was given to babies to make them sleep (*see* QUIETNESS). The ancient Greeks also knew of the poppy and celebrated its narcotic properties by linking it to Thanatos, god of death, Nyx, goddess of night, Hypnos (q.v.), god of sleep, and Morpheus (q.v.), god of dreams (q.v.). Miraculous temple cures owed much to the use of the poppy. Hippocrates (q.v.) advised that a wine should be made of it and used medicinally. Most of the Greek and Roman medical writers mentioned the poppy, either praising its properties or suggesting caution in its use. The Romans employed opium to poison their enemies and to commit suicide (q.v.). Hannibal (q.v.) wore a hollow ring in which the opium that he used to commit suicide was secreted. Galen (q.v.) found it invaluable in the treatment of many disorders, including melancholia (q.v.). Avicenna (q.v.) recommended opium enthusiastically. It is said that he died of a mixture of opium and wine. Opium was introduced to the East and to the West by the Arabs. The Chinese were converted to smoking it, especially after the emperor Tsung Cheng made tobacco smoking illegal in 1644. Paracelsus (q.v.) is said to have been addicted to opium, which he carried in the hollow pommel of his sword. Honoré Balzac (q.v.), in one of his plays, included morphine (q.v.), a derivative of opium, in the devil's list of the causes for overpopulation in hell. In various forms, opium has claimed many addicts among the famous as well as the unknown, including Thomas de Quincey, George Crabbe, and Samuel Coleridge (qq.v.).
Bibliography: Scott, J. M. 1969. *The white poppy: a history of opium.*

OPORINUS (1507-1568). The Latin name adopted by Johann Herbst. He was a Swiss professor of Latin and Greek, one-time secretary to Paracelsus (q.v.), and a printer. After losing faith in Paracelsus and trying teaching, he became a printer of scholarly books. Andreas Vesalius' (q.v.) *Fabrica* was beautifully printed by him, and he printed *De Praestigiis Daemonum* (q.v.) by Johann Weyer (q.v.).
Bibliography: Pachter, H. M. 1951. *Paracelsus.*

OPPENHEIM, HERMANN (1858-1919). A German neurologist. His work on traumatic neuroses (*see* NEUROSIS), published in 1889, suggested that psychic disorders following trauma were caused by molecular changes in the brain. He went on to theorize that the neurosis was then perpetuated by the changes in the psyche. This theory was opposed by Jean Martin Charcot (q.v.) and others. Oppenheim also wrote on brain surgery and syphilitic (*see* SYPHILIS) diseases of the brain. *Amyotonia congenita* was described by him and is now known as Oppenheim's disease.
Bibliography: Oppenheim, H. 1894. *Lehrbuch der Nervenkrankheiten.*

OPPENHEIMER, FRANZ (1864-1943). A German sociologist. He was a champion of liberal socialism and regarded society as an organism in a state of normality when justice was observed. In his opinion, value judgments about structures in a society were possible if they were compared with norms defined by history, sociology, and psychology. He was the author of several books.

Bibliography: Oppenheimer, F. 1922-1929. *System der Soziology.*

ORACLES. The answer given by a god and spoken through a priest who asked a question on behalf of a worshipper. Oracles are linked with prophecy and can be found throughout history. They often have been associated with temples of healing in which the sick seek treatment guidance. The strong element of suggestion involved in oracular practices sometimes is aided by drugs in the form of herbal drinks that cause intoxication and hallucinations (q.v.). In many ancient cultures, for example Egypt, Greece and Rome, the affairs of the state were regulated by the official oracle's prophesies, and no important decision was taken without consulting him. In more recent times, the government of Tibet consulted its state oracle. The oracle was a monk, who, in a state of deep trance, uttered answers to the questions posed to him by the consulting cabinet minister. The ceremony took place in the Nechung Monastery, in an atmosphere of mystery and gloom that was increased by eerie music. A god was believed to speak through the mouth of the possessed (*see* POSSESSION) monk. If the policy of these answers constantly was opposed to that of the government, the oracle was liable to be replaced.

See also DELPHI and PYTHIA.

Bibliography: Hall, A., and King, F. 1978. *Mysteries of prediction.*

ORCHIS. *Orchis maculata*, a flowering tuberous plant found in damp ground. In Turkey, Arabia and Persia the roots are dried in the sun and made into a flour that is mixed with honey, milk, and hot water. The mixture is said to cure nervous disorders, tremors, and nightmares (q.v.).

Bibliography: de Bairacli Levy, J. 1974. *The illustrated herbal handbook.*

ORDER OF SERAPHIM, THE. In Sweden a religious order that had charge of the hospitals until 1876. The mentally ill also came under its care.

Bibliography: Retterstøl, N. 1975. Scandinavia. In *World history of psychiatry*, ed. J. G. Howells.

ORENDA. (Iroquois). A term from the Iroquois Indian religion. It conveys the idea that certain objects are sacred and have special powers, including the power to bring sickness or health.

Bibliography: Drever, J. 1956. *A dictionary of psychology.*

ORESTES. In Greek mythology (q.v.), the son of Agamemnon and Clytemnestra (q.v.). During her husband's absence, his mother lived with Ae-

gisthus. On Agamemnon's return the two murdered him. Orestes, persuaded by his sister Electra (q.v.), murdered his mother and was driven mad by the avenging Furies (q.v.). There are two accounts of his cure. One claims that after taking refuge in the temple of Athena in Athens he was acquitted by the court of Areopagus and recovered. The other claims his recovery occurred after stealing the statue of Artemis from Taurus. In psychiatry, the Orestes complex is a son's wish to murder his mother.
Bibliography: Hammond, N.G.L., and Scullard, H. H., eds. 1973. *The Oxford classical dictionary.*

ORGANISMIC THEORY. A theory of personality developed by Kurt Goldstein (q.v.). It stresses the need for an holistic and phenomenological approach to the study of personality and asserts that the individual must be investigated in his or her totality.
Bibliography: Misiak, H., and Sexton, V. S. 1966. *History of psychology.*

ORGANS. In many cultures throughout history, certain organs have been associated with personality characteristics and have been regarded as the center of various emotions. The heart (q.v.) has been given particular significance as the seat of the soul and has been associated with the capacity to love. The liver (q.v.) was associated with courage and lust; a small or poorly functioning liver was blamed for cowardice. The spleen (q.v.) was believed responsible for spite, anger, and rage. Shakespeare's plays offer many examples of this belief in the relationship between organs and feelings: "My knight, I will inflame thy noble liver, And make thee rage." (Henry IV, Part 2, V, v); "I have no spleen against you." (Henry VIII, II iv); etc.
See also BRAIN, CONCEPTS OF and STOMACH.

ORGONE THERAPY (VEGETOTHERAPY). A therapeutic approach developed by Wilhelm Reich (q.v.). It involved the dissipation of sexual tensions by the attainment of a full orgasm. Reich believed that there was a connection between sexuality (q.v.), anxiety, and the vegetative system.
Bibliography: Reich, W. 1942. *The discovery of the orgone.*

ORIBASIUS (c.323-403). A Byzantine physician. He compiled medical writings based on the works of Aristotle, Asclepiades, and Soranus (qq.v.) and wrote on melancholia (q.v.) in Galenic terms. Galen (q.v.) was so much his model that he was termed "the ape of Galen."
Bibliography: Temkin, O. 1973. *Galenism.*

ORIGEN (186?-?254). A Christian writer and teacher, born in Alexandria (q.v.). His asceticism was pathological. Fearing that his chastity was in danger, he castrated himself.
Bibliography: Fedden, H. R. 1938. *Suicide*.

ORILLIA, ONTARIO. The site of the first institution for the feebleminded in Canada. It was founded in 1876.
Bibliography: Barr, M. W. 1904. *Mental defectives*.

ORLANDO FURIOSO. A poem by the Italian poet Ludovico Ariosto (1474-1533), first published in 1516. Orlando, a knight of Charlemagne, loses his sanity through unrequited love for Angelica and runs naked through the woods destroying all he meets on his path. Eventually he returns to the camp and is cured of his madness when his friend Astalfo journeys to the moon and brings back his wits.
Bibliography: Ariosto, L. *Orlando Furioso*, trans. J. Harrington, and ed. R. Gottfried.

ORMUZD (*or* AHURA MAZDA). The Persian god of goodness and cre-ator of the world. According to the myth he assigned medicine to a special angel, Thraetona, who, was therefore, regarded by the Persians as the orig-inal physician.
Bibliography: Elgood, C. 1951. *A medical history of Persia and the Eastern caliphate*.

ORPHAN COMPLEX. A feeling of inferiority found in individuals who have lost their parents early in life. It is prominent in Japan, where there is a traditional prejudice against orphans. It is believed that because of their parental deprivation, the consequent lack of supervision in their upbringing, and their own insecurity, they are not reliable. Many employers will not accept orphans, who frequently grow up with the feeling, not wholly un-justified, that they are discriminated against and persecuted.
Bibliography: Iga, M., and Yamamoto, J. 1973. The chrysanthemum versus the sword in suicide. *Life Threatening Behavior* 3: 198-212.

ORPHEUS. In Greek legend, the son of the muse Calliope and Apollo (q.v.). He was said to play the lyre so well that even rocks and rivers were moved, and dragons were lulled to sleep by his song. When his beloved wife Eurydice died, he tried to rescue her from the infernal regions, but failed. In his grief, he would not respond to the advances of the Thracian women, who, enraged, tore him to pieces. His followers were associated with sorcery, magic (q.v.), and mysterious practices. Orphicism developed

as a religion in the sixth century B.C. It believed in the transmigration of the soul and retribution in another life.
Bibliography: Guthrie, W. K. C. 1952. *Orpheus and Greek religion.*

ORTA, GARCIA DA (fl. 1563). A sixteenth-century Portuguese physician who emigrated to India to escape the Inquisition (q.v.). In 1563 he wrote a book in Portuguese that described the properties of cannabis indica (q.v.) and opium (q.v.). He noted that the Indian opium-eaters could remain lucid after ingesting large quantities of opium and that it relieved mental and physical sufferings. The author added that he did not experiment personally with these drugs.
Bibliography: Orta, Garcia da. 1574. *Aromatum et simplicium aliquot medicamentorum apud Indos nascentium historia.*

ORWELL, GEORGE (1903-1950). The pseudonym of the British novelist Eric Arthur Blair. Educated at Eton, he served in the Indian Police in Burma, experienced a period of poverty, fought in the Spanish Civil War, and used his varied experiences as a basis for his writing. Ill with tuberculosis (q.v.) and completely disillusioned, be became identified with despair and honesty. He felt that the world was moving toward fear, hatred, and unrelieved cruelty, and refused to mask with platitudes his inexorable political pessimism and his disgust with what he called "centralised economy." "Power," he wrote, "is in inflicting pain and humiliation. Power is in tearing human minds to pieces and putting them together again in new shapes of your own choosing." In his novel *Nineteen Eighty-Four* he pictured the horrors and perversions brought about by totalitarianism.
Bibliography: Woodcock, G. 1966. *Crystal spirit: a study of George Orwell.*

OSA-KAFFIRS. A primitive society in South Africa. In it a tribesman may assume the role of witch doctor only after falling into a trance, often accompanied by convulsions, during which it is revealed to him that he has been chosen by the deities.
Bibliography: Alexander, F. G., and Selesnick, S. T. 1966. *The history of psychiatry.*

OSCILLATION. Vibration. Plato (q.v.) wrote that "all bodies are benefited by shakings, and motion by swings. . . ." Celsus (q.v.) advocated movement, such as the motion of a ship, a litter, a carriage, or the suspension of the bed to relieve mental disorders. It was still prescribed in the nineteenth century, but it fell into disrepute after the death of a patient at the Charité (q.v.) in Berlin.
Bibliography: Whitwell, J. R. 1946. *Analecta psychiatrica.*

O'SHAUGHNESSY, SIR WILLIAM BROOKE (1809-1889). A British physician and surgeon in the Bengal army. Although he is better remembered

for his introduction of the electric telegraph in India, he was also the first physician to undertake clinical tests with cannabis sativa (q.v.), which he regarded as the most effective agent in the treatment of convulsions, delirium tremens (q.v.), chronic rheumatism, hydrophobia, cholera, and tetanus. He discussed his findings in a book entitled *On the Preparations of the Indian Hemp or Gunjah (Cannabis Indica)* which was published in the 1840s.
Bibliography: 1842. *Bengal dispensatory.*

OSKAR DIETHELM HISTORICAL LIBRARY. An extensive collection of works on the history of psychiatry and the behavioral sciences. It is located in the New York Hospital, a part of Cornell University Medical College in New York. The collection was originally part of the library of the department of psychiatry but became a separate library in 1953. It was named after its founder, Dr. Oskar Diethelm, on his retirement in 1962.
Bibliography: Annual Report. 1978. *Friends of the Oskar Diethelm Historical Library.*

OSLER, SIR WILLIAM (1849-1919). A Canadian-born physician, medical historian, and teacher, equally well known in the United States and Great Britain. He was the first professor of medicine at the newly founded Johns Hopkins University and later became Regius Professor of medicine at Oxford University. It was thought that he lacked sympathy for patients suffering from mental disorders, but in fact he supported the founding of the Henry Phipps Psychiatric Clinic (q.v.) at Johns Hopkins. He bequeathed his magnificent collection of more than 7,500 books to McGill University.
Bibliography: Belt, W. R. 1952. *Osler.*

OSORIO, MIGUEL ANGEL. *See* BARBA-JACOB,PORFIRIO.

OSPEDALE DEI PAZZERELLI. An Italian institution established in Turin in 1727 by Vittorio Amedeo II (1666-1732), king of Piedmont. It was dedicated to the care of the mentally ill and supervised by laymen. *Pazzerelli*, the diminutive of *pazzi* (the insane), reflects the paternalistic attitude towards those in need of protection.
Bibliography: Mora, G. 1975. Italy. In *World history of psychiatry*, ed. J. G. Howells.

OSPIZIO DI SAN LAZZARO. An Italian institution situated in Reggio Emilia. In 1754 Francesco III d'Este (1698-1780) proclaimed that it would be used exclusively for the care of the mentally ill.
Bibliography: Mora, G. 1975. Italy. In *World history of psychiatry*, ed. J. G. Howells.

OTHELLO. The hero of the play *Othello* by William Shakespeare (q.v.). He is the prototype of the jealous man who is destroyed by his own anxiety,

which is fanned by his enemies. The term "Othello syndrome" refers to morbid jealousy (q.v.).
Bibliography: Mowat, R. R. 1966. *Morbid jealousy and murder.*

OTHO, MARCUS SALVIUS (c. A.D. 31-69). A Roman emperor for a few months. He was incompetent and led a dissolute life. After his defeat by the generals of Aulus Vitellius, (A.D. 15-69), he committed suicide (q.v.). His widow, Poppaea Sabina (A.D. 65), married Nero (q.v.).
Bibliography: Suetonius, *The twelve Caesars*, trans. R. Graves.

OTIS GROUP INTELLIGENCE SCALE. A pioneer intelligence test (q.v.) devised by the American psychologist A. S. Otis and first published in 1918. It was developed for the use of the United States Army at the beginning of World War I but found wider uses in schools and industry. It has been reprinted many times and is still used in schools.
See also ALPHA TESTS and BETA TESTS.
Bibliography: Misiak, H., and Sexton, V. S. 1966. *History of psychology.*

OTTO I (1848-1916). A king of Bavaria and the younger brother of Ludwig II (q.v.). Even as a child his behavior had given rise to anxiety. In 1870 Ludwig had hoped to abdicate in his favor, but Otto was already displaying marked symptoms of instability. He was often depressed and given to fits of weeping accompanied by pathological fears. His behavior in public became scandalous, and in 1875 he was declared insane and deprived of his liberty. Ludwig, who was to follow the same course to insanity, visited his brother regularly until the strain became too great. He was the only one who could calm Otto's violent outbursts. On Ludwig's death in 1886, Otto became nominal king of Bavaria until 1913, when his cousin, Ludwig III (1845-1921) assumed the crown.
Bibliography: Blunt, W. 1970. *The dream king: Ludwig II of Bavaria.*

OUIJA BOARD. A board with letters and numbers and a planchette (q.v.). It is used by mediums (q.v.) who purport to receive messages from the spirits of the dead through it.
Bibliography: Pearsall, R. 1972. *The table-rappers.*

OUTPATIENT DEPARTMENTS IN MENTAL HOSPITALS. The first outpatient department for the mentally ill in the United States was opened in 1885 at the Pennsylvania Hospital (q.v.) in Philadelphia. Hoping to prevent more serious disorders, it offered free treatment to those suffering from "incipient mental disease." In England the establishment of outpatient departments for the mentally ill had been suggested as early as 1868. Around

1890 the first outpatient departments were opened at Saint Thomas' Hospital in London, and at the Wakefield Asylum (q.v.).
Bibliography: Deutsch, A. 1949. *The mentally ill in America.* Hunter, R., and Macalpine, I. 1963. *Three hundred years of psychiatry.*

OVARIOTOMY. The surgical removal of the ovaries. In the nineteenth century, it was often performed on hysterical (*see* HYSTERIA) patients. Jean Martin Charcot (q.v.) was primarily responsible for this practice as he promoted the belief in the sexual aspect of hysteria.
Bibliography: Charcot, J. M. 1887-1888. *Leçons sur les maladies sur le système nerveux.* Vol 1.

OVID (PUBLIUS OVIDIUS NASO) (43 B.C.-c. A.D. 17). A Latin poet. He was born into a rich family and studied and practiced law before dedicating himself to poetry. His life was gay, licentious, and often offensive to the Roman authorities, who eventually exiled him. His *Ars Amatoria* and *Remedia Amoris* deal with sexual problems, and many of his works show particular insight into human nature. He was aware of the dangers of isolation and warned "beware of solitude and of lonely places." Aware of the sensibility of the unbalanced he wrote, "A sick mind cannot endure harshness."
Bibliography: Frankel, H. 1945. *Ovid, a poet between two worlds.*

OVINUS HIBERNUS. The name given by Carolus Linnaeus (q.v.) to a "wild," or feral child (q.v.) discovered among sheep in Ireland.
See also FERAL CHILD.
Bibliography: Barr, M. W. 1904. *Mental defectives.*

OWEN, ROBERT (1771-1858). A British social reformer. He believed that the environment is important in the formation of character. He rose from humble origins to the position of cotton mill manager at the age of nineteen. In 1800 he founded an industrial community at New Lanark, Scotland, that provided good housing and schools for the families of cotton mill workers. Similar villages were established in many other places after his experiment attracted the interest of European sociologists. He was the first to institute schools for infants. The Factory Act of 1819, which he ardently advocated, improved the conditions of the workers. After many years of enthusiastic preaching for reforms, at the age of eighty-two, he became a fervent spiritualist (*see* SPIRITUALISM).
Bibliography: Cole, M. 1953. *Robert Owen of New Lanark.*

P

PACCHIONI, ANTONIO (1665-1726). An Italian anatomist. He described the clusters on the surface of the dura mater that are formed by small arachnoid elevations (Pacchionian bodies). He wrongly believed that the depressions produced on the inner surface of the cranium were lymph-producing glands. He wrote about his findings in 1705.
Bibliography: Garrison, F. H. 1929. *An introduction to the history of medicine.*

PACIFICK MEDICINES. The eighteenth-century equivalent of tranquilizers. Under this term Sir Richard Blackmore (q.v.) listed opium (q.v.). In his *A Treatise of the Spleen and Vapours* (1725), he wrote that it "calms and sooths the Disorders and Perturbations of the animal Spirits. . . ."
Bibliography: Hunter, R., and Macalpine, I. 1963. *Three hundred years of psychiatry.*

PACKARD, E.P.W. An American woman. In 1860 she was admitted as a patient to the state insane asylum in Jacksonville, Illinois. She was kept there until 1893, when she finally succeeded in proving that she had been wrongly committed by her husband, a Presbyterian minister. She then sued the medical superintendent of the hospital, Dr. McFarland, who was forced to resign because of the publicity given to the case. Mrs. Packard was a forceful woman, who proceeded to write about her experiences in a melodramatic and sentimental way in her book *The Prisoners' Hidden Life; or Insane Asylums Unveiled* (1868). Her sensational allegations aroused public feeling and eventually led to the enactment of a state law designed to protect people from being declared insane wrongly. It ruled that individuals could not be committed without a trial by jury. The legislation was opposed by the psychiatric profession because it left diagnosis in the hands of laymen.
Bibliography: Grob, G. N. 1973. *Mental institutions in America.*

PACKING. A method used in the past for treating the insane. The patient was wrapped in sheets saturated with water to which mustard was often

added. He was then left packed for some time. It was a variation of the baths (q.v.) therapy.
Bibliography: Tuke, D. H. 1892. *A dictionary of psychological medicine.*

PADDED ROOM. A small room lined with rubber and cork. It was invented by Ferdinand Autenrieth (q.v.), a German professor. Violent mental patients were confined to it until their fury was spent. By the nineteenth century most asylums (q.v.) had a padded room, which was an improvement on the more severe forms of restraint (q.v.) previously used.
Bibliography: Burrows, G. M. 1828. *Commentaries on insanity.*

PALACE IN THE VALLEY. The euphemistic term by which the inhabitants of the Kip Valley near Greenock, Scotland, referred to the Smithson Poor Law Institute and Parochial Asylum, a mental hospital built in 1876 to replace an older institution. During World War II it became the "Niobe" and was used for the sailors of the Canadian navy as a shore establishment, but it returned to its original purpose after the war and was named Ravenscraig Hospital.

PALMA DE MALLORCA (MAJORCA). A general hospital was built in Mallorca in 1456. The Spaniards of this period believed that an increase in luxury, ambition, and vanity had contributed to a corresponding increase in sickness of the soul, therefore the new hospital contained a section for mental patients. Its pleasant and comfortable surroundings were a part of the treatment.
Bibliography: Chamberlain, A. S. 1966. Early mental hospitals in Spain. *Am. J. Psychiat.* 123: 143-49.

PALMISTRY. *See* CHIROMANCY.

PAN. In Greek mythology (q.v.) the pastoral god of fertility. He was believed to make flocks and herds fertile and wandered the countryside playing the syrinx, his own special pipes that at night raised frightening echoes. He startled those who came upon him suddenly and was said to make cattle bolt in terror. The word "panic" is derived from his name.
Bibliography: 1978. *Brewer's dictionary of phrase and fable.*

PANACEA. In Greek mythology (q.v.) the name of the daughter of Aesculapius (q.v.), the god of medicine. The term came to be applied to any medicine that cures all. In the Middle Ages (q.v.) those dabbling in alchemy (q.v.) searched for a substance that would cure all things and make man invulnerable to all ills.
Bibliography: 1978. *Brewer's dictionary of phrase and fable.*

PANNENBORG, H. J. *and* W. A. Two German brothers. In the early part of the twentieth century, they put forward the hypothesis that creative personalities fell into certain typological groups. For example, according to them, sculptors were serious men who were reliable despite their natural reserve, while painters were less reliable and more likely to be discontented with their environment.

Bibliography: Pannenborg, H. J., and W. A. 1917. Die Psychologie des Zeichners und Malers. *Zeitschrift für angewandte Psychologie* 12: 230-75.

PANNETIER, ODETTE. A French journalist. By pretending to seek treatment she managed to interview Sigmund Freud (q.v.) in 1936, when, because of ill health and old age, he had ceased to grant interviews to journalists. Despite her reputation for sarcastic comments, she showed Freud as a friendly and good-humored individual.

Bibliography: Pannetier, Odette. 1936. Appointment in Vienna. *The living age* 351: 138-44.

PAPEZ, JAMES WENCESLAUS (1883-1958). An American neurologist and professor of anatomy at Cornell University, in Ithaca, New York. His studies on the importance of the hippocampus and its significance in the mechanism of emotion were valuable contributions to the field of neurology (q.v.) and neuropathology. To his many scientific papers he added a volume of poetry entitled *Fragments of Verse*, published in 1957.

Bibliography: Haymaker, W., and Schiller, F. 1970. *The founders of neurology*. 2d. ed.

PAPPENHEIM, BERTA. *See* ANNA O.

PARACELSUS, PHILIPPUS AUREOLUS (1493?-1541). The pseudonym proclaiming superiority to Celsus (q.v.) assumed by Theophrastus Bombastus von Hohenheim, a Swiss physician. He was a colorful, turbulent, and imaginative man whose progressive ideas often were rejected because of his fanciful and wild statements. He regarded man as a microcosm of the universe, and believed each organ paralleled a planet. According to him, life was directed by a pervading principle that he called the *archeus* (q.v.). He threw the canon of Avicenna (q.v.) on a bonfire, condemned Aristotle (q.v.), and put forward theories that his contemporaries found strange. His temper and impetuosity caused him much trouble. He became professor of medicine at Basel but had to leave. He then spent many years wandering in poverty, full of bitterness, but still unrepentent and scornful of those physicians who adhered to the old teachings. He wrote and lectured in the vernacular rather than in the accepted Latin, which shocked the medical profession. His many books include one on mental disorders which was published posthumously in 1567 and entitled *Diseases that Deprive Man of His Reason*. He rejected the beliefs of the demonologists and stated that mental disorders were caused by excesses of heat (q.v.) or cold (q.v.), which could be regulated by scarify-

ing the patient's fingertips or drilling small holes in his skull. Poisons, the moon (q.v.), and heredity were also listed by him as causes of madness, which he believed arose from the brain, the seat of reason. He regarded the heart as the seat of the soul. He advised some harsh treatments for the insane but asserted with much insight that spiritual diseases called for spiritual remedies, counseling, and suggestion. He called Saint Vitus' dance (q.v.) "chorea lasciva" (q.v.), thus linking hysteria (q.v.) with sexual disorders, a concept that was not accepted until four hundred years later under Sigmund Freud (q.v.). Like his father, Paracelsus was also an alchemist (*see* ALCHEMY) and compounded his medical remedies from strange mineral substances.
Bibliography: Hargrave, J. 1951. *The life and soul of Paracelsus.*

PARADIS, MARIA THERESA VON (1758?-?). The daughter of a wealthy Austrian civil servant. She had been blind from early childhood, but, despite her disability, she was a gifted musician. Her patron was the Empress Maria Thérèsa (1717-1780) of Austria, who paid for her musical education. At the age of eighteen Paradis became a patient of Franz Mesmer (q.v.), who treated her by magnetism (q.v.). He claimed to have cured her blindness, but both the court physician and the ophthalmologist who examined her could not agree that there was any improvement in her condition. Mesmer's anger and abuse of his detractors caused such a scandal that he was forced to leave Vienna.
Bibliography: Franke, L. A. 1876. *Maria Theresa von Paradis.*

PARAKEETS. Small, long-tailed parrots. In the 1960s, when the island of Cyprus was divided by hostility between the Greek and Turkish communities, the raising of these birds became a mass hobby for the Cypriot Turks. The birds became a symbol of freedom, and the excessive importance given to them acted as a psychological safety valve.
Bibliography: Volkan, V. D. 1972. The birds of Cyprus. *Am. J. Psychother.* 26: 378-83.

PARALYTIC INSANITY. *See* INSANITY, PARALYTIC.

PARANOIA. A term derived from the Greek meaning "folly," or "madness." Hippocrates (q.v.) used the term in his classification to denote an illness characterized by mental deterioration. In 1764 Rudolph August Vogel introduced the term to indicate *morbus mentis* in general into medicine. In the sense of a specific psychosis (q.v.), paranoia was used for the first time in 1863 by Karl Kahlbaum (q.v.) and in 1883 by a New York neurologist, Edward Charles Spitzka (q.v.). Prior to Kahlbaum, Johann Christian Heinroth (q.v.) had given a description of paranoid states in 1818, but had used the term *Verrüchtheit* to describe them. Other German clinicians of the same

period studied the phenomenology of paranoia in detail and caused it to be included in classifications of mental disorders as a separate disease entity.
Bibliography: Retterstøl, N. 1966. *Paranoid and paranoiac psychoses.*

PARAPATHY. Wilhelm Stekel (q.v.) used this term in his book *Parapathie und Phimose* in 1931 to describe disordered emotions. He objected to the term "neurosis" (q.v.) because he felt that it emphasized the functions of the nervous system.
Bibliography: Sketel, W. 1931. *Parapathy und Phimose.*

PARAPHRENIA. A term used to refer to a group of psychoses (*see* PSY-CHOSIS) marked by delusions (q.v.). Joseph Guislain (q.v.) originally defined it as "folly." Emil Kraepelin (q.v.) included paraphrenia in his 1912 classification, but the term had been suggested some years previously by Karl Kahlbaum (q.v.). Sigmund Freud (q.v.) used it in reference to schizophrenia (q.v.) or dementia praecox (q.v.).
Bibliography: Henderson, D. K., and Gillespie, R. D. 1950. *A textbook of psychiatry.* 5th ed.

PARAPHRONSYNIAS. A term under which François de Sauvages (q.v.), in 1771, classified those mental disorders characterized by ecstasy (q.v.) leading to false perceptions. John B. Erhard (q.v.) used the same term in his classification.
Bibliography: Zilboorg, G. 1941. *A history of medical psychology.*

PARAPRAXIS. An erroneous performance caused by unconscious conflict. In 1901, Sigmund Freud (q.v.) investigated disorders connected with parapraxis, which gave rise to the expression "Freudian slip" referring to the same phenomena.
Bibliography: Freud, S. 1901. *The psychopathology of everyday life.*

PARCHAPPE, J.B.M. (1800-1866). A French physician. He was opposed to psychology and considered the psychological manifestations in mental disorders secondary to physical lesions of the brain. According to him, a satisfactory psychiatric classification should be based on physical findings. He introduced the term "paralytic insanity" to describe general paralysis of the insane (q.v.), which he associated with softening of the cortex of both hemispheres. He based his findings on the postmortem examinations of 322 cases of the disease.
Bibliography: Parchappe, J.B.M. 1838. *Recherches sur l'encephale.*

PARDOUX, BARTHOLOMY (1545-1611). A French physician. He believed that the functions of the body could be affected by emotion. In his book *De Morbis Animi,* published in Paris in 1639, he discussed the pathology of love (q.v.). He believed that an excessive desire for sexual intercourse could affect the brain and cause madness and thought that nymphomania (q.v.) could be caused by a hot climate, wine, spicy food, an overly leisurely life, and over stimulation of the imagination (q.v.) by books and plays, when these stimuli were associated to a bilious constitution and moist humors. He advised a cooling diet (q.v.) that included cold drinks and cold baths (q.v.), purging (q.v.), bleeding (q.v.), and, for women, pious reading. He advised patients suffering from love-sickness to possess the loved one, whenever possible. If this was impractical, he suggested that the patient should be treated as a "melancholicus," kept busy and diverted, given religious advice, and starved and beaten. Other suggested treatments included travel (q.v.), purging, enemas, bleeding and sedatives. He thought that vilification of the loved one and/or presenting a new and more beautiful subject for affection could be therapeutic.

Bibliography: Rather, L. J. 1965. *Mind and body in eighteenth-century medicine.*

PARÉ, AMBROISE (c.1510-1590). A French barber-surgeon. He became the first advocate of experimental methods in medicine. His pleasant personality and his manual and verbal skills attracted many admirers and followers, who were fascinated by his operations and his autopsies. Although he is considered the father of modern surgery, the scientific side of his personality was at variance with his belief in witchcraft (q.v.) and his intolerance of those accused of practicing it. He believed in demoniac possession (q.v.) and took it into consideration in diagnosis. He also employed music therapy (q.v.) after surgical operations, maintaining that it improved the rate of healing.

Bibliography: Hamby, W. B. 1967. *Ambroise Paré.*

PARGETER, WILLIAM (1760-1810). An English physician and naval chaplain. In 1792 he wrote a book entitled *Observations on Maniacal Disorders* in which he asserted that the classification of mental disorders was not as important as the management of the mentally ill. He emphasized the need for rapport between physician and patient; the latter's attention was to be engaged by catching his eye; gaining the patient's confidence would lead to better management without need of physical restraint (q.v.) or "stupifying liquor." His observations were so insightful that it has been suggested that they were based upon personal experience of mental disorder.

Bibliography: Leigh, D. 1961. *The historical development of British psychiatry.*

PARHON, C. I. (1874-1969). A Rumanian psychiatrist. He was the first holder of the chair of neurology and psychiatry at the University of Iasi. He studied and later worked with Georges Marinescu (q.v.). In 1909 in collaboration with M. Goldstein he published what is believed to be the first treatise of endocrinology. In it he theorized that certain psychiatric disorders had an endocrinological aetiology. He founded a psychiatric society in Iasi.

Bibliography: Predescu, V., and Christodorescu, D. 1975. Rumania. In *World history of psychiatry*, ed. J. G. Howells.

PÂRIS, FRANÇOIS DE (1690-1727). A French Jansenist theologian, better known as Diacre Paris. After his death, his followers continued to meet. As they gathered around his tomb in the Saint Médard Cemetery in Paris, scenes of mass hysteria (q.v.) leading to convulsions developed (see Plate 11). Those affected were called *convulsionaires* and were often the victims of severe beatings by unsympathetic onlookers.

Bibliography: Pelicier, Y. 1975. France. In *World history of psychiatry*, ed. J. G. Howells.

PARKINSON, JAMES (1755-1824). A British physician, surgeon, and paleontologist. He studied under John Hunter (q.v.). In his *Essay on the Shaking Palsy*, published in 1817, he gave the first description of a type of paralysis that is now known as Parkinson's disease. In his work *Medical Admonitions to Families* he discussed with insight on hysterical (*see* HYSTERIA) affections, stating that they were usually symptomatic of other disorders. Hypochondria (q.v.) received a similar sympathetic explanation. In 1811 he wrote a progressive volume on the management of the insane, entitled *Observations on the Act for Regulating Madhouses*. He was not popular with the British government as he often attacked it in pamphlets published under the pseudonym of "Old Hubert." He voiced the grievances of the people with such revolutionary fervor that he was brought before the Privy Council on the unlikely charge that he had plotted to assassinate George III (q.v.) with a poisoned dart. He escaped prison, but his writings became mellower.

Bibliography: Critchley, M., ed. 1955. *James Parkinson, 1755-1824*.

PARMIGIANINO (GIROLAMO FRANCESCO MARIA MAZZOLA) (1503-1540). An Italian painter who provides a clear example of neurotic obsession (q.v.). Giorgio Vasari (1511-1574) described how Parmigianino neglected his work when he became obsessed with alchemy (q.v.). Vasari wrote:

In the end, having his mind still set on his alchemy, Parmigianino, like so many others, grew quite crazy. He changed from a fastidious and gentle person into an almost savage and unrecognizable man with a long beard and unkempt hair. Being so reduced and having grown melancholic and eccentric, he fell a prey to a severe fever and a cruel flux, which in a few days caused him to pass to a better life. And in this way he found relief from the torments of this world, which he never knew

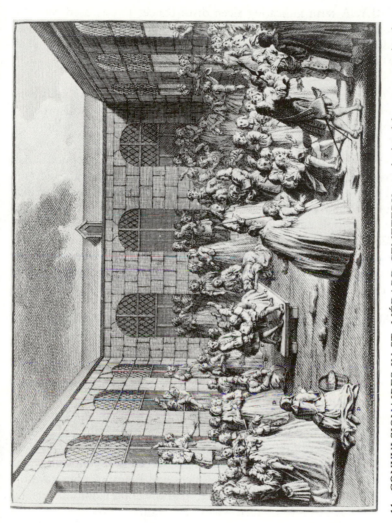

11. CONVULSIONAIRES IN ST. MÉDARD CEMETERY, as depicted by an engraving by Bernard Picard for *Histoire générale des ceremonies*, Paris, 1741. This shows the mass hysteria of the convulsionaires around the tomb of *Francois de Paris*. By courtesy of the Wellcome Trustees, Wellcome Institute for the History of Medicine, London.

but as a place full of troubles and cares. He was buried naked, as he had directed, with a cross of cypress wood upright on his chest.

Bibliography: Vasari, G. 1963. *Lives of the most eminent painters, sculptors and architects*, trans. W. Gaunt.

PARONIRIA. A term indicating sleep disturbance. It was used by John Mason Good (q.v.) in his classification of mental disorders. He placed it as a sub-division under the class Neurotica.

See also ALUSIA, APHLEXIA, ECPHRONIA, and EMPATHEMA.

PARSLEY. An herb related to the carrot. Russian folk healers used concoctions of parsley as remedies for epilepsy (q.v.) and nervous disorders.

Bibliography: Kourennoff, P., and St. George, G. 1970. *Russian folk medicine*.

PARSONS, ELIZABETH (1749-1807). The daughter of the deputy parish clerk of Saint Sepulchre in London. When she was eleven years old, she convinced people that a ghost existed in her house by producing mysterious noises. She attracted a great deal of attention and was visited by a number of fashionable people, including the Duke of York and Horace Walpole (1717-1797). Eventually her fraud was detected, and Samuel Johnson (q.v.) published a paper in the *Gentlemen's Magazine* describing the investigations into the imposture, thus putting an end to the mass suggestibility that she had generated. William Hogarth (q.v.) ridiculed the episode in a plate entitled *Credulity, Superstition and Fanaticism*.

Bibliography: Mackay, C. 1973. *Selections from extraordinary popular delusions and the madness of crowds*.

PASCAL, BLAISE (1623-1662). A French writer, philosopher, and mathematician. When he was a year old he became involved in an accusation of witchcraft. His illness at that time was said to have been caused by a spell cast by a woman whose case his father, a lawyer, had refused. She was forced to confess and agreed to transfer the spell to a cat. She prescribed a poultice, made from nine leaves of three plants and gathered before sunset by a seven-year-old child, to be applied on the abdomen at seven in the morning. The treatment brought no immediate improvement and Pascal's father gave the woman a beating, whereupon she promised that the child would be well by midnight. He was. His mother died when he was three years old and when he was seven, his father gave up his occupation to devote himself completely to the education of his two daughters and Blaise, his only surviving son. The program for his education was carefully drawn. The curriculum covered every branch of knowledge; reason, judgment, and evaluation of facts were the principles on which the teaching was based. Pascal was so precocious that he finished his father's program and begged for more advanced teaching. He remained detached from all people, isolated and lonely because of his

superior intellect. He contested the views of René Descartes (q.v.) on human reason because he believed that man's intelligence was not capable of solving metaphysical problems. He was greatly influenced by the Jansenists, a body of religious thinkers who opposed the Jesuits. His famous *Pensées* included the following: "Men are so necessarily mad, that not to be mad would amount to another form of madness."
Bibliography: Mortimer, E. 1959. *Blaise Pascal.*

PASSIFLORA. A climbing herb better known as the passion flower because the flower resembles the instruments of the crucifixion. The juice of its leaves and flowers has been used as a sedative by herbalists.
Bibliography: Thomson, W.A.F., ed. 1978. *Healing plants.*

PATCH. A term that has come to denote a fool (q.v.). It is probably derived from Sexton (fl. 1520), the jester of Thomas Wolsey (q.v.), who was called "patch" from the Italian *pazzo*, meaning "fool." It is also possible that the term is derived from the patches on the dress worn by licensed fools in the sixteenth century.
Bibliography: 1978. *Brewer's dictionary of phrase and fable.*

PATHICS. A term derived from the Greek word *pathos*, meaning "disease." It was used by Caelius Aurelianus (q.v.) in referring to homosexual men. Although homosexuality (q.v.) was seldom discussed in Roman medical texts, Caelius Aurelianus and Soranus (q.v.) described effeminate men and their sexual practices. They regarded homosexuality as "an affliction of a diseased mind" and thought it to be incurable.
Bibliography: Veith, I. 1964. The infancy of psychiatry. *Bull Menninger Clinic* 28: 189-97.

PATHONEUROSES. A term used by Sandor Ferenczi (q.v.) to indicate psychological reactions occurring in physical diseases. These later were known as psychosomatic disorders.
Bibliography: Hallos, S., and Ferenczi, S. 1925. *Psychoanalysis and the psychic disorder of general paresis*, trans. Barnes and Keil.

PAUL, SAINT (c.A.D. 67). Originally known as Saul of Tarsus, one of the Apostles, born at Tarsus in Cilicia. He actively supported the persecution of the Christians until he was converted by a vision on the road to Damascus. His hallucinations (q.v.) have been attributed to a discharging lesion on the occipital cortex. He was said to suffer from bouts of severe depression.
Bibliography: Pollock, J. C. 1969. *The Apostle: A life of Paul.*

PAUL I (1754-1801). An emperor of Russia, and the son of Peter III (q.v.) and Catherine the Great (q.v.). His mother disliked him intensely and it is possible that his real father was one of Catherine's many lovers. He was ugly, a weakling, unintelligent, fickle, and given to violent outbursts of rage, during which he gave vent to terrible cruelty. He had an obsessional (*see* OBSESSION) interest in military drill, uniforms, and petty regulations. His intolerable behavior led to a palace rebellion, and he was strangled by his own principal officials.

Bibliography: Ireland, W. W. 1885. *The blot upon the brain: Studies in history and psychology.*

PAUL OF AEGINA (625-690). A Greek physician of great repute, especially in the areas of surgery and obstetrics. Like his contemporaries, he was not an innovator but followed the teachings of Galen (q.v.). He suggested that hysteria (q.v.) should be treated by ligature of the limbs and mania (q.v.) by tying the patient to a mattress placed within a wicker basket and suspended from the ceiling. He also recommended baths (q.v.), wine, special diets (q.v.), and sedatives for the mentally ill. He described the following mental disorders: phrenitis (q.v.), which he felt was caused by inflammation of the brain meninges; delirium (q.v.), arising from the stomach (q.v.); lethargus; melancholia (q.v.); mania; incubus (q.v.); lycanthropy (q.v.); and epilepsy (q.v.). It was Paul of Aegina who gave the first known description of lead poisoning in his *De Re Medica*.

Bibliography: Adams, F. 1844-1847. *The seven books of Paulus Aegenita.*

PAUSANIAS (?-c.470 B.C.). A Spartan general. Jean Esquirol (q.v.) cited him as an example of a sufferer of hallucinations (q.v.) caused by intense guilt. He killed a young female slave that had been given to him and thereafter claimed he was followed by her spirit wherever he went.

Bibliography: Esquirol, J.E.D. 1845. Reprint. 1965. *Mental maladies: A treatise on insanity.*

PAVESE, CESARE (1908-1950). An Italian novelist and poet. His father died when he was six years old, and his mother was a rigid, cold woman who could give him no love. He was imprisoned by the Fascists and became a Communist as an act of solidarity with the people he liked. His writings reflect the feeling of purposelessness and disillusionment prevalent under a totalitarian political system. At the height of his success and in full possession of his creative powers, he took the excuse of a failed love affair with an insignificant American actress to commit suicide (q.v.) with an overdose of sleeping tablets. He said, "No one ever lacks a good reason for suicide." The best known of his books in English translation is *The Moon and the Bonfire*, which clearly shows his state of mind.

Bibliography: Pavese, C. 1974. *The moon and the bonfire*, trans. L. Sinclair.

PAVILION F. A ward for the detention and care of mental patients at the Albany Hospital, in New York. It was established in 1902 and became the

first psychopathic (see PSYCHOPATHY) ward in an American general hospital that offered treatment as well as custody and observation. Dr. J. Montgomery Mosher was responsible for its inception and functioning.
Bibliography: Deutsch, A. 1949. *The mentally ill in America.*

PAVLOV, IVAN PETROVICH (1849-1936). A Russian physiologist. He was the son of a peasant priest and was himself destined for the priesthood but turned to medicine. His many contributions to medicine include the evidence that established the importance of the autonomic nervous system. He studied conditioned reflexes in dogs and associated the reflexes with definite areas of the cortex. In gratitude to the animals he used, he erected in the courtyard of the Institute of Experimental Medicine a stone monument representing a dog. When he became interested in psychiatric disorders, he applied his theories of nervous activity to them. According to him, schizophrenia (q.v.) resulted from a state of inhibition of the cerebral cortex. His discovery of the conditioned reflex (q.v.) for which he received the Nobel Prize in 1904 especially influenced the field of learning. His career, although sponsored by the government and by many members of the Russian aristocracy, suffered because of conflict between the political climate of his country and his own inability to compromise by accepting the czarist policies. The Soviet government treated him more generously than the czarist authorities. His life was regular to the extreme, and he kept routine habits to the end. In his last years he suffered from insomnia especially after the death of his son who served in the White Army.
Bibliography: Babkin, B. P. 1949. *Pavlov.*

PAYNE WHITNEY PSYCHIATRIC CLINIC. A clinic attached to the New York Hospital at White Plains. It opened on October 1, 1932. Its building cost over $2 million, and the clinic provides an extensive psychiatric service with inpatients and outpatients departments.
Bibliography: Deutsch, A. 1949. *The mentally ill in America.*

PAZZARELLA. A mental hospital founded in Rome, Italy, toward the end of the fourteenth century by two Spaniards. The name meant "place for mad people." An account published in Oxford, England, in 1687 states that it was supported by charity and endowed with the entire estate of a Venetian noblewoman. According to the account, the hospital received "crazed persons of whatever nation they be; and at their first entrance care is taken by the physicians to restore them to their right mind, by hellebore or any medicines proper to that efect. If the madness prove incurable, then they are kept there during life, having food and raiment, necessary to the miserable condition they are in, charitably provided for them."
Bibliography: Burdett, H. C. 1891. *Hospitals and asylums of the world.*

PÉAN, JULES ÉMILE (1830-1898). A French surgeon. He introduced the ovariotomy (q.v.) in France in 1864. In 1882 he performed the operation

on a hysterical (*see* HYSTERIA) woman in the belief that removal of the ovary would cure hysteria.
Bibliography: Cesbron, H. 1909. *Histoire critique de l'hystérie.*

PEARSON, KARL (1857-1936). An English scientist. He worked with Francis Galton (q.v.) and, in 1911, became director of the eugenics laboratory at University College in London. He established the present mathematical foundation for the theory of correlation between mental traits. He also investigated the normality of biological distribution and established new methods of statistical investigation for psychological problems. He was a cofounder of *Biometrika*, a journal dedicated to mathematical research in biology and psychology. He was also the biographer of Galton.
Bibliography: Boring, E. G. 1950. *A history of experimental psychology.*

PEAS THERAPY. An early form of treatment for lunacy (*see* LUNATIC) that involved the insertion of dried peas in a head wound intentionally inflicted for this purpose. It was reasoned that the peas would cause suppuration, which was regarded as a counter-irritant that would combat the irritation within the skull. Peas therapy was still in use in the nineteenth century. Augustin Prichard (1818-1896), a surgeon, the son of J. C. Prichard (q.v.) noted that his father had devised a technique for inserting a string of peas in a cut made on the forehead.
Bibliography: Prichard, A. 1896. *A few medical and surgical reminiscences.*

PEDAGOGICAL SEMINARY, THE. See JOURNAL OF GENETIC PSYCHOLOGY.

PEDILUVIA. Plunging the legs of mental patients in water containing an irritant. It was a form of treatment used in the nineteenth century.
Bibliography: Esquirol, J.E.D. 1845. Reprint. 1965. *Mental maladies: a treatise on insanity.*

PEEPING TOM. A term that popularly refers to a voyeur, or a person who finds sexual satisfaction through looking at nudity or watching the sexual activity of others. The term is derived from the name of the Coventry tailor who was said to have watched Lady Godiva (c. 1040-1080) as she rode naked through the city.
Bibliography: Hinsie, L. E., and Campbell, R. J. 1960. *Psychiatric dictionary.*

PELECANICIDIUM, or CHRISTIAN ADVERTISER AGAINST SELF-MURDER. A work written in 1653 by Sir William Denny (?-1676). It was intended as an answer to *Biathanatos* (q.v.) by John Donne (q.v.).

The title *Pelecanicidium* referred to the belief that pelicans committed suicide (q.v.) by feeding their young with their own blood.
Bibliography: Fedden, H. R. 1938. *Suicide.*

PELIZAEUS, FRIEDRICH (1850-1917). A German neurologist. In 1885 he described a congenital, familial anomaly caused by degeneration of cerebral white matter and characterized by mental retardation, poor coordination, and marked speech disorders. It is now called Pelizaeus-Merzbacher's disease.
See also LUDWIG MERZBACHER.
Bibliography: Kanner, L. 1964. *A history of the care and study of the mentally retarded.*

PELLAGRA. A deficiency disease. It has been called the disease of the four "d's": diarrhea, dermatitis, depression, and dementia. It was first described in the eighteenth century as occurring in Italian and Spanish peasants. In 1817 Sir Henry Holland (q.v.) wrote a paper on his observations of patients in Northern Italy:

These unhappy objects seem under the influence of an invincible despondency; they seek to be alone; scarcely answer the questions put to them; and often shed tears without any obvious cause. Their faculties and senses become alike impaired; and the progress of the disease, where it does not carry them off from debility and exhaustion of the vital powers, generally leaves them incurable idiots, or produces occasionally maniacal affections, which terminate eventually in the same state. . . . The mania consequent upon pellagra is often of a very violent kind. . . . Attempts at suicide are frequent. . . .
[Holland, H. 1817. On the pellagra, a disease prevailing in Lombardy. *Medico-Chirurgical Transactions* 8: 317-48.]

Many unexplained mental disorders and strange forms of behavior in the Middle Ages (q.v.) have now been explained by the lack of vitamins which produced pellagra.
Bibliography: Roe, D. A. 1973. A plague of corn: the social history of pellagra.

PENFIELD, WILDER GRAVES (1891-1976). A naturalized Canadian neurosurgeon, born in the United States. His work helped to locate the functional areas of the cerebral cortex. He also developed the surgical treatment of epilepsy (q.v.) and demonstrated that the stimulation of human interpretive cortex produces vivid recollections of early childhood events. Among the many recognitions of his work that he received are the Order of Merit from Great Britain and the Companion of Canada. His books

include *The Cerebral Cortex of Man* (1950) and *Speech and Brain Mechanisms* (1959).
Bibliography: Penfield, W., and Jasper, H. 1954. *Epilepsy and the functional anatomy of the human brain.*

PENNSYLVANIA HOSPITAL. The first general hospital in America to admit mental patients for treatment. It was founded in 1750, after a petition to the Provincial Assembly drawn up by Benjamin Franklin (q.v.). Originally patients were kept in cells in the basement of a private house. In 1756, when a new building for the whole hospital was erected, mental patients were transferred to it but still relegated to cells scattered in the lower parts of the hospital. They were treated little better than prisoners; rigid rules regulated their duties, and treatment consisted of purging (q.v.), bleeding (q.v.), and blistering. They were kept in chains and released only to perform menial duties. Visitors flocked to the hospital to view the lunatics, seeking entertainment well worth the small admission fee. The practice of viewing patients persisted as late as 1822. In 1841, the mental patients, who had been transferred to a separate wing in 1796, were finally given a whole new building on the outskirts of Philadelphia. This separate institution was named the Pennsylvania Hospital for the Insane. Dr. Thomas S. Kirkbride (q.v.) was its first superintendent. Despite its shortcomings, the hospital was advanced for its time and provided occupational therapy (q.v.) for its patients, not only in the form of productive work but also in the form of recreational activities, which were an essential aspect of the nineteenth-century moral medicine (q.v.).
Bibliography: Morton, T. G. 1895. Reprint. 1973. *The history of the Pennsylvania Hospital, 1751-1895.*

PENNSYLVANIA LABORATORY. A psychological laboratory (q.v.) founded in 1888 by James McKeen Cattell (q.v.) at the University of Pennsylvania.
See also PSYCHOLOGICAL LABORATORY.
Bibliography: Flugel, J. C. 1945. *A hundred years of psychology.*

PENNY GATES. The gates to Bethlem Royal Hospital (q.v.) at which visitors were charged a penny entrance fee to be admitted to the hospital to be amused by the antics of the inmates. The penny fee was abolished in 1770, but it had contributed considerably to the institutional income. The money was collected in boxes held by two painted wooden figures representing gipsies, that stood in niches on either side of the gates. The figures had been donated by a merchant, Charles Foot, who had become a governor

of Bethlem in 1676. They are now in the Wellcome Historical Medical Museum in London.
Bibliography: Allderidge, P. 1976. *The Bethlem Historical Museum.*

PENSION. A term suggested by Johann C. Reil (q.v.) in lieu of "asylum" (q.v.) to describe a hospital for nervous disorders. His suggestion appeared in an article in the first issue of *Archiv für die Physiologie*, which he had founded in 1796.

PENTECOSTAL CHURCHES. Religious groups begun in the United States at the beginning of the twentieth century. They emphasize Christian perfection and the second coming of Christ. Their members practise glossolalia (q.v.); motor automatism and sometimes bizarre practices also characterize their worship.
Bibliography: Clark, E. T. 1957. *The small sects in America.*

PENTHEUS. A central figure in the drama *Bacchanals* (q.v.) by Euripedes (q.v.) as the women of Thebes were seized with a madness sent by Dionysus (q.v.) when Pentheus forbade his worship. Pentheus, dressed in women's clothes, spied on their orgies and was killed by the women, including his own mother, while they were in a frenzy.
Bibliography: Way, A. S., trans. 1912. *Euripides*, Vol. 3.

PEONY. Paeonia, a plant considered medically important from early times. The name is derived from the Greek Paean, a physician of the gods. Its root, hung round the neck, was believed to prevent or to cure epilepsy (q.v.). It also could be taken by mouth in powder form. Galen (q.v.) advised that a root of peony should be worn as an amulet (q.v.) to ward off disease. In the *Anglo-Saxon Herbal* (q.v.), it is suggested that peony can cure insanity: "For lunacy if a man lays the wort peony over the lunatic as he lies, soon he lifts himself up well: and if he has it with him, the disease never again approaches him." In the thirteenth century the Salerno Medical School (q.v.) listed the peony in its pharmacopoeia. John Gerard (q.v.) wrote in his herbal in 1597: "The black grains (that is the seed) [of peony] to the number of fifteen taken in wine or mead is a special remedie for those that are troubled in the night with the disease called the Night Mare, which is as though a heavy burthen were laid upon them and they oppressed therewith, as if they were overcome with their enemies or overprest with some great weight or burthen, and they are also good against melancholic dreames."
Like the mandragora (q.v.) the peony had to be uprooted by a dog.
Bibliography: Rohde, E. S. 1974. *The old English herbals.*

PEPPERELL PRIVATE ASYLUM. A private mental institution in Pepperell, Massachusetts. It developed from the practice of Dr. Nehemiah Cut-

ter (q.v.). He so successfully treated mental patients in his own home that his house had to be enlarged to accommodate their increasing numbers. Eventually a completely new building became necessary. The new asylum (q.v.) was well accepted, despite the general distrust in private mental institutions prevalent at the time. It was destroyed by a fire in 1853 and never rebuilt.
Bibliography: Deutsch, A. 1949. *The mentally ill in America.*

PEPPERMINT. A fragrant perennial herb of the mint family. It was known to the ancient Egyptians, to the Greeks and to the Romans and was mentioned in the pharmacopoeias of Iceland in the thirteenth century. Although employed mostly in remedies for gastric or respiratory disorders, in folk medicine an infusion of peppermint leaves is used as a stimulant and believed to relieve depression. It is also used to induce sleep and to break shock.
Bibliography: le Strange, R. 1977. *A history of herbal plants.*

PEPYS, SAMUEL (1633-1703). An English diarist and official of the Admiralty. His diary is an outstanding record of the years 1660-1669 and offers descriptions of the Great Plague, the Fire of London and many lesser events of human interest. He was also a governor of Bethlem Royal Hospital (q.v.). When a tax of two shillings per chimney threatened the hospital, he interceded and obtained an exemption from payment. He was a friend of Dr. Thomas Allen (q.v.) physician to Bethlem from 1667 to 1684. Pepys' diary contains frequent references to people connected with the hospital, as well as references to asylum visiting (q.v.). The entry for January 21, 1668, relates the attempted suicide (q.v.) of his cousin's husband, who had thrown himself into a pond in a fit of depression and risked the loss of his estate to the Crown because, by law, the estates of suicides were confiscated. Pepys discussed the case with the king, who promised to help. Another entry of psychiatric interest concerns arrangements made for a blood transfusion (q.v.) as an experimental treatment for insanity; the patient came from Bethlem Hospital.
Bibliography: Latham, R., and Matthews, W., ed. 1971. *The diary of Samuel Pepys.*

PERCEVAL, JOHN THOMAS (1803-1876). An English military man, the fifth of the twelve children of Spencer Perceval (q.v.). In 1830 Perceval left the army and became involved in a religious evangelical cult. The same year he began to behave erratically and to suffer from delusions (q.v.) and hallucinations (q.v.). Eventually he became a patient of Dr. Edward L. Fox (q.v.) at Brislington House (q.v.). Perceval commented adversely on the asylum, saying that he had been humiliated and ill-treated there. He spent some time also in Ticehurst Asylum (q.v.), which he liked better. In 1834 he was released and married Anna Gardner, by whom he had four children. His experiences in the asylums were related in a work published in 1838

and entitled *A Narrative of the Treatment Experienced by a Gentleman, during a State of Mental Derangement*. He also tried to explain the reasons for his mental illness and why it manifested itself in particular symptoms. His reactions to hallucinations and the anguishing stress he suffered are recounted by him with insight. He was one of the founders of The Alleged Lunatics' Friend Society (q.v.).
Bibliography: Bateson, G. 1962. *Perceval's narrative: a patient's account of his psychosis.*

PERCEVAL, SPENCER (1762-1812). An English politician. In 1809 he became prime minister. He was assassinated in the House of Commons by a lunatic (q.v.), John Bellingham, who had a grudge against the government. The assassination and the subsequent hanging of Bellingham brought about greater public awareness of insanity. Perceval's son, John Perceval (q.v.) became a champion of the rights of the insane.
Bibliography: Parry-Jones, W. Ll. 1972. *The trade in lunacy.*

PERCIVAL, JAMES GATES (1795-1856). An American poet, who studied medicine, geology, botany, and languages. He became professor of chemistry at West Point, and was considered an eccentric genius, but he lacked consistency of purpose. He was feeble and nervous and toward the end of his life, his eccentricity became pathological, and he was considered mad.
Bibliography: Winslow, L.S.F. 1898. *Mad humanity: its forms, apparent and obscure.*

PERCY'S RELIQUES OF ANCIENT ENGLISH POETRY. A collection of ancient English verses, ballads, and sonnets. It was published in 1765 by Thomas Percy (1729-1811), bishop of Dromore. He stated in the volume that the English have more ballads on the subject of insanity than any other people.
Bibliography: Percy, T. 1765. *Reliques of ancient English poetry.*

PERDICCAS. Son of Amyntas III, king of Macedonia. As a young man he developed a hectic fever, and Hippocrates (q.v.) correctly diagnosed that the illness was caused by a psychological factor, that is Perdiccas' love for Phyla, one of his father's concubines.
Bibliography: Esquirol, J.E.D. 1845. Reprint. 1965. *Mental maladies: a treatise on insanity.*

PÉREIRÉ, JACOB RODRIGUE (1715-1780). A Spanish Jew. He became the first educator of deaf-mutes in France and evolved a sign language for them.
Bibliography: La Rochelle, E. 1877. *Jacob Rodrigue Péreiré.*

PERFECT, WILLIAM (1737-1809). A British physician. He started his career in general practice, but his interest in insanity led to his dedication

to mental patients. He started a private asylum, known as Malling Place, in Kent. He treated his patients with resourceful and humane methods. In 1778 his first book was published. Entitled *Methods of Cure, in Some particular Cases of Insanity. . . . and Nervous Disorders*, it contained a large number of case histories and a distillation of the author's factual experience. The book was widely read and ran into seven editions with variations in its title.
Bibliography: Parry-Jones, W. Ll. 1972. *The trade in lunacy.*

PERIWINKLE. A herb found in most parts of the world. The Anglo-Saxons believed it possessed great curative properties in cases of demoniac possession (q.v.). The fifth-century herbal of Apuleius Platonicus recommended it for the treatment and prevention of many illnesses, including "devil sickness and demoniacal possessions" and for "envy and for terror."
Bibliography: Rohde, E. S. 1974. *The old English herbals.*

PERKINS, ELISHA (1741-1799). An American physician and follower of Franz Mesmer (q.v.). He invented the Perkins tractors (*see* METALLIC TRACTORS). They consisted of two metallic rods that he claimed were charged with a force that could treat mental and physical disorders. His son introduced the tractors to England, and a Perkins Institute was established in London in 1796. However, the treatment fell into disrepute when it was proven that they were no more effective than rods made from any material.
Bibliography: Alexander, F. G., and Selesnick, S. T. 1966. *The history of psychiatry.*

PERRINE, THOMAS (?-1774). An American sailor. In 1765 he became deranged and was admitted to the Pennsylvania Hospital (q.v.). He was a difficult and, at times, violent patient. Because he did not like his underground cell, he escaped and rushed to the top of the house, where he barricaded himself in the cupola. Nobody could bring him down and eventually it was accepted that he should live up there. He remained in his cramped quarters for nine years, summer and winter, with no fire even in the coldest days.
Bibliography: Morton, Thomas G. 1897. *History of the Pennsylvania Hospital.*

PERSECUTORY CHILD REARING. In the nineteenth century, especially in Germany, child-rearing practices often verged on persecution. Special devices were designed to tie children in bed, strap them to chairs, keep their shoulders back, and, in general, prevent them from assuming relaxed positions. Cold baths, unheated bedrooms, self-denial, and almost total suppression of pleasurable activities were advised for their upbringing. A series of books elaborating this calculated repressive system was written by

Dr. Gottlieb Moritz Schreber (1808-1861), the father of Daniel Paul Schreber (q.v.).
Bibliography: Schatzmann, M. 1973. *Soul murder: Persecution in the family.*

PERSIAN GALEN. The appellative sometimes applied to Avicenna (q.v.).

PERSONAL EQUATION. A theory introduced by the Prussian astronomer Friedrich W. Bessel (1784-1846). Indignant over the unjust dismissal of the astronomer royal in 1796, he proved by studies of time factors that divergences in observational reports were due to individual differences in the speed of reaction.
Bibliography: Flugel, J. C. 1945. *A hundred years of psychology.*

PERTH ROYAL MENTAL HOSPITAL. (*See* MURRAY ROYAL HOSPITAL).

PERTURBATIONES. The term used by Cicero (q.v.) to describe what is now known as emotional disorders. He clearly differentiated them from mental diseases.
Bibliography: Cicero. *Tusculan Disputations,* trans. J. E. King.

PESTALOZZI, JOHANN HEINRICH (1746-1827). A Swiss educational reformer. He believed that a child's observations and spontaneous interest were more important than formal instruction. He devoted his life to the education of poor children for whom he established a farming community. This venture lasted for five difficult years and was followed by other educational establishments that also failed because of Pestalozzi's inability to manage the practical aspects of their administration. His ideas eventually were accepted and stimulated greater interest in devising new methods of teaching the mentally retarded.
Bibliography: Heafford, M. 1967. *Pestalozzi: His thought and its relevance today.*

PETER I *or* **PETER THE GREAT** (1682-1725). A czar of Russia. His psychopathology was multisymptomatic. He suffered from headaches, nightmares (q.v.), and insomnia. When he slept, his head was covered and pressed against the naked belly of a male servant who was expected to remain motionless. His fears were said to have begun when he was ten years old and witnessed an invasion of the palace by the militia, which resulted in murder, pillage, and a threat to his own life. He also suffered from alcoholism, epilepsy, syphilis (qq.v.), and, possibly, insanity.
Bibliography: Graham, S. 1929. *Peter the Great.*

PETER III (1728-1762). A czar of Russia, grandson of Peter the Great (q.v.). As a child he was prone to fainting fits and convulsions. A strict and, at times, cruel system of education that included whipping and humiliations turned him into a suspicious, restless, and frightened young man. In 1745, he married Sophie of Anhalt-Zubst later known as Catherine the Great (q.v.). The marriage was unhappy, and Catherine plotted against him and headed a conspiracy to dethrone him. He was too weak and dimwitted to protect himself. He was said to have been strangled by the conspirators who sided with his wife.

Bibliography: Bain, R. N. 1902. *Peter III.*

PETER OF HANOVER (?-1785). A child found in the forest near Hameln, Hanover, Germany, in 1724. A year after his father had abandoned him in a forest, he had tried to go back to his home, but he had been turned away by his stepmother. He returned to the forest and lived by eating plants and the bark of trees. By the time he was captured, he had become wild. He never fully adjusted to social living and never learned to talk. He was presented to King George I (1660-1727) of England who had him taken to a farm in Hertfordshire and placed under the care of Dr. John Arbuthnot (q.v.). He was the subject of much interest, as at the time the mind of the "savage" was a topical subject. He lived to old age.

See also FERAL CHILD.

Bibliography: Malson, L. 1972. *Wolf children.*

PETER PAN. The central character in a play written by Sir James M. Barrie in 1904. He is a little boy who does not wish to grow up. In psychiatry, the Peter Pan syndrome refers to those immature individuals who refuse to take on responsibilities commensurate with their age. A statue of Peter Pan is in Kensington Gardens, London, placed there by Barrie in 1912.

Bibliography: Barrie, J. M. 1937. *Peter Pan.*

PETITES MAISONS. Special institutions for the care of the mentally ill. They were founded in France in 1645 by Madame Louise Le Gras (q.v.). The nurses of the petites maisons were perhaps the first trained mental health nurses.

Bibliography: Burdett, H. C. 1891. *Hospitals and asylums of the world.*

PETITES PERCEPTIONS. A term used by Gottfried Leibniz (q.v.) to describe a concept that was later called the unconscious (q.v.).

Bibliography: Flugel, J. C. 1945. *A hundred years of psychology.*

PETRARCA, FRANCESCO (1304-1374). One of the earliest and greatest Italian poets and humanists. Despite his popularity in the courts of Italy, he longed for solitude, and his mood often changed from elation to despair. He suffered from depression, his sleep was disturbed by nightmares (q.v.), and he often was unable to shake off melancholia (q.v.) that tormented him night and day: "For me this is a time without light or life. It is an inferno

and most bitter death." His constant and pure love for Laura (1308?-1348), inspired most of his poetry. His approach to human problems was influenced by the philosophy of Cicero (q.v.) and strongly rejected the mediaeval methods of deductive reasoning.
Bibliography: Bishop, M. 1963. *Petrarch and his world.*

PETRUS HISPANUS (c.1200-1277). A Portuguese physician, principal of a school in Lisbon, and archbishop of Bragga. He wrote a treatise in which psychology was treated as a separate subject and given a complete chapter on its history. Anticipating by several centuries the findings of psychosomatic medicine (q.v.), he thought that passions were the main causes of emotional disorders and that even bodily illness could be linked to them. For epilepsy (q.v.), he advised the gall of a dog, or the liver of a vulture, killed at the exact moment the epileptic fell into a fit. In 1276, he was elected pope with the name of John XXI (q.v.), but his papacy was brief, as he was killed eight months after his election by a falling ceiling. It was said that his mode of death was retribution for having sold his soul to the devil in exchange for knowledge, but Dante's (q.v.) *Divina Commedia* mentions him as the only contemporary pope in Paradise.
Bibliography: Castiglioni, A. 1946. *A history of medicine*, trans. and ed. E. B. Knumbhaar.

PEYOTE. *Lophophora williamsii*, a cactus found primarily in Mexico. A narcotic drug that produces intoxication with vivid visual hallucinations (q.v.), withdrawal from reality, and heightened perception can be obtained by fermenting its juices. Mexican and American Indians have known and used it since the Aztec era. Originally its use usually was restricted to ritual religious ceremonies because divinatory properties were attributed to it. Later it was employed as a therapeutic agent for many disorders and sometimes taken simply for its intoxicant effect. In the sixteenth century the Spanish conquistadors brought it back to Europe. Bernardino de Sahagún (1499?-1590) first described its effects in 1560: "Those who eat or drink it see visions either frightful or laughable." He added that they remained intoxicated for two or three days. Mescaline (q.v.) was abstracted from the peyote in 1896; subsequent research demonstrated the bewildering hallucinations, confusion, and disorientation that it produces. Havelock Ellis (q.v.) wrote of its effect on the appreciation of colors; D. H. Lawrence (q.v.) described mescal intoxication in *The Woman Who Rode Away* (1928), and Aldous Huxley (q.v.) reported the effects from his personal experience in *Doors of Perception* (1956).
Bibliography: Emboden, W. 1972. *Narcotic plants.*

P FACTOR. A factor isolated by Charles E. Spearman (q.v.) in his factorial analysis of performance. It manifests itself as a general inertia that prevents the subject from passing rapidly from one mental operation to another and compels his perseveration in the same operation.

See also G FACTOR, O FACTOR, and W FACTOR.

Bibliography: Spearman, C. E. 1927. *Abilities of man, their nature and measurement.*

PFISTER, OSKAR (1873-1956). A Swiss educator and pastor. As a child he witnessed a teacher striking a sick pupil, and this act of brutality, which he never forgot, prompted him to become a teacher who would show kindness to his charges. His pastoral work with adolescents provided him with first-hand knowledge of their problems, which he used in his lectures and writings. He was a friend and follower of Sigmund Freud (q.v.) and introduced psychoanalysis (q.v.) to Switzerland with his first book *The Psychoanalytic Method* (1913). His psychoanalytic theories of education led to the development of child analysis. With Eugen Bleuler (q.v.) he was the founder of the Swiss Society for Psychoanalysis (q.v.). Many of his works, which combined psychoanalytic principles and Christian doctrine, were translated into several languages.

Bibliography: Alexander, F., Eisenstein, S., and Grotjahn, M., eds. 1966. *Psychoanalytic pioneers.*

PHAEDRA. In Greek mythology (q.v.), the wife of Theseus. She fell in love with her stepson, Hippolytus, who rejected her. His action so enraged her that she told her husband Hippolytus had tried to rape her. Theseus asked the gods for his destruction, and Phaedra, overcome with guilt, strangled herself. In psychiatry the Phaedra complex refers to a mother's sexual attraction for her son.

Bibliography: Graves, R. 1960. *The Greek myths.*

PHAGYI-DAU (?-1845). A king of Burma. He was dominated by his queen, a plain woman who was said to use sorcery to influence him. He was an hypochondriac (*see* HYPOCHONDRIA) and became insane in 1837, when he was deposed and imprisoned. His brother, Tharrawaddy, succeeded him, but he too was deposed because of insanity.

Bibliography: Ireland, W. W. 1889. *Through the ivory gate.*

PHAIRE, THOMAS (or FAIER, PHAER) (1510?-1560). English physician and solicitor. He wrote the first book on pediatrics written in the English language. It was also one of the earliest medical books to be printed. In the *Boke of Chyldren*, first published in 1545 as an addition to *The Regiment of Life*, the author stressed the importance of psychological as well as physical elements in child raising. He advised that a nurse should be chosen with care and that she should be "sobre, honeste and chaste" and "amyable and chearfull, so that she may accustome the infant into mirth." For epilepsy (q.v.) in children he recommended various herbs, such as chicory, rosemary

(q.v.), sea thistle, and peony (q.v.), made into concoction and taken internally. Sapphires, emeralds, and red coral (qq.v.) are among his external prescriptions. For enuresis (q.v.) he suggested a powder made from the windpipe of a cock, or from the feet of a goat.
Bibliography: Phaire, T. reprint. 1957. *The boke of chyldren*.

PHALLUS. A model of the erect male organ of reproduction. In ancient Greece it was used in religious ceremonies connected with fertility rites. Two such models, 54 meters high, stood outside the temple of Aphrodite at Hierapolis. Many other religions have similar symbols and practices.
Bibliography: Scott, G. R. 1951. *Phallic worship*.

PHENOMENOLOGY. A movement initiated in Germany in the nineteenth century by the philosopher Edmund Husserl (q.v.). It advocated the description and understanding of phenomena through immediate experience and claimed that all science, including psychological phenomena, should rest on these principles.
Bibliography: Spiegelberg, H. 1965. *The phenomenological movement*.

PHENYLKETONURIA. A metabolic disorder, also called phenylpyruvic acid oligophrenia, that causes mental deficiency. Its discovery in 1934 by Ivor Følling (q.v.) gave new impetus to biological studies of mental deficiency and brought new hope that the effects of inborn errors of metabolism could be reversed through diet (q.v.).
Bibliography: Kanner, L. 1957. *Child psychiatry*. 3rd ed.

PHII BAH. In Thailand (q.v.) a spirit that can assume a human form and has the power to drive people mad by possession (q.v.). The term "Phii Bah" literally means "crazy ghost." It is applied to those individuals who are believed to be insane or possessed. *Phii Pob* is the term applied to the person who is the originating host of the spirit. The spirit comes and goes from his body, transferring itself to other people who go mad. The spirit may be inherited from an ancestor. In Thai society such possessions are a socially acceptable way of solving conflicts; those affected are diagnosed as hysterical neurotics (*see* NEUROSIS) or even psychotics (*see* PSYCHOSIS) and are treated in mental hospitals.
Bibliography: Sangsingkeo, P. 1975. Thailand. In *World history of psychiatry*, ed. J. G. Howells.

PHILIP II (1527-1598). A king of Spain, son of Charles V (q.v.). He was taught to hate heretics and to rely on the Inquisition (q.v.) to protect Spain from them. His grandmother was the mad Joanna of Castille (q.v.); his two younger brothers, who died in infancy, were subject to seizures that were said to be caused by evil spirits. He was married at sixteen to Maria Manoela

(1527-1545) of Portugal, who died soon after giving birth to their son, Don Carlos (q.v.). Philip sought comfort in his mistresses who provided him with healthy but illegitimate sons. His marriage to Mary I (q.v.) of England proved emotionally disastrous; she was his senior by nine years and failed to give him an heir. For his third wife he took Elizabeth of Valois (1545-1568), the daughter of the king of France. She had been betrothed to his son Carlos. Carlos was eventually incarcerated and possibly murdered on his orders. His fourth wife was his niece, Anne of Austria (1549-1580) who gave him a son and heir. His bigotry and despotism have obscured his good qualities: he searched for affection from his early years, but a deprivatory upbringing prevented him from expressing warmth.

Bibliography: Grierson, E. 1974. *King of two worlds: Philip II of Spain.*

PHILIP V (1683-1746). The first of the Bourbon kings of Spain, grandson of Louis XIV (1638-1715) of France. He was a weak individual who was greatly influenced by his confessor, his wife, Maria Luisa of Savoy (1688-1714) through her formidable lady in waiting, and, after her death, by his second wife, Isabella Farnese (1692-1766). He had no personal friends due to his inability to sustain close relationships. Philip was morbidly religious; his two primary interests outside his devotions were music and hunting. During periods of melancholy (*see* MELANCHOLIA) music was his only solace, and his melancholy was eased by the singing of Carlo Farinelli (q.v.) who would sing the same few tunes for him night after night, while the king shouted the words in a tuneless voice. As he grew old, Philip became deranged, neglected his appearance, and stood dazed and open-mouthed at audiences. He was afraid of being poisoned and would wear no garment other than his wife's chemise. He let his hair and beard grow untidily and spent long periods in bed without uttering a word. The affairs of government were largely controlled by his wife.

Bibliography: Baudrillart, H.M.A. 1890-1900. *Philippe V et la court de France.* 5 vols.

PHILOLAOS OF CROTON. A fifth-century B.C. Greek philosopher, mathematician, and astronomer, born in southern Italy. He was a disciple of Pythagoras (q.v.) whose teachings he recorded. According to Philolaos, sensory functions were localized in the brain, animal functions in the heart, and vegetative functions in the navel. He regarded the soul as a harmonious mixture of the bodily parts.

Bibliography: Diels, H., and Kranz, W. 1954. *Fragmente der Vorsokratiker.* Vol. 1.

PHILOSOPHER'S STONE. A substance searched for by alchemists (*see* ALCHEMY) from early Egyptian times to the seventeenth century. It was believed that it could purify base metals until the *materia prima*, which was

thought to be gold, was obtained. The search for the philosopher's stone, sometimes termed the elixir of life, was associated with astrologers (*see* ASTROLOGY) and magicians (*see* MAGIC) who were regarded as physicians skilled in the treatment of mental and physical ills.
Bibliography: Jung, C. J. 1968. *Psychology and alchemy.*

PHILOSOPHICAL TRANSACTIONS, THE. A journal recording the transactions of the Royal Society (q.v.). It was founded in London in 1665 to report on the whole field of scientific knowledge. Medical matters were among the issues discussed by the members of the Royal Society, who were expected to adopt "a close, naked, natural way of speaking; positive expressions; clear senses; a native easiness."
Bibliography: Hartley, H. ed. 1960. *The Royal Society: its origins and founders.*

PHILOSOPHIE DE LA FOLIE. A book by Joseph Daquin (q.v.) published in France in 1791. The author dedicated the first edition of it to "humanity" and the second to Philippe Pinel (q.v.). It was an important work in which the problems of mental disorder were approached from a new angle; direct observation of the patient was presented as the basis of diagnosis and subsequent treatment. Daquin believed that the insane should not be kept under constant restraint (q.v.) and that violent measures were unnecessary and harmful. He pleaded for humane treatment and suggested that mental patients should be employed as a part of the plan of therapy. Pinel was influenced greatly by this work, which, to some extent, changed the history of psychiatry.
Bibliography: Daquin, J. 1791. *Philosophie de la folie.*

PHILOSOPHISCHE STUDIEN. A journal established by Wilhelm Wundt (q.v.) in 1881. It published reports of the experimental work conducted at Wundt's laboratory in Leipzig. For this reason, it is considered the first purely psychological journal. In 1903 Wundt renamed it *Psychologische Studien.*
Bibliography: Misiak, H., and Sexton, V. S. 1966. *History of psychology.*

PHILOSOPHY OF THE UNCONSCIOUS. A book written in 1869 by Karl von Hartmann (q.v.), who arrived at a formulation of the unconscious (q.v.) through a process of abstract reasoning. It preceded Sigmund Freud's (q.v.) concept of the unconscious.
Bibliography: Hartmann, E. von. 1869. *Philosophie des Unbewussten.*

PHI-PHENOMENON. A term used by Max Wertheimer (q.v.) to describe movement, which implies the perception of both time and space.
Bibliography: Flugel, J. C. 1945. *A hundred years of psychology.*

PHIPPS CLINIC. *See* HENRY PHIPPS PSYCHIATRIC CLINIC.

PHOBIAS. In a parody of William Cullen's (q.v.) classification of mental diseases, his former teacher, Benjamin Rush (q.v.) wrote *On the Different*

Species of Phobias (1798), a humourous nosology of phobias. He divided them into eighteen categories, each named after the particular situation or thing feared. However, his nosology was taken seriously and adopted in many textbooks.
Bibliography: Runes, D. D., ed. 1947. *The selected writings of Benjamin Rush*.

PHRAN BOON LARNG NUER. A holy well (q.v.) in central Thailand (q.v.). The mentally ill drink its water or bathe in it in the belief that they will be cured.
Bibliography: Sangsingkeo, P. 1975. Thailand. In *World history of psychiatry*, ed.
    J. G. Howells.

PHRA SRI MAHABHODI. A mental hospital in the Ubol province of Thailand (q.v.). It is named after the sacred bhodi tree, which was originally brought from Ceylon.
Bibliography: Sangsingkeo, P. 1975. Thailand. In *World history of psychiatry*, ed.
    J. G. Howells.

PHRENITIS. A term first used by Hippocrates (q.v.) to describe inflammation of the brain. Later authors, for example, Celsus (q.v.), used it in their classification of mental disorders. They frequently recognized three types of phrenitis: those states of delirium (q.v.) due to fever, melancholia (q.v.) caused by black bile (q.v.), and states characterized by hallucinations (q.v.). It was originally related to the diaphragm (q.v.) (*phrenos*), which was believed to be the seat of at least a part of the mind and was called by some Greek medical writers "the temple of the body." The term "frenzy" is derived from it. As late as the nineteenth century, the term "phrenitis" was used to refer to delirious states.
Bibliography: Veith, I. 1957. Psychiatric nosology: from Hippocrates to Kraepelin.
    Am. J. Psychiat. 114: 385-91.

PHRENOLOGICAL JOURNAL. A publication founded in 1824 by Andrew and George Combe (q.v.). From Britain it was transferred to the United States, where it ceased publication in 1911 after producing 124 volumes.

PHRENOLOGY. A term derived from the Greek *phrenos* (q.v.) and used with different meanings by nineteenth-century writers. Benjamin Rush (q.v.) used the term as early as 1805 to designate "the science of the mind," which today would be called psychology (q.v.). The term was used by Thomas Forster (q.v.) in 1815 to describe a theory of personality based on the belief that bumps on the skull are related to specific areas in which certain psychological qualities are located. Franz J. Gall (q.v.) applied this definition to his beliefs that the brain was divided into areas subserving psychological faculties. His theories were adopted and then developed independently by

Johann Spurzheim (q.v.) in 1818. Spurzheim used the term "phrenology" in place of the discarded terms "craniology" and "cranioscopy." Phrenology came to be regarded as a new "science of the mind" and gained popularity during the first half of the nineteenth century. Maps and models of the head were devised showing the areas in which each faculty was localized. Thirty-seven such areas were recognized. Some educators and enthusiastic laymen practiced phrenology, claiming to be able to recognize genius (q.v.) or mental defect from the bumps. The more gullible were taken in by charlatans, who were quick to see the possibility of financial gain. They offered special lotions that would develop this or that faculty if rubbed on the appropriate part of the head. Some unfortunate mental patients had leeches (q.v.) and mustard plasters applied to their shaven heads; others were submitted to trepanation (q.v.). A number of journals were dedicated to phrenology in Britain and in the United States. The Ohio State Phrenological Society continued its activities until 1938.

Bibliography: Noel, P. S., and Carlson, E. T. 1970. Origins of the word "phrenology." *Am. J. Psychiat.* 127: 694-97.

PHRENOS. A Greek word originally meaning "diaphragm." It came to be used as a term for the mind as this was believed to be located in the diaphragm (q.v.), called by the stoic philosopher Aristo (fl. 250 B.C.) "the temple of the body."

Bibliography: Phillips, E. D. 1973. *Greek medicine.*

PHRYGIA. A country in Asia Minor famous for the orgies of Dionysus (q.v.). After it was conquered by the Persians, its inhabitants were regarded as proverbially stupid.

Bibliography: 1978. *Brewer's dictionary of phrase and fable.*

PHYSIOGNOMY. The correlation of personality and outward appearances, especially facial features. Aristotle (q.v.) and earlier Greek writers observed gestures, growth of hair, and skin, as well as other characteristics, and tried to deduce the character of a person from them. *Physiognomica*, a book attributed to Aristotle, suggests that people have the temperament of the animals they resemble and that the same broad principles can be applied to a whole race of people. Socrates (q.v.), the Stoics (q.v.), and, later, the gymnasts of the second century A.D. emphasized these assumptions. The belief continued into the Middle Ages (q.v.). In the sixteenth century, Giovanni Della Porta (q.v.) compared human facial expressions to animal faces and deduced personality traits from his comparisons; Johann Lavater (q.v.) dedicated his work *Physiognomic Fragments* to the study of physiognomy, but his conclusions were sharply criticized by Franz Gall (q.v.). In the nineteenth century, the foremost exponent of this doctrine was Carl Gustav Carus (q.v.). Cesare Lombroso (q.v.) also applied the principles of phy-

siognomy to the study of criminals and believed that certain features — close set eyes, a low forehead, or pointed ears — were particularly significant. He called them "stigmata of degeneracy." During the early part of the twentieth century physiognomy remained in vogue and personnel selection was sometimes based on its principles.
Bibliography: Paterson, D. G. 1930. *Physique and intellect.*

PHYSIOLOGICAL PSYCHOLOGY. The psychology of organic sensations. The first systematic treatise on physiological psychology appeared in *Handbuch der Physiologie des Menschen,* a textbook on physiology by Johannes Müller (q.v.), which was published between 1833 and 1840.
Bibliography: Boring, E. G. 1950. *A history of experimental psychology.*

PIAGET, JEAN (1896-1980). Swiss psychologist, professor of experimental psychology (q.v.) at the University of Geneva. His primary concern was the intellectual and perceptual development of children. He wrote on reasoning, thinking, moral judgment, and language development of the child. His studies were based on methodical observations of children within his own immediate circle. Among his best known books are *The Child's Conception of the World* (1929), *The Language and Thought of the Child* (1932), and *Structuralism* (1970).
Bibliography: Murray, F. B., ed. 1979. *The impact of Piagetian theory on education, philosophy, psychiatry and psychology.*

PIBLOKTOQ. A term used to describe an emotional disorder in Eskimo women. Admiral Robert E. Peary (1856-1920) observed its manifestations during his arctic exploration toward the end of the nineteenth century. He described how the women would be seized by uncontrollable excitement that culminates in collapse and unconsciousness. The condition was believed to be caused by the women's anxiety and insecurity within the Eskimo society.
See also ARCTIC HYSTERIA.
Bibliography: Goldenson, R. M. 1970. *The encyclopedia of human behavior.*

PICA. A term derived from medieval Latin, meaning "magpie," a bird believed to eat anything. It refers to the consumption of substances such as clay, ashes, dirt, and sand. Primitive African tribes encouraged their warriors to eat earth taken from their home ground in the belief that this would strengthen them on long journeys. In China (q.v.) a similar belief existed as early as the fifth century A.D. Many religious ceremonies in primitive cultures included the eating of clay, which at times has been associated with curative practices. Pica is still found as a practice among some American

Negroes, especially in pregnant women, who believe that if they eat earth, clay or starch their children will be strong.
Bibliography: Cooper, M. 1957. *Pica*.

PICK, ARNOLD (1851-1924). A Czech psychiatrist and director of a hospital for mental diseases at Dobřan. In 1892 he became the first to describe presenile dementia caused by lobar atrophy (now known as Pick's disease). He also contributed to a better knowledge of cerebral function localization and neuropathology.
Bibliography: Haymaker, W., and Schiller, F. 1970. *The founders of neurology*. 2d. ed.

PICKWICK PAPERS, THE. A novel by Charles Dickens (q.v.) published between 1836 and 1837. It contains a melodramatic self-description of a madman, who is the author of a manuscript lent to Pickwick. Pickwick finds the description so vivid that he is frightened when he reads it alone in his bedroom.
Bibliography: Dickens, C. 1837. *The Pickwick papers*.

PICO DELLA MIRANDOLA (1463-1494). An Italian philosopher of encyclopedic knowledge. He once challenged anyone who was interested to debate any of his nine hundred theses concerning the reconcilation of Christianity with Platonic philosophy. The pope considered some of these disputations heretical and banned them. According to Pico della Mirandola, man was free to determine his own destiny and had the capacity to realize his ideals.
Bibliography: Dulles, A. 1941. *Princeps concordiae*.

PIERCE, ROBERT (1620-1710). A British physician. In 1697 he published *Bath memoirs*, a collection of the case histories of patients treated primarily by the mineral waters of Bath. Among the histories he related were those of two young women. One of them had become addicted to laudanum (q.v.), which she took to relieve pain that may have been the result of hysteria (q.v.), and the other was suffering from "hysteric passion" and other psychosomatic symptoms. Both were said to have recovered after taking the waters of Bath. One of them left the city to have a child and the other to get married. These events may have contributed to their cure.
Bibliography: Hunter, R., and Macalpine, I. 1963. *Three hundred years of psychiatry*.

PIERO DI COSIMO (1461-1521). An Italian painter. His behavior led people to think that he was deranged. Giorgio Vasari (1511-1574) described how he simplified his domestic chores by hard-boiling fifty eggs at a time when he was heating his glue; he would then eat them over several days. He could not bear the crying of children, the coughing of men, the jingling

of bells, the chanting of friars, and the noise of thunder. In his old age he became very eccentric and would not accept any help even when he was no longer able to hold his brushes.
Bibliography: Wittkower, R., and Wittkower, M. 1963. *Born under Saturn.*

PIÉRON, HENRI (1881-1964). A French psychologist. His father had wanted him to become a mathematician, but Piéron became interested in searching for a better means of understanding the human mind. He studied philosophy and biology and, for a time, was secretary to Pierre Janet (q.v.). He subsequently undertook research in techniques for measuring mental functions, in problems related to sleeping and dreaming, and in comparative studies of animal psychology. He eventually concentrated his efforts on psychophysiology, especially of the senses. In 1928 he created the Institute of the Study of Work and Professional Guidance in Paris. He is considered the initiator of a French school of behaviorism (q.v.), "psychologie du comportement."
Bibliography: Piéron, H. 1952. *The sensations.*

PIERROT. A character in French pantomime. He is a pathetic figure who is lovelorn, ludicrous, amoral, and greedy. He is eternally disappointed yet remains hopeful.

PIKE. A freshwater fish. Its head, dried, reduced to a powder, and taken in a glass of warm water, was used as a remedy for enuresis (q.v.) in old Russia, especially northern Siberia.
Bibliography: Kourennoff, P. M., and St. George, G. 1970. *Russian folk medicine.*

PILLSBURY, WALTER BOWERS (1872-1960). An American psychologist. He was the author of several books, including *Essentials of Psychology* (1911), which became one of the most popular textbooks in America. Although he defined psychology as "the science of behavior" he stressed that behavior must be studied "through the consciousness of the individual and by external observation." His *History of Psychology* was published in 1929.
Bibliography: Pillsbury, W. B. 1911. *Essentials of psychology.*

PINDAR (c.518-438 B.C.). The greatest of the Greek lyric poets. In one of his poems he writes about Aesculapius (q.v.) and states that the god often used incantations (q.v.) to heal the sick. The poem provides an early example of suggestion to produce improvement in an illness.
Bibliography: Bowra, C. M. 1964. *Pindar.*

PINEL, PHILIPPE (1745-1826). A French psychiatrist and one of the founders of modern psychiatry (q.v.). As an adolescent he considered a career in the church or mathematics. Eventually he followed in his father's footsteps and qualified in medicine at the University of Toulouse. In 1778 he moved to Paris, where he taught mathematics, translated medical works into French, and frequently visited a private asylum (q.v.) belonging to J. E. Belhomme (q.v.), who was responsible for stimulating his interest in mental disorders. Pinel's decision to devote himself to psychiatry was prompted by the tragic death of a friend who became insane, ran into a forest, and was devoured by wolves. In 1793 Pinel was appointed head physician at the Bicêtre (q.v.), where one of his first innovations was to remove the chains and fetters from the insane. His actions met with opposition from the officers of the Commune, who regarded the patients as "wild animals." Moreover, they distrusted Pinel and suspected that he was hiding enemies of the French Revolution in his hospital. Once he was seized by an angry crowd and would have been hanged if one of his own patients, Chevigné (q.v.), had not rescued him. In 1795 Pinel became head of the Salpêtrière (q.v.), where he introduced the same enlightened changes. He reorganized both hospitals and based his new methods of treatment on kindness, respect, and encouragement and discouraged the indiscriminate use of drugs (q.v.). In his psychosocial approach to mental illness he was influenced by English and Scottish medicine. Moral medicine (q.v.) and the classification of mental disorders were his two major interests. His most important books were *Nosographie Philosophique* (1798) in which he classified mental disorders into mania (q.v.), melancholia (q.v.), dementia and idiocy (*see* IDIOT), and *Traité médico-philosophique sur l'alienation mental ou la manie* (1801) in which he discussed his theories of aetiology and advocated moral medicine in addition to some physical treatment. He recognized the influence of the environment and heredity on mental disorders. His career spanned a period of drastic changes in France. He served under Louis XVI (1754-1793) and was forced to attend in full military dress his execution; he then worked under the French Revolution and the Reign of Terror; he was consultant physician to Napoleon (q.v.) and saw his downfall and the restoration of the Bourbons. Because of his high position he was in contact with all these regimes, yet he managed to remain detached, above intrigues, and courageously faithful to the task of caring for the mentally ill. His distinguished friend and pupil, Jean Esquirol (q.v.), succeeded him and continued his work. Pinel's son, Scipion, and nephew, Casimir also became leading psychiatrists. In 1850, Pinel's treatise on insanity was still so popular that it was copied by hand for the use of physicians in mental hospitals of Lima, Peru.

Bibliography: McKown, R. 1961. *Pioneers in mental health*.

PINELESS, FRIEDRICK (1868-1936). A German physician. He was the

first to distinguish sporadic cretinism from endemic cretinism (q.v.) associated with goiter. His findings were published in 1902.
Bibliography: Schmidt, J. E. 1959. *Medical discoveries: who and when.*

PINE NEEDLE BATHS. Baths (q.v.) in water in which pine needles and cones had been boiled were prescribed in Russian folk medicine for nervous disorders, including insomnia.
Bibliography: Kourennoff, P. M., and St. George, G. 1970. *Russian folk medicine.*

PINEYS. The fictitious name of a family clinically investigated because of the high number of mental defectives among its members. Like other genetic studies of the time, it attempted to demonstrate that mental deficiency was hereditary.
See also EUGENICS.
Bibliography: Kite, E. S. 1913. *The Pineys.*

PINI, PAOLO. A sixteenth-century Italian painter. In 1548 he wrote a book of discussions on art, entitled *Dialogo di Pittura* in which he mentioned melancholia (q.v.) as a common trait among artists. He believed that melancholy was dependent upon the stars but recommended exercise, sport, and good company to combat it.
Bibliography: Wittkower, R., and Wittkower, M. 1963. *Born under Saturn.*

PINNING. The practice of pinning down the body of a suicide (q.v.). It dates from very early times and is mentioned by Cornelius Tacitus (55?-?117 A.D.). The idea was probably to prevent the spirit of the dead from returning to harm the living.
Bibliography: Rosen, S. 1971. History in the study of suicide. *Psychol. Med.* 1: 267-85.

PIRANDELLO, LUIGI (1867-1936). Italian dramatist and novelist. After an initial period of literary activity, a financial crisis forced him to become a teacher. This period of anxiety is said to have caused his wife's mental illness, which in turn had an effect on his work when he returned to writing. His plays and novels present many facets of the human mind, a field which had become popular in literature and in the theatre. His irony alternated with compassion for the solitude of man and the incoherence and instability of society. He saw the world as disintegrating and dominated by formal relationships, laws based on convention, and illusions. As he aged, he became more and more pessimistic and critical of all human actions and thoughts, which he regarded as relative, neither true nor false, rational or irrational, normal or insane. Many of his characters display a kind of "lucid insanity." One of his best-known plays, *Six Characters in Search of an Author* (1922) is of great psychiatric interest; the characters, with no drama, force the actors to create one for them and thus the story of a family beset by guilt and hostility, which leads to death and suicide (q.v.), evolves. The characters are fascinated by the drama but in the end they do not recognize themselves in it.

Bibliography: Guidice, G. 1974. *Pirandello: a biography*, trans. A. Hamilton.

PIRANESI, GIOVANNI BATTISTA (1720-1778). An Italian etcher, draughtsman, and architect. He was a precocious child who was able to draw the architecture of Venice at the age of eight. He was said to be vain and susceptible to flattery. One of his friends, Robert Adam, described him as a difficult man, with a "furious and fantastic expression" and whose "ideas in locution were so ill ranged" that it was difficult to follow his conversation. Piranesi was unpredictable and, at times, truculent. His many controversies are reflected in the number of names erased from title pages and dedications. His unbound imagination (q.v.) and fantastic representations have led to speculations about his mental health. His *Carceri d'Invenzione*, a series of etchings of imaginary prisons, have an hallucinatory (*see* HALLUCINATION) quality reminiscent of drawings of schizophrenics (*see* SCHIZOPHRENIA). They show enormous staircases leading nowhere, gigantic instruments of torture, and human figures dwarfed by the surrounding architectural details.

Bibliography: Samuel, A. 1910. *Piranesi: a critical study of his life and works.*

PIRATA, IL. The second opera (q.v.) by the Italian composer Vincenzo Bellini (c.1802-1835). The pirate Gualtiero is captured and condemned to death. His mistress Imogene becomes mad at the thought of his death and imagines she can see the scaffold on which her lover must die. She begs the sun to conceal itself and not shed light on this tragic scene: "Oh! s'io potessi: Col sorriso d'innocenza (Act. 2).

PISANI, PIETRO (1760-1837). An Italian nobleman and scholar. After the death of his son, he dedicated himself to philanthropic work. In 1824 in Palermo, Sicily, he opened the Real Casa dei Matti (q.v.), a mental hospital in which he introduced many innovations. He also wrote a book of regulations for the hospital in which he outlined a humanitarian program of treatment. "In spite of their mental disorders," he wrote, "patients respond to a frank and sincere approach and are able to experience feelings of confidence, benevolence, friendship and pride." New patients were handed a guide which explained Pisani's methods of treatment and the philosophy upon which they were based.

Bibliography: Pisani, P. 1827. *Istruzioni per la novella Real Casa dei Matti in Palermo.*

PITHIASTISME. A term coined by Josef Babinski (q.v.) from two Greek words meaning "persuasion" and "curable." He used it in place of Jean Martin Charcot's (q.v.) concept of hysteria (q.v.) because he believed that hysterical manifestations could be cured by persuasion without the more drastic measure of hypnotizing (*see* HYPNOTISM) the patient.

Bibliography: Zilboorg, G. 1941. *A history of medical psychology.*

PITRES, JEAN ALBERT (1848-1928). A French physician. He developed techniques for the study of the cortical motor centers. In 1884 he gave the first classic account of agraphia, the loss of the ability to express oneself in writing. In 1895 he published an interesting study on aphasia in polyglots.

Bibliography: McHenry, L. C., ed. 1969. *Garrison's history of neurology.*

PITT, WILLIAM, EARL OF CHATHAM (1708-1778). An English statesman known as the Elder Pitt. He was famous for his brilliant and stormy political career. He suffered from gout, and it is said that the remedies administered to him for this disorder caused him to become insane. He could not hear a child's voice or the lightest allusion to a parliamentary debate without going into a frenzy. From 1767 to 1768 he was so incapacitated that he was unable to continue his political activities. During that period, he was a patient in Bethlem Royal Hospital (q.v.), and spent his days sitting at a table with his head between his hands, not speaking to anyone. He occupied two rooms in the hospital; the anteroom had a small hatch where his servant placed his food and retired. The patient then would open the door to the hatch and remove the food. He returned to political activity in 1770. In 1778, while vehemently protesting in the House of Lords against the withdrawal of English forces from America, he fell backward in a seizure and died a month later.

Bibliography: Ayling, S. 1970. *The Elder Pitt.*

PIUS IV (1499-1565). The name assumed by Giovanni Angelo Medici when he became pope. Unlike others of his time who regarded the insane as sinners, he believed that the insane should be protected, not punished and rejected. In a papal edict dated 1561, he authorized the foundation of a mental hospital in Rome saying that "the poor, in as much as they are deprived of intellect, need a roof over their head, a bed and means for survival" (139. *Bullarium Romanum.* 1561.)

PLACEBO. In medicine, an innocuous substance that may have an effect on the patient through suggestion. It is derived from the first antiphon of

the vespers for the dead, which begins "Placebo Domino in regione vivorum" (I shall be pleasing to the Lord in the land of the living). "Sing placebo" came to mean "be flattering," because those hoping to receive some remunerations from the family of a deceased person would attend the service.
Bibliography: 1978. *Brewer's dictionary of phrase and fable.*

PLANCHETTE. A board employed in the recording of automatic writing during seances. It was devised in the middle of the nineteenth century when trance sessions were fashionable and mediums (q.v.) purported to receive messages from the spirits of the dead. The planchette would rest on a smooth surface or be suspended over it.
Bibliography: Pearsall, R. 1972. *The table-rappers.*

PLANETS. Planets were believed to have special influence on the destiny and character of men. Carrying the names of the Greek gods, each planet was assumed to possess the failings and virtues of its god. In time, these characteristics came to be applied also to men. Certain planets were associated with particular characteristics: Mars was linked to energy and aggression, Jupiter to good health, Mercury to intelligence, and Saturn (q.v.) to melancholia (q.v.). Astrologers (*see* ASTROLOGY) believed the position of the planet in the sky at the time of birth was especially significant. Those born under Saturn were considered particularly prone to mental disorders. These beliefs were widespread in the Middle Ages (q.v.) and even survived until much later.
See also ZODIAC.
Bibliography: Graubard, M. 1953. *Astrology and alchemy.*

PLANTAIN. *Plantago*, a genus of herbaceous plants known and used in medicine since antiquity. One of its species, the weybroed, was considered sacred by the Anglo-Saxons. Plantains are mentioned in most of the old herbals as a remedy for a multitude of ills, including epilepsy (q.v.). To its medico-magical properties was added the supposed power of divination (q.v.).
Bibliography: Grigson, G. 1958. *The Englishman's flora.*

PLATER (*or* PLATTER), FELIX (1536-1614). A Swiss physician and anatomist. He studied medicine at the universities of Montpellier and Paris and traveled widely before settling in Basle. His interest in mental disorders caused him to observe the mentally ill in the dungeons where they were kept. His observations resulted in a system of classification that replaced the one proposed by Paracelsus (q.v.) but remained faithful to the principles of Galen (q.v.). Plater distinguished two types of mental disorders: natural and unnatural. He classified natural disorders according to observable symptoms and listed them as: *mentis imbecilitas* (mental deficiency), *mentis con-*

sternatio (cerebral vascular accidents, epilepsy [q.v.]), *mentis alienatio* (psychosis [q.v.]), and *mentis defatigatio* (sleep disturbances). Unnatural disorders included delusions (q.v.) and hallucinations (q.v.), which he attributed to the devil and claimed should be left to the clergy. In the aetiology of the natural disorders he emphasized heredity, lesions of the brain, rising vapors, poison, excess of blood, humoral imbalance (*see* HUMORAL THEORY), and dryness of the brain. He advised a multitude of remedies, including the lung of a pig, the blood of a tortoise applied to the head, precious stones (q.v.) worn round the neck, purgatives, massage, exercise, persuasion, and threats. For the very disturbed he recommended chains to restrain them. He believed that acute attacks of insanity were linked with particular days of the months or with the seasons. Despite his erroneous beliefs, his work was of great significance because it was the first modern attempt to classify mental disorders systematically and according to the nature of the disease, rather than the part of the body. His *Praxis Medica* (q.v.), published in 1602, was translated into English in 1662 and was followed in 1664 by a translation of his *Observationum Libri Tres*, which contains psychiatric case histories. Robert Burton (q.v.) frequently cited him.
Bibliography: Diethelm, O., and Heffernan, T. 1965. Felix Platter and psychiatry. *J. Hist. Behav. Sci.* 1: 10-23.

PLATH, SYLVIA (1932-1963). An American poet. Her first poems were published when she was eight years old. After her father's death when she was nine years old, her mother made enormous sacrifices to give her a good education. Although she achieved academic success, she became desperately depressed and attempted suicide (q.v.). She described her feelings of disintegration and her fear of and fascination with schizophrenia (q.v.) in a novel entitled *The Bell Jar* (1962). She married, but her depression increased following a miscarriage and general poor health. Thoughts of death were never far from her mind. She constantly mourned her father and even the birth of her children did not bring a reconciliation to life. Her poems, like "Death & Co.," invoked death. She committed suicide in London by gassing herself.
Bibliography: Butscher, E. 1977. *Sylvia Plath: method and madness.*

PLATNER, ERNST (1744-1818). A German physician, anthropologist and philosopher. He believed that each separate organ is imbued with its own vital force, or soul.
Bibliography: Zilboorg, G. 1941. *A history of medical psychology.*

PLATO (427-347 B.C.). A Greek philosopher, a disciple of Socrates (q.v.) and admirer of Hippocrates (q.v.). He held clear views on the brain, soul and mind. Like his contemporaries, he believed that the brain was of the same nature as the bone marrow. He placed the immortal soul in the head and endowed it with three qualities: intelligence, science, and true opinion. The mortal part of the soul he seated in the thorax and desires in the neighborhood of the umbilicus. His attitude to disease was governed by the humoral theory (q.v.), but he suggested that mental disorders were partially somatic, partially moral, and partially divine in origin. Referring to the types of mental disorder he wrote:

But disease of the soul resulting from the habit of the body, are as follows: we must admit that disease of the soul is folly, or privation of intellect; and there are two kinds of folly, the one madness and the other ignorance! [Timaeus.]

In *Alcibiades*, he offered a classification of diseases arising from the body, or natural conditions: (1) mania (q.v.), (2) stupor or dementia, (3) imbecility. In addition to natural madness, he recognized a divine madness arising from great trouble or from the Muses. He advocated a mixture of psychotherapeutics, incantations (q.v.), and drugs (q.v.). The doctor-patient relationship was given due importance:

But the doctor. . .enters into discussion with his patient, and is at once getting information and also instructing him: at last, when he has brought the patient more and more under his persuasive influences, and set him on the road to health, he attempts to effect a cure. [*Laws.*]

And therefore if the head and body are to be well, you must begin by curing the soul; that is the first thing. And the cure, my dear youth, has to be effected by the use of certain charms, and these charms are fair words; and by them temperance is implanted in the soul, and where temperance is, there health is speedily imparted, not only to the head, but to the whole body. [*The Charmides.*]

He interpreted dreams (q.v.) and believed that they were expressions of the mind's frustrated desires. He also believed that a patient who was not responsible for his behavior, should not be punished, but should be required to pay for whatever damage he had caused. He claimed that relatives should care for the insane and be fined if they failed in their duties. He viewed crime as the product of adverse childhood circumstances and not a matter of wilful misbehavior. He also believed that emotion and desire dominate all men, with the possible exception of philosophers, and that intrapsychic harmony based on reason was necessary to control primitive impulses. Social order should have as its objective the fulfilment of needs and the opportunity for all men to realize their potentiality. To protect the state, Plato felt that those affected by incurable diseases ought not to be allowed to live. All his writings have been preserved, although their chronological order has remained a matter for debate.

Bibliography: Taylor, A. E. 1960. *Plato: the man and his work.*

PLATONIC LOVE. Spiritual love without sensual desire between members of the opposite sex. Marsilio Ficino (q.v.) was probably the first to use the term, but he used it to refer to love between men.

Bibliography: 1933. *Oxford English dictionary.*

PLINY THE ELDER (GAIUS PLINIUS SECUNDUS) (A.D. 23-79). A Roman naturalist. His lifelong observations were collected into a volume entitled *Historia Naturalis.* Twelve books of it are concerned with medicine. The work contains many items of psychiatric interest. Among other things, it mentioned the belief that henbane (q.v.), used as a remedy for earache, could cause mental disorders if poured in the ear. This belief is also found in *Hamlet* by William Shakespeare (q.v.). For melancholia (q.v.) Pliny advised, among other remedies, calf's dung boiled in wine. He referred to the soporific effects of the juice of poppy seeds and also warned against its abuse. To rouse those fallen into a coma he suggested the fumes of burnt goat's hair or horn. Descriptions of epilepsy (q.v.) and the mental disorders caused by fauni (q.v.) are given, as well as a description of the application of electric eels (*see* ELECTROICHTHYOLOGY) to the head for the treatment of intractable headaches. Pliny believed that man is superior to other creatures through his ability to reason and had the right to take his own life if he so wished. His curiosity about all natural phenomena cost him his life, as he was suffocated by the sulphurous fumes of Vesuvius, when he observed its eruption too closely. His works were read throughout the Middle Ages (q.v.) and, when printing was invented, went through some eighty editions. Their influence unfortunately perpetuated many errors for a long time.

Bibliography: Pliny. *Natural History.* 10 vols. Trans. H. Rackham, W.H.S. Jones, and D. E. Eichholz.

PLOTINUS (c.204-269). A Greek philosopher born in Egypt. He was the author of fifty-four treatises under the general title of *Enneads* that covered a number of subjects including psychology. According to him reason is an uncertain source of knowledge. Furthermore, ecstasy (q.v.) and absolute unity cannot be fully understood and explained by man. Plotinus believed in a form of mysticism above the reality of the senses. He felt that the study of mental activity was the only logical method of understanding the soul.

Bibliography: Rich, A.N.M. 1963. Body and soul in the philosophy of Plotinus. *J. Hist. Philosophy* 1: 1-15.

PLUTARCH (A.D. c. 46-120). A Greek philosopher and historian. Of great interest to psychiatry is his *Parallel Lives* in which he gave pen portraits of various individuals and displayed their characters in revealing details, words, or actions. He was not a physician but was conscious of the issues raised by mental disorders. He gave an accurate clinical description of the emotional disorder in a man affected by religious melancholia (q.v.):

To such a man every little evil is magnified by the scaring spectres of his anxiety. He looks on himself as a man whom the gods hate and pursue with their anger. A far worse lot is before him; he dares not employ any means of averting or of remedying the evil, lest he be found fighting against the gods. The physician, the consoling friend, is driven away. "Leave me," says the wretched man, "me the impious, the accursed, hated of the gods, to suffer my punishment." He sits out of doors, wrapped in sackcloth or in filthy rags. Ever and anon he rolls himself, naked, in the dirt confessing about this and that sin. He has eaten or drunk something wrong; he has gone some way or other which the Divine Being did not approve of. The festivals in honor of the gods give no pleasure to him, but fill him rather with fear and affright. He proves in his own case the saying of Pythagoras to be false, that we are happiest when we approach the gods, for it is just then that he is most wretched. Temples and altars are places of refuges for the persecuted; but where all others find deliverance from their fears, there this wretched man most fears and trembles. Asleep or awake, he is haunted alike by the spectres of his anxiety. Awake, he makes no use of his reason; and asleep, he enjoys no respite from his alarms. His reason always slumbers; his fears are awake. Nowhere can he find an escape from his imaginary terrors.

Bibliography: Turner, P., ed. 1963. *Plutarch's lives.*

PNEUMA. For the Greeks pneuma represented breath, or air. Hippocrates (q.v.) believed that the pneuma reached the brain through the mouth and was involved with the process of thinking and feeling. He believed that all organs were permeated with the pneuma, which was necessary for the maintenance of life. Galen (q.v.) thought that the pneuma became natural spirit, which promoted growth, vital spirit, which promoted movement, and animal spirit, which promoted thought. According to him plants had only natural spirit, animals had vital spirit, and man had all three.

Bibliography: Watson, R. I. 1963. *The great psychologists.*

POBOUH LANG. A West African illness. Its symptoms are compulsive geophagia, pallor, weakness, edema, depression, anxiety, and social isolation. Some features of the illness probably are related to nutritional deficiencies, but others may depend on cultural attitudes and social pressure.

Bibliography: Beiser, M., et al. 1974. Pobouh Lang in Senegal. *Soc. Psychiat.* 9: 123-29.

PODMORE, FRANK (1855-1910). An English writer on psychical phenomena. He believed that many phenomena attributed to spiritualistic (*see* SPIRITUALISM) causes could be explained in terms of psychological theories.

He was one of the founders of the Fabian Society and is believed to have suggested its name.

Bibliography: Tinterow, M. M. 1970. *Foundations of hypnosis: from Mesmer to Freud.*

POE, EDGAR ALLAN (1809-1849). An American poet and writer. His father was Scots-Irish and his mother English. His only sister was a mental defective and his brother an alcoholic (*see* ALCOHOLISM). Orphaned when he was three years old, he was adopted by a wealthy merchant, John Allen (1780-1834). His adolescent love of gambling and drinking caused frequent quarrels with his foster father. He ran away from home when he was eighteen years old and started to write poetry. A reconciliation with his foster father lasted for only one year. He became addicted to opium (q.v.), which he took to relieve recurrent attacks of depression. At twenty-six, he married his thirteen-year-old frail and delicate cousin, who died of tuberculosis (q.v.) ten years later. As an alcoholic he was unable to resist drink, which gave him a respite from his depression. By nineteenth-century standards, he was considered highly-strung, nervous, and suffering from what was then called "moral insanity" (q.v.). Paranoid (*see* PARANOIA) delusions made it difficult for him to continue publishing the journal he had bought. In 1848, he tried to commit suicide (q.v.) by drinking laudanum (q.v.). He survived this attempt but died shortly after of cerebral edema brought about by alcoholism. His writings are famous for their weird and fantastic content. Impressed by magnetism (q.v.), he wrote *The Facts in the Case of Mr. Valdemar* (1845) in which he related how the spirit of a dying man was kept in his body through the practices of a magnetizer.

Bibliography: Symons, J. 1978. *The tell-tale heart: The life and works of Edgar Allan Poe.*

POEM OF THE RIGHTEOUS SUFFERER. The title given to a Babylonian document probably written by a mental patient. All the priestly writings in it have Sumerian titles and deal with delirium (q.v.), loss of libido (q.v.), projection, delusion (q.v.), and depression as well as other emotional problems.

Bibliography: Kinnier Wilson, J. V. 1967. Mental diseases of ancient Mesopotamia. In *Diseases in antiquity*, ed. D. Brothwell and A. T. Sandison.

POLICRATES (535-513 B.C.) A tyrant of Samos. He was so successful in all things that he feared the envy of the gods. To appease them he threw a precious ring that he treasured into the sea. The ring, however, was restored to him during a meal in the stomach of a fish he was preparing to eat. His guests regarded this as a bad omen, as the gods had returned his sacrifice, and immediately left him. He faced his punishment alone. He met death by crucifixion. Johann Schiller (q.v.) wrote a poem about this episode, *The*

Ring of Policrates. In psychiatry the term "Policrates complex" was suggested by J. C. Flugel in 1945 to indicate those individuals who are afraid of their success and anxiously anticipate a reversal of fortunes.
Bibliography: Flugel, J. C. 1945. *Man, morals, and society.*

POLISH PSYCHIATRIC ASSOCIATION. The official professional body of Polish psychiatrists. It was founded in 1920 and its first president was Witol Chodzko. It published a number of journals including, *Psychiatric Annals* (1923-1939), *Psychiatric Hygiene,* and *Psychiatria Polska.*
Bibliography: 1968. *World Psychiatric Association Bulletin,* Winter: 25-26.

POLLICH VON MELLERSTADT, MARTIN (?-1513). A German physician. He was the author of an early work on syphilis (q.v.). He was torn between science and religious ideas and solved the dilemma by attributing mental illness to just punishment sent by God to those who had sinned. Sinful thought and actions he accepted as originating in the brain, but he thought that a more virtuous way of life could be encouraged by the right diet (q.v.).
Bibliography: Zilboorg, G. 1941. *A history of medical psychology.*

POLTERGEIST. A term derived from two Greek words meaning noise and spirit. The term was coined in the nineteenth century, when interest in spiritistic manifestations was at its peak. It was believed that the poltergeist was a spirit that particularly enjoyed throwing things about to annoy and startle people.
Bibliography: Peasall, R. 1972. *The table-rappers.*

POLYGAMY. A marriage in which either spouse may have more than one mate. Polygamous marriages were expressly recognized in the Old Testament (Deut. 21: 15), and there is no direct condemnation of them in the New Testament. Some of the Merovingian kings, for example, Clotaire I, Childibert I, and Pepin I, although Christian, were polygamous, and the church did not oppose their practices.
Bibliography: Cairncross, J. 1974. *After polygamy was made a sin: the social history of Christian polygamy.*

POLYPSYCHISM. A term coined by Joseph P. Durand de Gros (q.v.) to indicate his theory that the human body was divided into anatomical segments. Each section, according to him, had its own psyche (q.v.), which was subject to a general psychic ego, the conscious. All the subegos together constituted the unconscious (q.v.). According to Durand de Gros, it was possible that on some occasions, for example, during hypnosis (*see* HYP-

NOTISM) or anesthesia, only a few of the subegos were involved in psychic activity.
Bibliography: Ellenberger, H. F. 1970. *The discovery of the unconscious.*

POMBO, RAFAEL (1833-1912). A Colombian poet, who spent many years in the United States. From his adolescence on, he experienced periods of deep depression. In his twenties he wrote poems under the pseudonym of Edda. They were so feminine in content that his readers were easily convinced that he was a woman. He was excessively dependent on his mother and his habits were very childish. His house was so crammed with art objects, books, and papers that it was difficult to move from one room to the other. He spent two decades in this disorder, usually in bed, deteriorating physically and mentally. His best known poem is *Hora de Tinieblas.*
Bibliography: Rosselli, H. 1968. *Historia de la psiquiatria en Colombia.*

POMPADOUR, JEANNE ANTOINETTE POISSON, MARQUISE DE (1721-1764). The mistress of the French king Louis XV (q.v.). Despite an almost perfect relationship with her royal lover, she was said to be frigid. She tried to remedy this by taking elixirs and submitting to a diet of vanilla, truffles, and celery, all of which were said to "heat the blood." Although she longed to have a child by the king, her pregnancies ended in spontaneous abortions. A sufferer of insomnia, poor health often confined her to bed with fevers and attacks of asthma, probably of psychogenic origin.
Bibliography: Mitford, N. 1954. *Madame de Pompadour.*

POMPANAZZI, PIETRO (POMPONATIUS) (1462-1525). An Italian philosopher and physician. He followed the teachings of both Aristotle (q.v.) and Averröes (q.v.) and was intrigued by the relationship of mind and body. He believed that the mind could not function without the physical equipment of the body but then asserted that reason could exist independently. In his *De Immortalitate Animi* (1516), he wrote that only those phenomena that he could understand through personal experience were of interest to him. As he could not hope to understand the soul, which was outside the perception of the senses, it was of no concern to him. His writings bear witness to the fact that hypnotic (*see* HYPNOTISM) phenomena and practices similar to psychotherapy (q.v.) were known in his time. He believed that lycanthropy (q.v.) was a clinical entity.
Bibliography: Alexander, F. G., and Selesnick, S. T. 1966. *The history of psychiatry.*

PONTIUS PILATE (fl. 1st century A.D.). The Roman procurator of Judea who tried Jesus Christ. The province grew restless under his rigid and rapacious rule and in 36 A.D. he was called by the emperor Tiberius (42 B.C.-A.D. 37) to explain his conduct. According to the church historian

Eusebius of Caesarea (260?-?340) he committed suicide (q.v.), overcome by guilt.

Bibliography: Franzero, C. M. 1945. *The memoirs of Pontius Pilate.*

PONTORMO, JACOPO DA (1494-1556). An Italian painter. He began painting at the age of eleven and was a pupil of Piero di Cosimo (q.v.). The death of his parents while he was still a child may have contributed to his personality disorders. He was a hypochondriac (*see* HYPOCHONDRIA) and an obsessional (*see* OBSESSION). He left a diary recording his smallest indispositions and the remedies he used to combat them. Giorgio Vasari (1511-1574) described Pontormo as an eccentric and solitary man. To reach his bedroom he had a ladder, which he would pull up after him so that no one could follow him. Vasari further noted that "he was so afraid of death that he could not bear to hear it mentioned, and he fled from the sight of corpses. He never went to festivals, or to any place where people gathered, so as not to be caught in the crowd; and he was solitary beyond belief."

Bibliography: Wittkower, R., and Wittkower, M. 1963. *Born under Saturn* .

POPPY. *See* OPIUM.

PORK. In medieval England it was believed that eating the marrow of pork bones would cause madness.

Bibliography: 1973. *The Reader's Digest folklore myths and legends of Britain.*

PORPHYRIA. A metabolic disorder. Its symptoms include mental derangement. The term is derived from the Greek word meaning purple and is a reference to the color of the urine in those suffering from porphyria. A study conducted by Ida Macalpine and Richard Hunter in 1969 has traced the path of the disease in the descendants of Mary, Queen of Scots, among whom are James I of England and VI of Scotland, George III, and Frederick the Great of Prussia (qq.v.).

Bibliography: Macalpine, I., and Hunter, R. 1969. *George III and the mad-business.*

PORTA, GIOVANNI BATTISTA DELLA (1535-1615). An Italian scientist, philosopher, and dramatist, born in Naples. He was the chief exponent of physiognomy (q.v.), which he tried to elevate to a science. In his *De Humana Physiognomia* (1586) he compared the facial features of men to those of animals and then related them to moral characteristics.

Bibliography: Porta, G. B. Della, 1586. *De humana physiognomia.*

PORTMANTEAU WORD. A term invented by Lewis Carroll (q.v.). In *Through the Looking Glass* (1872) he explained a portmanteau word as a word that included two meanings closely combined, or "packed" into it.

In psychiatry portmanteau words are often found in the vocabulary of schizophrenics (see SCHIZOPHRENIA); for example, "steamsail" blends the idea of a steamship and a sailing ship.

POSEIDONIUS. A Byzantine writer and physician of the fourth century A.D.. He paid special attention to functional damage after brain injury and related the area of the injury to the loss of sensory perception, memory (q.v.), or reason, among other things. He recognized the following mental disorders: phrenitis (q.v.), carus (sleeping sickness), coma, lethargus (stupor), vertigo, incubus (q.v.), nightmares (q.v.), epilepsy (q.v.), melancholia (q.v.), and mania (q.v.).
Bibliography: Menninger, M. A. et al. 1977. *The vital balance; the life process in mental health and illness.*

POSITIVISM. A philosophical approach devised by Auguste Comte (q.v.). The term referred to phenomena immediately observable, basic, and undebatable, as opposed to inferences and speculations.
Bibliography: Fletcher, R. 1966. *Auguste Comte and the making of sociology.*

POSSESSION. The occupancy of a human being by supernatural power. In the past, aggressive and destructive behavior, frenzy, trance, paralysis, or any condition that could not be explained and attributed to natural causes was believed to be the result of possession. Possessions could be of two kinds: one destructive and causing harm to the possessed, and the other beneficial and an honor accorded to those who were chosen by the gods to reveal their wishes or predict coming events. The belief caused the mentally ill to be regarded with fear or respect, depending upon whether their "possession" was viewed as punishment or privilege. Although classic Greek literature offers many examples of mortals possessed by an offended divinity and driven to perform dreadful deeds against others or themselves, it also includes the possessions of the oracles (q.v.). Epilepsy (q.v.) was known as the "sacred disease" because it was believed to be the result of divine possession. In early Christian times, demoniac possessions (q.v.) often were considered responsible for physical and mental illness, and exorcism (q.v.) was used to bring about a cure. The belief still persists in some primitive cultures, and magic (q.v.) ceremonies are performed by the healer, who is frequently believed to be possessed himself, to free the sick individual from the evil spirits that are causing the illness.
Bibliography: Sargeant, W. 1973. *Mind possessed: physiology of possession, mysticism, and faith healing.*

POSTPARTUM PSYCHOSIS. Depression following childbirth. As a clinical syndrome it was first described by Charles Lepois (q.v.) in the sixteenth

century. He believed that the mental disorders he observed in women who had given birth recently were due to an excess of dark humors (q.v.).
Bibliography: Galdston, I. 1967. *Historic derivations of modern psychiatry.*

POTABLE GOLD. Also called *aqua mirabilis*, it was believed to be an elixir of life that would confer immortal youth and cure all diseases, including insanity, amnesia (q.v.), and depression. The search for it was linked with the idea of the transmutation of metals. It was most popular in the seventeenth century.
Bibliography: Garrison, F. H. 1929. *An introduction to the history of medicine.*

POUND, EZRA LOOMIS (1885-1972). An American poet, critic, and translator. In 1924 he settled in Italy and became a vocal supporter of fascism. After World War II, he was taken back to the United States and tried for treason, but he was found to be mentally unfit to answer the charges. He was admitted to Saint Elizabeth's Hospital (q.v.) in Washington, D.C. In 1958 he was adjudicated sane and released. He had an illegitimate daughter, Mary, by Olga Rudge, the violinist who was his constant companion. Neither parent had any idea of how to raise a child. Mary was placed with foster parents, a peasant family in northern Italy, and throughout her childhood shuttled between foster and natural parents. At the end of the war, she married a Russian-Italian nobleman, the Prince de Rachewiltz. Her biographical recollections provide insight into the life of her father and make more comprehensible much of his more obscure poetry.
Bibliography: Rachewiltz, Mary de. 1971. *Discretions.*

POWNALL, JAMES (fl. 1853-1859). An English physician and the proprietor of an asylum (q.v.) known as Northfield House in Wiltshire. In 1853, prior to acquiring Northfield House, he had suffered several attacks of mania (q.v.) and had been a mental patient in various asylums. The commissioners in lunacy (q.v.) reported his mismanagement of the establishment after they had found that he had shot a patient. Northfield House was closed down, and Pownall was sent to Northwoods Asylum in Gloucestershire. His state did not improve, and, in 1859, he murdered a girl by slashing her throat with a razor.
Bibliography: Parry-Jones, W. Ll. 1972. *The trade in lunacy.*

PRAGMATISM. A doctrine that asserts that the value of ideas must be measured in their practical consequences upon human purposes and interests. Its foremost supporter and organizer was William James (q.v.), who wrote two books on this subject, *Pragmatism* (1907) and *The Meaning of Truth* (1909).
Bibliography: Ayer, A. J. 1968. *The origin of pragmatism.*

PRAISE OF FOLLY, THE. The English translation of *Encomium Moriae*, a satire by Desiderius Erasmus (q.v.). In this work Erasmus regarded mad-

ness as the essence of reason and truth; the medical profession was criticized and derided, and theologians were attacked. The book was written at the suggestion of Sir Thomas More (q.v.).
Bibliography: Kaiser, W. 1963. *On the problem of "folly" in the Renaissance: praisers of folly.*

PRANA. An oriental concept discussed in the Ayur-Veda (q.v.). It is identical to the pneuma (q.v.) of Hippocrates (q.v.) in that prana was believed to pervade all organs of the body, reach the brain, and serve as the source of thought and feelings.
Bibliography: Keith, A. B. 1925. *Religion and philosophy of the Vedas.*

PRAXIS MEDICA. A book written by Felix Plater (q.v.) in 1602. It was the first seventeenth-century medical textbook to discuss in detail mental disorders and their aetiology, course, treatment, and classification.
Bibliography: Diethelm, O., and Heffernan, T. 1965. Felix Platter and psychiatry. *J. Hist. Behav. Sci.* 1: 10-23.

PRECIOUS STONES. In ancient times gems were used in medicine for diagnosis and therapy. They were regarded as particularly pure substances because of the long, gradual process of purification and crystallization that resulted in their formation. Originally they were worn to ward off evil influences. The Chinese believed that pearls were obtained from the brains of dragons. Paracelsus (q.v.) believed that gems gave off special radiations in the form of light, heat, and energy. A sick person's reaction to a particular stone was a clue to his disorder; thus agate (q.v.) , for example, made epileptics (*see* EPILEPSY) uncomfortable. Red coral (q.v.) was efficacious against melancholia (q.v.). Robert Burton (q.v.) in his *Anatomy of Melancholy* (q.v.) wrote at length about the relationship between certain precious stones and mental disorders. According to him garnets (q.v.) and topaz (q.v.) would "allay anger, grief, diminish madness, much delight and exhilarate the mind"; he quoted Girolamo Cardano (q.v.) as having cured many madmen with such stones and added other examples from the past. Many superstitions were associated with precious stones; opals (q.v.) in particular were believed to bring bad luck.
See also AGATE, AMBER, AMETHYST, ARMENIAN STONE, BERYL, CRYSTAL, DIAMOND, EMERALD, GALACTITE, GARNET, JACINTH, JASPER, JET, LAPIS LAZULI, ONYX, RUBY, SAPPHIRE, SARDONYX, SELENITE, SMARAGDUS, AND TOPAZ.
Bibliography: Evans, J. 1922. *Magical jewels.*

PRECOCITY. According to Cesare Lombroso (q.v.), precocity is a characteristic shared by genius (q.v.) and insanity. He quoted the examples of Dante Alighieri, Michelangelo, Johann Wolfgang von Goethe, and Ludwig von Beethoven (qq.v.). He added that children of insane parents are often

precocious and recalled the proverb, "A man who has genius at five is mad at fifteen."
Bibliography: Lombroso, C. 1891. *Man of genius.*

PRECORDIAL ANXIETY. Anxiety producing cardiac symptoms. The term was first introduced in medicine in the nineteenth century by Carl F. Flemming (q.v.).
Bibliography: Flemming, C. F. 1859. *Pathologie und therapie der psychosen.*

PREISWERK, HÉLÈNE. The eleventh child of Rudolph Preiswerk, the maternal uncle of Carl G. Jung (q.v.). As an adolescent Hélène Preiswerk was a medium (q.v.) and was subject to fits of somnambulism (q.v.). Jung, who was then twenty-three years old, performed many experiments with her and took copious notes, which he later used in his medical dissertation.
Bibliography: Brome, V. 1978. *Jung: man and myth.*

PREISWERK, SAMUEL (1799-1871). A Swiss theologian, the maternal grandfather of Carl G. Jung (q.v.). After the death of his first wife by whom he had one child, he married again and had thirteen more children. He was said to have visions, during which he would talk with invisible beings who, according to him, appeared behind him when he was writing sermons. To protect his writings from them, he made his daughter sit behind him. He kept a special chair in his study for the spirit of his first wife whose weekly visits were a source of great annoyance to his second wife. She, however, had her own special qualities in the form of "second sight".
Bibliography: Jung, C. G. 1962. *Erinnerungen, Träume, Gedanken.*

PREPSYCHOTIC PERSONALITY. The basic premorbid personality of an individual. The first clinical description of prepsychotic personality traits probably was provided by Aretaeus (q.v.), who wrote that those who become "furious" or "manic" are usually prone to violent outbursts, have superficial feelings, and are childish, while those who become "melancholic" (*see* MELANCHOLIA) show early signs of depression.
Bibliography: Trélat, U. 1839. *Recherches historiques sur la folie.*

PRÉVOST, EUGENE MARCEL (1862-1941). A French novelist. His writings reflect the nineteenth-century preoccupation with psychological problems. His novel *Le Jardin Secret* (1897) concerns a woman who acquires a new personality when she marries. After some years she finds the diary she kept as a young girl, and, reading it, she discovers her previous personality. She then reevaluates her life and her present behavior. Another novel, *The Autumn of a Woman* (1893), tells the story of a young man, Maurice, who has an affair with a frustrated, middle-aged woman whose deep religious feelings cause her to feel guilt stricken. Her daughter Claire

is in love with Maurice and does not want to marry the steady, older gentleman chosen for her. Claire's depression develops into a serious psychosomatic illness, and she is treated by a Dr. Daumier, who is modeled on Pierre Janet (q.v.). The insightful physician discovers the situation, treats the whole group, and rearranges the psychic forces. Maurice marries Claire, her mother is sent to confession, and the older gentleman is advised to become a priest.
Bibliography: Prévost, E. M. 1893. *L'automne d'une femme.*

PREYER, WILHELM THIERRY (1841-1897). A German physiologist and psychologist, born in England. He studied in Bonn and in Paris with Claude Bernard (q.v.), before becoming professor of physiology at Jena and then in Berlin. His main field of study was that of child development and behavior, and his work is considered the beginning of modern child psychology (q.v.). His account of the development of early functions was based on his systematic observations of his son from birth to the age of three. Preyer's interest extended also into the field of color vision, hearing, and hypnotism (q.v.). Gustav Fechner (q.v.) and Wilhelm Wundt (q.v.) were his friends.
Bibliography: Preyer, W. T. 1882. *The mind of the child.*

PRIAPUS. A god of fertility in Greek mythology (q.v.). Representing the natural generative force, he was believed to be the son of Dionysus (q.v.) and Aphrodite. Shepherds, fishermen, and farmers worshipped him. He was symbolized by a phallus (q.v.). His cult eventually degenerated, and he was later represented as a misshapen, short, fat man with enormous genitals. His comical statue was placed in gardens to protect the plants and scare off the birds.
Bibliography: Herter, H. 1932. *De priapo.*

PRICE, WILLIAM (1800-1893). A Welsh physician, the son of a clergyman who was said to have been periodically insane. Price believed that he was a direct descendent of the Druids and dressed in what he thought was their garb, which he adapted to be as decorative and colorful as possible. On moonlight nights he would dance naked and chanting incantations (q.v.) on a hill overlooking the town of Pontypridd. He was against formal marriage and believed in free love, which provided him with a number of fertile liaisons. When he was eighty-four years old he became the father of a boy who died at the age of five months. Price would not entrust the child's body for burial by the clergy and burned it on a pyre. His action aroused great hostility, and he was arrested but subsequently acquitted. He left instructions for a similar disposal of his own body after death. He is regarded as the pioneer of the practice of cremation in modern times.
Bibliography: Nicholas, I. A. 1972. *Llantrisant Welsh heretic: Dr. William Price.*

PRICHARD, JAMES COWLES (1786-1848). A Scottish physician. His parents were Quakers (q.v.). His early education, which he received at home, included foreign languages, a dominant interest of his for the remainder of his life. Despite opposition from his father, he became a physician after writing a thesis entitled *De Generis Humani Varietate*. He later expanded it into five volumes entitled *Natural History of Man* (1843). In 1812 he became physician to Saint Peter's Hospital (q.v.) in Bristol, where he came into contact with a number of psychiatric patients. He was an enthusiastic supporter of bleeding (q.v.) and purging (q.v.). His work in psychiatry, which was influenced heavily by French writers, is contained in three books: *A Treatise on Diseases of the Nervous System* (1822), *A Treatise on Insanity* (1835) and *Different Forms of Insanity in Relation to Jurisprudence* (1842). In this last book he introduced the term "moral insanity" to describe a new concept in medico-legal practice that became extremely important. Prichard was even more eminent in ethnology and anthropology than in psychiatry. His home in Bristol was a meeting place for the intellectuals of the time. He was happily married; his ten children left him time not only for hard work, but also for much social activity. In 1845 he was appointed one of the commissioners in lunacy (q.v.).

Bibliography: Leigh, D. 1955. James Cowles Prichard, M.D., 1786-1848. *Proc. Roy. Soc. Med.* 48: 586-90.

PRICHARD, THOMAS OCTAVIUS (1808-1847). A British psychiatrist. He was the first medical superintendent of the Northampton General Lunatic Asylum (q.v.), where he implemented the practice of nonrestraint. Among his patients was the poet John Clare (q.v.).

PRICKERS. Assistants who accompanied the inquisitors (*see* INQUISITION) in their search for heretics. Their function was to prick suspected persons in various parts of the body to see whether or not the devil had made them insensitive to pain. Hysterical anesthesia (q.v.), therefore, could cost a person his life.

Bibliography: Veith, I. 1965. *Hysteria: the history of a disease.*

PRICKLY LETTUCE. *Lactuca scariola*, a plant that grows wild in Pakistan, where it is used as a sedative and as a hypnotic. The Anglo-Saxons cultivated a similar plant which was known to them as sleepworth (*Lactuca virosa*), a reference to its narcotic properties. The Chinese prepare a liquid, which they call *Ku-chin-kan*, from its milky juice and use it in the treatment of insomnia.

Bibliography: Leyel, C. F. 1949. *Hearts-ease.*

PRIESTS. The physicians of antiquity were priests; examples are found in the literature of ancient Babylonia, of India, of Greece and of most primitive cultures. They treated physical and mental afflictions that were blamed on evil spirits and often were mentally ill. Their hallucinations (q.v.)

were believed to be revelations from the gods, who would guide them in diagnosis and therapy. Early Christian priests also claimed to heal patients through divine intervention and these miraculous cures form part of the traditional literature of Christianity.

Bibliography: Alexander, F. G., and Selesnick, S. T. 1966. *The history of psychiatry*.

PRIG, BETSEY. The disreputable nurse in *Martin Chuzzlewit* (1843-1844) by Charles Dickens (q.v.). She had nursed "many lunacies, and well she knows their ways."

Bibliography: Dickens, C. 1843-44. *Martin Chuzzlewit*.

PRINCE, MORTON (1854-1929). An American psychiatrist and neurologist. After receiving his medical degree from Harvard Medical School, he studied in Europe with Pierre Janet, Ambroise-August Liebeault, Hippolyte-Marie Bernheim, and Jean Martin Charcot (qq.v.). On his return to Boston he became a physician of nervous disorders at a number of hospitals. His special interests were hysteria (q.v.), multiple personality, and hallucinations (q.v.). He developed his own concepts about these disorders and modified some of Janet's ideas, as well as some of Sigmund Freud's (q.v.) teachings. Prince believed mental illness was caused by a number of factors that cause dissociation and conflict. He felt therapy should try to resolve conflict and substitute for it a new dynamic integration of the personality. His account of the case of Christine Beauchamp (q.v.) exemplified these theories. He treated her with his own brand of psychotherapy (q.v.), which included hypnotism (q.v.). In 1906 he founded the *Journal of Abnormal Psychology*, and he served as editor of it until his death. At the beginning of World War I, he wrote a book entitled *The Psychology of the Kaiser* (1915), which was used extensively in anti-German propaganda. In 1927 he founded the Harvard Psychological Clinic, which was dedicated to the study of abnormal and dynamic psychology.

Bibliography: Prince, M. 1906. *Dissociation of personality*.

PRINCESSE DE CLÈVES, LA. A novel by Madame de La Fayette (1634-1693) written in 1678. It describes life at the court of Henry II (1519-1559) of France and the love of the duke of Nemours for the princess of Clèves. It is considered one of the earliest psychological novels and remains a subtle study of the emotions.

Bibliography: Madame de la Fayette. 1678. *La Princesse de Clèves*.

PRINGLE, SIR JOHN (1707-1782). A Scottish physician greatly influenced by Hermann Boerhaave (q.v.) during his training at the University of Leyden. Pringle served in the British army in Europe in the struggle against France and worked strenuously to make the treatment of soldiers and prisoners more humane through the work of neutral groups, forerunners

of the Red Cross. He is considered the founder of modern military medicine. He was interested in mental disorders, especially melancholia (q.v.), which he firmly associated with black bile (q.v.). He was president of the Royal Society (q.v.) and physician to George III (q.v.).
Bibliography: Pettigrew, T. J. 1840. *Medical portrait gallery*. Vol. 2.

PRINGLE, JOHN JAMES (1855-1922). A British dermatologist. He contributed to the clinical understanding of some forms of mental deficiency. In 1890, expanding the description given by Friedrich D. von Recklinghausen (q.v.), he presented a case of congenital *adenoma sebaceum* (q.v.), later more commonly known as tuberous sclerosis (q.v.).
Bibliography: Pringle, J. J. 1890. A case of congenital adenoma sebaceum. *Brit. J. Dermatol.* 2: 1-14.

PRIORY IN BARNWELL. An Augustinian monastery in England. During the Middle Ages (q.v.), it made special provisions for those members who became ill because of the stresses of monastic life. It provided them with a period of rest that included exercise in the open air and a wholesome diet (q.v.).
See also MONASTERIES.
Bibliography: Clarke, J. W. 1897. *Observances of Priory of Barnwell*.

PRISON CLINICS. The first prison psychiatric clinic was established in the United States at Sing Sing State Prison in Ossining, New York, following a project begun in 1917 to elucidate the incidence of mental conditions among prisoners. The project was sponsored by the National Committee for Mental Hygiene and was directed by Dr. Bernard Glueck. Research conducted by the clinic resulted in a better classification of prisoners and in special institutions for certain classes of criminals.
Bibliography: Deutsch, A. 1949. *The mentally ill in America*.

PRIVATE MADHOUSES. Privately owned madhouses established for the care of the more prosperous mentally ill. They were common in Britain in the eighteenth century, although earlier examples can be found at the beginning of the seventeenth century. Some of these madhouses provided board and lodgings only and were known as "free houses" (q.v.). Often the same family owned several establishments and remained involved in their operation for generations as the licence could be transferred to a relative. Although some establishments accepted a number of insane paupers, others, such as Dunnington House, restricted their clientele to "persons of distinction." A few private madhouses were used by the government for the confinement of the criminally insane. In 1774 the government established legal provisions for their regulation. They were subjected to regular inspections that determined the renewal of their license. Despite these in-

spections, an official investigation held in 1877 revealed some irregularities, especially in regard to the wrongful detention of patients, who were unlawfully deprived of personal liberty. Fishponds Private Lunatic Asylum (q.v.), near Bristol, and Brooke House (q.v.), in Clapton, London, are examples of early private madhouses in Britain.
See also ASYLUMS.
Bibliography: Parry-Jones, W. L. 1972. The trade in lunacy.

PROBATIONARY ASYLUM. A type of preventive establishment advocated in the 1870s by Dr. B. Stout, of San Francisco, California. His idea was to provide "quick and prompt intervention in the incipiency of mental disorders," and thus arrest its development. He drew up a bill for the provision of such an asylum, but it was not accepted by the legislature.
See also ASYLUMS.
Bibliography: Stout, B. 1871-1873. Report on probationary asylums. Second biennial report of the State Board of Health of California.

PROCHASKA, GEORGE (1749–1820). A Czech physiologist. He introduced the concept of vis nervosa, or nervous power, to replace the idea of a hypothetical fluid that was believed to be the force behind the functioning of the nervous system. He thought that all impressions passing to individual nerve centers were coordinated by a section of the cortex, which he called sensorium commune (q.v.). In 1784 he wrote a book entitled De Functionibus Systematis Nervosi Commentatio.
Bibliography: Riese, W. 1959. History of neurology.

PROCHAZKA, HUBERT (1885–1935). A Czech psychiatrist and professor of psychiatry in Prague. He was an expert in forensic psychiatry and died in the service of his profession when he was shot by one of his patients.
Bibliography: Vencovsky, E. 1975. Czechoslovakia. In World history of psychiatry, ed. J. G. Howells.

PROETUS. In Greek mythology (q.v.) the king of Argos. His three daughters were stricken with madness by either Dionysus (q.v.) whom they had slighted or by Hera for presuming their beauty to be equal to hers. The entire female population of Argos became affected and roamed about believing themselves to be cows. They eventually were cured by Melampus (q.v.).
Bibliography: Hammond, N.G.L., and Scullard, H. H. 1970. The Oxford classical dictionary.

PROGNOSIS. The forecast of the course of an illness. Hippocrates (q.v.) and his followers used prognosis in medicine to arrive at a diagnosis. The same method was followed by Emil Kraepelin (q.v.) in the diagnosis of

mental disorders. This attitude caused a weakening of therapeutic efforts in psychiatry. The progress of a mental disease was regarded with fatalism as its outcome was anticipated and determined the disease's classification. This method was later rejected mostly through the work of Eugen Bleuler (q.v.).
Bibliography: Zilboorg, G. 1941. *A history of medical psychology.*

PROPHETS. In antiquity prophets were respected and powerful members of many communities. They were believed to speak with the gods and had the gift of predicting the future. Their utterances were usually delivered while in a state of trance or frenzy, often induced by drugs (q.v.), self-hypnosis, or mental disorders. Their odd behavior was not only tolerated and explained but also rewarded.
Bibliography: Rosen, G. 1968. *Madness in society.*

PROTAGORAS OF THRACE (c.480-410 B.C.). A Greek philosopher who believed that there were no absolute standards of truth and that "man is the measure of all things." He felt that individuals could achieve a happy and useful life by the correct use of their reasoning powers. His philosophy was practical and aimed at producing good citizens by emphasizing the importance of the individual. He is said to be the first to teach for payment.
Bibliography: Burnet, J. 1914. *Greek philosophy: Thales to Plato.*

PROTOPHALLIC. A term coined by Ernest Jones (q.v.). He used it to describe a phase of childhood that is marked by the child's assumption "that the rest of the world is built like itself and has a satisfactory male organ — penis or clitoris, as the case may be."
Bibliography: Jones, E. 1927. *The early development of female sexuality.*

PROUST, MARCEL (1871-1922). A French novelist, of half-Jewish blood. As a child he was delicate, sensitive, and overly dependent on his parents, especially his mother. He suffered from sleeping difficulties, asthma, and indigestion, which were precipitated by anxiety. His moods were unpredictable and would rapidly swing from elation to depression. His appearance was so effeminate that his schoolmates rejected him and threatened to thrash him when he tried to make friends. In youth he seems to have been physically attracted to heterosexual men. His lifelong ill health contributed to his dependence on his mother. He was thirty-four years old at the time of her death, which precipitated his withdrawal from society. He retreated into introspection in the isolation of a soundproof flat. His writings reflect his preoccupation with emotional life and human morbidity, which he described in medical terms that he probably learned from his father, a professor in

public health, and his brother, a surgeon. Nearly all his characters are drawn round their illnesses.
Bibliography: Shattuck, R. 1974. *Proust*.

PSALMS. The songs to God in the nineteenth book of the Old Testament. Most of them are attributed to David (q.v.). They contain many examples of emotional stress, for example, the two following, which refer to deep depression:

. . . for I have had my fill of woes,
and they have brought me to the threshold of Sheol.
I am numbered with those who go down to the abyss
and have become like a man beyond help.

[Ps. 88: 3,4.]

My thoughts went back to times long past,
I remembered forgotten years;
all night long I was in deep distress,
as I lay thinking, my spirit was sunk in despair.

[Ps. 77: 5,6.]

PSAMMETICHOS (? - 610 B.C.). A king of Egypt (q.v.). He was reported by Herodotus (q.v.) to have isolated two infants for two years. It was thought that whatever language the children spoke spontaneously would be the first language that had ever been spoken and would prove the Egyptian claim to greater antiquity than Phrygia. The children were cared for among a herd of goats, but no one ever spoke to them or in their presence. The only word the children could utter when released was *bekos*, Phrygian for bread, and the Egyptians had to admit the greater antiquity of the Phrygians. It later was explained that *bekos* was an imitation of the bleating of the goats that had fed the children during their captivity.
Bibliography: Galdston, I. 1967. *Historic derivations of modern psychiatry*.

PSELLUS, MICHAEL CONSTANTINE (1018-1078?). A Byzantine philosopher and writer. He was subject to hallucinations (q.v.), which may have been a source of his writings on demons. He included a detailed classification of their hierarchy in the medical section of his encyclopedic work and attributed the troubles and corruptions that plague the human soul to them.
Bibliography: Hussey, J. M. 1937. *Church and learning in the Byzantine empire, 867-1185*.

PSEUDOCYESIS. False pregnancy. The term is derived from two Greek words. It was introduced into medical nomenclature by John Mason Good

(q.v.) in his *Physiological System of Nosology* in 1823, but the clinical condition had been recognized as early as 300 B.C. by Hippocrates (q.v.) who described its occurrence in twelve women. A classic example of pseudocyesis is provided by Mary I (q.v.). Anna O. (q.v.) presented an hysterical (*see* HYSTERIA) childbirth as the culmination of her pseudocyesis, which she had attributed to her psychiatrist, Joseph Breuer (q.v.), who was profoundly shocked by the event.
Bibliography: Brown, E., and Barglow, P. 1971. Pseudocyesis: A paradigm for psychophysiological interactions. *Arch. gen Psychiat.* 24: 221-29.

PSEUDOLOGIA FANTASTICA. A term derived from two Greek words and meaning "elaborate false speech." It refers to a clinical condition characterized by pathological lying linked with truths. Examples of this are provided by the poet Thomas Chatterton and the painters Guiseppe Balsamo and Henricus van Meegeren (qq.v.).
Bibliography: Fenichel, O. 1939. *Zur Oekonomie der Pseudologica Phantastica.*

PSYCHASTHENIA. A term introduced by Pierre Janet (q.v.) in his *Les obsessions et la psychasthénie* in 1903. It refers to the concept of exhaustion of the nervous system.
Bibliography: Janet, P. 1903. *Les obsessions et la psychasthénie.*

PSYCHE. A term meaning "breath" in Greek. The concept of the soul is derived from it. At various stages, the term has been represented as a bird, as a kind of ghostly double of the dead person, as a butterfly, and finally as a beautiful maiden. According to the Greek myth, Psyche was loved by Cupid, who secretly visited her at night but was never seen by her until she lit a lamp, woke him up, and caused him to abandon her. After much suffering she was forgiven and made immortal. To early philosophers *psyche*, the soul, represented a vital force in charge of all functions of the body, including the senses. They believed the force was capable of development, thus having a biological basis. As different theories were evolved by philosophers and poets, the psyche became dematerialized, eternal, and the seat of the passions.
Bibliography: Swahn, J. Ö. 1955. *The tale of Cupid and Psyche.*

PSYCHEDELIC EXPERIENCES. An expression originating in the United States in the 1960s. It was used to describe the effect produced by certain hallucinogenic drugs when combined with pop music, dancing, and flashing lights at gatherings of people who considered themselves different from orthodox society.
Bibliography: 1978. *Brewer's dictionary of phrase and fable.*

PSYCHIATRIC SOCIAL WORK. Before it was recognized as a profession in the 1920s, social work in the psychiatric field was undertaken by vol-

unteers who were usually wealthy women with an urge to "do good." The advent of child guidance clinics (q.v.) resulted in the emergence of the professional psychiatric social worker. Later, this type of work was extended to hospitals, outpatients clinics, and community services embracing all ages.
Bibliography: Woodroofe, K. 1974. *From charity to social work: in England and the United States.*

PSYCHIATRY. The diagnosis and treatment of mental disorders. The term evolved from *psychiaterie*, a word first used by Johannes Christian Reil (q.v.) in his *Rhapsodies in the Application of Psychic Methods in the Treatment of Mental Disturbances*, published in 1803. Johann Christian Heinroth (q.v.) used the term *psychiatrie* in 1818, and Ernst von Feuchtersleben (q.v.) coined the term *psychiatrics*.
Bibliography: Hunter, R., and Macalpine, I. 1963. *Three hundred years of psychiatry.*

PSYCHICAL PHENOMENA. Phenomena that include divination (q.v.), premonitory dreams (q.v.), telepathy (q.v.), apparitions, and contact with the dead. A belief in these phenomena can be found in all cultures. Both the early philosophers of Greece and Rome and today's modern psychologists have demonstrated their interests in psychical phenomena. Around the middle of the nineteenth century Europe and America experienced a revival of interest in the psychical field, especially as it was presented by mediums (q.v.). Meetings, societies, congresses, research, and literature were dedicated to paranormal experiences. Telepathy was studied, and experiments were designed to find evidence of its existence. In 1886 *Phantasms of the Living* by Edmund Gurney (1847-1888), Frederick W. Myers (q.v.), and Frank Podmore (q.v.) added weight to the belief in psychical phenomena. In 1892 at the Second International Congress of Psychology in London, papers on psychical research outnumbered all others, but this emphasis caused a reaction away from the subject in subsequent congresses.
Bibliography: Rao, K. R. 1966. *Experimental parapsychology.*

PSYCHIC ENERGY. That part of the mind's force employed in any mental activity. A concept introduced by Sigmund Freud (q.v.) in 1900 in his *The Interpretation of Dreams*. He built the basic explanation of mental life and instinct theory on it.
Bibliography: Freud, S. 1900. *The interpretation of dreams.*

PSYCHIC PAIN. Pain caused by unconscious conflict. A concept introduced by Sigmund Freud (q.v.) as a working hypothesis.
Bibliography: Zilboorg, G. 1941. *A history of medical psychology.*

PSYCHOANALYSIS. A method of therapeutics developed by Sigmund Freud (q.v.). As Freud developed it, it consisted of analyzing and inter-

preting what his patients had told him during free association talks. He named this method "psychoanalysis" in 1896 and dropped the term "psychological analysis," which had been coined by Pierre Janet (q.v.).
Bibliography: Fine, R. 1979. *A history of psychoanalysis.*

PSYCHOANALYTICAL CONGRESS. The first psychoanalytical congress was held in 1908 in Salzburg, Austria.
Bibliography: Flugel, J. C. 1945. *A hundred years of psychology.*

PSYCHOANALYTIC POLICLINIC (LATER BERLIN INSTITUTE). The first center for psychoanalytic education. It was opened in Berlin in 1920. The financial means for this venture were provided by Max Eitingon (q.v.).
Bibliography: Alexander, F. G., and Selesnick, S. T. 1966. *The history of psychiatry.*

PSYCHOBIOLOGY. A psychological concept originated and systematized by Adolf Meyer (q.v.). It denies the duality of body and mind, and regards the individual as the total product of his life experience.
Bibliography: Lief, A., ed. 1948. *The commonsense psychiatry of Adolf Meyer.*

PSYCHODRAMA. A psychiatric technique used in group treatment. It was developed by Jacob L. Moreno (q.v.) and evolved from his theatre of spontaneity, which he had founded in Vienna in 1921. Moreno introduced the technique to the United States in 1925, where it is used most frequently to elucidate family disorders. Individual family members act out their problems in front of a therapist.
Bibliography: Moreno, J. L. 1946. *Psychodrama.*

PSYCHOLOGICAL ABSTRACTS. Systematic summarized accounts of all the important literature on psychology. They have been published since 1927 by the Clark University Press in the U.S.A.
Bibliography: Flugel, J. C. 1945. *A hundred years of psychology.*

PSYCHOLOGICAL CORPORATION. A professional body organized in 1921 in New York by James Cattell (q.v.). Its purpose was stated as the "advancement of psychology and the promotion of the useful applications of psychology."
Bibliography: Watson, R. I. 1963. *The great psychologists.*

PSYCHOLOGICAL LABORATORY. The first psychological laboratory was probably that organized by Francis Galton (q.v.) in 1884. It was called the Anthropometric Laboratory (q.v.) and was opened in London on the occasion of the International Health Exhibition. The laboratory collected the personal data of 9,337 persons. The first laboratory for experimental psychology (q.v.) was founded by Wilhelm Wundt (q.v.) in Leipzig, Germany, in 1879. Although the first premises consisted of only a few rooms in an old building, an entire school of psychologists was trained there. Better quarters were obtained in 1897.

Bibliography: Flugel, J. C. 1945. *A hundred years of psychology*. Forrest, D. W. 1974. *Francis Galton: the life and work of a Victorian genius*.

PSYCHOLOGICAL MEDICINE, CERTIFICATE IN. A British qualification founded by the Royal Medico-Psychological Association (q.v.) in 1885. In 1948 it was superseded by the diploma in psychological medicine, which then was transferred to the examining body of the Royal College of Physicians and Surgeons in 1954. The Royal College of Psychiatrists was founded in 1971. The Royal College now has instituted a more advanced examination for membership in the college.

PSYCHOLOGICAL REALITY. A concept introduced by Sigmund Freud (q.v.) to refer to irrational fantasies that are real to the patient.

Bibliography: Freud, S. 1933. *New introductory lectures in psychiatry*.

PSYCHOLOGICAL REVIEW. A journal founded in 1894 by James Cattell (q.v.) in collaboration with James M. Baldwin (q.v.).

PSYCHOLOGICAL TYPES. The question of psychological typology has been discussed since antiquity. From the humoral theory (q.v.) to the typology of Ernst Kretschmer (q.v.) and Carl G. Jung (q.v.) types of personality, or temperament, have been linked to constitutional characteristics or to kinds of mental activity. When increasing interest in the description of personality types occurred during the 1920s, it resulted in the development of a special branch of psychology, typological psychology, which attempted to interrelate the psychological and physiological aspects of man and emphasized the influence of heredity on character. In modern times, Carl G. Jung has been regarded as the outstanding exponent in this field. In 1921 he produced his classic *Psychological Types*. Jung broadly classified people into extrovert (q.v.) and introvert (q.v.) categories and added to this a description of the four basic psychological functions: thinking, feeling, sensation, and intuition.

Bibliography: Hull, R.F.C., ed. 1971. *The collected works of C. G. Jung*. Vol. 6. Trans. H. G. Baynes.

PSYCHOLOGISCHE FORSCHUNG. The official journal of Gestalt psychology (q.v.). It was founded in Germany in 1921 by Max Wertheimer, Wolfgang Köhler and Karl Koffka (qq.v.) in association with two psychopathologists, Kurt Goldstein and Hans Gruhle (qq.v.). It was a forum for the new trends of German psychology, which were represented by the

Gestalt school. Despite the Nazi regime, it lasted until 1938, and, in its last years, Köhler edited it from the United States, where he had taken refuge. In all twenty-two volumes were published.

PSYCHOLOGY. In 1590, Rudolf Goeckel (1547-1628), a German philosopher, wrote a book entitled *Psychologia—Hoc est de Hominis Perfectione, Anima, Ortu*. In it he discussed human behavior and its improvement. This is probably the earliest use of the term "psychology" in the modern sense of science of human behavior, although the sentence "psichiologia de ratione animae humane" is found in an earlier manuscript by the Yugoslavian Marko Marulić (q.v.). Other authors who are also credited with coining the term are Philip Melanchthon (q.v.) and Otto Casmann (1562-1607). It was popularized in the 1730s by Christian von Wolff (q.v.) who distinguished between empirical and rational psychology.
See also ACT PSYCHOLOGY, APPLIED PSYCHOLOGY, BEHAVIORISM, CHILD PSYCHOLOGY, EXPERIMENTAL PSYCHOLOGY, GESTALT PSYCHOLOGY, INDIVIDUAL PSYCHOLOGY, METAPSYCHOLOGY, SOCIAL PSYCHOLOGY, and STRUCTURAL PSYCHOLOGY.
Bibliography: Boring, E. G. 1966. A note on the origin of the word psychology. *J. Hist. Behav. Sci.* 2: 167.

PSYCHOLOGY AS A PROFESSION. Francis Galton (q.v.), in 1882, established a psychological laboratory in London where clients were tested and a report of the results given to them on payment of a fee. Galton can thus be regarded as the first practitioner of psychology.
Bibliography: Forrest, D. W. 1974. *Francis Galton: the life and work of a Victorian genius.*

PSYCHOMETRY. A term referring to a psychical phenomenon (*see* PSYCHICAL PHENOMENA) whereby some people claim to possess the ability to relate facts about the history of an object by holding it in their hands. It is related to telepathy (q.v.).
Bibliography: Hettinger, J. 1940. *The ultra-perceptive faculty.*

PSYCHONEUROSIS. A term introduced by Paul Charles Dubois (q.v.) to indicate mental disorders of psychological aetiology.
Bibliography: Dubois, P. 1905. *The psychic treatment of nervous disorders*, trans. W.A. White and S. E. Jeliffe.

PSYCHOPATHIC HOSPITAL. The first psychopathic hospital in the United States that functioned as a department of a state hospital was opened in Boston, Massachusetts, in 1912. Attached to the Boston State Hospital, it was directed by Dr. Elmer E. Southard (q.v.) until his death in 1920. Between 1912 and 1943 similar hospitals were opened in Iowa City, Iowa,

Denver, Colorado, New York, New York, Galveston, Texas, Chicago, Illinois, Pittsburgh, Pennsylvania, and San Francisco, California.
Bibliography: Deutsch, A. 1949. *The mentally ill in America.*

PSYCHOPATHY. Psychic morbidity. The concept and term of "psychological pathology" was introduced by Jeremy Bentham (q.v.) in 1817. It was shortened into "psychopathy" by Ernst von Feuchtersleben (q.v.) in 1845. He used it in the modern sense of the word of psychic morbidity associated with antisocial behavior.
Bibliography: Werlinder, H. 1978. *Psychopathy: a history of the concepts.*

PSYCHOSIS. The term was first introduced into psychiatry in 1845 by Ernst von Feuchtersleben (q.v.) to indicate a mental disorder that was distinguished from neurosis (q.v.), or functional disease of nerves.
Bibliography: Hunter, R., and Macalpine, I. 1963. *Three hundred years of psychiatry.*

PSYCHOSOMATIC MEDICINE. Although they did not understand the mechanisms involved, early physicians did accept the relationship between the mind and the body. After the sixteenth century, medicine concentrated on physical phenomena, but the mind-body question continued to puzzle medical practitioners. The father of surgical anatomy, Joseph Lieutaud (q.v.), asserted that "the mind and the body exercise on one another a reciprocal power, the extent of which we do not know." The term "psychosomatic" was used for the first time in 1818 by Johann Heinroth (q.v.).
Bibliography: Margetts, E. L. 1950. The early history of the word "psychosomatic."
   Can. Med. Assn. J. 63: 402.

PSYCHOSURGERY. Surgery involving the opening of the skull. It has been practiced since antiquity to relieve symptoms of insanity that have been variously attributed to devils, vapors (q.v.), or humors (q.v.) trapped in the head. In the twelfth century, Rogerius Frugardi (q.v.) of the school of Salerno, believed that mania (q.v.) could be cured by cutting holes in the skull and allowing the poisonous vapors to escape. Marcus Aurelius Severinus (1580-1656) performed the same operation five hundred years later. Toward the end of the nineteenth century, Gottlieb Burckhardt, a Swiss physician, excised pieces of cortex to calm psychotic (*see* PSYCHOSIS) patients. In the twentieth century, the pioneer of psychosurgery has been Egas Moniz (q.v.).
Bibliography: Moniz, E. 1936. *Tentatives opératoires dans le traitement de certaines psychoses.*

PSYCHOTHERAPY. Healing through the psyche (q.v.). It is uncertain when the term was first used or who coined it. Walter Cooper Dendy (q.v.) wrote a paper entitled "Psychotherapeia, or the Remedial Influence of the

Mind," which was published in 1853 in the *Journal of Psychological Medicine and Mental Pathology*. The term was certainly used by the Nancy School (q.v.) and was employed extensively by the end of the nineteenth century, after it was made popular by a book, published in 1890, entitled *Hypnotism, or Psychotherapeutics* by Felkin. The term had been preceded by such terms as "psychological methods of treatment" and "moral medicine" (q.v.). All these terms, although innovative, covered a practice that goes back to the dawn of recorded history. Healers and medicine men, primitive shamen and witch doctors, Greek thinkers and Hindu philosophers, Chinese sages and western Christian theologians, magnetizers and alienists, psychoanalysts and dynamic psychiatrists, whether by magic or science, have all followed the same well-trodden path trying to bring about health, physical or mental, through psychological means.

Bibliography: Ehrenwald, J., ed. 1976. *The history of psychotherapy*.

PUCCINI, GIACOMO (1858-1924). An Italian composer. During his early music lessons he was kicked on the shin every time he struck the wrong note. From this treatment, he acquired a permanent reflex whereby his foot would jerk up whenever he heard a false note. He was a flamboyant man who loved women, fast cars, and shooting and yet remained a depressive all his life. Liu, a character in his opera *Turandot*, is said to be based on Doria, a maid who aroused his wife's jealousy (q.v.) and was so hounded by her that she committed suicide (q.v.). Puccini was so affected by the event that every year he would take flowers to Doria's grave on the anniversary of her death.

Bibliography: Jackson, S. 1973. *Madam Butterfly: the story of Puccini*.

PUEPERAL INSANITY. *See* INSANITY, PUEPERAL.

PULSE. The observation of the pulse reaction was first used by Erasistratus (q.v.) to diagnose love sickness. It was later used by Galen, Paul of Aegina (q.v.), Avicenna and Felix Plater (qq.v.). In the diagnosis of insanity the pulse was still an important consideration at the end of the nineteenth century. Daniel Hack Tuke (q.v.) allowed it twenty columns in his *Dictionary of Psychological Medicine* (q.v.).

Bibliography: Tuke, D. H. 1892. *Dictionary of psychological medicine*.

PURCELL, HENRY (1659-1695). An English composer. Among his dramatic song scenes, there is one entitled *Mad Bess of Bedlam*, which deals with an insane woman.

PURCELL, JOHN (1674-1730). An English physician. In 1702 he wrote a book of psychiatric interest entitled *A Treatise of Vapours, or Hysterick Fits* in which he discussed the causes, symptoms, and cures of such disorders.

Using what he called "the newest and most rational principles" and breaking away from "the Galenick old-fashion'd doctors, who explicate all things by hidden qualities," he claimed vapors (q.v.) arising in the stomach reached the brain and caused "hysterick fits." The more violent of these he regarded as "epilepsies" (*see* EPILEPSY). He thought that some patients were troubled with seizures brought on by "anger, passion or disturbance of the mind" and recommended that the physician discover what troubled the patient. Treatment then should include the avoidance of "all concerns, anxieties, and passions," and diversion in the form of plays, merry company, and walks.
Bibliography: Leigh, D. 1961. *The historical development of British psychiatry.*

PURGING. The belief that bodily and mental disorders were due to noxious matters, poisons, or humors (q.v.) led to the use of purgatives to cleanse the body. Until the nineteenth century purgative herbs were used widely in the treatment of mental diseases, although over the years hellebore (q.v.) gave way to more sophisticated medications. In the sixth century, Alexander of Tralles (q.v.) found armenian stone (q.v.) to be superior to hellebore. Felix Plater (q.v.) also enthusiastically prescribed purging for mental patients and, as late as the second half of the nineteenth century, Sir John Bucknill and Daniel Hack Tuke (qq.v.) in their *Manual of Psychological Medicine* recorded that "the purgative treatment of insanity by hellebore is the oldest on record, and it still enjoys some traditional favor." Not for nothing was a quack doctor in Molière's 'Le Malade Imaginaire' called "Purgon"!
Bibliography: Zilboorg, G. 1941. *A history of medical psychology.*

PURITANI, I. An opera by the Italian composer Vincenzo Bellini (1801-1835). In the mad scene of this opera, Elvira believes that Arturo, her husband-to-be, has eloped with another woman on her wedding day. She is shocked into madness and cries out in despair "Give me back my hope, or let me die." She recalls that he promised to be faithful, then went away and their mutual joy is destroyed. In a state of hallucination (q.v.), she believes that Arturo is near and calls him back to her: "Que la voce sua soave: Vien, diletto" (Act 2.).

PURKYNĚ (*or* PURKINJE), JAN EVANGELISTA (1787-1869). A Czech physiologist. He was the son of peasants. After his father's death, he was educated by monks and spent three years in a religious order. He intended to become a priest, but his scientific interest led to a career in medicine. As a student, he experimented on himself with drugs that caused symptoms similar to epilepsy (q.v.) and observed the signs of vertigo in those using the swings and roundabouts in Prague's park. He was the first to draw attention to the individuality of fingerprints. His greatest contributions were in the field of neurology (q.v.) and included his observations on nerve cells and his description of the visual phenomena that bear his name. His two volumes on visual phenomena were dedicated to Johann Wolfgang von Goethe (q.v.). He also wrote on dreams (q.v.), which he believed were an index of personality. He wrote poetry and translated into Czech poems by William Shakespeare, Tasso, and Johann Schiller (qq.v.). He was a leading figure in the movement for Czech nationalism.

Bibliography: John, H. J. 1959. *Jan Evangelista Purkyně.*

PUSHKIN, ALEXANDER SERGEYEVICH (1799-1837). A Russian poet and prose writer who laid the foundation of realism in Russian literature. His parents, rich and cultured society people, paid little attention to his emotional needs, but he received all the affection he needed from his grandmother and his nurse. At the age of twelve he went to a boarding school, which he enjoyed. As an adolescent he led a life of pleasure, but his unconventionality and the sentiments expressed in his *Ode to Liberty* aroused official disapproval and he was exiled by Alexander I (1777-1825). Nicholas I was more lenient with him but still restricted his work, which caused him much distress and bitterness. His marriage to a society woman of little intellectual interest brought him more suffering, and he isolated himself while a campaign of slander was launched against him and his writings. Anonymous letters involving his wife finally pushed him to a duel to defend her honor and he was fatally wounded by his adversary.

Bibliography: Troyat, H. 1974. *Pushkin.*

PUSSIN, JEAN-BAPTISTE (1746-1809). A French male nurse. He was chief male nurse at the Bicêtre (q.v.), where he had been a patient in his early manhood. His nursing assistants were usually chosen from the ranks of former patients, and his wife, a resourceful and witty woman, helped him in his work by presiding over the female staff. He was kindly and sympathetic to his charges and replaced chains with straitjackets. Philippe Pinel (q.v.) met him on becoming physician at the Bicêtre and approved of his methods. Both of them subsequently worked together at the Salpêtrière (q.v.). Pinel wrote about him in his *Traité Médico-philosophique*, and praised his devotion and skill, while acknowledging the guidance he had received from him.

Bibliography: Weiner, D. B. 1979. The apprenticeship of Philippe Pinel: a new document, "Observations of Citizen Pussin on the insane." *Am. J. Psychiat.* 136: 1128-34.

PUTNAM, JAMES JACKSON (1846-1918). An American psychiatrist and professor of neurology at Harvard University. The first use of the term "psychoanalysis" (q.v.) in a psychological journal is attributed to him. He used the term in an article published in 1906 in the *Journal of Abnormal Psychology*. He introduced psychoanalysis to the United States as a form of treatment and, after meeting Sigmund Freud (q.v.) in 1909, gave it his

enthusiastic public support. The first American Psychoanalytic Society was organized by him in 1910, and he became the first president of the American Psychoanalytic Association, founded by Ernest Jones (q.v.) in 1911.
Bibliography: Quen, J. M., and Carlson, E. T. 1978. *American psychoanalysis: origins and development.*

PUYSÉGUR, AMAND-MARIE-JACQUES DE CHASTENET (1751-1825). A French pupil of Franz Mesmer (q.v.). He brought magnetism (q.v.) back to respectability after it had fallen into disrepute. Modifying previous practices, he introduced the trance state, which he called "artificial somnambulism" and abandoned induced convulsions. Many of his experiments were conducted on his gardener, Victor Race (q.v.), who, under mesmerism (q.v.) changed from a shy young man to a talkative individual. Puységur's "magnetizing tree" was touched by a large number of patients who had traveled great distances to come under the influence of the "magnetic fluid" that they believed impregnated it. Numerous cures were attributed officially to him by a commission of civil servants and physicians. He also was said to have been able to magnetize animals. In 1785 he founded in Strasbourg a training school for mesmerism called the Society of Harmony (q.v.). In 1807 he published his primary work on mesmerism, *Du Magnétism Animal.*
Bibliography: Tinterow, M. M. 1970. *Foundations of hypnosis: from Mesmer to Freud.*

PUZZLE BOX. A mental testing device used by Edward L. Thorndike (q.v.) in 1898 to assess the intelligence of cats, dogs, and chickens. The animals were enclosed in boxes from which they could escape only by a series of complicated movements. He later used the same technique with children.
Bibliography: Flugel, J. C. 1945. *A hundred years of psychology.*

PYGMALION. Legendary king of Cyprus and sculptor. He carved in ivory the image of a girl and, despite his hatred of women, fell in love with his creation. He prayed to Aphrodite to give life to the statue, and, when his wish was granted, he married her. Pygmalionism is a term derived from this legend indicating a form of fetishism (*see* FETISH). From Ovid (q.v.) to George Bernard Shaw (q.v.) the story of Pygmalion has provided material for writers.
Bibliography: Berest, J. J. 1971. Fetishism: three case histories. *J. Sex. Res.* 7: 237-39.

PYKNIC TYPE. One of the four types distinguished by Ernst Kretschmer (q.v.). It referred to a short, broad individual resembling an orangutang.
See also ATHLETIC TYPE, ASTHENIC TYPE.
Bibliography: Kretschmer, E. 1944. *Körperbau und Charakter.*

PYRRHO (c.365-272 B.C.). A Greek philosopher who believed that virtue was the only good and all other things were unimportant. According to him, human cognition was insufficient to attain certainty. Because good is eternal and truth is impossible to recognize, judgment must be suspended, which leads to a state of tranquillity and happiness. His philosophy was adopted by a school of thought called skepticism.

Bibliography: Zeller, E. 1962. *Stoics, Epicureans, and Skeptics.*

PYTHAGORAS (fl.c.530 B.C.). A Greek thinker who invented the term "philosopher." He may have been the first philosopher to state definitely that the brain was the central organ of intellectual activity. He stated that the soul of man was in a condition of absolute imperfection. It had three elements, reason, intelligence, and passion. Although intelligence and passion could be found in men and animals, reason was the distinguishing feature of man. Pythagoras taught that sense perceptions were fused together in the brain. They combined into memories; memories into inferences; and these into reason. He attributed mental diseases to disorders of the brain and attributed health to the correct balance between the elemental qualities— heat, cold, moisture, and dryness.

Bibliography: Guthrie, C. 1967. *A history of Greek philosophy.* Vol. 1.

PYTHIA. The priestess of Apollo (q.v.) who had a temple at Delphi (q.v.). When possessed (*see* POSSESSION) by the god she became frenzied, and, in a state of trance, she would deliver utterances that were considered to contain advice, judgments or prophesies. Her trance was probably brought about by self-suggestion and firm belief in the power of Apollo aided by the sulphurous vapors issuing from the ground within the temple.

See also ORACLES.

Bibliography: Parke, H. W. 1939. *A history of the Delphic oracle.*

Q

QAT. *See* KAT.

QUAIL. A bird that was believed to have an inordinate sexual appetite. For this reason the term was applied to courtesans. The belief was most common in the sixteenth century.
Bibliography: 1978. *Brewer's dictionary of phrase and fable.*

QUAKERS. Originally a derogatory term for the Religious Society of Friends. The term was used as early as 1647 to indicate the followers of George Fox (q.v.) because they were said to tremble under the influence of the Holy Ghost. In trance-like states, they were inspired to preach by the "Spirit." During periods of persecution, they were accused of drawing people into their movement and causing them to behave strangely. The Quakers later became identified with good works and enterprise. They pioneered social reforms and were responsible for founding the Pennsylvania Hospital (q.v.) and the York Retreat (q.v.).
Bibliography: Clark, R. A., and Elkinton, J. R. 1978. *The Quaker heritage in medicine.*

QUATERNITY. An archetypal image of the self represented by a square or any shape related to the number four. It was linked by Carl G. Jung (q.v.) to the process of individuation. He found it in seventy-four out of four hundred dreams (q.v.) he analyzed.
Bibliography: Jung, C. G. 1937. *Psychology and religion.*

QUEEN OF HUNGARY'S WATER. An infusion of rosemary (q.v.) and spices in spirits. It is said to have been invented by Saint Elizabeth, queen of Hungary, in the thirteenth century. It was regarded as a cure-all. Madame Marie de Rabutin-Chantal de Sévigné (1626-1696), the noted French woman

of letters, used it frequently and found it "good against sadness," as she wrote to a friend in 1675.
Bibliography: Focault, M. 1967. *Madness and civilization.*

QUENTAL, ANTERO TARQUINIO DE (1842-1891). A Portuguese poet. He suffered from fits of acute depression and anxiety. At one point in 1877, mental anguish prevented him working, and he consulted Jean Martin Charcot (q.v.) in Paris. After a period of treatment, he improved enough to write again. Eventually he was forced to abandon his political involvements because of his health. He retired to a house near Oporto and dedicated himself to raising the two orphan girls he had adopted. In 1891 he undertook a long visit to his family in Ponta Delgada. This visit caused him considerable emotional strain and precipitated an episode of deep depression that culminated in suicide (q.v.). His works show a dark pessimism and reflect conflict within himself and his disillusionment with an existence that never reached his expectations.
Bibliography: Carreiro, J. B. 1948. *A. de Quental, subsídios para a sua biografia.*

QUERULANTENWAHN. A German term applied to individuals who have a pathological wish to go to law in order to redress imaginary wrongs that they believe have been done to them. Daniel Hack Tuke (q.v.) described these patients in his *Dictionary of Psychological Medicine* (q.v.) as predisposed to this disorder by egoism. Their paranoia (q.v.) prevents them from seeing the real state of affairs, and they become a "plague to the courts of justice, and a terror to judges and lawyers, as well as to friends and neighbours."
Bibliography: Tuke, D. H. 1892. *A dictionary of psychological medicine.*

QUETELET, LAMBERT ADOLPHE JACQUES (1796-1874). A Belgian statistician and astronomer. His statistical researches into the development of man's physical and intellectual qualities culminated in 1835 with the publication of *Sur l'Homme et le Dévelopment de ses Facultés ou Essai de Physique Sociale* (Man and the development of his faculties or essay on social constitution), which contains the theory of the "average man." Quetelet was the first to demonstrate that the normal curve can be used to describe the distribution of human characters. He is regarded as the founder of modern statistics and a pioneer of sociology.
Bibliography: Boring, E. G. 1950. *A history of experimental psychology.*

QUEVEDO Y VILLEGAS, FRANCISCO GÓMEZ DE (1580-1645). A Spanish writer and poet. He was a passionate and complex man who lived life to the full, combining a high sense of morality with a need to experience what low life could offer. He had several illegitimate children, served as the

king's secretary, performed diplomatic missions and was imprisoned for a time. His public and private life was a cause of tension and guilt in him. He was obsessed (*see* OBSESSION) with crudeness that caused him disgust and poured his intense emotional feelings into strong and dignified verse full of psychological insight into human nature.
Bibliography: Astrana Marin, L. 1945. *La vida turbulenta de Quevedo.*

QUIETISM. A form of passive mysticism in which the will is completely subjugated and the individual abandons himself to total contemplation of God. The doctrine was originated in the seventeenth century by a Spanish priest, Miguel de Molinos (q.v.), who was persecuted and imprisoned by the Inquisition (q.v.) for his teachings. In France it was advocated by Madame Jeanne Marie de la Motte Guyon (1648-1717) but found few followers.
Bibliography: Knox, R. A. 1950. *Enthusiasm.*

QUIETNESS. The popular name for a preparation of opium (q.v.) often used by working mothers in nineteenth-century England. Heavy doses of this narcotic were given to babies in order to quieten them while their mothers worked in cotton mills or other employment. Many children wasted away and died.
Bibliography: Sanders, W. B., ed. 1970. *Juvenile offenders for a thousand years.*

QUIMBY, PHINEAS PARKHURST (1802-1866). An American watchmaker who became interested in magnetism (q.v.) after attending a public demonstration given by Charles Poyen, a French follower of Franz Mesmer (q.v.). Quimby began to practice magnetism and was so convinced that it was an electric phenomenon that he would perform during thunderstorms. When he was proved wrong, he observed what happened more critically and concluded that it was not magnetic fluids or special powers that achieved results but rather the unquestioning faith of the subjects. He then called the treatment "mind cure." His successes made him famous throughout the United States. In the latter part of his life he tried to systematize his theories into a religious philosophy and a scientific explanation of health and happiness. After his death, his doctrines formed the basis of a movement called New Thought. Among his patients was Mary Baker Eddy (q.v.), the founder of Christian Science (q.v.).
Bibliography: Dresser, H. W., ed. 1921. *The Quimby manuscripts.*

QUINCKE, HEINRICH IRENÄUS (1842-1922). A German physician and neurologist. He contributed to the understanding of central nervous system diseases by introducing the spinal puncture (q.v.). He arrived at this diagnostic technique while searching for a method of relieving the tension produced by hydrocephalus in children. He made his findings known in

1891 at the Wiesbaden congress of Medicine, but it was some years before the value of his technique was realized.

Bibliography: Haymaker, W., and Schiller, F. 1970. *The founders of neurology*. 2d. ed.

QUNUBU (*or* QUNNABU). A term used by the Assyrians to indicate hemp (q.v.). They burned its seeds and inhaled the vapors to produce joyous and noisy intoxication. Herodotus (484-424 B.C.) reported that the Scythians followed this practice.

Bibliography: Herodotus. *Histories*, trans. 1920-24 by A. D. Godley.

R

RABELAIS, FRANÇOIS (1494-1553). A French satirist, physician, and humanist. He was educated by monks and took religious orders. While in the monastery, he had access to the classics and learned Greek, Hebrew, and Arabic. He also read books on medicine, astronomy, and other sciences. Jealousy (q.v.) on the part of the monks caused him to be deprived of his books and led to his hatred of the monastery, which he left. He then studied medicine at Montpellier and practiced as a physician in a hospital in Lyons. He later combined medicine with ecclesiastical offices and spent time in Rome and Paris. In his writings he directed his bitter and destructive satire against charlatans, the old traditions of the medical profession, and the hypocrisy of the church. Henricus Agrippa (q.v.) was one of the victims of his satire and was called by him "Herr Trippa." Rabelais rejected the old ways and adopted a realistic approach that revealed the natural basic impulses of man and the falsity of repressing them. Contradictory, exuberant, at times cruel, but always resourceful, his characters reflect his own peculiar personality.
Bibliography: Screech, M. A. 1979. *Rabelais*.

RACE, VICTOR (fl. 1784). A French peasant and gardener to Armand-Marie-Jacques Puységur (q.v.), who in 1784 used him for his first magnetizing (*see* MAGNETISM) experiments. In his normal state, Race was shy and rather dull, but, when hypnotized, he became a fluent conversationalist and displayed a bright and interesting personality.
Bibliography: Tinterow, M. M. 1970. *Foundations of hypnosis from Mesmer to Freud*.

RACHMANINOFF, SERGEI VASILIEVICH (1873-1943). A Russian composer and pianist. He fled the Russian revolution and settled in the United States. After the disastrous failure of his First Symphony in 1897, he suffered a nervous breakdown that prevented him from composing for

three years. In 1900 he was treated by a practitioner of medical hypnosis (*see* HYPNOTISM), Dr. Nicolai Dahl. After a series of relaxing sessions, Rachmaninoff recovered and continued his successful musical career.
Bibliography: Norris, G. 1976. *Rakhmaninov.*

RADO, SANDOR (1890-1972). A Hungarian psychiatrist. After graduating in political science from the university in Budapest, he became interested in the work of Sigmund Freud (q.v.) and consequently became a pupil of Sandor Ferenczi (q.v.). Rado graduated in medicine in 1915 and, until 1931, worked as a psychiatrist at the Psychoanalytic Institute (q.v.) in Berlin. He then emigrated to the United States where he became a professor of psychiatry at Columbia University. He systematized education methods in psychoanalysis (q.v.) and revised methods of treatment. He came to believe that after the process of regression during analysis the patient must be brought back to an adult level, where he can best cooperate with the therapist and adapt to the actual situation. Rado also formulated the concept of traumataphobia (q.v.) or avoidance of further trauma by an already traumatized person.
Bibliography: Rado, S. 1922 and 1956. *Psychoanalysis of behavior.* Vols. 1 and 2.

RAHERE (?-1144). An English court jester, divine, and founder of the Royal Hospital of Saint Bartholomew (q.v.). He was born of a poor family and as a youth frequented the houses of nobles to amuse them. Later he turned to religion and made a pilgrimage to Rome to expiate his sins. When he fell ill, he promised that if he got better and was allowed to return home, he would found a hospital for the poor. On his return journey, he had a vision of Saint Bartholomew, who told him to build and dedicate a church to him. Henry I (q.v.) granted him a site at Smithfield in London, and in 1123, he built Saint Bartholomew's Church and hospital. The hospital treated the mentally ill as well as those physically ill.
Bibliography: Medvei, V. C., and Thornton, J. L. 1973. *The Royal Hospital of Saint Bartholomew 1123-1973.*

RAILWAY BRAIN. A term used in nineteenth-century medico-legal reports. It covered obscure nervous disorders that were then attributed to railroad accidents.
Bibliography: Tuke, D. H. 1892. *A dictionary of psychological medicine.*

RAILWAY SPINE. A disorder described and named by Jonathan Erichsen (q.v.). He mistook a multitude of hysterical (*see* HYSTERIA) symptoms for neurological damage, which he ascribed to concussion of the spine. According to him, chronic meningitis could result from railway accidents.

Furneaux Jordan and Herbert Page opposed Erichsen's theories and eventually proved them false.
Bibliography: Trimble, M. R. 1981. *Post-traumatic neurosis: from railway spine to the whiplash.*

RAKE'S PROGRESS, THE. The title of a series of eight engravings by William Hogarth (q.v.), published in 1735. They depict the downfall of Thomas Bakewell, a young, irresponsible, pleasure-seeking gallant, who ends his days in a madhouse. Hogarth used the wards of Bethlem Royal Hospital (q.v.) as his model and depicted the rake as one of its inmates. He is shown with a shaven head, vacant expression, and wearing irons and chains. He is surrounded by wretched people who have reached the same stage of degradation. Visitors, society ladies, are looking on with a total lack of compassion, but with much mirth. In the eighteenth century visiting madhouses was an accepted and fashionable form of entertainment. In 1951, the same theme was chosen by Igor Stravinsky (1882-1971) for an opera (q.v.).
Bibliography: Burke, J., and Caldwell, C. 1968. *Hogarth: the complete engravings.*

RAMAYANA. An epic poem of ancient India. It is attributed to the sage Valmiki. Parts of it date from 500 B.C. It is the story of Rama, a hero who is the reincarnation of the god Vishnu. It contains many medical and psychological ideas and reflects the ancient Indian beliefs in these fields.
Bibliography: Shastri, H. P. trans. 1962-1970. *The Ramayana of Valmiki.* 3 vols.

RAMAZZINI, BERNARDINO (1633-1714). An Italian physician and author of the first book on occupational diseases, entitled *De Morbis Artificum Diatriba* (1713). Among other things he discussed the depression and "melancholic fits" (*see* MELANCHOLIA) that often plague painters. He attributed them to a physical cause, "the injurious qualities of the colours they use."
Bibliography: Koelsch, F. 1912. *Life of Ramazzini.*

RAMPTON HOSPITAL. An institution in Nottinghamshire, England. It was founded in 1914 as a criminal lunatic asylum. In 1920 it became a state institution for mental defectives with dangerous propensities. When it was taken over by the Ministry of Health in 1960, it was designated as a special hospital for the treatment of subnormal mentally ill patients under compulsive detention.
Bibliography: McGrath, P. G. 1966. Hospital care of the mentally abnormal offender. *Proc. Roy. Soc. Med.* 59: 699-700.

RANK, OTTO (1884-1939). An Austrian psychoanalyst. His original name was Rosenfeld, but he changed it to Rank in 1901. His father was a violent, alcoholic (*see* ALCOHOLISM) man, and it was his mother, a gentle and loving

woman, who kept the family together. At the age of sixteen, he and his brother, ceased to speak to their father, although they continued to live in the same house. Rank was never physically strong, and his diaries show him as depressed and even suicidal (*see* SUICIDE). As a young man he could not bear physical contact and would wear gloves to shake hands. He was a great admirer of Friedrich Nietzsche (q.v.) and had a life-long interest in the arts and creative powers. In 1906 he met Sigmund Freud (q.v.). Although they later disagreed, Rank was greatly helped and liked by Freud. He became a pioneer of psychoanalysis (q.v.) but developed a new psychology based on his belief that humanity was controlled by two contradictory impulses, life fear and death fear. According to him, a successful individual achieved independence by resolving the conflict and becoming free to create. Rank called such a man an "artist." His methods of therapy were based on a process of transference (q.v.), rather than psychoanalytical free association, and attempted to give the patient independence. Among his most important books are *The Artist* (1907), *The Myth of the Birth of the Hero* (1909) and *The Trauma of Birth* (1924) in which he argued that the terror experienced during the birth process shapes future development. From 1906 to 1915 Rank was secretary of the Vienna Psychoanalytic Society. He was a co-founder of *Imago* (q.v.).
Bibliography: Taft, J. 1958. *Otto Rank*.

RANSON, STEPHEN WALTER (1880-1924). An American anatomist. He greatly contributed to the revival in neurological studies in the United States. His investigations included research on the structure of the peripheral nervous system and on the function of the hypothalamus.
Bibliography: Haymaker, W., and Schiller, F. 1970. *The founders of neurology*. 2d. ed.

RASPUTIN, GRIGORI (1872-1916). A Russian self-styled holy man, the son of peasants. His name means "dissolute," and was given to him when he was a young man in his native village. Even as a child he had such insight into other people's minds that he was immediately aware if one of his friends had pilfered something; he had such "magnetism" that he could easily dominate those around him. He was only fifteen years old when he discovered his own sexual irresistibility. At twenty he had a vision of the Virgin and devoted himself to religion. He gained enormous ascendancy over the czar and the czarina and interfered in matters of government and national policy. His debauchery became notorious: he seduced women and asserted that contact with him was purifying. He was unkempt, dirty, and smelled like a goat. He was murdered by a group of noblemen who wanted to liberate Russia from his evil influence.
Bibliography: Minney, R. J. 1972. *Rasputin*.

RAT-MAN. A patient of Sigmund Freud (q.v.). He had suffered from an obsessional neurosis (q.v.) since his childhood. His symptoms became acute

after hearing that prisoners in the Far East were subjected to a form of torture involving rats. The patient improved greatly after eleven months of psychoanalysis (q.v.). Freud presented his case history at the First International Congress of Psychoanalysis in Salzburg in 1908 and published it in 1909.
Bibliography: Freud, S. 1909. *Notes upon a case of obsessional neurosis.*

RATZEL, FRIEDRICH (1844-1904). A German geographer and anthropologist. His importance to anthropological psychology rests on his studies of human settlements and their social structure and customs, which he believed were dictated by the environment. He refuted the theory that all primitive societies develop on parallel lines.
Bibliography: Ratzel, F. 1882-1891. *Anthropogeographie.* 2 vols.

RATZENHOFER, GUSTAV (1842-1904). An Austrian sociologist. His concept of politics was based on the belief that various groups undergo periods of conflict and adjustment to further their interests. He developed the theory of accommodation, which postulates that individual behavior is changed to achieve a degree of adjustment with society.
Bibliography: Ratzenhofer, G. 1908. *Soziologie.*

RAUCH, FREDERICK AUGUSTUS (1806-1841). A German philosopher and educationalist. He is considered the first personalist. As a young man he emigrated to the United States, qualified for the ministry, and became professor of biblical literature. In 1840 he published a book entitled *Psychology or a View of the Human Soul, including Anthropology,* which met with immediate success. In his book, he tried to amalgamate German and American views about man and his environment. Rauch believed that "the person is not only the centre of man, but also the centre of nature." From this postulate he developed an original point of view.
Bibliography: Roback, A. A. 1962. *History of psychology and psychiatry.*

RAULIN, JOSEPH (fl.1758). An eighteenth-century French physician. In 1758 he wrote a book on psycho-sexual disorders, entitled *Traité des Affections Vaporeuses du Sexe.* Among the substances prescribed by him for mental disorders were honey (q.v.), saffron (q.v.), soot, woodlice, and powdered lobster claws.
Bibliography: Focault, M. 1967. *Madness and civilization.*

RAUWOLFIA SERPENTINA. One of the 110 species of the genus Rauwolfia. It was called serpentina, or snakeroot, because it was believed to be an antidote to the bite of poisonous snakes. The term "Rauwolfia" was devised by Charles Plumier (1646-1704) a French botanist monk, in honor of Leonard Rauwolf (?-1596) who visited parts of Africa and Asia to study

those plants cited by ancient Greek and Arab medical writers. Plumier was the first to describe the plant, which is found in tropical regions. It was known in ancient Indian medicine as the "herb of folly," because an infusion of its root was used for mental disorders. Holy men, including Mahatma Gandhi (1869-1948), used the root to promote meditation and introspection. In the 1930s five alkaloids were isolated from *Rauwolfia serpentina*, and two Indian doctors, Ganneth Sen (q.v.) and Katrick Bose (q.v.) described the sedative properties of the plant. Some twenty years later its usefulness in cases of high blood pressure and psychoses (*see* PSYCHOSIS) was recognized in the West, and the compound derived from it took the name of Reserpine.
Bibliography: Emboden, W. 1972. *Narcotic plants.*

RAVEN'S PROGRESSIVE MATRICES. An intelligence test (q.v.) for children devised by the British psychologist J. C. Raven in 1951.
Bibliography: Raven, J. C. 1956. *Guide to the standard progressive matrices.* (Revised ed.)

RAY, ISAAC (1807–1881). An American psychiatrist. He was a humane, thoughtful, scholarly man. He began his career in general practice in East-port, Maine, but, once his interest was aroused in mental disorders, he turned to psychiatry and became the medical superintendent of the state mental hospital. In 1845 he became head of the Butler Asylum in Providence, Rhode Island for which he had helped to plan the new building. He was considered the foremost authority in forensic psychiatry and was the author of the first book in the English language in this field. It was entitled *Treatise of the Medical Jurisprudence of Insanity* and published in 1838. In 1863 in his book *Mental Hygiene*, he defined mental hygiene as "the art of preserving the health of the mind against all the incidents and influences calculated to deteriorate its qualities, impair its energies and derange its movements." Even though he was an enlightened man, he was against the abolition of restraint (q.v.) but also understandably critical of the exaggerated claims of cures made by many asylums (q.v.). He wrote a guide for psychiatrists entitled *Ideal Characters of the Officers of a Hospital for the Insane* after dreaming that he was reading a manuscript entitled *The Good Superintendent*. Ray was one of the thirteen original founders of the American Psychiatric Association (q.v.).
Bibliography: Ray, I. 1863. Reprint. 1968. *Mental hygiene.*

RAYMOND, FULGENCE (1844-1910). A French neurologist. He produced important work on nerve and mental pathology as well as neurasthenia (q.v.). He was the author of several books.
Bibliography: Raymond, F. 1894-1903. *Clinique des maladies du système nerveux.*

RAYNER, HENRY (1842–1926). A British physician. He was the medical superintendent of Hanwell Asylum (q.v.) and physician to Saint Thomas's

Hospital. He organized the first outpatient department for psychiatric disorders at a London teaching hospital in 1893.
Bibliography: Hunter, R., and Macalpine, I. 1974. *Psychiatry for the poor.*

RAYNESFORD. A courtier to Henry VII (1457–1509) of England. He became insane, and the king paid for him to be kept in Bethlem Royal Hospital (q.v.).
Bibliography: O'Donoghue, E. G. 1914. *The story of Bethlehem Hospital.*

REACTION EXPERIMENTS. A series of experiments conducted by Wilhelm Wundt (q.v.) in the 1880s to ascertain the influence of stimulus intensity upon reaction time, word perception, and other things.
Bibliography: Watson, R. I. 1963. *The great psychologists.*

READE, CHARLES (1814–1884). An English novelist and dramatist. He was an irascible and cantankerous man but an enthusiastic reformer. His works were based on documentary information that he collected and classified for future reference. He wrote about these methods in a novel entitled *A Terrible Temptation* (1871). In it he also described how a man was incarcerated in an asylum by an unscrupulous cousin. The story was used to show the unsatisfactory legal position of those facing certification. In his best novel *Hard Cash* (1863), he attacked asylums (q.v.), Dr. John Conolly (q.v.) (under the name of Dr. Wycherley), and the commissioners in lunacy (q.v.). *Hard Cash* was first serialized in *All the Year Round*, a periodical edited by Charles Dickens (q.v.), who, with Reade, had to bear the wrath of the *British Medical Journal* for their so-called irresponsibility in casting "diabolical charges upon the character of all medical men connected with the management of lunatics. . . ." Dickens replied that the views expressed belonged solely to the author and continued to publish instalments of the novel.
Bibliography: Burns, W. 1961. *Charles Reade.*

REAL CASA DEI MATTI. An institution for the mentally ill opened in 1824 in Palermo, Italy, by Pietro Pisani (q.v.). It was an unusually advanced institution; restraint (q.v.) was abolished, each patient's history was carefully compiled on admission, relatives and staff cooperated in the treatment, worktherapy, as well as emotional supports, was employed, and patients were allowed a voice in the running of the institution. The official guide to the Casa dei Matti was written by one of the patients while convalescing and a copy of it was handed to each new patient. The institution attracted many observers who reported favorably on it.
Bibliography: Mora, G. 1975. Italy. In *World history of psychiatry*, ed. J. G. Howells.

REBECCA OF BEDLAM (fl. 1780). An eighteenth century London maidservant. In 1780 she fell in love with her employer's friend, who had given her a golden guinea. Her infatuation developed into an obsession (q.v.), and she became deranged. She was admitted to Bethlem Royal Hospital (q.v.), where she spent the rest of her life clutching the golden coin. When she died a keeper prised open her fingers and took the money. According to legend, since the theft, Rebecca's ghost has haunted the corridors of the hospital searching for her lost treasure.

Bibliography: Ludlam, H. 1969. *A casebook of ghosts.*

RECKE-VOLMERSTEIN, ADALBERT VON DER (1791–1876). A German philanthropist. In the 1860s in Düsseldorf, Germany, he built a special institution for handicapped children that also accepted mentally retarded children. Contributions to the building fund came from King Frederick William IV of Prussia, Napoleon III (q.v.), and England.

Bibliography: Kanner, L. 1964. *A history of the care and study of the mentally retarded.*

RECKLINGHAUSEN, FRIEDRICH DANIEL VON (1833–1910). A German pathologist. In 1863 he described for the first time a condition that received more attention later, when called tuberous sclerosis (q.v.) by Désiré-Magloine Bourneville (q.v.).

Bibliography: Kanner, L. 1964. *A history of the care and study of the mentally retarded.*

RECOVERABLE PSYCHOSES. Emil Kraepelin (q.v.) devised a classification of mental disorders based on prognosis (q.v.). Those disorders that were not regarded as chronic were grouped together in a category of their own.

Bibliography: Zilboorg, G. 1941. *A history of medical psychology.*

RECOVERY WITH DEFECT. A term introduced by the German physician K. G. Neumann (1774–1850) to describe those mental patients whose personality remained changed after recovery from their basic disorder.

Bibliography: Zilboorg, G. 1941. *A history of medical psychology.*

RED WOOL. Ancient herbals often prescribed binding the herbs for mental disorders to the patient with red wool. It was thought to add to their effectiveness.

Bibliography: Rohde, E. S. 1974. *The old English herbals.*

REED, ANDREW (1787–1862). A British Congregational minister and philanthropist. He was the founder of several orphanages. In 1847 he visited the Abendberg Institution (q.v.), which inspired him to help the feeble-minded. With the support of John Conolly (q.v.), he launched an appeal for the foundation of a public institution. The motto of the appeal committee was "We plead for those who cannot plead for themselves." Thus, Park House (q.v.), the first English public institution for the mentally retarded was founded at Highgate in 1847 and opened in 1848. In 1855 it moved to Earlswood in Surrey.

Bibliography: Kanner, L. 1964. *A history of the care and study of the mentally retarded.*

REES, JOHN RAWLINGS (1890–1969). A British psychiatrist. He was one of the seven children of a Wesleyan Methodist minister. He began his medical career hoping to become a missionary, but he was drawn towards psychiatry during his service in World War I, when he witnessed the psychological afflictions of soldiers in active service. On the retirement of Dr. Hugh Crichton-Miller in 1932 he became director of the Tavistock Clinic (q.v.) and introduced many innovations. During World War II he was appointed consultant psychiatrist to the army at home and brought about a new approach to military psychiatry. His book *The Case of Rudolf Hess* (1947), was the result of his personal experience with Rudolf Hess (1894–) in Britain. In 1949 he became the founder/president of the World Federation for Mental Health. He was the author of several books and the editor of *Modern Practice in Psychological Medicine.* He gave discreet but active support to the movement to found a Royal College of Psychiatrists. (*See* ASSOCIATION OF MEDICAL OFFICERS OF ASYLUMS AND HOSPITALS FOR THE INSANE)

Bibliography: Rees, J. R. 1945. *The shaping of psychiatry by war.*

REEVE, JOHN (1799-1838). An English actor and comedian. He was subject to fits of depression during which he could not appear on the stage without the help of powerful stimulants. He was a heavy drinker and at times could not learn his parts, but he was such a favorite of the public that managers engaged him despite his problems. Off stage he was often irritable, nervous, and moody, even during the middle of a show. When this occurred, he would be treated with a mixture of aromatic spirits of ammonia in camphor, which seemed to enable him to go back on stage.

Bibliography: Clarke, J. F. 1874. *Autobiographical recollections of the medical profession.*

REGIMEN SANITATIS SALERNITANUM. An eleventh-century poem that encompasses the teaching of the Salerno Medical School (q.v.). It was originally dedicated to a king of England whose identity has not been established. For several centuries this work was memorized by most physicians. It was translated into several languages and published in over 100 editions. As well as containing remedies for physical ills, it offers advice on mental health. It claims, for example, that the brain of chickens or capons are good for the memory (q.v.) while certain fruits, such as peaches, apples,

and pears, engender melancholia (q.v.), as do milk, cheese, and certain kinds of meat, especially from four-legged animals. Conversely, its authors stated that wine was good for melancholy as it helped to expel the black humors (q.v.) from the body,.
Bibliography: Harrington, J. 1920. *Regimen sanitatis salernitanium.*

REGINALD OF BATH (?–1255). An English physician. He was physician to the wife of Henry III, Eleanor of Provence (d. 1291), and attended the members of her household. In 1255 the queen sent him to Edinburgh, Scotland, to her daughter Margaret (q.v.) to report on her state of health. In his report, he underlined the fact that the young queen's depression was due to the stresses she was undergoing. His too bold report, however, upset the court of Scotland, and Reginald is said to have been poisoned.
Bibliography: Talbot, C. H., and Hammond, E. A. 1965. *The medical practitioners in medieval England.*

REGISTERED HOSPITALS. Under nineteenth-century English legislation, hospitals for the mentally ill that catered for paying patients as well as a small number of patients accepted without cost. They were independent, charitable institutions, most of which were begun in the 1860s.
See also ASYLUMS.

REICH, WILHELM (1897–1957). An Austrian psychiatrist. Both his parents died when he was an adolescent. His mother committed suicide (q.v.) after an unhappy love affair with his tutor, and his father died of tuberculosis (q.v.) three years later. Reich quickly became famous in psychoanalytic circles, but his ideas were not approved by Sigmund Freud (q.v.), who refused to analyze him. Freud's refusal precipitated a period of depression. His ambition to combine Marxism with psychoanalysis (q.v.) resulted in his expulsion from the Communist party and the International Psychoanalytic Association (q.v.). He overemphasized the importance of sexual potency and satisfaction and became renowned for his orgone therapy (q.v.), but this too met with hostility by the profession and the public. Almost the only person he did not quarrel with was Alexander S. Neill (q.v.). Reich's clinical work was investigated, and complaints were made. He was ludicrously prosecuted by the Food and Drug Administration for violation of the Food and Drug Act and contempt of court, found guilty, and sent to prison, where he died of bronchopneumonia, having refused medical treatment. His paranoia (q.v.) was perhaps justified. Both his third wife and his son, Peter, have written biographies of him.
Bibliography: Reich, P. 1973. *A book of dreams.*

REID, HENRY (1736–1816). An Irish physician who practiced in Downpatrick. He accepted wealthy patients with psychiatric disabilities in his

private asylum (q.v.). His association with United Irishmen led him and his family to seek temporary refuge in South Carolina. On his return to Ireland (q.v.), he continued to run the asylum, which, after his death, was managed by his widow and then his son. No other mental hospital existed in Downpatrick until 1869, when the Downshire Hospital (q.v.) came into existence.
Bibliography: Parkinson, R. E. 1969. *Historical sketch of Downshire Hospital.*

REID, JOHN (1776–1822). A British physician who practiced in London. In 1808 he stated in his *Report on Diseases* that "madness strides like a Colossus in the country" and that "more people are mad than are supposed to be. There are atoms, or specks of insanity, which cannot be discerned by the naked or uneducated eye." In his *Essay on Insanity, Hypochondriasis, and Other Nervous Affections*, written in 1816, he presented his observations on the influence of psychological events on mental derangement. He believed that institutional life was often harmful because of the isolation, prolonged confinement, and humiliating treatment the patients underwent. He called asylums (q.v.) "nurseries of madness." He was aware of the mind's influence on the body and dedicated a chapter in his book to its discussion.
Bibliography: Hunter, R., and Macalpine, I. 1963. *Three hundred years of psychiatry.*

REID, THOMAS (1710–1796). A Scottish professor of philosophy at the University of Aberdeen and the University of Glasgow. He descended from a line of Presbyterian ministers. In 1763 he published a book entitled *An Inquiry into the Human Mind on the Principles of Common Sense* to refute the writings of David Hume (q.v.) on the mind. He believed that, based on observation and induction an "anatomy" of the mind, similar to that of the body, was possible and would be achieved by introspection and the methods advocated by Jeremy Bentham (q.v.).
Bibliography: Grave, S. A. 1960. *The Scottish philosophy of common sense.*

REIL, JOHANN CHRISTIAN (1759–1813). A German physician, one of the first to dedicate himself completely to psychiatry. He was health director of the University of Halle. In his later life he became a neuroanatomist and produced many revolutionary ideas in the field of psychiatry. He was a follower of Immanuel Kant (q.v.) and regarded the relationship between mind and body as one of mere interaction. He fought against punitive methods of treatment for the insane and strived to establish what he considered to be a more humanitarian approach that employed "psychic methods to cure mental derangement." These, however, included throwing patients into cold water, firing cannons to startle them, shutting them in dark cells, and organizing plays in which angels, the dead out of their graves, judges, and other fear-inspiring figures were used to shock the patients. He called this method "non-injurious torture" (q.v.). Yet, according to Johanna Wolfgang von Goethe (q.v.) who was one of his patients, he was a kind and

considerate physician. In 1806 Napoleon I (q.v.) closed the University of Halle, and Reil dedicated himself fully to the study of cerebral structures, doing many dissections. He was an ardent patriot in the war of liberation. After the retreat from Moscow, he was in charge of field hospitals and wrote angry reports about the inadequate conditions. He died of typhus contracted in the lazarets after the battle of Leipzig. His ideas typified a period of transition, and his writings reflect the struggle to relate mental and physical events. Among his best remembered works of interest to psychiatry are *Memorabilia Clinica* (1792), *Tractatus de Polycholia* (1783), and *Rapsodien* (1803), which deals with German asylums (q.v.) and describes their appalling conditions. It also shows how nebulous and speculative the theory of psychiatry was at that time. The *Magazin fur psychishe Heilkunde*, one of the first psychiatric journals, was founded by Reil in 1805.
Bibliography: Neuburger, M. 1913. *Johann Christian Reil: Gedenkrede*.

REIMARUS, HERMANN SAMUEL (1694–1768). A German scholar and philosopher. He was an independent thinker, and his writings on the life and purposes of Jesus, published posthumously and anonymously as *Fragments of an Unknown*, were denounced as derogatory. His systematic writings on comparative animal psychology, emphasized the difference between man and beast and led him to approach a theory of evolution.
Bibliography: Roback, A. A. 1962. *History of psychology and psychiatry*.

REISCHENBÖCK, ERNST (1923–?). An Austrian painter. His psychopathological (*see* PSYCHOPATHY) characteristics culminated in a frenzy of activity that produced a series of seven hundred paintings in the space of three months. All the paintings have an erotic-religious content and he called the theme depicted in them "Christ above eroticism." According to his philosophy, the salvation of mankind and its liberation from base motives is achieved through orgasm in an exalted interrelationship.
Bibliography: Müller-Thalheim, W. K. 1972. Sexus und Religion: Der Maler Ernst Reischenböck. *Confinia Psychiat.* 15: 91-98.

RELIGIO MEDICI. The most famous work of Sir Thomas Browne (q.v.), written in 1635 and published in 1643. John Aubrey (q.v.) referred to it as the book "which first opened my understanding." In it, Browne presented his belief in two truths, one arrived at by reason and the other by faith or intuition. A grasp of psychological motivations is apparent throughout the work, which covers many aspects of religious thought. Browne's erudition and tolerance did not, however, prevent him from believing in spirits and witches (*see* WITCHCRAFT) as the cause of mental disorders. He wrote: "I hold that the Devil doth really possess some men, the spirit of Melancholy others, the Spirit of Delusion others . . . " Good spirits, according to him, were responsible for "courteous revelations." In writing about sleep, he

maintained that individuals often dream of themselves as they would like to be: "we are somewhat more than our selves in our sleeps . . . ", a concept reminiscent of Freudian theories.
Bibliography: Keynes, G. 1968. *Sir Thomas Browne: selected writings.*

REMAK, ROBERT (1815-1865). A German physician, born in the ghetto of the Polish city of Poznan. He was a neurocytologist who published important papers on the histological structure of the nervous system. His lectures on embryology were outstanding, and his ideas stimulated further studies in his pupils, among them Wilhelm His (q.v.) and Rudolf von Kölliker (q.v.). In the clinical field, he was a pioneer in the use of electrotherapy in nervous diseases and introduced such changes as the use of induced current in place of galvanic current.
Bibliography: Haymaker, W., and Schiller, F. 1970. *The founders of neurology.* 2d. ed.

REMBRANDT HARMENSZ VAN RIJN (1606-1669). A Dutch painter. He began to study painting as an adolescent and became famous when he was still a young man. His marriage to Saskia van Ulyenburgh was saddened by the death of three of their four children. After her death in 1642, he formed a relationship with a trumpeter's widow. When Hendrickje Stoffels became his mistress, the widow sued him for breach of promise. She was eventually declared insane and sent to an asylum (q.v.). Rembrandt never married Hendrickje because he would have lost the income granted to him by his wife's will. After Saskia's death, his style changed. Shadows and darkness in his painting made him unfashionable and led to his bankruptcy. His numerous portraits of old people are particularly sensitive and moving and display his fascination with the old and the sick. He had a narcissistic (*see* NARCISSISM) need to paint himself over and over again. He left nearly 100 self-portraits that document his transformation from an exuberant youth to a sorrowing old man. He died in poverty a year after the death of his only son, Titus (1642-1668).
Bibliography: Rosenberg, J. 1964. *Rembrandt: life and work.*

RENDU, HENRI JULES LOUIS (1844-1902). A French physician. In 1888, he became the first to describe a form of hysterical (*see* HYSTERIA) tremor precipitated or aggravated by volitional movements. This disorder is now known as Rendu's tremor.
Bibliography: Schmidt, J. E. 1959. *Medical discoveries: who and when.*

RENI, GUIDO (1575-1642). An Italian painter. He was a compulsive gambler who was chronically attracted to gambling by the risks involved in it. Because he gambled away most of his considerable earnings, he was forced to produce carelessly executed pictures to pay his debts. His downfall was

aided by some of his associates who exploited him. His own nephew added to his constant state of anxiety by selling copies of his works, often before the originals were finished.
Bibliography: Wittkower, R., Wittkower, M. 1963. *Born under Saturn.*

REPERSONALIZATION. A term suggested in 1926 by Morton Prince (q.v.) to replace "hypnotism" (q.v.).
Bibliography: Prince, M. 1926. Society transactions. *Arch. Neurol. Psychiat.* 15: 800-802.

REPORT OF SELECT COMMITTEE ON MADHOUSES. A short report of only eleven pages produced in England in 1763. It recommended "the interposition of the legislature" in the control of madhouses and led to an act of Parliament to that effect in 1774. (*see* INSPECTION OF MADHOUSES).
Bibliography: Jones, K. 1972. *A history of the mental health services.*

REPORT OF THE METROPOLITAN COMMISSIONERS IN LUNACY. The first report to cover the state of the mental health provisions in England and Wales. It was prepared by a committee under the chairmanship of Lord Ashley (q.v.) (1801-1885). It produced suggestions for changes in the law that led to the reforms enacted in 1845.
Bibliography: Jones, K. 1972. *A history of the mental health services.*

REPUBLIC, THE. A book by Plato (q.v.) written in the form of a dialogue and describing the ideal state. It contains a discussion of the personality of men in relation to their political institutions. Plato observed that childhood experiences within the family influence the mature personality. Family dynamics and their resultant emotions are also discussed.
Bibliography: Plato. *The Republic*, trans. A. D. Lindsay.

REST CURE. A form of therapy for nervous disorders. It was first formulated in 1877 by the American neurologist Silas Weir Mitchell (q.v.). It consisted of complete rest, good food, seclusion from those surroundings that have contributed to the illness, massage, and electrotherapy.
Bibliography: Mitchell, S. W. 1877. *Fat and blood.*

RESTRAINT. The prevention of abnormal behavior that would cause violence against the self or others. Methods of restraint have varied little over the ages. Primitive cultures and early civilizations were, on the whole, more humane than the seventeenth, eighteenth, and nineteenth centuries in the way they treated the insane. Their tolerance was rewarded by less extreme forms of behavior. The coercive measures of the later centuries were abused

and misused; they humiliated and antagonized patients, who responded with as much aggression as their weakened and exhausted bodies would allow. Special garments, cages, restraining cots, and similar devices were invented by physicians who did not stop at starving the patient in an effort to repress symptoms. (See Plate 12). Benjamin Rush (q.v.) was among those who believed in such methods. Then came an era of "gentler" management: leather thongs in place of iron chains, padded cells in place of dungeons. Vicenzo Chiarugi, John Conolly, and Philippe Pinel (qq.v.), as well as many other enlightened physicians, brought about a change in the feelings toward restraining violent patients. Physical restraint, however, has not been abolished; the chains have now been replaced by chemical products and surgery.
Bibliography: Conolly, J. 1856. Reprint. 1973. *Treatment of the insane without mechanical restraints.*

RÉTIF (*or* RESTIF) DE LA BRETONNE, NICHOLAS EDME (1734-1806). A French novelist, the author of over 250 educational novels. His work, although now considered valuable as a description of working class life in the eighteenth century, was frowned upon because of its coarseness and frequent obscenity. He was said to suffer from a sexual deviation, that consisted of seeking gratification from women's shoes, therefore, this form of fetishism is often termed "rétifism."
Bibliography: London, L. S., and Caprio, F. S. 1951. *Sexual deviations.*

RETREAT, THE (*see* YORK RETREAT).

RETREAT GAZETTE. An American intramural periodical, published at the Hartford Retreat (q.v.) in 1837. The editor, who was the mainspring of the project, was a newspaper man who had become mentally ill. When he recovered and left the Retreat, the journal ceased publication.
See also JOURNALS BY PATIENTS.
Bibliography: Deutsch, A. 1949. *The mentally ill in America.*

RETZ, (*or* RAIS) GILLES DE LAVAL, SEIGNEUR DE (1404-1440). A French marshal and supporter of Joan of Arc (q.v.). He was interested in necromancy (q.v.) and kidnapped and killed more than 100 children. In French folklore (q.v.) he is associated with Blue Beard.
Bibliography: Benedetti, J. 1971. *Gilles de Rais.*

RETZIUS, GUSTAF (1842-1919). A Swedish physician and neurologist. His studies of prehistoric crania contributed to the field of physical anthropology. He also added to the knowledge of the sensory organs and the nerve terminations and presented accounts of the comparative morphology of the nervous system. He was not only a scientist but also a biographer and poet with several volumes to his credit. His brain, bequeathed to scientific re-

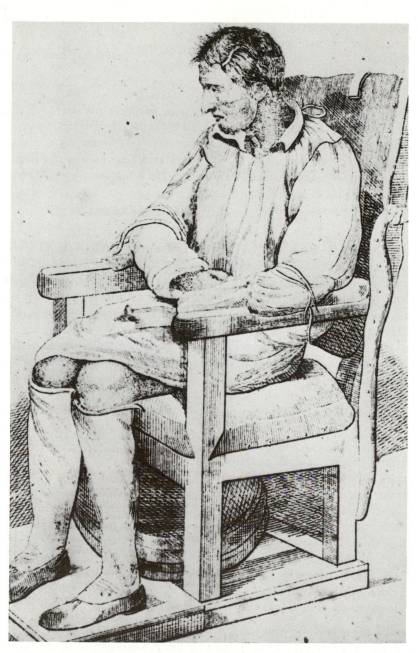

12. A RESTRAINING CHAIR FOR MENTAL PATIENTS. This model, more humane than earlier contraptions, was used in Poland in the nineteenth century. By courtesy of the Department of Medical Illustration, Ipswich Hospital.

search, is now preserved in the Museum of Pathology of the Caroline Institute, where he had been a teacher.

Bibliography: Haymaker, W., and Schiller, F. 1970. *The founders of neurology*. 2d. ed.

REVESZ, GEZA (1878-1955). A Hungarian psychologist. Because of the political situation in Hungary he emigrated to Holland and in 1932 he became the first professor of psychology at the University of Amsterdam, where he established a psychological institute. With David Katz (1884-) he founded an international journal, *Acta Psychologica*. He wrote on a variety of psychological topics in several languages.

Bibliography: Robeck, A. A. 1962. *History of psychology and psychiatry*.

RHAZES (ABÛ-BAKR MUHAMMAD IBN-ZAKARIA-Y-AL-RÂZI) (c.865-925). A Persian physician. He studied medicine in Baghdad and became the chief physician at the hospital of Raj in Tabaristan near Teheran before returning to Baghdad as a teacher. He is said to have become blind when beaten on the head with his own book; the ruler of Bokhara had ordered that he should be so punished until either the book or his head broke because some of Rhazes's chemical experiments had failed. As well as writing extensively on medicine, he wrote on philosophy, astronomy, mathematics, and religion. His medical encyclopedia, completed by his pupil after his death, was known in the West under the title of *Liber Continens*. It discussed the practical issues of diagnosis and therapy. It was translated into Latin by the order of Charles of Anjou, king of Sicily, by a Jewish physician, Farag ben Salem, in 1279. The printed edition of 1486 is literally the most weighty of all incunabula, tipping the scales at twenty-two pounds. Rhazes followed the principles of Galen (q.v.) and was indeed called the Persian Galen. He accepted the Aristotelian (*see* ARISTOTLE) classification of three souls, vegetative, animal, and rational, and attributed disorders to a lack or excess of one or other of them. His approach to mental illness was enlightened for the time. In addition to purgatives, he advocated confrontation with the patient to stir him out of his melancholia (q.v.). He described various mental disorders and discussed alcoholism (q.v.). His books, more than two hundred of them, were referred to until the seventeenth century.

Bibliography: Elgood, C. 1951. *A medical history of Persia*.

RHEINAU PSYCHIATRIC INSTITUTE. A Swiss institution for chronic psychiatric patients. Situated in picturesque surroundings in a remote corner of the Zürich canton, it is self-supporting and in some respects resembles the Gheel Colony (q.v.). Discharged patients often stay on in the village and are looked after in the homes of local families. Eugen Bleuler (q.v.) was

director of the institution from 1886 to 1898, and it was there that he gathered most of the material for his monograph on schizophrenia (q.v.).
Bibliography: Finkelstein, B. A. 1971. Eugen Bleuler and the Psychiatric Institute Rheinau. *Am. J. Psychiat.* 128: 5.

RHINE, JOSEPH BANKS (1895-1980). An American parapsychologist. His research on psychical phenomena (q.v.) made the field acceptable to the scientific world. The term "extra-sensory perception" (ESP) (q.v.) was coined by him. In 1927 he established the parapsychology laboratory at Duke University in Durham, North Carolina. There, he conducted experiments in many aspects of extra-sensory perception. The Foundation for Research on the Nature of Man was formed by him after his retirement from Duke University.
Bibliography: Rhine, D. B. 1973. *New frontiers of the mind: story of the Duke experiments.*

RIBOT, THÉODULE ARMAND (1839-1916). A French psychologist and a pioneer in experimental psychology (q.v.). He introduced into France the concepts that had been developed by English and German psychologists. His *La Psychologie Anglaise Contemporaine* appeared in 1870 and was followed nine years later by a companion volume on German developments, entitled *La Psychologie Allemande Contemporaine.* In 1885 he was appointed head of a course in experimental psychology at the Sorbonne, and in 1888 he became professor of experimental and comparative psychology at the Collège de France. Pierre Janet (q.v.) was one of his pupils. He wrote on disorders of memory (q.v.), will, and personality and was the first to employ the concept of anhedonia (q.v.). He also devised a classification of sexual disorders according to their aetiology.
Bibliography: Flugel, J. C. 1945. *A hundred years of psychology.*

RICHARD III (1452-1485). A king of England. As duke of Gloucester, he was appointed regent after the death of his brother Edward IV (1442-1483), but he imprisoned the young Edward V and his brother. According to the description of his character appearing in *Richard III* by William Shakespeare (q.v.), he was physically deformed, bitter, and cruel. His birth was a difficult breech presentation. Moreover he was said to have been born with congenital teeth and therefore superstitiously regarded as evil. Unloved, even by his own mother, and unloving, he represents the classic psychopath, selfish and self-centered as a result of unsatisfactory experiences, which, in this case, started as early as in the prenatal period.
Bibliography: Cheetham, A. 1972. *The life and times of Richard III.*

RICHARDSON, DOROTHY MILLER (1873-1957). An English novelist. Her life was terribly dreary. After spending some years as a paid companion,

she married Alan Odle, an artist, fifteen years her junior, who was so ill that he was expected to live for only a few months, but he survived for another twenty-five years. She was accident prone, for instance her love affair with Herbert G. Wells (q.v.) ended in pregnancy and a miscarriage. Her books never sold despite the fact that their importance was recognized. Between 1915 and 1938 she wrote a sequence of novels with the collective title of Pilgrimage; in them she originated the "stream of consciousness" technique that influenced the writings of Virginia Woolf (q.v.) and James Joyce (q.v.) among others.
Bibliography: Rosenberg, J. 1973. *The genius they forgot.*

RICHELIEU, ARMAND JEAN DU PLESSIS, DUC DE (1585-1642). A French cardinal and statesman, renowned for his ascendency over Louis XIII (q.v.) and the way in which he made France the most important European power of his time by destroying internal democracy, using immoral and inhuman methods to achieve his ends. He was the center of intrigues, plots, and espionage. He suffered from epilepsy (q.v.), and during seizures he believed that he was a horse. He would gallop round the room kicking and neighing. He was also the founder of the French Academy.
Bibliography: Auchincloss, L. 1973. *Richelieu.*

RICHET, CHARLES ROBERT (1850-1935). A French physiologist. He was interested particularly in hypnotic (*see* HYPNOTISM) phenomena and their application in therapy. His interest led him to point out that Armand-Marie-Jacques Puysegur (q.v.) had made the earliest discoveries in that field. He was one of the founders of the Societé de Psychologie Physiologique and one of the first workers to investigate the clinical possibilities of hypnotism. Jean Martin Charcot (q.v.) not only accepted Richet's judgment that hypnotic phenomena were genuine but also was greatly influenced by his work on somnambulism (q.v.).
Bibliography: Watson, R. I. 1963. *The great psychologists.*

RICHMOND DISTRICT LUNATIC ASYLUM. The first public asylum (q.v.) in Ireland (q.v.). It was opened in 1815 in Dublin, following a government inquiry into the needs of the insane. The institution accepted patients from all of Ireland and was the only organized asylum outside of Saint Patrick's Hospital (q.v.), founded by Jonathan Swift (q.v.).
Bibliography: Letchworth, W. P. 1889. *The insane in foreign countries.*

RICKMAN, JOHN (1891-1951). A British psychoanalyst. He was one of the founders of the London Psychoanalytic Society. In 1928 he published

his *Index Psychoanalyticus*, a bibliography of works on psychoanalysis (q.v.) appearing between 1893 and 1926. It contained nearly 5,000 titles.
Bibliography: Rickman, J. 1928. *Index psychoanalyticus.*

RIDDELL, HENRY SCOTT (1798-1870). A Scottish poet, son of a shepherd. He was a solitary man, who showed signs of mental instability and excessive excitability even in his early years. Placed in an asylum, he talked about his sufferings and quoted his own poetry. After a brief remission, he relapsed into a state of deep confusion, which he remained in for the rest of his life.
Bibliography: Winslow, L.S.F. 1898. *Mad humanity: its forms, apparent and obscure.*

RIEDEL, JOSEPH GOTTFRIED VON (1803-1870). A physician born in Friedland, Bohemia. He was director of the mental hospital in Prague. In 1851, he became the first director of the newly built mental hospital in Vienna. He was a progressive man and introduced many humane innovations in the treatment of mental patients in Austria and in Germany.
Bibliography: Mora, G. 1971. Anniversaries. *Am. J. Psychiat.* 127: 901-7.

RIEGER, CONRAD (1855-1939). A German psychiatrist and pioneer in psychological testing. He devised tests for the assessment of defects that were a result of brain injuries. His earlier work had been with patients suffering mental deterioration as a consequence of general paralysis of the insane (q.v.).
Bibliography: Bondy, M. 1974. Psychiatric antecedents of psychological testing (before Binet). *J. Hist. Behav. Sci.* 10: 180-94.

RIGA INSTITUTION FOR THE FEEBLEMINDED. An institution founded in Riga, then the capital of Livonia, in 1854 by Friedrich Platz. It was the first of its kind in Russia.
Bibliography: Barr, M. W. 1904. *Mental defectives.*

RIGGS, AUSTEN FOX (1876-1940). An American physician. He may be regarded as the originator of the therapeutic community as it is known today. After graduating from the College of Physicians and Surgeons of Columbia University, he studied under Sir William Osler (q.v.). In 1907 he was stricken with tuberculosis (q.v.). During the subsequent period of enforced rest, he became interested in the influence of mental states on bodily functions. His first paper on neurasthenia (q.v.), published in 1908 in the *Medical Record*, was written after observing a patient with conversion hysteria (q.v.). By 1913 he developed a fully integrated conceptual system of ego psychology. In 1919 he designed and founded the Austen Riggs Center in Stockbridge, Massachusetts. It was a highly organized therapeutic community for the reeducational treatment of neuroses (*see* NEUROSIS). Riggs also was active

in the field of student mental health, child guidance (q.v.), community psychiatry, and psychosomatic medicine (q.v.).
Bibliography: Kubie, L. S., ed. 1960. *The Riggs story.*

RIGOLETTO. The fool (q.v.) in the opera (q.v.) entitled *Rigoletto* by Giuseppe Verdi (1813-1901). He exemplifies the pathetic figure of the court jester, who was forced to assume a cloak of folly to amuse his master, with licencious behavior and words, while his emotions remained those of a sensitive man.
Bibliography: Harewood, ed. 1969. *Kobbe's complete opera book.*

RIMBAUD, JEAN NICOLAS ARTHUR (1854-1891). A French poet. His family was poor, the father, an army officer, deserted his family, and Rimbaud was brought up very strictly by a stern mother. Discipline and religion played an important part in his early childhood. A quiet and pensive child, he was a brilliant student, who won a prize for Latin poetry at the age of thirteen. When he was fifteen years old, he rebelled and ran away to Paris, where he was arrested for traveling without a ticket. Defiant and unruly, he immersed himself in the study of the occult and mysticism. He believed that suffering and a dissolute life would fit him for the role of a poet-seer, who had an important message for the world. He was a member of a group of artists known as "the symbolists," who now are regarded as the forerunners of surrealism (q.v.). Rimbaud's poetry was full of daring drama based on eccentric and imaginative thinking that possessed a hallucinatory quality. He lived in Paris and then in London with Paul Verlaine (q.v.) with whom he shared drugs (q.v.), drink, and debaucheries. Their mutual influence and their passionate relationship was so intense that when Rimbaud wanted to leave Verlaine, Verlaine shot and wounded him and was imprisoned for attempted murder and for immorality. At the age of nineteen, Rimbaud tired of poetry and poets, set fire to his papers, and spent the rest of his short life wandering as a soldier, a circus manager, and, finally, a trader in Africa, trafficking in arms and slaves. He died after an unsuccessful operation to amputate an infected leg. At the end he was a frustrated and unhappy individual, vainly searching for attention.
Bibliography: Starkie, E. 1961. *Arthur Rimbaud.*

RIMSKY-KORSAKOV, NICOLAI ANDREYEVICH (1844-1908). A Russian composer and friend of Modest Petrovich Moussorgsky (q.v.). He was the victim of depression that was aggravated by the death of two of his children. He was said to have suffered from cerebrospinal neurasthenia (q.v.).

It was considered the cause of a period of crisis from 1892 until 1895 during which he was unable to compose or listen to music.
Bibliography: Rimsky-Korsakov, N. A. 1942. *My musical life*. 3rd. ed., trans. J. A. Joffe.

RINGSEIS, JOHANN NEPOMUK VON. (1785-1880). A German physician. As a Catholic mystical philosopher he belonged to a group that worked toward an integration of magnetism (q.v.) and the teaching of the church.
Bibliography: Galdston, I., ed. 1967. *Historic derivations of modern psychiatry*.

RIO DE JANEIRO. The first Brazilian psychiatric hospital, the Hospicio Pedro II, opened in 1852 in Rio de Janeiro, following the efforts of Dr. José Clemento Pereira and Dr. Jose Da Cruz Jobim. Its opening marked the approval of the first legislative measures for the care of the mentally ill. The hospital was considered exceptionally well appointed, even in comparison with contemporary hospitals in Europe.
Bibliography: Leon, C. A. and Rosselli, H. 1975. Latin America. In *World history of psychiatry*, ed. J. G. Howells.

RIOLAN, JEAN (1577-1657). A French physician. He was chief physician to Marie de' Medici (1573-1642). His attitude to mental disorders was enlightened for his times, as he believed that hysteria (q.v.) was a clinical condition rather than a form of behavior induced by demonaic (q.v.) possession. He affirmed this belief in the case of Martha Brossier (q.v.).
Bibliography: Trevor-Roper, H. R. 1969. *The European witch-craze of the sixteenth and seventeenth centuries*.

RIVERS, WILLIAM HALSE (1864-1922). A British anthropologist. He pioneered the genealogical method of social research. His work resulted in several books that linked anthropology and psychology. Among his best-known works are *Instinct and the Unconscious* (1920), *Psychology and Politics* (1923), *Conflict and Dream* (1923) and *Psychology and Ethnology* (1926). He also studied the effects of drugs (q.v.) and alcohol on mental activity.
Bibliography: Rivers, W. H. 1926. *Psychology and ethnology*.

RIVIÈRE, LAZARE (RIVERIUS) (1589-1655). A French physician. As a follower of Galen (q.v.), he believed in a humoral theory (q.v.) of melancholia (q.v.) and advocated the use of purgatives (*see* PURGING) in its treatment. He was the first to teach chemistry at Montpellier. In his book *Praxis Medica*, (1660) he included chapters entitled "De Hysterica Passione" and "De Furore Uteris," in which he linked hysterical (*see* HYSTERIA) disorders with excessive sexuality in women.
Bibliography: Zilboorg, G. 1941. *A history of medical psychology*.

ROBERTSON, DOUGLAS ARGYLL (1837-1909). A Scottish ophthalmic surgeon. Conducting experiments on himself with the African calabar bean,

he searched for a substance that would contract the pupil. The alkaloid eserin was isolated from the calabar bean, and the further studies derived from this discovery led to important chemical research in neurology (q.v.).
Bibliography: Haymaker, W., and Schiller, F. 1970. *The founders of neurology*. 2d. ed.

ROBESPIERRE, MAXIMILIEN DE FRANÇOIS MARIE ISIDORE

(1758–1794). A French revolutionary and leader of the radical party during the French Revolution (q.v.). His mother died when he was nine years old, which left his father, a doctor, so distraught that he abandoned his practice and his family and wandered through Europe. Robespierre was brought up by pious aunts and grew into a bitter, unattractive, and self-possessed individual. It is said that he never forgave Louis XVI and Marie Antoinette for canceling a visit to his school where he was to recite an ode of welcome to them and that this was one of the reasons he insisted on their death during the Reign of Terror, which he instigated. His integrity and imagination (q.v.) were clouded by his dourness and lack of humor. Although he fought for the common people, he never understood them. Like most dictators, he was the product of rejection and humiliation and felt that he was basically despised by those around him. To him the guillotine was the only real deterrent. His psychopathic (*see* PSYCHOPATHY) behavior led to a revolt, and he too died by the guillotine.
Bibliography: Carr, J. L. 1973. *Robespierre*.

RODIA, SABATINO

(1878-1965). An Italian immigrant to the United States who supported himself in various labouring jobs. He led a lonely life in a shack that was poorly constructed, cold, and unfurnished but enobled by a complete set of the *Encyclopaedia Britannica*. When he was forty-three years old, he began to construct a strange sculpture of concrete and steel. The work became an obsession (q.v.), and he spent all his meagre earnings on ornamental materials for his creation, which also claimed all his free time. After thirty-three years of daily, compulsive work he was satisfied that his sculpture was sufficient to assure his immortality. He presented it to the neighborhood and left the locality. The Rodia Towers of Watts, California, were proclaimed of historical interest and protected as a work of art deserving to be kept for posterity.
Bibliography: Wayne, G. J. 1971. A creative obsession. The quest for immortality. In *Proceedings fifth world congress of psychiatry*.

ROELANS, CORNELIUS

(1450-1525). A Flemish medical writer. In 1483 he wrote a book on pediatrics entitled *De Aegritudinis Infantum* in which

he referred to sleep disorders in children, including insomnia and nightmares (q.v.) originating from fear.
Bibliography: Still, G. F. 1965. *The history of paediatrics.*

ROGER OF SALERNO (ROGERIUS FRUGARDI). A twelfth-century Italian surgeon of the Salerno Medical School (q.v.). He advocated trephining (*see* TREPANATION) for mania and melancholia (qq.v.) and cauterization (q.v.) of the occiput for epilepsy (q.v.). His writings also include a reference to the use of seaweeds in the treatment of goitre; this was a remarkable precedent in the use of iodine, which is present in certain algae.
Bibliography: Castiglioni, A. 1947. *History of medicine*, ed., and trans. E. B. Krumbhaar.

ROHEIM, GEZA (1891-1953). A Hungarian psychoanalyst and anthropologist who emigrated to the United States. He was influenced by the work of Karl Abraham (q.v.), and forged a link between psychoanalysis (q.v.) and anthropology. Applying the tenets of psychoanalysis to his field work in anthropology, he studied the mythological, cultural, and sexual aspects of a number of primitive tribes in Somaliland and Australia.
Bibliography: Roheim, G. 1943. *The origin and function of culture.*

ROLANDO, LUIGI (1773-1831). An Italian physician. He was personal physician to the king of Savoy and traveled with him to Sardinia when Napoleon I (q.v.) invaded Piedmont. He taught medicine at the University of Sassari and there, with limited facilities, pursued his studies of the brain and its functions. He believed the cerebellum secreted a fluid that was conducted by the nerves and stimulated the muscles of locomotion. He compared the cerebellum to the battery of Alessandro Volta (1745-1827) and its secretion to galvanic fluid because it increases and straightens the voluntary movements that the cerebrum initiates. In his view the cerebral hemispheres were "the principal seats of the immediate cause of sleep, of dementia, of apoplexy, of melancholia and of mania." Several structures of the brain, for example the fissure of Rolando, are named after him. His essay on the structure of the brain represents a milestone in the history of neurology (q.v.).
Bibliography: Riese, W. 1959. *A history of neurology.*

ROLFE, FREDERICK WILLIAM *See* CORVO, BARON.

ROMANES, GEORGE JOHN (1848-1894). An English biologist and physiologist. He was a friend and a follower of Charles Darwin (q.v.) and applied the Darwinian theory of evolution to the development of the mind. In 1882 he wrote a book entitled *Animal Intelligence*, which is regarded as the first published work on comparative psychology. He reported in it the

results of a wide investigation into animal behavior, and he provided much of the material that laid the foundation for subsequent research. He followed this book with *Mental Evolution in Animals* (1883) and *Mental Evolution in Man* (1887).
Bibliography: Romanes, E. 1896. *Life and letters of John Romanes.*

ROMANTICISM. A new feeling, rather than a movement, that originated in France at the beginning of the nineteenth century. It pervaded the arts and influenced intellectuals in all fields. It followed the emotional and physical upheaval of the French Revolution (q.v.) and was characterized by general restlessness, swings of mood from the deepest melancholy (*see* MELANCHOLIA) to elation, and brooding, as well as a freer expression of emotions. The doctrines of romanticism pushed the sublime to the point of the grotesque. The morbid interest in death deteriorated into a desire to shock, best exemplified by lurid tales of vampirism, ghosts, and evil doings by supernatural beings. Psychological speculations led to a new wave of interest in psychiatric disorders. Although interest was focused on the illness, rather than on the patient as a person, the importance of the emotions was again recognized.
Bibliography: Furst, R. 1970. *Romanticism in perspective.*

ROMBERG, MORITZ HEINRICH (1795-1873). A German pathologist and neurologist. He was the first physician to relate clinical manifestations to the alteration of nerve structures. He translated into German the work of Charles Bell (q.v.) and was greatly influenced by him. In 1840 Romberg wrote his *Hehrbuch der Nervenkrankheiten* which became a classic in the field of neurology (q.v.). It was reprinted several times and translated into English. He was also the first physician to give a clinical description of tabes dorsalis, now termed Romberg's syndrome.
Bibliography: Romberg, M. H. 1853. *A manual of the nervous diseases of man.*

ROMULUS. The legendary founder of Rome, one of twin sons born to the vestal virgin Rhea Sylvia, who was put to death because of her illicit relationship with the god of war, Mars. The children were exposed in a forest but survived because a she-wolf fostered them. Unlike later examples, they did not lose their human qualities (*see* WOLF CHILDREN). According to legend, Romulus killed Remus when the latter, deriding his efforts, jumped over the furrow that marked where the walls of Rome were to be erected. Romulus was made immortal by his father and became the Roman god Quirinus. The story compounds many facets of Roman thinking, including loyalty to the state before family ties.
See also FERAL CHILD).
Bibliography: Bloch, R. 1960. *The origins of Rome.*

RONDELET, GUILLAUME (1507-1566). A French physician and professor of medicine at Montpellier. He was a friend and a coworker of Fran-

çois Rabelais (q.v.). In his work *Metodus de Materia Medicinali et Compositionem Medicamentorum*, he discussed the aetiology of melancholia (q.v.), which he believed to be caused primarily by a defect in the brain, or secondarily by disorders of the body in general, or corrupted fluids rising from the stomach. This latter disorder he called "melancholia hypochondriaca." He also wrote on the structure of the nerves, which he discovered were separate strands.
Bibliography: Lewis, A. 1967. *The state of psychiatry.*

RORSCHACH, HERMANN (1884-1922). A Swiss psychiatrist. His father was an artist. While training in psychiatry under the supervision of Eugen Bleuler (q.v.), Rorschach in collaboration with Konrad Gehring, an art teacher, undertook a project that attempted to ascertain whether or not successful students produced more works based on fantasy than less gifted students. For the first time, he recorded people's reactions to inkblots. He was introduced to psychoanalysis (q.v.) by Bleuler and Carl G. Jung (q.v.) and became the vice-president of the Swiss Psychoanalytic Society. In 1921, after fourteen years of experimentation on 300 mental patients and 100 normal controls, he published the results of his research with the inkblots in a volume entitled *Psychodiagnostik*. The Rorschach test, a selection of ten inkblots, has become one of the most widely used projection tests. The ambiguous inkblots stimulate thoughts that reveal personality traits. Rorschach died the year following the publication of his work.
Bibliography: Rorschach, H. 1949. *Psychodiagnostics*, trans. P. Lemkau and B. Kronenberg.

RORSCHACH RESEARCH EXCHANGE. An organization founded in 1936 and administered by Bruno Klopfer. Originally it was concerned with the standardization of the inkblot test devised by Hermann Rorschach (q.v.). It later became the International Rorschach Institute. Its purpose then became the organization of research and the training of medical and educational workers in the administration of the tests.
Bibliography: Alexander, F. G., and Selesnick, S. T. 1966. *The history of psychiatry.*

RÖSCH, HEINRICH KARL (1808-1866). A German physician. He was entrusted by Wilhelm I (1781-1864) king of Würtemberg, with the task of organizing Mariaberg (q.v.), the first German state institution for retarded children. Rösch was a liberal and enlightened man who dedicated all his energies to the new institution of which he was director. Unfortunately, his ideas were opposed, and he was removed from that position. This disappointment and his lack of sympathy with the political climate of the time, caused him to emigrate to the United States, where he spent the remainder

of his life. In 1850 he founded a journal entitled *Beobachtungen über den Cretinismus* (q.v.).
Bibliography: Kanner, L. 1964. *A history of the care and study of the mentally retarded.*

ROSE. A large genus of flowering plants. From early times, rose petals have been thought to possess special curative properties for a number of illnesses, including hysterical (*see* HYSTERIA) disorders and disorders of the nervous system. Even the perfume of the rose was said to relieve worry and anxiety. Andrew Boorde (q.v.), who was among the supporters of the medicinal properties of the rose, recommended bathing the heads of manic patients in rosewater and vinegar to calm them.
Bibliography: Mayhew, A., and Pollard, M. 1979. *The rose: myth, folklore and legend.*

ROSEMARY. *Rosmarinus officinalis*, a plant known since antiquity. The Greeks thought it stimulated the mind, and the Moors introduced it into Spanish pharmacopoeia. It was reputed to cure insanity and was believed to strengthen the memory (q.v.), as Shakespeare (q.v.) reminds us in *Hamlet*: "Rosemary, that's for remembrance," says Ophelia. Rosemary tea was used to cure migraine (q.v.) and to promote sleep in insomniac patients. It was mentioned in the Saxon herbal, *The Leech-book of Bald*, as possessing the ability to "tempereth, comforteth and sootheth the brayne and all the head." The *Great Herbal* of the sixteenth century recommended rosemary for "weakness of the brain and cold thereof." After it was soaked in wine, it was to be placed under the nose of the patient, who, was to keep his head warm. Richard Banckes's herbal of 1525 advised: "put the leaves under thy bedde and thou shalt be delivered of all evil dreames." The herbal of John Gerard (q.v.) also recommended the herb; Gerard believed that a garland of rosemary worn on the head "comforteth the brain, the memory, the inward senses and comforteth the heart and maketh it merry."
Bibliography: Rohde, E. S. 1974. *The old English herbals.*

ROSENBACH, OTTOMAR (1851-1907). A German physician. He observed that neurasthenics (*see* NEURASTHENIA) are unable to close their eyes immediately and completely on command. This phenomenon is known as the Rosenbach's sign.
Bibliography: Garrison, F. H. 1929. *History of medicine*, 4th ed.

ROSSETTI, CHRISTINA GEORGINA (1830-1894). An English poet. She was the daughter of an Italian writer and poet and the sister of Dante Gabriel Rossetti (q.v.). She was so committed to her Anglican religious beliefs and to her widowed mother that she broke off her engagement to a Roman Catholic artist. This renunciation cost her a great effort and accounts for her constant state of depression and for the melancholic (see MELAN-CHOLIA) nature of her verses. She wrote with intense feeling and never deviated from the canons of the Pre-Raphaelite brotherhood which rejected modern art forms and relied on mystical symbolism. In 1874 she developed Graves disease, a disorder of the thyroid gland, and remained an invalid and a recluse for the rest of her life.

Bibliography: Packer, L. M. 1963. *Christina Rossetti.*

ROSSETTI, DANTE GABRIEL (1828-1882). An English poet and painter and one of the founders of the Pre-Raphaelite brotherhood, which sought to recapture the Italian artistic spirit of the fifteenth century. In 1860, he married Elizabeth Siddal (q.v.) after a long and troublesome engagement. Her death from an overdose of laudanum (q.v.) left him depressed and so guilt ridden that he enclosed in her coffin the only complete copy of his poems. Seven years later, in 1869, he agreed to its exhumation. A mistress and an infatuation with the wife of a friend then filled his emotional life. In 1872 he attempted suicide (q.v.). Neuralgia, depression, and insomnia contributed to his addiction to chloral, morphia, laudanum (q.v.), and whisky. He suffered from paranoia (q.v.) to the point of accusing his psychiatrist, Henry Maudsley (q.v.), of posing as a physician in order to injure him. Delusions (q.v.) and hallucinations (q.v.) persisted, his bitterness isolated him, and he died a recluse.

Bibliography: Grylls, R. 1965. *Portrait of Rossetti.*

ROSSOLIMO, GREGORY IVANOVICH (1860-1928). A Russian neu-rologist, the son of Greek parents. He was the first to describe the plantar flexion of the toes, which becomes exaggerated in certain cerebral lesions. It is now known as Rossolimo's reflex.

ROTATORY MACHINES Apparatus in use in the nineteenth century. Using the rationale that shock would improve circulation and circulation disorders caused insanity, mental patients were subjected to rapid gyration by rotary machines (see Plate 13). The most famous of these machines was the one invented by Erasmus Darwin (q.v.). Dr. Joseph M. Cox (q.v.) was one of the physicians who used it extensively. Jean Esquirol (q.v.) wrote about the accidents caused by the practice and stated that patients "fell into a state of syncope, and had also copious evacuations both by vomiting and purging, which prostrated them extremely." He, however, continued to believe that the treatment could be useful to insane persons "who present symptoms of gastric derangement." The machine eventually was abandoned as too dangerous.

Bibliography: Esquirol, J.E.D. 1845. Reprint. 1965. *Mental Maladies: a treatise on insanity.*

ROUAULT, GEORGES (1871-1958). A French painter and engraver. As he matured, serenity and joy replaced the anguish in his earlier work. Hid-

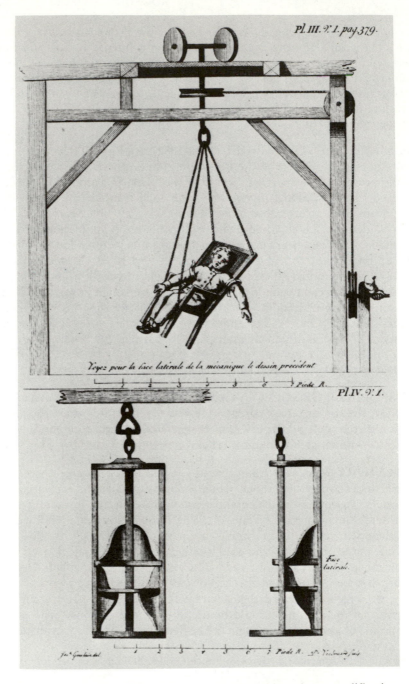

Pl. III. 9.ᵉ1. pag. 379.

Voyez pour la face latérale de la mécanique le dessin précédent

Pl. IV. 9.ᵉ1.

Face latérale.

13. A rotatory machine of German origin with a later modification (below). From J. Guislain, *Traité sur l'aliénation mental et sur les hospices des aliénés*, 1826. By courtesy of the Department of Medical Illustration, Ipswich Hospital.

eous portraits of prostitutes, repulsive rich men, and tragic clowns gave way to graceful paintings of female figures and landscapes glowing with color.
Bibliography: Venturi, L. 1959. *Rouault: biographical and critical study.*

ROUÉ. A French term meaning literally "broken." It has come to mean "a rake," or "a profligate." It was first used in this sense by the duke of Orleans (1674-1723), regent of France, in the 1720s. He boasted that he and his companions led such worthless and depraved lives that they deserved to be broken on the wheel.
Bibliography: 1978. *Brewer's dictionary of phrase and fable.*

ROULET. A sixteenth-century Frenchman who, with his brother and cousin, was arrested for having murdered many children. They claimed they had rubbed their bodies with a magic ointment, that had changed them into wolves and compelled them to run in the fields, devouring children. They were not punished but sent to a hospital for the insane. Their case was quoted by Jean Esquirol (q.v.) as an example of lycanthropy (q.v.).
Bibliography: Esquirol, J.E.D. 1845. Reprint 1965. *Mental maladies: a treatise on insanity.*

ROUSSEAU, JEAN-JACQUES (1712-1778). A French writer and philosopher, born in Geneva, Switzerland. His mother died at his birth. In his *Confessions* (q.v.) (1781-1788) written after he was savagely attacked by Voltaire (q.v.), Rousseau claimed that his behavior and character had been deteriorating ever since his uncle, who cared for him after his father had deserted him, had unjustly punished him with a beating. From then on, he became furious if he was confronted with an act of injustice. In early manhood he was devoted to Madame Louise de Warens, who was separated from her husband and some years older than Rousseau. He referred to her as "Mamma." During the time that her relationship with him remained asexual she maintained a sexual relationship with a male servant, Claude Anet. Later, faced with Rousseau's increasing interest in women, Madame de Warens encouraged him into a sexual relationship, which was distasteful to him. The three of them then lived in a close triple relationship until the death of Anet. After his death, Rousseau and de Warens shared a happy partnership for a number of years, but, when she took a second lover, Rousseau refused to share her, and they reverted to a mother-son relationship. Increasing strain caused him to leave her. In his working life, he entered twelve different occupations and abandoned them all. He was an anxious and taciturn man, given to frequent periods of moodiness and depression and likely to fall physically ill in response to anxiety. His actions often showed a total lack of moral principle. If, for example, he felt he had been unjustly treated, he would resort to stealing. For twenty-five years he lived with Thérèse Le Vasseur, an illiterate kitchen maid, by whom he had five children. He left them all in a foundling hospital. His novel *Julie, ou La*

Nouvelle Héloise (1761), written after he had become famous, reflects his revolt against the accepted social order and his belief that all evil stemmed from society. He emphasized the importance of the family; Rousseau believed if man returned to nature, he would again be happy and good; therefore, he felt all artificial elements should be banned from life. In *Emile, ou Traité de l'Education* (q.v.) he set forth his views on education; they were so advanced that he had to leave Paris and Switzerland and seek refuge in England. His political work, *Le Contrat Social* (1762) offended the government and the church, as well as contemporary philosophers, and added to his unpopularity. Because he was suspicious of everyone, his friends soon turned into enemies, persecution mania (q.v.) never left him, and his guilt, delusions and hypersensitivity made him miserable. He found happiness only when he was able to escape to an imaginary world. In 1775, he felt that even God had rejected him when he tried to put his work on the high altar in Notre Dame but found that a metal grille made the altar unreachable. He is said to have been insane for at least the last decade of his life.

Bibliography: Guéhenno, J. 1966. *Jean-Jacques Rousseau*, trans. J. Weightman and
   D. Weightman.

ROUSSY, GUSTAVE (1874-1948). A Swiss neurologist who studied and worked in Paris, where he filled several important academic positions. His research contributed to a better understanding of the anatomy, physiology, and pathology of the thalamus. He also wrote on the psychoneurosis (q.v.) of war, on the degeneration of the cerebral cortex, and on injuries of the spinal cord. His work on endocrinology, *Traité de Neuroendocrinologie*, was published in Paris in 1946.

Bibliography: Haymaker, W., and Schiller, F. 1970. *The founders of neurology.* 2d.
   ed.

ROWLANDSON, THOMAS (1756-1827). An English artist. He was famous for his vigorous and at times crude caricatures. He liked women and alcohol and was a compulsive gambler. He lost the entire fortune left him by a doting French aunt through gambling. He had a phobia (*see* PHOBIAS) of doctors, which he expressed by pouring savage ridicule on them in his drawings. He depicted them as corrupt, uncaring, lecherous, ignorant, and greedy. His work provides a fascinating documentary of the social life of his time, as well as an insight into his own preoccupations. His anxiety about old age and death, which appears in many drawings, reflects his dislike for a medical profession that could not prevent either event. After a gay and comfortable life, his old age was lonely. He was forgotten by the public, and his fear of death made his last years more miserable than they need have been.

Bibliography: George, D. M. 1963. *Hogarth to Cruickshank: social change in graphic satire.*

ROWLEY, WILLIAM (1742-1806). An English physician. He taught medicine in London and specialized in obstetrics. In 1788 he wrote a book entitled *Treatise on Female Nervous, Hysterical, Hypochondriacal, Bilious, Convulsive Diseases.* Apoplexy and palsy, as well as "thoughts on madness, suicide, etc.," were also discussed in the volume, which purported to explain their aetiology and nature and to offer new methods of treatment.

Bibliography: Hunter, R., and Macalpine, I. 1963. *Three hundred years of psychiatry.*

ROYAL ASYLUMS. Seven asylums (q.v.) in Scotland founded primarily, but not exclusively, for the benefit of pauper patients. Established through private enterprise, they derive the title "royal" from the royal charter of incorporation granted to each of them. They were founded at Montrose (1781); Aberdeen (1800); Dundee (founded in 1805, opened in 1820); Edinburgh (1813); Glasgow (1814); Perth (Murray Royal Asylum) (1826); and Dumfries (Crichton Royal Institution) (1839), and covered practically the whole of Scotland. When provisions were made by the Lunacy Act (Scotland 1857) for the erection of district asylums, the royal asylums tended to exclude pauper patients, who became the responsibility of the counties. The asylums began to cater more to middleclass patients who were unable to pay the higher rates demanded by private asylums.

See also ABERDEEN ROYAL MENTAL HOSPITAL, CRICHTON ROYAL HOSPITAL, DUNDEE LUNATIC ASYLUM, EDINBURGH LUNATIC ASYLUM, GLASGOW ASYLUM FOR LUNATICS, MONTROSE ROYAL MENTAL HOSPITAL, and MURRAY ROYAL HOSPITAL.

Bibliography: Henderson, D. K. 1964. *The evolution of psychiatry in Scotland.*

ROYAL EARLSWOOD HOSPITAL. An institution for the mentally retarded founded in 1847 by the Reverend Andrew Reed (q.v.), opened in 1848, and still in existence. Originally known as Park House and located in Highgate, it was the first institution of this type in England. It came into existence after Reed had visited similar institutions on the continent and read accounts of the work of Edouard Séguin (q.v.) in Paris. Support was provided by John Conolly, Alexander Sutherland, and the commissioners in lunacy (qq.v.). When the premises became inadequate, a new branch was opened at Colchester, and this was followed by a new asylum (q.v.) in Earlswood, Surrey. Albert, the prince consort, laid the foundation stone in 1852, and the first patients were admitted in 1855. The retarded were trained to the maximum of their capabilities, and some of them were able to find gainful employment. The institution provided a stimulus for further work and legislation concerning mental deficiency.

Bibliography: Royal Earlswood Institution. 1947. *Royal Earlswood Institution 1847-1947*. Pamphlet printed by patients.

ROYALE ISLAND. An island in the archipelago of Iles de Salut, French Guiana. It housed the notorious prison mental hospital. From 1852, until 1945, it was part of a French penal settlement that included Devil's Island and Saint-Joseph Island. Saint-Joseph Island was also called the Island of Silence because prisoners there were kept in solitary confinement. Many committed suicide (q.v.), or went mad and were transferred to the Maison des Fous on Royale Island. The last convict was released in 1946, but some ex-convicts, mainly tramps and alcoholics, still live on the islands.

Bibliography: Charriere, H. 1970. *Papillon*, trans. P. O'Brian.

ROYAL HOSPITAL OF SAINT BARTHOLOMEW, A hospital in London founded by the court jester Rahere (q.v.) in 1123. Four Augustine nuns originally cared for the patients. Mental patients were accepted along with others. John Stow (q.v.) in his *Survey of London* (1598) wrote that "St. Bartlemew, in Smithfield, an hospital of great receipt and relief for the poor, was suppressed by Henry VIII, and again by him given to the city, and is endowed by the citizens' benevolence." Timothy Bright (q.v.) was a physician there from 1585-1591. The hospital was rebuilt by public subscription in 1730.

Bibliography: Medvei, V.C., and Thornton, J.L. 1973. *The Royal Hospital of Saint Bartholomew 1123-1973*.

ROYAL MEDICO-PSYCHOLOGICAL ASSOCIATION. *See* ASSOCIATION OF MEDICAL OFFICERS OF ASYLUMS AND HOSPITALS FOR THE INSANE.

ROYAL SOCIETY. The oldest scientific organization in Great Britain. It developed from the Philosophical Society, which was founded in 1645. In 1662 it was granted a royal charter as the Royal Society of London for Improving Natural Knowledge. It met in London and provided a forum for scholars in all fields of knowledge. Scholars were expected to express their views in "a close, naked, natural way of speaking; positive expressions; clear senses; a native easiness." A number of distinguished physicians were among its members. The society's investigations into natural phenomena helped to dispel many misconceptions concerning mental disorders. It investigated, for example, such activities as the "stroking" of Valentine Greatrakes (q.v.) and reported in its journal, *The Philosophical Transactions* (q.v.), such ex-

periments as a blood transfusion (q.v.) from an animal to a madman and the effects of Indian hemp (q.v.).
Bibliography: Sprat, T. 1966. *History of the Royal Society*.

ROYAL TOUCH. *See* KING'S TOUCH.

ROYCE, JOSIAH (1855–1916). An American philosopher and psychologist. He was an exponent of philosophical idealism. His ideas on the human mind, which he believed to be part of an absolute mind capable of perceiving truth, inspired Pierre Janet (q.v.). To Royce, the community was all important and individual life was no more than an epitome of social life. He believed that mental pathology resulted when the individual was displaced in social life. His *Outline of Psychology* was published in 1903, and he produced numerous other books that covered religion, logic, and immortality, among other things.
Bibliography: Ellenberger, H. F. 1970. *The discovery of the unconscious*.

RUBIN, EDGAR (1886–1951). A Danish psychologist, and pupil of Georg E. Müller (q.v.) at his laboratory at Göttingen. His studies on visual perception revealed that attention is usually focused on a figure or an object. Surrounding details, or ground, are of secondary importance to the viewer, who sees them as ambiguous and less well-defined images. The results of his investigations were published in 1915 and were subsequently translated in a number of languages.
Bibliography: Boring, E. G. 1950. *A history of experimental psychology*.

RUBY. A precious stone that was considered a remedy for many diseases. The Hindus linked its color to inextinguishable fire. Although associated with passion, it was also believed to preserve the mental health of those who wore it.
See also PRECIOUS STONES.
Bibliography: Hodges, D. M. 1972. *Healing gems*.

RUDDIGORE (THE WITCH'S CURSE). An operetta by the English composer Arthur S. Sullivan (1842–1900) on a libretto by William S. Gilbert (1836–1911), first presented in 1887. The characters include Mad Margaret, who was driven to insanity by the faithless Sir Despard.
Bibliography: Baily, L. 1952. *The Gilbert and Sullivan book*.

RUE. (*Ruta gravolens*), an herb cultivated in the Orient for protection against evil influences. In ancient cultures it was highly regarded, and the Arabs (q.v.) still cherish it as the only herb to have been blessed by Mohammed (q.v.), who was said to have been miraculously cured of a dangerous illness by it. It was believed to be efficacious in the treatment of insanity, epilepsy (q.v.), hysteria (q.v.), and convulsions in children. it as also one of

the components of mithridate (q.v.), the antidote to poison used by Mithridates, king of Pontus. The volatile, acrid oil of rue was used medicinally. The plant was known as the "herb of grace" and associated with sorrow and repentance (rue). It was one of the herbs in mad Ophelia's posy in Shakespeare's play 'Hamlet'. It was also believed that witches used it in their brews.
Bibliography: le Strange, R. 1977. *A history of herbal plants.*

RUFUS OF EPHESUS (fl. c. A.D. 100). A Greek physician and leading authority on obstetrics and pediatrics. He was among the first medical writers to believe that the nervous system was instrumental in mediating voluntary movement and sensation. The optic chiasma, which he believed had a life of its own, was discovered by him during his anatomical studies of the brain. He stressed the importance of interrogating the patient and taking a history of both physical and mental disorders. He gave a detailed account of melancholia (q.v.) and frequently was quoted by Galen (q.v.).
Bibliography: Whitwell, J. R. 1936. *Historical notes on psychiatry.*

RUMINATION. Rumination in humans was first described by Fabricius ab Aquapendente (1537–1619) in 1618. Its aetiology is believed to be linked with anxiety, and it can occur as early as in infancy when the infant fails to thrive because of emotional deprivation.
Bibliography: 1971. Rumination. (Editorial.) *Brit. med. J.*, 4: 3.

RUMPF, THEODOR (1862–1923). A German physician. He observed that in neurasthenic (*see* NEURASTHENIA) patients, pressure over a painful point will quicken the pulse from ten to twenty beats per minute. This phenomenon has become known as Rumpf's sign.
Bibliography: Hinsie, L. E., and Campbell, R. J. 1960. *Psychiatric dictionary.*

RUSH, BENJAMIN (1745?–1813). The first American psychiatrist. His ancestors came to America with William Penn (1644–1718) after fighting under Oliver Cromwell (1599–1688). His father and his grandfather, although Quakers (q.v.), were gunsmiths. His father died when he was a young child, and he was brought up by his mother, who had to sell her husband's tools and the family's slave to support herself and her seven children. His uncle, a Presbyterian minister, instilled in him a sense of duty and responsibility. He graduated when he was fifteen years old from the University of New Jersey, became a medical apprentice for six years, and in 1768 obtained a medical degree from the University of Edinburgh, a rare achievement for an American at that time. He was greatly influenced by William Cullen (q.v.). Rush rapidly became prominent and lent his intelligence, enthusiasm, and enormous energy to many humanitarian causes.

He was one of the signitories of the Declaration of Independence and became the leading physician at the Pennsylvania Hospital (q.v.). He considered knowledge of the human mind the most important branch of all the sciences. In 1812, he wrote the first American textbook of psychiatry (q.v.), *Medical Enquiries and Observations upon the Diseases of the Mind,* which influenced American psychiatry for over seventy years. He believed that mental illness could be caused by somatic disorders or by sexual excesses, and that certain emotional states such as anxiety, anger, and sadness, indirectly caused mental pathology by affecting the blood vessels of the brain. He advocated shock treatment, ducking in cold water, tranquilizing the patient with blinkers and strapping him in a special chair of his invention, or spinning him to make the blood rush to his head, bleeding (q.v.), and emetics and purgatives. He also advised kind treatment and occupational therapy (q.v.). He suggested that patients should write down their own thoughts as a form of abreaction (q.v.). Although he was criticized and resented and made many enemies because of his dogmatism, he is regarded as the father of American psychiatry. His profile appears on the seal of the American Psychiatric Association (q.v.) and is reproduced on the medallion worn by its president, which was donated by the Royal Medico-Psychological Association (q.v.) in 1968 at a joint meeting held in Boston. Rush had a personal link with the mentally ill, as his son John became insane at the age of thirty and his condition was so severe that the family could not manage him; he was admitted to the Pennsylvania Hospital under the classification of "lunatic" (q.v.). He died there twenty-seven years later. In addition to his medical, political, and military activities, Rush was director of the Philadelphia mint.
Bibliography: Goodman, N. G. 1934. *Benjamin Rush: physician and citizen.*

RUSH, JAMES (1786–1869). An American physician and psychologist, the son of Benjamin Rush (q.v.). He conducted extensive research on the human voice and devised a new system of vocal training. The results of his work were published at his own expense because no publisher would handle the material, which was considered too independent from current theories. He thought that the brain worked like a mirror and "reflected" images, that were not only the cause of thought but thought itself. He advocated the study of animal behavior and is considered the first American behaviorist psychologist. Continuous opposition to his ideas and his own intransigence turned him into a bitter and disillusioned man.
Bibliography: Roback. A. A. 1962. *History of psychology and psychiatry.*

RUSKIN, JOHN (1819–1900). An English author and critic, born in London. His overly religious parents brought him up in fear of hellfire. As a child, he was not allowed toys or companions and was made to read the Bible (q.v.) to his mother every day. When he went to Oxford University, his mother moved there for the three years of his residence and saw him every day. Under these circumstances, he never loved his parents nor had any capacity for a close relationship. His own marriage remained unconsummated, and, after six years, his wife eloped with the painter John Millais (1829-1896). Ruskin then became infatuated with Rose La Touche (1848–1875) a precocious and melancholic (*see* MELANCHOLIA) child of ten. The entanglement lasted until her premature death and was frowned upon by her parents. Her death devastated him. Among his most famous writings are *Modern Painters* (1843–1860) and his incomplete biography *Praeterita* (1885–1889). He also wrote poetry and many articles on art, social reform, economics, education, and science. He initiated industrial experiments and participated in philanthropic ventures that dissipated the fortune left to him by his father. He believed that emotional and spiritual participation in the world's miseries was necessary to those who wished to alleviate mankind of its sufferings. He suffered from periods of psychosis and was insane for the last ten years of his life.

Bibliography: Burd, V. A. 1980. *John Ruskin and Rose La Touche.*

RYE. A cereal crop plant. Infected rye, used to make bread, may have been responsible for the epidemics of mental disorders and convulsions occuring in the Middle Ages (q.v.). Those affected were said to be suffering from Saint Anthony's fire (q.v.). Ergot (q.v.) alkaloids have been isolated from grass and rye fungus and lysergic acid diethylamide (q.v.) is one of its derivatives.

Bibliography: Emboden, W. 1972. *Narcotic plants.*

S

SACHER-MASOCH, LEOPOLD RITTER VON (1836-1895). An Austrian lawyer and author of short stories and novels. Throughout his works eroticism is linked with torture, therefore his name became the origin of the term "masochism" (q.v.), which was coined by Richard von Krafft-Ebing (q.v.). Sacher-Masoch's own sexual deviations, which included a craving for humiliation, were described in several of his novels.
Bibliography: Sacher-Masoch, L. R. von. 1902. *Venus in furs.*

SACHS, BERNARD (1858-1944). An American neurologist and psychiatrist of German parentage, a pupil of Theodor Meynert (q.v.). He coined the term "amaurotic familial idiocy" (q.v.) to describe a condition caused by histiological changes in the cortex. His book *A Treatise of the Nervous Diseases of Children,* published in 1895, was the first of its kind in the United States and brought him immediate recognition.
Bibliography: Haymaker, W., and Schiller, F. 1970. *The founders of neurology.* 2d. ed.

SACHS, HANS (1881-1947). A German follower and pupil of Sigmund Freud (q.v.). He was one of the organizers of the first Psychoanalytic Training Institute in Berlin and was himself a training analyst there. With Otto Rank (q.v.) he helped to establish the journal *Imago* (q.v.), which linked psychoanalytic doctrines with mythology and the arts. He emigrated to Boston, Massachusetts and there founded another journal of the same title in 1939.
Bibliography: Alexander, F. G., and Selesnick, S. T. 1966. *The history of psychiatry.*

SACKVILLE-WEST, VICTORIA MARY (VITA) (1892-1962). English poet and novelist. She married Harold Nicolson (1886-1968), and, although fond of each other, they both loved people of their own sex. Their uncon-

ventional marriage survived infidelity, long absences, and sexual incompatibility. She never managed to establish close friendship with either of her sons. Toward the end of her life she withdrew from public life. Her writings, especially her diaries, reflect the contradictory emotions and stresses that shaped her life. They also provide insight into homosexuality (q.v.).
Bibliography: Nicholson, N. 1973. *Portrait of a marriage.*

SACRED DISEASE, THE. A discourse on epilepsy (q.v.) by Hippocrates of Cos (q.v.), written in the fifth century B.C. Hippocrates stated that he did not believe epilepsy was "divine" or "sacred" but rather resulted from a natural cause like any other disease. He substantiated this by asserting that an autopsy on the head of a dead epileptic would show the brain to be "humid" and diseased. He also wrote that the brain was the interpreter of consciousness and the regulator of complex processes.
Bibliography: Lloyd, G.E.R., ed. 1978. *Hippocratic writings.*

SACRED WELLS. *See* HOLY WELLS.

SADE, DONATIEN ALPHONSE FRANÇOIS COMTE DE (1740-1814). A French writer, member of an ancient and noble family. Cold parents, a Jesuit education, and a marriage of convenience marked his early life. After a spell in the army, he resigned his commission. Violent sexual excesses, and charges of blasphemy and indecency led to eight separate periods of imprisonment. He was in the Bastille from 1778 to 1790 and saw it stormed in 1789. Projecting his propensities, he wrote several novels in which he developed the theme of sexual satisfaction through aggression and violence. It is less well known that he also suggested social and penal reforms. As the aristocracy of his time was notorious for its way of life, it is likely that he was imprisoned and finally sent briefly to Bicêtre (q.v.) and then to Charenton asylum (q.v.) because of his political inconvenience rather than for his views on sexual aberrations or the death of a prostitute whom he had heavily drugged with an aphrodisiac. In the asylum he produced more novels and organized amateur theatricals. At the age of seventy-three he was still involved in sexual relationships, one of them with a fifteen year old girl. He died at Charenton, where he had been confined for eleven years. In all, he had spent fourteen years of his life in prison and thirteen in mental hospitals.
Bibliography: Hayman, R. 1978. *De Sade: a critical biography.*

SADISM. Richard von Krafft-Ebing (q.v.) introduced the term to denote

sexual pleasures associated with the infliction of physical pain. He derived it from the Donatien Alphonse François de Sade (q.v.) who indulged in cruel sexual practices and described them at length in his novels.
Bibliography: Krafft-Ebing, R. von. 1886. *Psychopatia sexualis.*

SAFFRON. *Crocus sativus*, a perennial native to south Europe. It is also cultivated in Turkey, Persia, India, and China. In Eastern medicine it is used as a sedative in nervous disorders and against melancholia (q.v.) and also as an aphrodisiac. The Greeks and the Romans used it as a nerve tonic and an opiate against hysteria (q.v.).
Bibliography: Lehner, E., and Lehner, J. 1973. *Folklore and odysseys of food and medicinal plants.*

SAGE. *Salvia*, a name derived from the Latin *salvere*, meaning to save. For centuries it has been thought to have many medical qualities and to exert a beneficial influence on human emotions. It was said that the memory (q.v.) could be improved by drinking an infusion of its leaves. John Gerard (q.v.) said that it "is singularly good for the head and brain, it quicknethe the senses and memory." Sage was also used in the treatment of neurotic disorders, insanity and epilepsy, (q.v.). As late as the nineteenth century, extravagant claims were made about its qualities.
Bibliography: Le Strange, R. 1977. *A history of herbal plants.*

SAINT. For canonized and uncanonized saints, *see* under proper name of person. For surnames and place names *see* in alphabetical position here.

SAINT-ANDRÉ, FRANÇOIS (fl. 1677-1725). A French physician. He courageously intervened when the parliament of Normandy sentenced a large number of people accused of witchcraft (q.v.) to death. He asserted that those who believed themselves to be involved in supernatural activities were the victims of mental disorders.
Bibliography: Zilboorg, G. 1941. *A history of medical psychology.*

SAINT ANNE'S HOSPITAL. A mental hospital near Paris. It was opened in 1867. Its position, close to the Bicêtre (q.v.) was selected by Guillaume Ferrus (q.v.), who inaugurated a program of occupational therapy (q.v.) in the form of farm work. Valentin Magnan (q.v.) was among the original staff of physicians, and his first lecture there was on general paralysis of the insane (q.v.). He was also instrumental in abolishing physical forms of restraint (q.v.) in the hospital.
Bibliography: Burdett, H. C. 1891. *Hospitals and asylums of the world.*

SAINT ANN'S HOSPITAL. A seaside psychiatric hospital in Dorset, England. It owes its existence to the success of Thomas Holloway (q.v.), who supplied the funds for it from the immense wealth he had accumulated selling

patent ointments and pills. The hospital was built after his death, between 1910 and 1912, as a branch of Holloway Sanatorium (q.v.).
Bibliography: Stevens, T. L. 1970. *A note on Saint Ann's Hospital, Canford Cliffs.*

SAINT ANTHONY'S FIRE. A disease consisting of gangrene accompanied by severe mental changes. It occurred in epidemic form during the Middle Ages (q.v.). It is believed to have been caused by ergot (q.v.) alkaloids present in infected rye (q.v.).

SAINT AUDRY'S HOSPITAL. A psychiatric hospital in the county of Suffolk in England. It was opened in 1767 as a "house of industry" for the poor of the hundreds of Loes and Wilford, a medieval division of the county. It became an asylum in 1827, when it was reconstructed and adapted to house 130 patients. It was further extended later in the century to accommodate over 1000 patients. The hospital is also the site of an extensive museum displaying furniture, clothing, instruments, and registers of the asylum.

SAINT AVERTIN'S DISEASE. Another term for insanity or epilepsy (q.v.). The French referred to lunatics (q.v.) as *avertineux* and regarded Saint Avertin as their patron saint.
See also HOLY WELLS.
Bibliography: Tuke, D. H. 1892. *A dictionary of psychological medicine.*

SAINT ELDRIN'S CHURCH. A church in Pembrokeshire, Wales, now in ruins. Its churchyard contained a well reputed to cure madness. It's power was said to have disappeared when its waters were used for washing clothes on a Sunday and the well dried up. The churchyard grass, however, acquired the reputation of protecting men and beasts from the bite of mad dogs.
Bibliography: Jones, F. 1954. *See also* HOLY WELLS.

SAINT ELIZABETH'S HOSPITAL. A beautifully located American mental hospital, founded in Washington, D. C., in 1852. It was first called the Government Hospital for the Insane. Dorothea Dix (q.v.) drafted its original bill for its establishment. The first superintendent was Dr. Charles H. Nichols, who remained in the post for twenty-five years. After World War II, Ezra Pound (q.v.) became a patient there.
Bibliography: Deutsch, A. 1949. *The mentally ill in America.*

SAINT FILLAN'S POOL. A pool in Perthshire, Scotland, believed to have special curative powers. Even as late as 1793, the pool was used for the treatment of the insane, who brought offerings and underwent special rituals in search of a miraculous cure. They were immersed in the water three times and bound hand and foot before spending the night in a nearby chapel. If they had managed to free themselves by the morning, it was considered a hopeful sign, otherwise they were believed to be incurable. On occasions the patients were found dead by morning. Sir Walter Scott (q.v.) mentions the pool in his poem *Marmion*:

Then to St. Fillan's blessed well,
Whose springs can frenzied dreams dispel,
An the craz'd brain restore.

See also HOLY WELLS.
Bibliography: Tuke, D. H. 1882. *History of the insane in the British Isles.*

SAINT GEORGE'S HOSPITAL. A psychiatric hospital in Staffordshire, England. It was founded in 1814 through the legacy of Isaac Hawkins Browne. It provided for three classes of patients. The first class included "persons of superior rank" who were charged "according to their pecuniary abilities." The charges imposed on the more affluent helped to pay for the care of less wealthy patients. Charges for pauper patients were subsidized by their respective parishes. Saint George's is one of the oldest county asylums (q.v.) in England.

SAINT GEORGE'S RETREAT. A private asylum (q.v.) opened in 1870 in Burgess Hill near Brighton, England, for the exclusive use of Roman Catholic patients.
Bibliography: Parry-Jones, W. L. 1972. *The trade in lunacy.*

SAINT GEORG INSANE ASYLUM. The first mental hospital in Germany. It was founded in Bayreuth by Johann G. Langermann (q.v.) who was its director from 1805 to 1810. It was an innovation of humanitarian methods of treatment and rejected restraint (q.v.) and punishment of patients.
Bibliography: Zilboorg, G. 1941. *A history of medical psychology.*

SAINT-GERMAIN, COMTE DE (c.1707-c.1784). A French adventurer at the court of Louis XV (q.v.). His claim that he had lived for many centuries and had known Jesus Christ deceived many people. Both the king and Madame de Pompadour (q.v.) seem to have believed his stories and befriended him. Pompadour even tried the elixir of eternal life that he was said to use. Eventually St. Germain had to leave France because of his dubious activities. He died in exile.
Bibliography: Mitford, N. 1968. *Madame de Pompadour.*

SAINT HANS HOSPITAL. The first modern mental hospital in Denmark. It was established in 1816 at Roskilde for the mentally ill of Copenhagen. Its first medical superintendent was Dr. H. Seidelin.
Bibliography: Retterstøl, N. 1975. Scandinavia. In *World history of psychiatry*, ed. J. G. Howells.

SAINT HILDEVERT DE GOURNAY. A shrine (q.v.) in France. Hospitals or towns often organized pilgrimages of the insane to it, in the hope that they would be cured.
Bibliography: Focault, M. 1967. *Madness and civilization.*

SAINT HUBERT'S DISEASE. A term used for hydrophobia. Saint Hubert, the patron saint of huntsmen, was believed to have the power to cure those bitten by a mad dog. The same power was attributed to his descendants.
Bibliography: Tuke, D. H. 1892. *A dictionary of psychological medicine.*

SAINT JAMES'S HOSPITAL. A general hospital with a psychiatric unit in Leeds, England. It was founded in 1846 as a "moral and industrial training school" to house and educate pauper children. A workhouse for adults was added in the 1850s. By 1870 its population primarily consisted of sick and senile patients, therefore, a part of the institution became a poor law infirmary. It was the first outside of London to be administered separately from the workhouse.

SAINT JOHN'S EVIL. Another of the many terms referring to epilepsy (q.v.).

ST.-JOHN'S-WORT. *Hypericum perforatum*, a wild herb that, when steeped in warm oil, was used frequently by the crusaders. It was believed to relieve pain, heal wounds, and cure nervous disorders. It was also considered a charm against all harmful eventualities. In the seventeenth century, after it was blessed and wrapped in "hallow paper," it was carried on the person and sniffed to keep the devil at bay, a superstition linked to the ancient Greek belief that evil spirits disliked the herb. In the nineteenth century it was used as a sedative in hysteria (q.v.) and nervous affections.
Bibliography: le Strange, R. 1977. *A history of plants.*

SAINT JOSEPH HOSPITAL. The first real mental hospital in Gibraltar. It was designed by Captain Buckle in 1886. Surmounted by twin towers, it looked like a fortress, and its function was mainly custodial. Before its

existence those mentally ill who were a public nuisance were confined in a military prison. Saint Joseph Hospital ceased functioning in 1971, when more modern premises were provided at King George V Hospital.
Bibliography: Montegriffo, C. 1978. History of medicine in Gibraltar. *Brit. med. J.* 2: 555.

SAINT LAWRENCE'S HOSPITAL. A psychiatric hospital in Bodmin, Cornwall, Great Britain. It perpetuates the tradition of caring for the sick that began in the village of Saint Lawrence in the eleventh century. It was then a hospital for lepers (*see* LEPROSY), who were admitted on condition that they paid a sum of money and brought with them a pot for their food and a purse to collect alms. The hospital received a charter in 1532. As leprosy declined, the hospital was left without patients, but in 1815 the revenues from its lands were expended to provide an asylum for the mentally ill.

SAINT LAZARE. An old hospital for leprosy (q.v.) in Paris. In the seventeenth century, it was adapted by Saint Vincent de Paul (q.v.) to serve as an asylum. The mentally ill within its walls were managed in a humane way and received whatever treatment was available at the time.
Bibliography: Whitwell, J. R. 1945. *Analecta Psychiatrica.*

SAINT LUKE'S HOSPITAL FOR LUNATICS. A mental hospital in London founded in 1751. It was established in part because of the abuses occuring in Bethlem Royal Hospital (q.v.). It was first located in Moorfields opposite Bethlem. The founders pledged that the patients would not be exposed to the public as spectacles of amusement. Dr. William Battie (q.v.) is regarded as one of its founders and its first physician. He taught that insanity was "manageable" and believed that the patients should receive treatment and not be shut up in "loathsome prisons." These beliefs were reflected in the management of St. Luke's. Physical means of restraint (q.v.) were used in its early days, but the hospital never caused the complaints that had been so common in other establishments of its time. In 1774 a second building was erected in Old Street. This building, despite being unsuitable, functioned until 1916, when the patients were moved to new premises. The old building was taken over by the Bank of England.
Bibliography: Leigh, D. 1961. *The historical development of British psychiatry.*

SAINT LUKE'S HOUSE. A private madhouse (q.v.) opened in Newcastle, England, in 1766. Its owner was Dr. John Hall (q.v.). On his death it was acquired by Dr. Stevenson who enlarged the premises and renamed it Bell-grove Retreat. It functioned until 1857.

Bibliography: Le Gassicke, J. 1972. Early history of psychiatry in Newcastle-upon-Tyne. *Brit. J. Psychiat.* 120: 419-22.

SAINT MAREE WELL. A pool in a small island on Loch Maree in Scotland. It was renowned for its treatment of lunatics. John Greenleaf Whittier (1807–1892), the American poet, wrote in a poem:

> O restless heart and fevered brain,
> Unquiet and unstable,
> That holy well of Loch Maree,
> Is more than idle fable.

See also HOLY WELLS.

Bibliography: Tuke, D. H. 1882. *History of the insane in the British Isles.*

SAINT MARTIN'S EVIL. A popular term for dipsomania (q.v.).

SAINT MATHURIN DE LARCHANT. A famous shrine (q.v.) in France. During the Middle Ages (q.v.), insane people undertook pilgrimages to it in the hopes of being cured.

Bibliography: Focault, M. 1967. *Madness and civilization.*

SAINT NUN'S POOL. A pool at Altarnun in Cornwall, England. It was famous in the past as a place of treatment for mental patients. The patients were plunged into the water backwards and forcibly kept in it until they were subdued. If they displayed signs of recovery, they were taken to the nearby church, in which prayers and gifts were offered in thanksgiving.

See also BOWSSENING.

Bibliography: Tuke, D.H. 1882. *History of the insane in the British Isles.*

SAINT PATRICK'S HOSPITAL. The first mental hospital in Ireland. It was founded in Dublin in 1745 with money bequeathed for its establishment by Jonathan Swift (q.v.). George II (q.v.) granted the hospital a charter, which incorporated the various regulations stipulated by Swift's will. Swift himself wrote about it:

> He gave the little wealth he had,
> To build a House for Fools and Mad;
> And show'd by one satyric touch,
> No Nation wanted it so much.

Bibliography: Burdett, H. C. 1891. *Hospitals and asylums of the world.*

SAINT PAUL DE MAUSOLE. The asylum at Saint Rémy in which Vincent Van Gogh (q.v.) was a patient. While there, he painted a large number of pictures of the house, the garden, and the view from his window, as well as the doctor, the attendants, the other inmates, and self-portraits.

SAINT PETER'S HOSPITAL. An asylum in Bristol, England. Founded in 1696 by John Carey, it was the first workhouse in England. It was established for the poor of the parish, who were to receive shelter and medical care. Dr. Thomas Dover (q.v.) was its first physician. The lunatic poor, or frenzied patients, were housed in the same building. James C. Prichard (q.v.) based his *Treatise of Insanity* (1835) on the case histories of the patients he had seen at Saint Peter's Hospital, where he was a physician. It later became the Bristol Lunatic Asylum. The hospital was totally destroyed by bombs in 1940.
Bibliography: Jancar, J. 1972. Fifty years of Brentry Hospital. *Bristol Med-Chirur. J.* 87: 23-30.

SAINT RONAN'S WELL. A spring near the Butt of Lewis in Scotland. Its water was believed to cure lunacy. The patients were sprinkled with it and then bound and placed on the altar of the nearby church for the night. If they slept, they were regarded as cured. A satirical novel entitled *Saint Ronan's Well* was written by Sir Walter Scott (q.v.) in 1823 and was based upon contemporary life at the Scottish spa of Saint Ronan's Well. Intrigue, seduction, gambling and impersonation cause such anxiety and unhappiness to the heroine, Clara Mowbray, that she becomes unhinged and eventually succumbs to the strain of it all.
See also HOLY WELLS.
Bibliography: Tuke, D. H. 1882. *History of the insane in the British Isles.*

SAINT ROSAMUND'S POND. A pond situated in Regents Park in London. It was a favorite spot for suicide (q.v.). Thomas Sydenham (q.v.) jokingly advised Hans Sloane (q.v.) to drown himself there rather than go to Jamaica.

SAINT VALENTINE'S HOSPITAL. A hospital founded in Alsace in 1486 for the care of epileptics (*see* EPILEPSY), who were subsequently said to be suffering from *morbus Saint Valentinii.*
Bibliography: Whitwell, J. R. 1936. *Historical notes on psychiatry.*

SAINT VITUS' DANCE. Another term for epilepsy (q.v.). It is probably derived from the tradition of taking epileptics to chapels dedicated to Saint Vitus in the hopes of a miraculous cure. It is also possible that the term is derived from the frantic dancing in front of the statue of the saint on his feast day. The custom was common in Germany in the seventeenth century when it was believed that it would bring good health for a year to the

dancers. Paracelsus (q.v.), who opposed attaching names of saints to diseases, suggested the term "chorea lasciva" (q.v.).
Bibliography: Temkin, O. 1971. *The falling sickness.*

SAINT WINIFRED'S WELL. A spring in Flintshire, Wales. It was renowned for its miraculous healing powers, including the ability to cure insanity. As early as the twelfth century Geraldus Cambrensis (1146?–1220?) (q.v.) referred to it in his *Topographia Hibernica.* It was so popular in the seventeenth century that James II of England was among its thousands of votaries.
See also HOLY WELLS.
Bibliography: Tuke, D. H. 1882. *History of the insane in the British Isles.*

SAKEL, MANFRED JOSHUA (1906–1957). An Austrian psychiatrist trained in Vienna. He emigrated to the United States in 1937. Following his experiences at the Lichterfeld Hospital in Berlin where he had observed that patients addicted to morphine became overexcited when abstaining, he experimented with insulin in the treatment of schizophrenia (q.v.). An initial enthusiasm for the Sakel's method (as the insulin coma treatment came to be known) followed the first reports of it in 1933, but the method was criticized later as ineffectual in chronic cases.
Bibliography: Alexander F. G., and Selesnick, S. T. 1966. *The history of psychiatry.*

SALAMMBÔ. A novel by Gustave Flaubert (q.v.) written in 1862. Salammbô is a priestess in the temple of the Carthaginians at the time of the first Punic War (264-241 B.C.). Her neurotic behavior is dictated by unconscious and repressed sexuality. Her symptoms disappear when she gives herself to Mathô, the enemy chief. This concept of hysteria (q.v.) reflects the opinions of medical men of the time. They regarded the condition as a manifestation of dual personality in women who behave seductively without realizing it.
Bibliography: Flaubert, G. 1862. *Salammbô.*

SALEM WITCHCRAFT TRIALS. A famous episode of mass hysteria (q.v.) in the village of Salem, Massachusetts, in 1692. It evolved from the activities of some young girls who engaged in fortune-telling and enjoyed ghost stories. The activity developed into an obsession with the supernatural. They became hysterical and were believed to be "bewitched." As their behavior became more dramatic, their screams, convulsions, and gibberish utterances so caught the imagination of the populace that the accusations of witchcraft (q.v.) were taken seriously. The trials resulted in 250 arrests. Fifty people were condemned, nineteen to death, and several persons were subjected to torture, which resulted in death in one case. The hysteria subsided when several prominent citizens came under suspicion, including the wife of the governor, William Phips (1651-1695), who had appointed a commission to try those accused of witchcraft. Many literary works have been

written aroud this episode; in modern times the most famous is "The Crucible", a play by Arthur Miller.
Bibliography: Boyer, P., and Nissenbaum, S. 1978. *Salem witchcraft papers.*

SALERNO MEDICAL SCHOOL. A school of medicine founded in the ninth century on the bay of Salerno in southern Italy by four physicians, a Greek, a Latin, a Jew, and an Arab. They taught medicine in their respective languages and drew on the knowledge of the ancient medical texts of their four countries of origin. Students came to this lay school from many countries. The work of the school included compilations intended for the practical instruction of students. Female doctors were among the teaching staff. The *Regimen Sanitatis Salernitanum* (q.v.) remained the basis of European medical teaching until the Renaissance and contained many prescriptions for psychiatric disabilities. The school was granted special privileges by Frederick II (q.v.), who gave to it a monopoly in conferring licences to practice medicine within the Holy Roman Empire. Toward the end of the thirteenth century it declined. It was finally suppressed in 1811 by a Napoleonic decree.
Bibliography: Harington, J. 1920 *The School of Salernum.*

SALICETTI, GUGLIELMO (c. 1210-1277). An Italian surgeon. He is better known by the name of Saliceto. He was a professor at the University of Bologna and wrote a number of textbooks on the theory and practice of medicine and surgery. In his treatise on practice he included a detailed and intelligent account of melancholia (q.v.).
Bibliography: Garrison, F. H. 1929. *An introduction to the history of medicine.*

SALMON, THOMAS WILLIAM (1876-1927). An American physician. During World War I, as a member of the National Committee for Mental Hygiene, he recommended to the Government that more impetus should be given to psychiatric services. He influenced the growth of psychiatry in America, especially in the field of military psychiatry.
Bibliography: Zilboorg, G. 1941. *A history of medical psychology.*

SALMONEUS. In Greek mythology (q.v.), a king of Elis. He was presumptuous to the point of imitating the thunder and lightning of Zeus, who punished him by casting him into the underworld. He is an example of exaggerated self-esteem.
Bibliography: Brothwell, D., and Sandison, A. T. 1967. *Diseases in antiquity.*

SALOME (A.D.14? -before A.D.62). The daughter of Herodias and stepdaughter of Herod Antipas. Herod, decadent and amoral, was in love with the unstable Salome. According to the Bible (q.v.), she demanded the head of John the Baptist as a price for her dancing. The story has been treated

with a number of variations by several dramatists, including Oscar Wilde whose version provided the libretto for the opera *Salome* by Richard Strauss (1864-1949).
Bibliography: Mark 6: 22.

SALPÊTRIÈRE, LA. A famous French hospital. La Salpêtrière was built in the sixteenth century as a saltpeter and gunpowder store. In 1656, Louis XIV authorized the organization of hospitals for the hundred homeless people who had converged on Paris from the country, following the devastation of recent wars. La Salpêtrière then was adapted to house destitute women, prostitutes, abandoned infants, and, in general, socially undesirable females. The diversity of inmates was reflected in the shape of the chapel, which had four naves facing the altar and four separate entrances, each reserved for a particular group. Saint Vincent de Paul (q.v.) devoted his life to the care of the women received there. During the French Revolution (q.v.) La Salpêtrière was used as a political prison, but eventually became a true hospital. The mentally ill remained there among the other sick women. Their management, however, did not improve, and, when Philippe Pinel (q.v.) became its physician, his first action was to remove the chains from the insane. Pinel was helped in his program of reorganization by Jean-Baptiste Pussin (q.v.). Jean Pierre Falret (q.v.) established a section there for mentally retarded women in 1831, and Jean Martin Charcot (q.v.) established a neurological clinic in 1878. It was at La Salpêtrière that Charcot developed his interest in hypnotism (q.v.), which led to the formation of a new school of psychopathology. Alfred Binet (q.v.) became the director of its psychological laboratory (q.v.) in 1890. Manon Lescaut (q.v.) in the famous novel (1731) by the Abbé Prévost was imprisoned in La Salpêtrière.
Bibliography: Guillain, G., and Matheiu, P. 1925. *La Salpêtrière.*

SALT. Salt sometimes was added to the holy water used in the healing of the insane because the devil was said to abhor it as the emblem of immortality.
Bibliography: Tuke, D. H. 1882. *History of the insane in the British Isles.*

SALUS. A goddess of healing and an attendant of Aesculapius (q.v.) in Roman mythology (q.v.). She was often represented on coins together with the sacred snake and was regarded as a deity of public health.
Bibliography: 1978. *Everyman's encyclopaedia.*

SALVARSAN. An arsenical preparation used as a specific remedy for syphilis (q.v.). It was discovered in 1907, in Germany by Paul Ehrlich (q.v.). After his report on it in 1910, it assumed an important role in therapy. Two years later preparations of salvarsan were injected directly into the cerebro-spinal fluid. The term was derived from the Latin words *salvare* and *sanitas,*

meaning "preserve" and "health" and thus carried the suggestion that it was a "health preserver."
Bibliography: Dennie, C. C. 1962. *A history of syphilis.*

SALVATION ARMY. An international religious organization founded in 1865 by an English Methodist preacher, William Booth (1829-1912). It was originally known as the Christian Mission. In 1878 it was designated the Salvation Army, and since then it has retained a quasi-military approach to its organization. It provides numerous centers in Great Britain, the United States, Canada, Australia, India, and Japan for the help of outcasts of society, including unbalanced or mentally ill people.
Bibliography: Sandall, R., and Wiggins, A. R. 1955. *The history of the Salvation Army.*

SAMKARA (788-820). An Indian saint and philosopher. He was the founder of a nondualistic school of philosophy. He interpreted the metaphysical treatises of the Vedic literature. His views on dreams (q.v.), which he regarded as a form of fulfilment, are close to psychoanalytical concepts.
Bibliography: Rao, A. V. 1975. India. In *World history of psychiatry*, ed. J. G. Howells.

SAM SIXTY. The ficticious name given to a family observed during a study on mental defect by Mary S. Kostir. Sixty was the average IQ of the family as measured on the point scale. Like other contemporary works, it arrived at the conclusion that mental defect was hereditary and that many social problems were caused by it.
See also EUGENICS, HILL FOLK, JUKES, KALLIKAK FAMILY, MARKUS FAMILY, NAM, PINEYS, and ZERO FAMILY.
Bibliography: Kostir, M. S. 1916. *The family of Sam Sixty, Ohio.*

SAMSON. A biblical figure, the last of the twelve judges. When he destroyed the Philistines by pulling down the temple of Dagon, he destroyed himself. His death wish is evident in his prayer "Let me die with the Philistines."
Bibliography: Judg. 16: 23-31.

SANBENITO. The garment worn by those condemned to the stake by the Spanish Inquisition (q.v.). It was made of black cloth on which were depicted demons, flames, and other symbols of evil, which were believed to possess (*see* POSSESSION) the heretics.
Bibliography: Harvey, P. 1966. *The Oxford companion to English Literature.*

SANCTA MARIA DELS INOCENTS. The name of the first institution in Europe built exclusively for the care of the mentally ill. It was founded in 1409 in Valencia, Spain, by Father Juan Gilabert Jofré (q.v.). The term *inocents* was used to describe the insane who cannot help their state, and the superintendent was known paternalistically as "el padre do los locos" (the father of the mad). An association of citizens provided the original funds to buy a house for the patients. The asylum (q.v.) enjoyed the protection of the antipope, Benedict XIII (1328?-?1423), who issued a bulla encouraging people to support it. It was granted a royal charter by King Martin I of Aragon. Although each patient had his own room, they shared day rooms, dining room, and gardens, which were built round a central patio. The males did maintenance and farm work, while the females were employed in weaving and domestic tasks. The patients were allowed out, received visitors regularly, and were involved with the staff in religious ceremonies, theatrical performances, and celebrations of feast days. All patients were legally protected by the hospital, and a plea of insanity was accepted even for homicides. In 1545, when the hospital was destroyed by fire, about thirty patients died in the flames. The disaster was attributed to the carelessness of carpenters, who had left wood shavings near a fire, and to the devil, who fanned the flames. The destruction of the hospital was accepted as punishment for sins, and a new building was erected. Later the hospital moved to another site and was amalgamated with other institutions for the physically ill to form a large general hospital. It continued to shelter the insane until 1876, when the patients were moved to a former monastery. Bibliography: Dominguez, E. J. 1963. The Hospital of Innocents: humane treatment of the mentally ill in Spain, 1409-1512. *Bulletin of the Menninger Clinic*. 5: 285-97.

SAND, GEORGE (1804-1876). The pseudonym of the French novelist Amandine Aurore Lucie Dupin, baronne Dudevant. Her mother was a dressmaker, and her father was a member of the French nobility. After his death she was brought up by her paternal grandmother and the nuns of a Paris convent. Her early marriage was unsuccessful, and, after eight years, she separated from her husband, Casimir Dudevant (1795-1871), who unsuccessfully petitioned Napoleon III (q.v.) for the Legion of Honor in recognition of his matrimonial tribulations. She then entered into a number of relationships with various famous artists. The poet Alfred de Musset (1810-1857) was followed, after a stormy parting, by Frédéric François Chopin (1810-1849). Although Sand affected male dress, smoked a pipe or cigars, and was notorious for her promiscuity, she had strong maternal feelings, which she exercised on her lovers as much as on her children. Her writings reflect her revolt against social restraints, her demand for the same freedoms for women that men had, and her rejection of the institution of marriage. In the latter part of her life she became interested in social reforms. Bibliography: Jordan, R. 1976. *George Sand: a biography*.

SANDBY, PAUL (1725-1809). English artist and draughtsman, known for his aquatints and etchings. He was one of many artists who attacked William

Hogarth (q.v.) for his *Analysis of Beauty* (1753). Sandby produced an etching entitled *The Author Run Mad* in which Hogarth is represented as a patient of Bethlem Royal Hospital (q.v.), confined in a ward for incurables, and engaged in absurd activities.

Bibliography: O'Donoghue, E. G. 1914. *The story of Bethlehem Hospital.*

SANDER, WILHELM (1838-1922). A German psychiatrist. He is remembered for his detailed description of paranoia (q.v.), which was published in 1868.

Bibliography: Sander, W. 1868. Originäre paranoia. *Archiv. für Psychiatrie.*

SANDOW, EUGENE (1867-1925). A German exponent of physical culture and a professional strongman. As a young boy he was a weakling but constant exercise made him strong. He is often quoted as an example of organ inferiority converted into superiority.

Bibliography: Flugel, J. C. 1945. *A hundred years of psychology.*

SANFORD, EDMUND CLARK (1859-1924). An American psychologist. He studied with Granville S. Hall (q.v.) at Johns Hopkins University and later became head of the new laboratory at Clark University in Worcester, Massachusetts. The first laboratory manual *Course in Experimental Psychology* was written by him. It was originally published as a series of papers in the *American Journal of Psychology* (q.v.) in 1891. It remained the standard reference manual for thirty years.

Bibliography: Sanford, E. C. 1898. *Course in Experimental Psychology.*

SAN HIPÓLITO HOSPITAL. The first mental hospital in Latin America. It was founded in 1567 by Bernardino Alvarez (q.v.) in Mexico. The Catholic church gave Alvarez permission for its establishment, and both the viceroy of Mexico and the king of Spain approved the project. The land was provided by friends, and the money for the construction came from gifts. The hospital was named after Saint Hyppolitus, the patron saint of Mexico City. At first, convalescents, old people, and the infirm, as well as the mentally ill, were accepted by the institution, which also took in illiterate children and anybody else who could not be cared for at home. Later it accepted mental patients only and built subsidiary hospitals in other parts of the country. Methods of treatment were well in advance of the times, and the patients led a peaceful communal life in pleasant surroundings. A religious order, the Hipólitos (q.v.), undertook all the work connected with the care of the patients. In the seventeenth century, the hospital admitted both Spaniards and Indians from a wide area. It was reconstructed in 1777 and was considered to be

superior to any found in Europe. The hospital continued to give uninter-
rupted service until 1910.
Bibliography: Rumbaut, R. D. 1971. Bernardino Alvarez: new world psychiatric
pioneer. *Am. J. Psychiat.* 127: 1217-221.

SAN PEDRO. The Peruvian name for the psychedelic cactus, *Trichocereus
pachanoi.* The cactus is employed by folk healers to divine illness. Both
healer and patient drink a potion made from boiled pieces of the cactus and
other plants that increase its purgative and emetic effects. Violent vomiting
is followed by hallucinations (q.v.) during which the patient is purified, and
the healer receives visions that enable him to diagnose the illness and to
prescribe appropriate treatment. Usually the patients are believed to have
been bewitched by a sorcerer employed by their enemies, or to have inhaled
evil air emanating from ancient sacred places or tombs. The stronger these
beliefs, the more likely that the San Pedro potion will result in a cure through
suggestion.
Bibliography: Emboden, W. 1972. *Narcotic plants.*

SAN SEVERO. A mental hospital in Barcelona, Spain. It was built in 1412
and cared for those members of the clergy who had become insane.
Bibliography: Chamberlain, A. S. 1966. Early mental hospitals in Spain. *Am. J.
Psychiat.* 123: 143-49.

SANTA CRUZ HOSPITAL. A general hospital established in Barcelona,
Spain, in 1229. In 1401 it began to admit some mental patients; by 1481,
the care of the mentally ill was an established part of the hospital's work.
In 1680 the hospital was rebuilt with special psychiatric wards.
Bibliography: Chamberlain, A. S.. 1966. Early mental hospitals in Spain. *Am J.
Psychiat.* 123: 143-49.

SANTA MARIA DELLA PIETÀ. A mental hospital founded in Rome,
Italy, in 1561 by the brothers of the Order of Charity. Special rules estab-
lished by the church stated that patients were to be treated with respect.
Most remarkable for that period, the hospital offered medical and nursing
care. At a later date, the mentally ill were housed in specially built wards.
Pilgrims and paupers also were accepted at the institution, but they were
separated from the mentally ill.
Bibliography: Mora, G. 1975. Italy. In *World history of psychiatry,* ed. J. G. Howells.

SANTA MARIA NUOVA. An ancient Italian hospital situated in Florence.
In the seventeenth century it began to accept the mentally ill.
Bibliography: Mora, G. 1975. Italy. In *World history of psychiatry,* ed. J. G. Howells.

SANTAYANA, GEORGE (1863-1952). A Spanish-born philosopher, educated in the United States. He became professor of philosophy at Harvard

University in 1889. After his retirement in 1912, he lived in England, France, and Italy. His complex philosophy was naturalistic and speculative and opposed German idealism. He believed that human thinking was a bodily function on a nonphysical plane and that reason was a logical activity based on facts. Religious concepts, according to him, were not about truth but about ideals that support mental well-being. His philosophy is expounded in *The Realms of Being* a series of four books published between 1923 and 1940.
Bibliography: Butler, R. 1955. *The life and work of George Santayana.*

SANTIAGO, MIGUEL DE (?-1673). A Latin American painter, born in Quito, Equador. He was said to have become insane and to have suffered from hallucinations (q.v.) after he severely attacked his model to produce a genuine expression of agony, which he wanted to reproduce in his work.
Bibliography: Leon, C. A., and Rosselli, H. 1975. Latin America. In *World history of psychiatry.* ed. J. G. Howells.

SANTORIO, SANTORIO (1561-1636). An Italian physician, professor of theoretical medicine in Padua and author of several books. He is also known as Sanctorius, the Latinized form of his name. In 1614 he wrote a collection of aphorisms entitled *Ars de Statica Medicina* in which he presented the findings of thirty years' experiments. He believed that the body lost water through the skin and attempted to measure the variations of this "perspiratio insensibilis" and to discover how the variations were influenced by physical activity, disease and emotional excitement—an early appreciation of psychosomatic phenomena. He also wrote commentaries on the works of Hippocrates, Galen, and Avicenna (qq.v.) and developed the clinical thermometer, as well as several other instruments.
Bibliography: Sigerist, H. E. 1933. *Great doctors.*

SAPPHIRE. A gem once believed to possess curative properties. Robert Burton (q.v.), in his *Anatomy of Melancholy* (q.v.), wrote: "It is the fairest of all precious stones of sky colour, and a great enemy to black choler, frees the mind, and mends manners."
See also PRECIOUS STONES.
Bibliography: Evans, J. 1922. *Magical jewels.*

SAPPHO (c.600 B.C.). The greatest of the early Greek lyric poets, born on the Greek island of Lesbos. She married Cercylas, by whom she had a daughter. According to legend, she threw herself into the sea because of her unrequited love for Phaon, a boatman who had been given youth and beauty by Venus (q.v.). Most of her poems were about love, tender or passionate,

at times for women. The term sapphism or lesbianism (q.v.) is now used to indicate an erotic attachment between women.
Bibliography: Bowra, C.M. 1961. *Greek lyric poetry*.

SARAGOSSA. *See* ZARAGOZA HOSPITAL.

SARDANAPALUS. An Assyrian king. He was extremely effeminate and lived in great luxury. Defeated in battle, he planned a spectacular suicide (q.v.). He had erected on the funeral pyre a chamber 100 feet long, which was furnished with golden couches and tables and packed with treasures. In this chamber he burned himself, his wife, and concubines to death. His name is used to indicate a selfish and extravagant tyrant.
Bibliography: Fedden, H. R. 1938. *Suicide*.

SARDONYX. A gem that medieval lapidaries believed was generated by the sun. Placed in the mouth or in close contact with the skin it was said to strengthen the intellect, improve understanding, sharpen the senses, and disperse angry and stupid thoughts.
See also PRECIOUS STONES.
Bibliography: Evans, J. 1922. *Magical jewels*.

SARRASIN DE MONTFERRIER, ALEXANDRE ANDRÉ VICTOR (1792-1863). A French mathematician, better known under his pseudonym "de Lausanne," which he used for his works on magnetism (q.v.). He believed in animal spirits (q.v.) and a personal magnetic fluid that could be employed in the treatment of various diseases. He was editor of the *Annales du Magnétism* and was one of the founders of the Société Parisienne du Magnétisme.
Bibliography: Tinterow, M. M. 1970. *Foundations of hypnosis: from Mesmer to Freud*.

SARTO, ANDREA DEL (1486-1531). A Florentine painter whose real name was Andrea d'Agnolo di Francesco. In spite of his undisputed genius he never achieved greatness because of the dominance of his wife. She changed his life to such an extent that he lost not only his spontaneous gaiety, but also his friends, who came to resent her. She was almost his sole model, she ran his workshop, and she dictated which commissions he was to accept: her apron-strings strangled his art. His infatuation for her is said to have been a defence for his homosexual inclinations.
Bibliography: Jones, E. 1951. The influence of Andrea del Sarto's wife on his art. In *Essays in Applied Psychoanalysis*.

SARTRE, JEAN-PAUL (1905-1980). A French philosopher and novelist, disciple of Martin Heidegger (q.v.) and exponent of a particular brand of

existentialism (q.v.). His long affair with Simone de Beauvoir (1908-) was both public and well documented by his contemporaries. His writings reflect his intense energy, his lack of sentimentality, and his aggression, which often ends in horrifying and disgusting events. According to him there is no God and man is condemned to freedom of choice, which leads him to despair and anguish. The existence of man and of the world is an absurdity with no justification. His bleak philosophy has had much influence on avant-garde thinking. In 1964 he was awarded the Nobel Prize for literature, but he refused to accept it on the grounds that it gives an author too much influence. Of his many works *The Words* (1964) is autobiographical.
Bibliography: Cumming, R. D., ed. 1965. *The philosophy of Jean-Paul Sartre.*

SASSOON, SIEGFRIED (1886-1967). An English poet and writer. His experiences in World War I convinced him of the hideous wastefulness of war. He rejected hypocrisy, especially as practiced in romanticism (q.v.) and expressed his feelings in vivid and satirical poetry. He wrote three semiautobiographical books; the third of the series, *Sherston's Progress* (1936), describes the protagonist in a military hospital suffering from shell shock. He recovers thanks to the care of Dr. William H. Rivers (q.v.) and returns to the battlefields, where he becomes known as "Mad Jack."
Bibliography: Corrigan, F. 1973. *Siegfried Sassoon: a poet's pilgrimage.*

SATANISM. A blasphemous attitude toward the Christian church. In me-dieval times, the Black Mass was a formalized denial of feelings of goodness and love and an exultation of hate as personified in Satan. Those involved in Satanism were regarded as heretics, but their attitudes toward society were often not a revolt against the established faith but rather a result of their own emotional states or organic disorders that produced distortions of thought and hallucinations (q.v.).
Bibliography: Rhodes, H.T.F. 1954. *The Satanic mass.*

SATORI. In Zen Buddhism (q.v.), an enlightening mystical experience ob-tained through successful intensive meditation during which man and the universe are united as a whole without distinction between inner and outer world. The organic whole embraces all opposites, and, according to Zen Buddhists those who personally experience satori will never see the world in the same way again.
Bibliography: Humphreys, C. 1975. *Buddhism.*

SATURN. During the Renaissance, when astrology (q.v.) reached its zenith of popularity, those born under the astrological sign of the planet Saturn were believed to be melancholic (*see* MELANCHOLIA). Depending on Saturn's conjunction with other planets (q.v.) at the time of birth, a "melancholic" could become either a sensible man, capable of poetic vision and artistic accomplishments, or he could be condemned to a life of inertia, depression, and possibly insanity. The term "saturnine" was applied to those possessing grave, dull, and phlegmatic dispositions; certain wrinkles on the forehead were called "Saturn-lines" by physiognomists, who believed them to be signs of a melancholic personality.

Bibliography: Wittkower, R., and Wittkower, M. 1963. *Born under Saturn*.

SATYRS. In classic mythology (q.v.), forest gods, usually attendants of Dionysus (q.v.). The term "satyriasis," pathological excessive sexual appetite, is derived from them as they were believed to be lascivious and were represented as half man and half goat, with little horns on their heads, goat-like ears, and a leering expression on their features.

Bibliography: Hammond, N.G.L., and Scullard, H. H., eds. 1970. *The Oxford classical dictionary*.

SAUCE, JEAN-LOUIS (1760-1788). A minor French painter. Just before his wedding he invited his future bride and some friends to a dinner. At the end of it, he threw himself on the girl, whom he shot and then killed with his sword. He then jumped out of the window and killed himself.

Bibliography: Wittkower, R., and Wittkower, M. 1963. *Born under Saturn*.

SAUCEROTTE, NICOLAS (1741-1814). A French physician. In 1772 he gave the first clinical description of a condition that was later termed "acromegaly."

Bibliography: Schmidt, J. E. 1959. *Medical discoveries: who and when*.

SAUL. The first king of the ancient Hebrews. His unusual personality is described in the Bible (q.v.). At an early age, (1 Sam. x) he fell into a state of ecstacy, probably epilepsy (q.v.), in which he made prophecies. After he became king, mounting problems led to a bout of depression that was cured by David's harp, (1 Sam. xvi 23): an early example of music therapy (q.v.). In another episode of depression and paranoia (q.v.), he attempted to kill David (1 Sam. xviii 9-11). In a later attack, during which he stripped himself naked, he tried to kill his son (1 Sam. xxviii 16). He finally committed suicide (q.v.) (1 Sam. xxxi. 4) by falling on his sword; his sword bearer imitated him. His madness was attributed to an evil spirit sent by the Lord, but his suicide is recorded in the Bible without criticism. The *Malleus Maleficarum* (q.v.), commenting on the events relating to Saul's illness, acknowledged that the music from David's harp had a calming influence but argued that the devil had fled from Saul's body because the harp and its

string provided the shape of a cross, effective against devils even ten centuries before Christ's crucifixion.
Bibliography: 1 Sam. 10-31.

SAUSSURE, HORACE BÉNÉDICT DE (1740-1799). A Swiss naturalist who traveled widely in the Alps. He believed that cretinism (q.v.) which he had seen in many Alpine regions, might be caused by geological factors that influenced the chemical composition of the water drunk by those affected.
Bibliography. Saussure, H. B. de. 1786. *Voyages dans les Alpes.* Vol. II.

SAUVAGES, FRANÇOIS BOISSIER DE (1706-1767). A French physician. He was called "le medicin de l'amour" because of his dissertation entitled *Whether Love Can Be Cured by Remedies Derived from Plants.* He became professor of botany at Montpellier and transferred botanical methods of classification to medicine. His book *Nosologie Methodique,* published posthumously between 1770 and 1771, consists of three volumes describing about two thousand diseases, arranged into classes, orders, and genera, in the same way as the botanical classification of Carolus Linnaeus (q.v.). Descriptions of mental diseases cover more than 300 pages and are divided into errors of reason, bizzare forms of behavior, deliria, and anomalies. He attributed delirium (q.v.) to cerebral pathology, recognized fourteen kinds of melancholia (q.v.), and thought that reason should be strong enough to control most manifestations of mental disorder. He advised physicians to treat patients kindly and gain their confidence. In spite of his conservative attitude, he was a severe critic of the belief in witchcraft (q.v.).
Bibliography: King, L. S. 1966. Boissière de Sauvages and 18th century nosology. *Bull. Hist. Med.* 40: 43-51.

SAVAGE, GEORGE (1842-1921). An English psychiatrist and author. He was physician superintendent at Bethlem Royal Hospital (q.v.) and a great believer in the therapeutic value of "counterirritation," the result of suppration by blistering, or the insertion of a foreign body under the skin of the shaved head.
Bibliography: Hunter, R., and Macalpine, I. 1963. *Three hundred years of psychiatry.*

SAVAGE, RICHARD (c.1697-1743). An English poet, a contemporary and acquaintance of Samuel Johnson (q.v.). Savage claimed to be the illegitimate son of nobility. He was rejected by his mother and brought up in humble surroundings. As an adolescent, he attempted to see his mother and was ejected from her house. Following a tavern brawl in which he killed a man, he was tried for homicide. His mother claimed that he had meant to kill her when he was ejected and tried to have him hanged, but he was reprieved. He took revenge on his mother in his poem *The Bastard* (1728) in which he exposed her cruelty. Johnson wrote a sympathetic account of

him in his *Life of the Poets*. His dissolute way of life and the stresses he endured hastened his death in a debtor's prison. He claimed that his best work was *The Wanderer* (1729).
Bibliography: Makower, S. U. 1935. *Richard Savage: A mystery in biography*.

SAVILL, THOMAS DIXON (1856-1910). An English physician. Before becoming physician to the West End Hospital for Diseases of the Nervous System in London, he obtained some of his training at Salpêtrière (q.v.). His books include *Lectures on Hysteria* (1909) and *Lectures on Neurasthenia* (1892) in which he gave a bibliography of 125 items on the topic. He was also the author of several papers on diseases of the nervous system. He is now best remembered for the first description of epidemic exfoliative dermatitis, now known as Savill's disease.
Bibliography: Savill, T. D. 1892. *Lectures on neurasthenia*.

SAYAGO, JOSÉ. A seventeenth-century carpenter who, with the help of his wife, founded the first South American mental hospital for female patients in Mexico City in 1687. It was called the Hospital Real del Divino Salvador, and it was so well managed that it soon acquired a worldwide reputation. It gave almost continuous care to mental patients from the day of its foundation until 1842.
Bibliography: Leon, C. A., and Rosselli, H. 1975. Latin America. In *World history of psychiatry*, ed. J. G. Howells.

SCABIES. A highly communicable parasitic skin disease. Infecting stuporose patients with scabies was one of the suggestions made by Johann C. Reil (q.v.), who thought the discomfort of the rash would bring them back to activity.
Bibliography: Zilboorg, G. 1941. *A history of medical psychology*.

SCALIGER, JULIUS CAESAR (1484-1558). An Italian philosopher and physician, who settled in France. He discovered the kinesthetic sense through which the position of parts of the body is registered and understood that movements are dependent on nerve impulses. Some of his assertions, such as his belief that instincts are inherited adaptive habits that influence behavior, later were proven accurate. He also emphasized the relation of muscular sense and emotion and gave the example of the brave man who reacts to an insult by striking out, as he feels it in the muscles used for striking, while the timid man reacts by speech or lack of it.
Bibliography: Brett, G. S. 1912. *A history of psychology*.

SCAPEGOAT. A term derived from the sacrificial goat that replaced human sacrifice in primitive religious ceremonies. The sins or illnesses of the worshippers are transferred symbolically to the innocent animal, which is then

sacrificed. Some primitive healing rituals make use of sacrifice of animals, usually a goat, indicating that the patient's uncleanliness causing physical or mental disorders is transferred to the goat. In psychiatry the scapegoat mechanism refers to the defense processes of resentful individuals who blame their own faults, frustrations, and difficulties on innocent people, usually within the family group.
Bibliography: Frazer, J. 1957. *The golden bough.*

SCARPA, ANTONIO (1747–1832). An Italian anatomist and surgeon. He was the author of several textbooks, as well as the first to describe accurately a number of anatomical features that now carry his name, such as Scarpa's ganglion. He conducted research on aneurisms and on the sense of smell. He was a skillful artist and illustrated his own books.
Bibliography: Castiglioni, A. 1946. *A history of medicine,* ed. and trans. E.B. Krambhaar

SCHAFFER, KAROLY (1864–1939). An Austrian neurologist who spent most of his life in Hungary. In 1890 he introduced the theory of virus propagation along nerves. His work includes important contributions to the field of neuropathology, as well as writings on hypnosis (*see* HYPNOTISM), the reflexes, and the psychological characteristics of certain prominent men.
Bibliography: Haymaker, W., and Schiller, F. 1970. *The founders of neurology.* 2d. ed.

SCHAUDINN, FRITZ RICHARD (1871–1906). A German bacteriologist. In 1904, in collaboration with Erich Hoffman (1868– ?) he discovered the *Spirochaeta pallida,* or *Treponema pallidum,* in primary genital lesions and recognized them as the causative agents of syphilis (q.v.). The discovery was published the following year.
Bibliography: Dennie, C. C. 1962. *A history of syphilis.*

SCHELLING, FREDRICH WILHELM JOSEPH VON (1775–1854). A German romantic philosopher. Like other philosophers of his time, he was preoccupied with a pantheistic view of the universe in which man and nature are parts of a whole. He believed that magnetism (q.v.) could provide a connection between the soul of the world and man.
Bibliography: Schelling, F. W. J. von. 1800. *System of transcendental idealism.*

SCHENK VON GRAFENBURG, JOHANN (1531–1589). A German physician and author of several extensive textbooks. He devised a classification of diseases based on their most likely causes. Unlike most of his contemporaries, he considered mental illness to be a pathological condition that had nothing to do with the devil.

Bibliography: Calmeil, L. J. 1845. *De la folie considérée sous le point de vue patholgique, philosophique, historique et judiciare.*

SCHIFF, MORITZ (1823–1896). A German physiologist who worked in Switzerland and Italy. His studies in the field of the physiology of the nervous system emphasized the autonomic influences and nerve regeneration. He thought that cretinism (q.v.) could be cured by transplanting the thyroid of an animal to the patient, but the operation proved unsuccessful.

Bibliography: Haymaker, W., and Schiller, F. 1970. *The founders of neurology.* 2d. ed.

SCHILDER, PAUL FERDINAND (1886–1940). An Austrian psychiatrist who emigrated to the United States in the 1920s. He was the first to describe an inflammation of the white matter of the cerebrum now known as Schilder's disease. Much of his work on behavior disorders in children was conducted in cooperation with his wife, Lauretta Bender (q.v.). He was a strong advocate of group therapy. A prolific writer, he wrote on hypnosis (*see* HYPNOTISM), psychoanalysis (q.v.), personality and psychotherapy (q.v.).

Bibliography: Sherman, M. H., ed. 1966. *Psychoanalysis in America: historical perspectives.*

SCHILLER, JOHANN CHRISTOPH FRIEDRICH VON (1759–1805). A German dramatist, poet, historian, and philosopher. He was closely associated with Johann Wolfgang von Goethe (q.v.). Both his life and his works are of great psychological interest. His early education was to prepare him for the church, but his patron, the duke of Württernberg, forced him to enter the military school. In 1780 he qualified as a military surgeon, but he wished to write poetry and drama. When he clandestinely attended a performance of his first play, he was arrested for having been absent without leave. He was ordered to abandon poetry and only write medical works. Schiller escaped from Stuttgart, went into hiding, and continued to write poetry and dramas. He found refuge and a respite from emotional and financial worries in Dresden. His love affairs caused him much unhappiness; he married in 1788. Overwork was blamed for the breakdown of his health in the following years, but, although he suffered from tuberculosis, he continued to write. His play *Mary Stuart* (1800) contains a subtle psychological study of the two queens, Elizabeth and Mary. The highly emotional content of a number of his dramas made them excellent subjects for operas (for example, *Mary Stuart*, *Wilhelm Tell* and *Don Carlos*). The Ninth

Symphony of Ludwig von Beethoven (q.v.) is Schiller's poem *An die Freude* (Ode to Joy) set to music.

Bibliography: Dewhurst, K., and Reeves, N. 1978. *Friedrich Schiller: medicine, psychology and literature.*

SCHIZOPHRENIA. The most important of the psychoses (*see* PSYCHOSIS). The term, derived from the Greek words "to split" and "mind," was coined in 1911 by Eugen Bleuler (q.v.) to replace dementia praecox (q.v.). Bleuler defined it as a split in psychic functioning, alterations in the thinking process, and disharmony of affect. Such disorders have been described with varying accuracy for over twenty centuries, but disagreements on aetiology, diagnosis, and classification are still widespread.

Bibliography: Bleuler, P. E. 1911. *Dementia praecox oder die Gruppe der Schizophrenien.*

SCHLEICHER, AUGUST (1821–1868). A German linguist. His investigations included a study on the speech development of children. He was probably the first individual to record methodically the speech development of a particular child. Schleicher also applied the theories of Charles Darwin (q.v.) to the study of Indo-European languages.

Bibliography: Dennis, W. 1949. Historical beginnings of child psychology. *Psychol. Bull.* 46: 224-39.

SCHLEIDEN, MATTHIAS JAKOB (1804–1881). A German botanist who studied plant and animal tissues. His microscopic studies led to the theory, which he evolved with Theodor Schwann (q.v.), that the cell is the basic structure of all living matter. He recognized the importance of the nucleus in the reproduction of the cell, which he regarded as a primordial protein substance. He accepted the theory of evolution evolved by Charles Darwin even though he was closely associated with the school of natural philosophy.

Bibliography: Alexander, F. G., and Selesnick, S. T. 1966. *The history of psychiatry.*

SCHNAUZKRAMPF. A German term coined by Karl L. Kahlbaum (q.v.). It refers to the protrusion of lips which resemble an animal snout, in catatonic schizophrenics (*see* SCHIZOPHRENIA).

SCHNEIDER, KURT (1887–1967). A German psychiatrist. His precise nosographic and diagnostic interpretations contributed greatly to German clinical psychiatry. He was a follower of Karl Jaspers (q.v.) and derived from him a phenomenological approach to mental disorders. He particularly studied delusions (q.v.) and the primary and secondary symptoms of schizophrenia (q.v.). He also explored psychopathology in his book *Psychopathic*

Personalities. According to him neuroses (*see* NEUROSIS) have their aetiology in constitutional abnormalities of personality.
Bibliography: Schneider, K. 1959. *Clinical psychopathology*, trans. M. W. Hamilton.

SCHNITZLER, ARTHUR (1862-1931). An Austrian physician, dramatist, and novelist. His works contain a deep understanding and masterly exposition of psychological situations and reflect his early studies in medicine and psychiatry. He was a pupil of Theodor Meynert (q.v.) and developed an interest in problems of hypnosis (*see* HYPNOTISM) and hysteria (q.v.), which he later used in his plays. His writing career began with papers in medical journals and reviews of medical books. The parallels between Schnitzler and Sigmund Freud (q.v.) led Freud to regard him almost as his own double. Amoral attitudes to erotic themes in his plays are usually contrasted to sadness at the declining morals of society. The material was often derived from his own stormy love affairs and the events of his life, including suicide (q.v.) of his only daughter. *Flight into Darkness*, published in 1931, is about a man's mental illness and traces the pattern of its persecution mania (q.v.).
Bibliography: Liptzin, S. 1932. *Arthur Schnitzler*.

SCHOLASTICISM. A philosophical system that took its name from the "schoolmen" of the Middle Ages (q.v.) who tried to derive a formula that would reconcile Christian doctrine and classical philosophy, faith and reason. Their basic approach to knowledge rested on the belief that the authority of the past needed to be reaffirmed, rather than reinterpreted. Pierre Abélard (q.v.) belonged to the early years of Scholasticism and Thomas Aquinas (q.v.) to its later period. Medicine was influenced by Scholasticism in its attitude toward the Greek medical writers, who were regarded as authoritative.
Bibliography: Jones, W. T. 1969. *The medieval mind*.

SCHOOLS, MEDICAL. The first schools dedicated solely to the teaching of medicine were opened in Europe in the thirteenth century. Medicine was taught at the following universities, which were founded between the thirteenth and fourteenth century: University of Paris (1205), Padua (1222), Lyons (1223), Naples (1224), Oxford (1249), Collegium Chirurgicum in Paris (1260), Cambridge (1284), Montpellier (1289), Lisbon (1290), Avignon (1303), Pisa (1339), Heidelberg (1346), Prague (1348), Cracow (1364), and Vienna (1364).
Bibliography: Garrison, F. H. 1929. *An introduction to the history of medicine*.

SCHOPENHAUER, ARTHUR (1788–1860). A German philosopher. His father was a ruthless, irritable, and violent individual, who showed extreme severity to his son; he drowned in a canal, and suicide (q.v.) was suspected. His mother was intellectual but cold and selfish; she refused to have her adolescent son living with her and could not avoid quarreling with him

during his brief visits. Schopenhauer spent most of his childhood away from his hostile parents and regarded the periods of separation as his happiest. He grew into a melancholic (*see* MELANCHOLIA) man who was given to brooding and possessed a morbid anxiety about death and illness. He slept with loaded pistols and his sword near him. He was so suspicious of others that he wrote his accounts in English and his business notes in Latin and Greek. After his death, the instructions in his will, which was written in Latin, were difficult to implement because he had hidden his more valuable possessions. His strong sexual drive filled him with guilt, and he hated women and people in general. His bad temper was proverbial: he once threw an old seamstress downstairs and so injured her that he had to pay damages to her until her death, which he greeted with relief. Although he was a hypochondriac, he remained active even in old age. His philosophy is pervaded with pessimism and based on the assumption that life consists of perpetual striving. His main work is *Die Welt als Wille und Vorstellung* (The World as Will and Idea), published in 1819 and translated in 1958.
Bibliography: Gardiner, P. 1963. *Schopenhauer.*

SCHREBER, DANIEL PAUL (1842–1911). A German magistrate. His record of his own mental illness provided Sigmund Freud (q.v.) with the material for his theory of paranoia (q.v.), although he never met Schreber. Schreber's father, Dr. Daniel Gottlieb Schreber (1808–1861) was an educationalist who had devised sadistic methods of child-rearing that included imprisoning children in a specially designed apparatus that prevented them from assuming relaxed postures. His methods which denied children the natural expression of their needs or any form of "childish" behavior were applied to his own children, who were terrified of him. The oldest child, Daniel Paul, shot himself but survived and achieved a distinguished legal career. At the age of forty-two however, he became mentally ill and was admitted to the psychiatric clinic of Paul E. Flechsig (q.v.) in Leipzig. After a spell in an asylum near Dresden, he recovered and returned to his work, but he suffered a second mental breakdown. In 1907 he suffered his third breakdown, which forced him back to an asylum for the rest of his life. His account of his mental illness contains descriptions of many psychosomatic disorders. The persecution he endured at the hands of his father was reflected in his paranoid symptoms. He believed that he was being transformed into a woman and was tortured by obsessions (q.v.) and compulsions. On several occasions he attempted suicide (q.v.).
Bibliography: Macalpine, I., and Hunter, R. 1955. *Daniel Paul Schreber: memoirs of my nervous illness.*
Schatzman, M. 1973. *Soul murder: persecution in the family.*

SCHRYVER, KONRAD (*or* SCRIBONIUS *or* GROPHAEUS) (1482–1558). A Dutch philosopher. He opposed the claims of Johann Weyer (q.v.),

who believed that witches (*see* WITCHCRAFT) were the victims of pathological imagination and drugs and Schryver accused Weyer of sorcery and claimed he was a mixer of poisons whose writings corrupted the people and enhanced the power of Satan.
Bibliography: Binz, C. 1885. *Doktor Johann Weyer*.

SCHUBERT, FRANZ PETER (1797–1828). An Austrian composer. In the words of his friend, Johann Mayrhofer "his character was a mixture of tenderness and coarseness, sensuality and candour." In spite of his emotionality, he was never able to become deeply involved with another person and never married. He enjoyed the carefree life of the Bohemian group to which he belonged, possibly as a rebellion against his father, a rigid schoolmaster, and found comfort in excessive drinking and unwise sexual adventures from which he contracted syphilis (q.v.). Although his short life was disordered, his compositions were exceptionally numerous. Edward Hitschmann (q.v.) included him in his pathographies.
Bibliography: Wechsberg, J. 1977. *Schubert: his life, his works, his time*.

SCHUBERT, GOTTHILF HEINRICH VON (1780–1860). A German physician and author. His book *Die Symbolik des Traumes* (The Symbolism of Dreaming) published in 1814, antedates Sigmund Freud (q.v.) by at least seventy-five years in its discussion of dreams (q.v.), symbolism, and the superego. He probably did not influence Freud, although Freud did quote him in his *Interpretation of Dreams* (1900).
Bibliography: D'Alessandro, A. J. 1968. An historical review of *Die Symbolik des Traumes*. *Psych. Quart.* 42: 337-43.

SCHÜLE, HEINRICH (1840–1916). A German psychiatrist. He devised a classification of mental disorders in which he combined some neuroses (*see* NEUROSIS) and psychoses (*see* PSYCHOSIS). He categorized some disorders as cerebropsychopathies, hereditary neuroses, and psychoneuroses.
Bibliography: Schule, H. 1878. *Handbüch der Geisteskrankheiten*.

SCHUMANN, FRIEDRICH (1863–1940). A German psychologist. At Göttingen he worked with Georg E. Müller (q.v.) on memory (q.v.), and in Berlin he worked with Carl Stumpf (q.v.). He also performed important work on visual space perception. In 1910 he went to Frankfurt, where he established a laboratory.
Bibliography: Boring, E. G. 1950. *A history of experimental psychology*.

SCHUMANN, ROBERT (1810–1856). A German composer. His father, who had encouraged his musical talent, died when he was sixteen years old, and his mother pressed him into legal studies for which he had no interest. With the excuse of widening his legal experience, he traveled in Italy and

Germany. He finally persuaded his mother to allow him to study music. Unwise, self-devised methods to straighten his fingers led to paralysis of his right hand and forced him to concentrate on composition rather than on playing the piano. Consequently, he became extremely depressed. After great opposition, including court proceedings, he married his teacher's daughter, Clara Wiech (1819–1896) who greatly encouraged his ambitions. Unfortunately, his original shyness increased; he became withdrawn and drank excessively. At times he was so lost in his own thoughts that he would continue to direct the orchestra even after the instrumentalists had stopped performing. His wife's tours as a concert pianist precipitated periods of depression. Her tour of Russia so upset him that he was ill and unable to compose for a year. He suffered from a number of psychosomatic complaints and was pathologically afraid of sickness, especially cholera, and of heights, particularly after attempting suicide (q.v.) by jumping from a fourth floor window. Paranoia (q.v.) and hallucinations (q.v.) of angels and devils dictating music to him became frequent. Although he begged to be admitted to an asylum (q.v.), it was not until 1853, when he attempted suicide by throwing himself in the Rhine, that his family had him admitted to the asylum at Enderich, where he died three years later. His death was accelerated by his refusal to take food. An autopsy revealed atrophy and partial ossification and degeneration of the brain. Other members of his family also suffered from mental disorders. His older sister committed suicide after a long period of withdrawal, and his son spent most of his life in an asylum. Bibliography: Walker, A., ed. 1972. *Schumann: the man and his music.*

SCHWAGELIN, ANNA MARIA (?-1775). A deranged German woman. She was accused of witchcraft (q.v.) and condemned to death. She was the last individual to be decapitated for witchcraft in Bavaria. Bibliography: Zilboorg, G. 1941. *A history of medical psychology.*

SCHWANN, THEODOR (1810-1882). A German neurologist. In collaboration with his friend Matthias Schleiden (q.v.) he established the theory that the cell is a universal unit of structure of animals and plants. Bibliography: Causey, G. 1960. *The cell of Schwann.*

SCHWARTZER, FERENCZ (1818-1889). A Hungarian psychiatrist. His psychiatric training took place in Vienna, but he also traveled throughout Europe, meeting the best psychiatrists of his time. On his return to Hungary he reported to the government his findings in other countries and made suggestions for the establishment of a mental hospital. Because of political unrest the project was postponed, but he was allowed to treat mental patients in his own home until a hospital was built in Buda in 1852. Bibliography: Horansky, N. 1975. Hungary. In *World History of Psychiatry*, ed. J. G. Howells.

SCHWEIK. The hero of *The Good Soldier Schweik* (1920-1923), a satirical novel by the Czech author Jaroslav Hašek (1883-1923). The good-hearted

Schweik's commonsense makes him a logical and rational figure in the mad world of World War I. Among his adventures there is an episode dealing with a lunatic asylum (q.v.) in which he enjoys his stay but complains that they threw him out without giving him lunch. His description of the inmates reflects the beliefs of many people at the time.
Bibliography: Hasek, J. 1973. *The good soldier Schweik*, trans. C. Parrott.

SCHWEIZER GESELLSCHAFT FÜR PSYCHIATRIE. A psychiatric association founded in Switzerland in 1850. In 1864 it was called Society of Medical Alienists, but it later changed its title.
Bibliography: Diethelm, O. 1975. Switzerland. In *World history of psychiatry*, ed. J. G. Howells.

SCOT (*or* SCOTT), MICHAEL(c.1175-1234). A Scottish scholar, physician, and astrologer (*see* ASTROLOGY). He was famous for his occult knowledge and was believed to be a magician (*see* MAGIC). In his *Liber Physiognomiae* he discussed how the predominant humor determined the content of a person's dreams (q.v.). He claimed that those with an excess of black bile (q.v.) had sad and frightening dreams; they were said to have a suspicious nature, to become depressed, anxious, irritable and stubborn easily. He also compared body features with personality. Dante Alighieri (q.v.) put him in the *Inferno*, and Giovanni Boccaccio (q.v.) wrote about him in the *Decameron*. He appears also in Sir Walter Scott's (q.v.) *Lay of the Last Minstrel*.
Bibliography: Thorndike, L. 1965. *Michael Scot*.

SCOT (*or* SCOTT), REGINALD (1538-1599). An English natural scientist and magistrate. His book *The Discoverie of Witchcraft* (q.v.) a treatise of about 200 folios, was published in 1584. The work was attacked by the bigoted James I of England and VI of Scotland (q.v.) in his *Daemonologie in the Forme of a Dialogue* (q.v.). Scot defended witches and bewitched and claimed that both were suffering from disorders of the brain. He called their hallucinations (q.v.) and feelings of persecution "unaccustomed sensations" and asserted that they were sick people in need of treatment. He did not deny that the devil took possession of their minds but argued that he was able to do so because they were old and sick and their "drousie minds" offered no resistance. He also made the important observation that self-accusation in criminal courts can not be relied upon and could be the result of delusions (q.v.).
Bibliography: Hunter, R., and Macalpine, I. 1963. *Three hundred years of psychiatry*.

SCOTT, SIR WALTER (1771-1832). A Scottish novelist and poet. His novels influenced Honoré de Balzac (q.v.) and Leo Tolstoy (q.v.). As a child he suffered from severe behavior problems, and his teachers found him unmanageable. He had a prodigious memory and would go about the house shouting poetry so loudly that other people could not make themselves heard. An attack of poliomyelitis left him lame and kept him from entering the army, causing him to take up writing. In some of his works he gives explanations of dreams (q.v.) and descriptions of mental disorders. David Do Little, a character appearing in *Waverley* (1814), is a masterly description of a mental defective, and Clara Mowbray, the heroine in *St. Ronan's Well* (1824), loses her reason as a result of her misfortunes. Scott was also one of the first writers to describe the feeling of "déjà vu" (q.v.), which he called "sentiment of pre-existence." In the last part of his life Scott suffered from dementia, and his memory (q.v.) deteriorated to the point where he could not recognize his own sonnets.

Bibliography: Oman, C. 1973. *The wizard of the north: the life of Sir Walter Scott.*

SCOTTISH SCHOOL. A school of philosophy. Its principal exponents, Thomas Reid (q.v.), Dugald Stewart (1753-1828) (q.v.), and Thomas Brown (1778-1820), were professors at Scottish universities. Regarding them as degrading to man, it rejected the doctrine of associationism (q.v.) and the physiological basis of behavior. It believed that common experience was all important in the understanding of the outside world.

Bibliography: Watson, R. I. 1963. *The great psychologists.*

SCOTUS, MICHAEL. *See* SCOT, MICHAEL.

SCRIBONIUS LARGUS (fl.c. A.D. 14-54). A Roman physician. He was the first to record the application of torpedo, or electric, fish to the head to treat intractable headache. Another strange remedy reported by him was the drinking of one's own blood. He was the author of a book on drugs and prescriptions entitled *Compositiones Medicamentorum* in which he described opium (q.v.) extractions. He visited Britain in A.D. 43.

See also ELECTROICH.

Bibliography: Scarborough, J. 1969. *Roman medicine.*

SCRIPTURE, EDWARD WHEELER (1864-1943). A German-American psychologist and pupil of Wilhelm Wundt (q.v.). George Ladd (q.v.) brought him to Yale University, where he worked as an instructor in experimental psychology (q.v.) for about ten years. He wrote *Thinking, Feeling, and Doing*, in 1895 and *The New Psychology* in 1897. The series of *Studies from the Yale Psychological Laboratory* was begun by him, and he was the chief contributor to it. After leaving Yale, he dedicated his studies to problems of speech and its defects. In 1906 he acquired a medical degree at Munich

and he was professor of experimental phonetics at Vienna from 1923 to 1933. The term "arm-chair psychology" was invented by him.
Bibliography: Murchinson, C., ed. 1936. *A history of psychology in autobiography.* Vol. 3.

SCROFULA. A tuberculous infection of the lymph glands. In England it was believed to respond to the king's touch (q.v.). Kings and queens held special ceremonies during which those affected were touched by the royal hand. Special coins or medals were struck for the occasion and often were worn around the neck. Samuel Johnson (q.v.) was taken by his mother to Queen Anne when he suffered from scrofula; he wore the coin she gave him round his neck for the rest of his life.
Bibliography: Bloch, M. 1973. *The royal touch: sacred monarchy and scrofula in England and France.*

SCULTETUS, JOANNIS (1595-1645). A German physician. He served as a military surgeon in the German army and wrote about his experiences in the *Armamentorium Chirurgicum,* published posthumously in 1653. The book was reprinted for over a hundred years. A large section of it deals with head injuries and their surgical treatment. One of the instruments illustrated, the modiolus, a kind of hand trephine, still finds favor with neurosurgeons performing leucotomies.
Bibliography: Bakay, L. 1971. *The treatment of head injuries in the Thirty Years War (1618-1648).*

SCYTHIANS. The inhabitants of an area west of the Himalayas, according to the ancient Greeks and Romans. Males of this race were said to become impotent between the ages of twenty and thirty. They developed some feminine sexual characteristics and even adopted female dress. At that point they would begin to live among females. Hippocrates of Cos (q.v.) commented on it and thought that the condition arose from excessive horse riding. It was also noted by Herodotus (q.v.). Similar conditions have been noted in the Kuban tribe of Nogays by Klaproth (*Reise in der Caucasus und nach Georgien.* Berlin, 1912) and in Pueblo Indians of New Mexico, who are termed *mujerados,* by Hammond (*Amer. J. Neur. & Psych.,* 1882).
Bibliography: Whitwell, J. R. 1936. *Historical notes on psychiatry.*

SEABROOK, WILLIAM. A contemporary American author. In 1935 he wrote a book entitled *Asylum,* which is an account of seven months he spent as an alcoholic (*see* ALCOHOLISM) in a large insane asylum (q.v.). His symptoms, reactions, and feelings, as well as some of the other patients, are vividly described in it.
Bibliography: Seabrook, W. 1935. *Asylum.*

SEAMAN, ELIZABETH. *See* BLY, NELLIE.

SEASHORE, CARL EMIL (1866-1949). A Swedish-born psychologist who emigrated to the United States as a boy. In his laboratory at the University of Iowa, he conducted a remarkable series of experiments in all branches of musical psychology. He was the originator of the Seashore Measures of Musical Talents in 1919. He also wrote on fatigue, mental work, and gifted students.
Bibliography: Seashore, C. E. 1939. *The psychology of music.*

SEASONS. The four divisions of the year were believed to have some influence on insanity. Hippocrates of Cos, Aretaeus of Cappadocia, and Celsus (qq.v.) believed that summer and autumn caused raging. Melancholia (q.v.) was said to be more common in the autumn, and dementia was thought to appear in winter.
Bibliography: Esquirol, J.E.D. 1845. Reprint. 1965. *Mental maladies: a treatise on insanity.*

SECHENOV, IVAN MIKHAILOVICH (1829-1905). A Russian physiologist. He is considered the father of Russian physiology because of his work on neurophysiology. His observations on reflexes later influenced Ivan Pavlov (q.v.). His main works were *Reflexes of the Brain* published in 1863, and *Who Must Investigate the Problems of Psychology and How*, published in 1870.
Bibliography: Haymaker, W., and Schiller, F. 1970. *The founders of neurology.* 2d. ed.

SECTOR THERAPY. A form of therapy devised by Felix Deutsch (q.v.). In it the chain of associations causing the emotional disorder is broken, and other patterns of thought are built up to help the patient toward a more constructive interpretation of events.
Bibliography: Deutsch, F. 1949. *Applied psychoanalysis: selected objectives of psychotherapy.*

SEDLEY, SIR CHARLES (1639?-1701). English courtier, dramatist, and poet. His wit and his debauchery were notorious. He is said to have joined the revolution in favor of James II's daughter in gratitude to the king, who had seduced his ugly daughter and made her a countess. He had a propensity for exhibitionism. In 1663 he was heavily fined, imprisoned for one week, and ordered to be of good behavior for three years, "for shewing himself naked in a balcony and throwing down bottles (pist in)" at Covent Garden. Samuel Pepys (q.v.) and Samuel Johnson (q.v.) recorded the event in detail.

Five years later Pepys again wrote about Sedley and claimed that he and some friends, had run naked through the street, caused a fight, and were beaten and imprisoned by the watch.
Bibliography: de S. Pinto, V. 1927. *Sir Charles Sedley.*

SEERESS OF PREVORST. *See* HAUFFE, FREDERICKE.

SÉGUIN, EDOUARD ONESIMUS (1812-1880). A French physician and psychologist known as "apostle of the idiots" because of his work for the mentally retarded. He was a pupil of Jean Esquirol (q.v.) and Jean Itard (q.v.), who inspired his interest in mental retardation. His work changed the previous custodial approach to the mentally deficient into a constructive program of rehabilitation and education. He based the program on what he described as a physiological method that consisted of exercises to develop the motor and sensory capacities. In 1842 he was appointed director of an institution for the mentally retarded in Paris, but eight years later French political situation forced him to leave the country. He continued his work in the United States. Of his numerous works, the most important is *Idiocy, Its Treatment by the Physiological Method* (1866). In Italy Maria Montessori (q.v.) was influenced by his work.
Bibliography: Murphy, G. 1956. *Historical introduction to modern psychology.*

SEILI HOSPITAL. An institution for lepers and for the mentally ill founded in Finland in 1623 by King Gustavus Adolphus. Patients were transferred to it from the hospital at Åbo (Turku) (q.v.), which was then over three hundred years old.
Bibliography: Retterstøl, N. 1975. Scandinavia. In *World history of psychiatry*, ed. J. G. Howells.

SELENIASMUS. An old term for lunacy (*see* LUNATIC) and epilepsy (q.v.). It was derived from Selene, the goddess of the moon (q.v.) in Greek mythology (q.v.).
Bibliography: Hinsie, L. E., and Campbell, R. J. 1960. *Psychiatric dictionary.*

SELENITE. A semiprecious stone, also known as a moonstone, which was worn to prevent attacks of epilepsy (q.v.). Dioscorides (q.v.) mentioned it in his *Materia Medica* and Marbode, bishop of Rennes between 1067 and 1081, wrote that it strengthened its wearers and brought about reconcilia-

tions between lovers. Girolamo Cardano (q.v.) wrote that it had drying properties, caused insomnia, and increased anxiety.
See also PRECIOUS STONES.
Bibliography: Evans, J. 1922. *Magical jewels.*

SELENOGAMIA. An obsolete term for somnambulism (q.v.) meaning "wedded to the moon" because the disorder was believed to be connected to phases of the moon (q.v.).
Bibliography: Hinsie, L. E., and Campbell, R. J. 1960. *Psychiatric dictionary.*

SELF-BURNERS. A group of religious fanatics who inflicted burns on their own bodies. Its followers still existed in Russia in the seventeenth century.
Bibliography: Zilboorg, G. 1941. *A history of medical psychology.*

SELMER, HARALD (1814-1879). A Danish physician known as the "father of Danish psychiatry." After observing German methods of treatment, he introduced many important reforms in the treatment of the mentally ill in Denmark. He was influenced further by the work of Philippe Pinel (q.v.), Jean Esquirol (q.v.), and James C. Prichard (q.v.), whose writings he translated. He advocated the establishment of new mental hospitals in which all matters concerning the patients would be decided by one person who would function as the physician and administrator.
Bibliography: Retterstøl, N. 1975. Scandinavia. In *World history of psychiatry*, ed. J. G. Howells.

SEMELAIGNE, RENÉ (1855-1934). A French psychiatrist. He was a follower of classical medicine. In the tradition of his father Armand Semelaigne who was a major psychiatric historian, and of his great-uncle Philippe Pinel (q.v.), he pursued research into the history of psychiatry.
Bibliography: Semelaigne, R. 1930-1932. *Les pionnieres de la psychiatrie Française avant et apres Pinel.*

SEMIRAMIS. Mythical queen of the Assyrians. She was said to be extremely beautiful and courageous. On the death of her husband, she assumed male dress, pretended to be her own son, and governed the country. She had many lovers, including her son. The invention of the chastity belt is attributed to her. She was said to have forced all her ladies to wear one so that they could not influence the men of the court with their charms. According to legend, she was killed by her son in a fit of anger.
Bibliography: Boccaccio, G. *De Mulieribus Claris.* 1967. ed. V. Zaccaria.

SEMMELWEIS, IGNAZ PHILIPP (1818-1865). A Hungarian physician. He was the first to realize that puerperal fever was caused by sepsis and

could be prevented. His views were ridiculed by the medical profession, and he was treated as a madman. His superior and his colleagues persecuted him and drove him from the Vienna general hospital. Bitter and broken in spirit, he became so depressed that he was thought to be insane and was admitted to an asylum where, ironically, he died of blood poisoning.
Bibliography: Slaughter, F. G. 1950. *Immortal Magyar*.

SEMON, FELIX (1849-1921). A German-born, English laryngologist. He recognized the link between myxoedema, cretinism and cachexia strumipriva, and found that their common cause is a loss of thyroid function. His findings were published in 1883.
Bibliography: Schmidt, J. E. 1959. *Medical discoveries: who and when*.

SEN, GANNETH. A contemporary Indian scientist. In 1931 in collaboration with Katrick Bose (q.v.), he described the use of *Rauwolfia serpentina* (q.v.) in the treatment of psychosis (q.v.), thus renewing interest in the drugs derived from this plant.
Bibliography: Morton, J. F. 1977. *Major medicinal plants*.

SENECA, LUCIUS ANNAEUS (c.4 B.C.-A.D.65). A Roman political philosopher and statesman born in Cordova, Spain, but educated in Rome. As a child, he was sickly and often incapacitated by asthmatic attacks. His father was an authoritarian narrowminded man, given to praising the past and condemning the present. He had little understanding of his son. Seneca, however, had a close relationship with his mother, who was about thirty years younger than her husband and a lively, well-educated woman. His character was full of contradictions: he was a Stoic philosopher, yet his way of life was not compatible with Stoicism (q.v.). He was selfish, acquisitive, and aggressive. When he was in his late thirties, he was exiled to Corsica as a result of an illicit love affair. He became tutor to Nero (q.v.), and, although he often helped him in his intrigues, he did have a beneficial influence on his pupil. In his old age he tried to change his personality and blamed his faults on his early upbringing. He lost favor with Nero, who tried to have him poisoned. When this failed, he was accused of conspiring against the emperor and ordered to commit suicide (q.v.). Seneca chose to open his veins in a warm bath. His writings include treatises on anger, tranquility of mind, and indolence; his *Epistolae* include a long and revealing letter to his mother. His tragedies focused on familial passions and incestuous (*see* INCEST) deeds. The philosophical thinkers of the Middle Ages (q.v.) were greatly influenced by him.
Bibliography: Rozelaar, M. 1973. Seneca—a new approach to his personality. *Psychiatry*. 36: 82-92.

SENESCENCE. Morbid changes in the mental faculties of old people. Aretaeus of Cappadocia (q.v.) wrote that these changes could not be arrested and were incurable. Rhazes (q.v.) remarked on the melancholia (q.v.) that assails the old, and Felix Plater (q.v.) was among those who noted the deterioration of memory (q.v.) in old people, who often forget names and faces of those near to them.

Bibliography: Howells, J. G., ed. 1975. *Modern perspectives in the psychiatry of old age.*

SENGELMANN, HEINRICH MATTHIAS (1821-1899). A German educationalist especially interested in feebleminded children. He established a special institution for them near Hamburg. In 1885 he wrote a textbook on the care of the idiot (q.v.) which was entitled *Idiotophilus,* and in 1874 he organized a conference of the directors of German institutions for mental defectives.

Bibliography: Kanner, L. 1964. *A history of the care and study of the mentally retarded.*

SENNERT, DANIEL (1572-1639). A German physician and professor of medicine and physics at the University of Wittenberg. The first volume of his *Institutiones Medical et de Origine Animasum in Brutes* appeared in 1611. The work contains a great deal of material on mental diseases, which he classified into two major groups: mania (q.v.) and melancholia (q.v.). He discussed the behavior of the insane and made some perceptive observations, although he believed that unusual mental phenomena were caused by the devil. He believed that lycanthropy (q.v.) was the real demoniacal transformation of a human being into a beast. He also wrote on the influence of the uterus (q.v.) on mental disorders. He tried to amalgamate the theories of Aristotle (q.v.) and Galen (q.v.) with the chemical doctrines of Paracelsus (q.v.). His therapy for mental disorders was based on diet (q.v.) and cathartics.

Bibliography: Zilboorg, G. 1941. *A history of medical psychology.*

SENSATION TYPE. The term used by Carl G. Jung (q.v.) for one of the four function types in his classification. The other three are thinking, feeling, and intuition types.

See also INTUITION TYPE and THINKING TYPE.

Bibliography: Jung, C. G. 1923. *Psychological types,* trans. H. G. Baynes.

SENSORIUM COMMUNE. A term first used by Aristotle (q.v.) for the heart (q.v.), which he regarded as the seat of all sensations.

Bibliography: Zilboorg, G. 1941. *A history of medical psychology.*

SENTIENT STATUE. Etienne Bonrat de Condillac (q.v.) used the example of an inanimate statue that could be endowed with a single sense at a time in his *Traité de sensations* (1754). According to him, with experience the

statue could acquire all the chief intellectual faculties. The concept illustrates the extreme sensualism and materialism of eighteenth-century philosophy.
Bibliography: Boring, E. G. 1950. *A history of experimental psychology.*

SENTIMENTS. William McDougall (q.v.) called sentiments the "complex and more or less permanent organizations of instincts." According to him, will and character were determined by what he called the "self-regarding sentiment."
Bibliography: McDougall, W. 1908. *Introduction to social psychology.*

SEPTIMANA MEDICALIS. In the teaching of Galen (q.v.) special medical importance was given to certain periods of the lunar calendar. The "septimana medicalis" (medical week) was the one week in the month considered most propitious for diagnosis and therapy.
Bibliography: Siegel, R. E. 1968. *Galen's system of physiology and medicine.*

SERENUS SAMMONICUS, QUINTUS (d. c. A.D. 212). A Roman poet, orator, and medical writer. In his writings on medicine he used the term "phrenitis" to cover all disorders of the mind including phrenitis, mania, and melancholia (qq.v.). According to him, in phrenitis either the mind is deceived as thought and judgment go astray, or imagination and perception are impaired. He regarded yellow bile (q.v.) as the cause of mania and black bile as the cause of melancholia. It was said that he had a library of 62,000 books. He was put to death by order of Caracalla (q.v.) because he had recommended amulets (q.v.) in the treatment of some disorders, a practice forbidden by the emperor.
Bibliography: Scarborough, J. 1969. *Roman medicine.*

SERER. A West African farming tribe of Senegal. They regard mental disorder as an "illness of the spirit." Their classification includes *o'bodah*, characterized by chronic disorders of speech and thinking, *o'dof*, characterized by violent behavior and hallucinations (q.v.), and *m'befedin*, similar to epilepsy (q.v.) but believed by the Serer to be contagious through the saliva of those affected. Ancestor spirits that have not been propitiated properly are regarded as the cause of illness and other misadventures.
Bibliography: Beiser, M. et. al. 1973. Illness of the spirit among the Serer of Senegal. *Am. J. Psychiat.* 130: 881-86.

SERIAL GROUPS, METHOD OF. A method elaborated early in the twentieth century by William McDougall (q.v.) as a modification of the method of minimal changes. A number of stimuli of the same intensity are presented in steps of ascending or descending order.
Bibliography: Flugel, J. C. 1945. *A hundred years of psychology.*

SERVETUS, MIGUEL (1511-1553). A Spanish physician and discoverer of pulmonary circulation. His theological opinions incurred the hostility of

John Calvin (q.v.). After traveling through the Holy Land he reported factually on its geographical features, including its barren areas. This upset the comfortable picture that his European contemporaries had drawn from biblical descriptions. He was accused of heresy and burnt at the stake.
Bibliography: Fulton, J. F. 1954. *Michael Servetus: humanist and martyr.*

SETH, SYMEON (fl. 1071-1078). A Byzantine physician who translated Arabic medical works, including a list of Arabic and Hindu herbal remedies, into Greek. This was the first time that a Western book contained information on Eastern medicine. Drugs affecting the mind were also listed. He later wrote a treatise on taste, smell, and touch.
Bibliography: 1968. *World who's who in science*, ed. A. G. Debus.

SEVEN DEADLY SINS. They are usually given as pride, lechery, envy, anger, covetousness, gluttony, and sloth. In medieval literature, paintings, and dramas, they were often personified and related to bodily characteristics. Certain animals were used sometimes as symbols of one or another sin.
Bibliography: 1978. *Brewers dictionary of phrase and fable.*

SEVILLE. The location of an institution for the mentally ill founded in the fifteenth century. In 1436 Marcos Sanches de Contreras bought a house in the city to give shelter to the mentally ill who roamed the street. With the help of other philanthropists, his house developed into a hospital consisting of a number of houses. It was informally called the hospital of the innocents and it was dedicated to Saint Cosmas and Saint Damian (q.v.). Marcos Sanches de Contreras oversaw its management for sixty-three years. The patients were well treated and records show that they were sometimes sent on pilgrimages to curative springs. In 1481 the hospital came under royal patronage. The buildings were improved in 1686. The hospital lasted until 1840, when the patients were transferred to new premises. Miguel de Cervantes Saavedra (q.v.) knew it well and used it as background for an episode in *Don Quixote* (q.v.).
Bibliography: Chamberlain, A. S. 1966. Early mental hospitals in Spain. *Am. J. Psych.* 123:143-49.

SEXUALITY. Many ancient civilizations have regarded expressions of sexuality more indulgently than later societies. In India, Greece, and the Roman empire, erotic trends and deviations were accepted and often encouraged and cultivated. With the advent of Christianity erotic behavior was discouraged and chastity became a virtue. Mental disorders and sexual excesses or perversions were linked to each other. When supernatural intervention was considered an aetiological factor in mental illness, the devil was believed to have had access to his victims, especially women, through sexual seduction. The *Malleus Maleficarum* (q.v.), the witch hunters manual, contains detailed descriptions of sexual pathology. It confirmed and encouraged the medieval belief that sex was sinful and injurious to mental health and that women were often in league with the devil to satisfy their lust. Even when these extreme points of view no longer prevailed, the concept of "love melancholy" as a pathological entity remained. In the eighteenth century the theory of "uterine furor" was fashionable. In the nineteenth century the interest in sexual matters was camouflaged: pseudoscientific works, with the more scabrous passages written in Latin, abounded. Sexual excesses, masturbation (q.v.), and such like were directly linked to insanity. Castration of males and females was an accepted method of therapy. The twentieth century has fared no better. Sigmund Freud (q.v.) continued the trend, encouraged by the work of Richard von Krafft-Ebing (q.v.), and his followers at the slightest excuse have scrutinized sexuality and declare mental health dependent on it.

Bibliography: Money, J., and Musaph, H., eds. 1977. *Handbook of sexology.*

SHAFTESBURY, ANTHONY ASHLEY COOPER, 7TH EARL OF

(1801-1885). English reformer and philanthropist. His extreme Protestantism originated from the naive beliefs of his mother's housekeeper, the only person to show him any kindness in his early life. His father neglected him and he, himself, described his mother as a fiend. When he was seven years old, he was sent to a harsh private school. At the age of twenty-six he became a member of Parliament, and as such he successfully agitated for a special committee to inquire into the public and private provisions for the care of the mentally ill. This resulted in changes in the law in 1845. He was chairman of the Commissioners in Lunacy (q.v.) and was the first president of the Mental After-Care Association (q.v.). He also was responsible for a number of Parliamentary Acts regulating working conditions in factories and banning the employment of women and children under the age of thirteen in the mines. His philanthropy, however, did not prevent him from hating almost all the prominent people who did not share his beliefs. He is commemorated by 'Ezos,' the statue in Piccadilly Circus, London.

Bibliography: Battiscombe, G. 1974. *Shaftesbury: a biography of the seventh earl, 1801-1885.*

SHAH DAULA.

A Muslim saint traditionally associated with insanity. Until the middle of the nineteenth century, in villages in the Punjab, poor families would offer their sons to him through the Muslim priest, or maulvi, who would fit them with iron caps that restricted the growth of the skull. Thus, they grew up with small heads and damaged brains and were called *Shah Daula ke Chuhe,* or mice of Shah Daula. They lived in association with holy mendicants. Their begging was profitable because, according to

superstition, those who refused them money would have mentally retarded children born to their families.
Bibliography: Mehta, Ved. 1972. *Daddyji.*

SHAKERS. Popular name for members of the United Society of Believers in Christ's Second Appearing. The sect originated from a Quaker (q.v.) revival in England in 1747. The name is derived from the trembling produced by religious fervor. The movement, which encouraged a rigid way of life, was begun in Manchester, England, in 1747 by James and Jane Wardley but it was Ann Lee, known as Mother Ann, who took the lead in its affairs and set out for America in 1774. A few Shakers still survive in the United States. In England a new group was started by Mary Anne Girling in the 1850s. This group practiced communal living in the New Forest but disbanded after the death of their leader.
Bibliography: Andrews, E. D. 1953. *The people called Shakers.*

SHAKESPEARE, WILLIAM (1564-1616). English dramatist. His plays contain several hundred passages of interest to psychiatry. His knowledge of abnormal psychology reflects the views of his contemporaries, but his acute sense of observation and mastery of language bring into focus essential features with an economy of words that vividly sharpens details. Many have conjectured where he acquired medical knowledge and have pointed to his son-in-law, Dr. John Hall (q.v.). It is almost certain that he was acquainted with *A Treatise of Melancholie* (q.v.) by Timothy Bright (q.v.), which would have given him more than a basic knowledge of sixteenth-century psychiatry.
See also AARON, EDMUND, HAMLET, IAGO, and LADY MACBETH.
Bibliography: Simpson, R. R.. 1959. *Shakespeare and medicine.*

SHAMANS. Members of primitive tribes who claim to have special powers of healing or curing illness through their links with the spirit world. They have great powers of suggestion, can induce states of trance in themselves and in others, and often indulge in behavior that would be considered abnormal in a more advanced culture. For example, some of them are transvestites, others homosexuals. Shamans have existed from the earliest times to the present day throughout the world.
Bibliography: Eliade, M. 1964. *Shamanism.*

SHAW, GEORGE BERNARD (1856-1950). Author and critic born in Dublin, Ireland. His home life was very unsettled and eccentric. His mother, a woman unbound by conventions, was twenty years younger than his father. The children were left in the care of the servants and spent their days in the basement kitchen. Shaw hated the servants, who often would strike him. His nurse took him to public houses in the slums. He never forgot how miserable his "devil of a childhood" had been and how he had been neglected by his mother. He did well at school, although he hated it. His impertinence caused one of his teachers to call him "the Devil incarnate." Later in life he described himself as "a disagreable little beast." He was an unorthodox man, often at variance with conventions. His difficulties with spelling caused him to invent an alphabet based on phonetic principles. He introduced his plays with challenging prefaces that were often as long as the play itself. His progressive ideas frequently were too advanced for the society of his time, and his belief in the futility of punishment and revenge was not universally accepted. He wrote "to punish is to injure." His dominating idea was the advancement of Socialism (he was a member of the Fabian Society). He was a nonsmoker, a teetotaller, a vegetarian, and, in general, a denier of physical pleasure. Women meant little to him. He saw a link between ugliness of environment and health. In his play *On the Rocks* he introduced a ghost from the future who runs a hospital in Wales in which the patients heal themselves by thought alone. The ghost claims that "bodily diseases are produced by half-used minds; for it is the mind that makes the body. . . ." — a psychosomatic approach taken to extremes. Shaw wrote over fifty plays, a number of novels, and critical articles on art, music, and drama. In 1925 he won the Nobel Prize for literature.

Bibliography: Brown, E. 1970. *George Bernard Shaw.*
Ervine, St. J. 1956. *Bernard Shaw: his life, work, and friends.*

SHAW, LEMUEL (1781-1861). An American jurist elected chief justice of the Massachusetts Supreme Court. He introduced the concept of irresistible impulse for cases in which crimes had been committed by individuals with diminished responsibility. It was the first serious attempt to reverse the harsh legal measures dealing with pathological mental states and criminal acts.

Bibliography: Weihofen, H. 1933. *Insanity as a defense in criminal law.*

SHAW, PETER (1694-1763). An English physician. Although he was aware of the influence of the emotions on physical complaints, he did not treat emotional disorders with the standard elixirs, pills, cordials, and powders of his time. His patients were advised to relieve depression through exercise, cheerful conversation, and the wise use of wine. He once prescribed oranges steeped in sherry for a hysterical (*see* HYSTERIA) patient. He believed that many diseases could be cured by pleasant expectations and that physical remedies brought about a cure because the patient believed in them, rather than because of their ingredients. He felt that a physician could kill or cure a patient by denying him hope or promising a better future and claimed that the first target of the physician was the imagination (q.v.) of the patient.

Bibliography: Hunter, R., and Macalpine, I. 1963. *Three hundred years of psychiatry.*

SHELDON, WILLIAM H. (1899-1977). An American psychologist. In the 1920s he correlated various psychoses (*see* PSYCHOSIS) with body types. He

used the term "ectomorphs" to describe very thin individuals who, according to him, appeared to be more prone to schizophrenia (q.v.) than "endomorphs," whom he described as fatter and more likely to develop manic-depressive psychoses (q.v.).
Bibliography: Sheldon, W. H. 1940. *Varieties of human physique.*

SHELLEY, PERCY BYSSHE (1792-1822). English poet and prose writer. His impetuous and passionate temperament were apparent even in his student days at Eton, where he vigorously opposed fagging. His temper was uncontrollable and he would fly into fits of rage, which earned for him the nickname of "Mad Shelley." At Eton his fellow students organized a "Shelley baiting society," the sole aim of which was to hunt him out and annoy him as much as possible. On his part, he experimented with gun powder, causing violent explosions, blowing up his desk in the classroom, and setting fire to trees and, on one occasion, killing the headmaster's pigs. At Oxford University, he became notorious for his anarchistic ideas and for the incredible untidiness of his room. He was expelled when he and his friend, Thomas Jefferson Hogg, published a pamphlet on atheism. His runaway marriage to Harriet Westbrook (1795-1816), a sixteen-year-old girl, was unhappy, and in 1814 Shelley left England for France with Mary Godwin (1797-1851). Harriet committed suicide (q.v.) in 1816, and he was denied legal custody of his two children. In 1818 he left England permanently. He suffered from illusions and visual hallucinations (q.v.). During one of these he believed that he could see his dead child arising from the sea, clapping his hands in joy. Eventually, rejected by English society, he isolated himself from the world and lived in Italy, putting into practice his theories of free love. He died on the sea when the small boat in which he was sailing foundered in a storm. His beautiful lyrics and his prose writings reflect the stirring political events of his time as well as his capacity for self-dramatization, self-pity, and self-deception.
Bibliography: Tomalin, C. 1980. *Shelley and his world.*

SHELL SHOCK. A term first used during World War I. The condition was believed to be an entirely new phenomenon and it was attributed to various causes, including separated synapses, punch form haemorrhages, or other damage to the cerebral centers, caused by the explosion of shells or bombs at close quarters. Only a small group of workers recognized it as a hysterical (*see* HYSTERIA) condition. Organic theories were abandoned eventually, and patients were treated by psychological methods. Its investigation and management aroused interest in psychopathology and led to the foundation of numerous hospitals and institutes for neuroses (*see* NEUROSIS) following the war.
Bibliography: Culpin, M. 1920. *Psychoneuroses of war and peace.*

SHEPPARD AND ENOCH PRATT HOSPITAL. A private mental hospital in Baltimore, Maryland. It was founded in 1853 by Moses Sheppard, a businessman and a member of the Religious Society of Friends. It was a progressive hospital from its beginnings; patients were treated with courtesy, consideration, and respect. Its founder considered every detail and even provided for chicken and ice cream to be served to patients twice a week. Donations by the Ford Foundation permitted extensive improvements in the building and its grounds. Harry Stack Sullivan (q.v.) was among the famous psychiatrists who worked there.

Bibliography: Forbush, Bliss. 1971. *The Sheppard and Enoch Pratt Hospital (1853-1970): a history.*

SHERRINGTON, CHARLES SCOTT (1857-1952). A British neurophysiologist. His early neurological studies on degeneration of spinal tracts were followed by research on reflex activity. In his book *Integrative Action of the Nervous System* (1906), he introduced the term and concept of "integrative action" in regard to the nervous system. *Man on His Nature* (1940), his last book, is a philosophical study of dualism. In 1932 he was awarded the Nobel Prize for his work on neural activity.

Bibliography: Eccles, J. C., and Gibson, W. C. 1979. *Sherrington: his life and thought.*

SHIP OF FOOLS. A painting by Hieronymus Bosch (q.v.) portrays a group of mad people, including a monk and a friar, enjoying worldly pleasures. Signs of madness are abundantly depicted in all the details of the picture, which is filled with symbols representing human folly. It was inspired by Sebastian Brant's (q.v.) *Narrenschiff* (q.v.).

Bibliography: Philip, L. B. 1956. *Hieronymus Bosch.*

SHIRLEY, LAWRENCE EARL FERRERS (1720-1760). An English nobleman. In a fit of temper he shot and killed his steward. The House of Lords tried him for murder, but, according to the law of the time, he was not allowed counsel. In pleading his own case he offered a plea of diminished responsibility (q.v.) because of insanity. His arguments were so well presented that it was decided that he could not be insane, and he was condemned to death.

Bibliography: 1900. *The dictionary of national biography.*

SHOLINGHUR. A small Indian town in the district of North Arcot, India. It has a famous shrine (q.v.) that is believed to have been visited by various legendary figures of ancient India, who wished to appease powerful divinities. Psychiatric patients visit the temple and stay within its precincts for several days. Their diet (q.v.) is restricted, no intoxicants are allowed, and they must circle the statue of the deity a hundred and eight times in the morning and evening on empty stomachs. If the god appears in their dreams (q.v.), they are considered cured.

Bibliography: Somasundaram, O. 1973. Religious treatment of mental illness in Tamil Nadu. *Indian J. Psychiat.* 15: 38-48.

SHORTHES HALL HOSPITAL. A school for mentally defective children in the West Riding of England. The site of its main building has a long history connected with a farm existing there in the thirteenth century. The term "shorthes" is derived from an old Norse word meaning "young plantation." The present building was originally a mansion, erected around 1791.

SHRINES. In the past, because illness in general, particularly mental illness, has been attributed to supernatural causes, supernatural intervention has been sought in treatment. Shrines dedicated to pagan and Christian divinities, saints, or holy men have had a long history of miraculous cures and are still the destination of many pilgrimages. In the Western world one of the most famous shrines for the mentally ill is that of Saint Dymphna (q.v.) in Belgium. *See also* TEMPLES.

Bibliography: Zilboorg, G. 1941. *A history of medical psychology.*

SHURPU. A Babylonian textbook similar to the *Maqlú* (q.v.) and divided into nine tablets. In it, psychopathic (*see* PSYCHOPATHY) behavior, obsessive-compulsive states, phobias (q.v.), and other neurotic disorders are described and somewhat classified.

Bibliography: Sigerist, H. E. 1951. *A history of medicine.* Vol. 1.

SIBERIAN TONIC. A herbal tonic for nervous children found in Russian folk medicine. It consists of an infusion of camomile flowers, marshmallow (q.v.) roots, licorice root, couch grass, and oats.

Bibliography: Kourennoff, P. M., and St. George, G. 1970. *Russian folk medicine.*

SICARD, JEAN ATHANASE (1872-1929). A French physician. His many contributions to neurology (q.v.) include the study of the cephalorhachidian fluid, the introduction of alcohol injections for trigeminal neuralgia, injections of sera for intracranial therapy, and milk injections for the treatment of migraine (q.v.).

Bibliography: Haymaker, W., and Schiller, F. 1970. *The founders of neurology.* 2d. ed.

SICK SOCIETY. Many ancient philosophers, including Cato the Elder (234-149 B.C.) and Aristotle (q.v.), have asserted that a whole community can have a sick collective mind and show collective symptoms. Robert Burton (q.v.) wrote that "kingdoms, provinces and politic bodies are likewise sensible and subject to this [melancholy] disease" and added that where one

sees general disorder, poverty, rebellions, or idleness "that kingdom, that country, must needs be discontent, melancholy, hath a sick body, and need be reformed."
Bibliography: Burton, R. 1621. *The anatomy of melancholy.*

SIDDAL, ELIZABETH ELEONOR (?–1862). English milliner's assistant and wife of Dante Gabriel Rossetti (q.v.). She modeled for all the members of the Pre-Raphaelite Brotherhood and learned to write poetry and to paint. She was consumptive and often depressed. She committed suicide (q.v.) with an overdose of laudanum (q.v.) a year after giving birth to a stillborn child. Her husband was so affected by her death that he enclosed the only complete manuscript of his poems in her coffin. Seven years later they were exhumed and published.
Bibliography: Gaunt, W. 1942. *The Pre-Raphaelite tragedy.*

SIDIS, BORIS (1867–1923). A Russian-born psychiatrist who practiced in the United States. He qualified in medicine at Harvard University and later became interested in psychology due to the influence of William James (q.v.). He popularized French psychopathology in the United States and inspired a psychological approach to insanity with his first book *The Psychology of Suggestion* (1899). His research on the emotional factors causing abnormal reactions, especially from the point of view of motivation, led to attempts to explain the subconscious (q.v.). He held numerous positions, wrote extensively, and was editor of two journals of psychiatry.
Bibliography: Sidis, B. 1916. *The causation and treatment of psychopathic diseases.*

SIGERIST, HENRY ERNEST (1891–1957). A French-born medical historian. In 1932 he emigrated to the United States and became the director of the Institute for the History of Medicine at the Johns Hopkins University. In 1947 he again emigrated and settled in Switzerland. He traveled widely, studying the medical and social systems of the countries he visited. Of his numerous books, *A History of Medicine* covers much of the history of psychiatry although it is made of only two of the eight volumes that the author originally had planned.
Bibliography: Sigerist, H. 1951–1961. *A history of medicine.* 2 vols.

SIGHELE, SCIPIO (1868–1913). An Italian psychologist and pupil of Cesare Lombroso (q.v.). Sighele stressed the importance of the irrational ele-

ments in the human mind that lead to abnormal behavior. He wrote on mass phenomena, the psychiatric aspects of criminology, and social psychology.
Bibliography: Sighele, S. 1891. *La folla delinquente.*

SIGIBALDUS. A ninth-century bishop of Metz. He founded two monasteries (q.v.) in Metz in which the monks undertook the care of the sick, including the mentally ill.
Bibliography: Walsh, J. J. 1920. *Medieval medicine.*

SIGMUND FREUD GESELLSCHAFT. An association founded in 1968 with the support of the Austrian government, which supplied funds for the restoration of the Vienna residence of Sigmund Freud (q.v.). The residence has been transformed into a center of study and research in psychoanalysis (q.v.). The formation of the association was inspired by American psychoanalysts. Freud's Vienna house was opened to the public in 1971.
Bibliography: Hacker, F. J. 1972. Freud [letter]. *Psychiatric News* 7: 2.

SIGURD I (1089?-1130). A king of Norway known as "the Crusader." He was said to have become insane, and the Norse sagas describe his extreme anxiety, swings of mood, hallucinations (q.v.), and delusions (q.v.). At times during his derangement he was violent and had to be restrained by his men.
Bibliography: Retterstøl, N. 1975. Scandinavia. In *World history of psychiatry*, ed. J. G. Howells.

SILLY. In old English, a term used to indicate someone innocent and happy. It was derived from the German *selig*, meaning "blessed." As an innocent is easily deceived, the term came to indicate someone who was gullible or foolish.
Bibliography: 1978. *Brewer's dictionary of phrase and fable.*

SILVA, JOSÉ ASUNCIÓN (1865–1896). A Columbian poet and founder of modernism in Latin America. A dominant mother and an excessive attachment to his sister shaped his early life. Some of his poetry vividly describes the symptoms of his constant depression and the futility of the physical treatment offered by his doctor. His autobiographical novel *Sobremesa* repeatedly cites the characteristics of his illness and lingers on descriptions of medical consultations and treatment. He was critical of the emphasis given to taxonomy, classification, and diagnosis in psychiatry,

rather than treatment. He committed suicide (q.v.) by shooting himself through the heart.
Bibliography: Rico, E. 1964. *La depresion melancholica en la vida, en la obra y en la muerte de José Assunción Silva.*

SILVANI. In Roman mythology (q.v.), spirits of the wood. They were believed to cause mental illness in humans.
Bibliography: Hammond, N. G. L., and Scullard, H. H. 1973. *The Oxford classical dictionary.*

SILVATICUS (SILVATICO), GIAMBATTISTA (1550–1621). An Italian physician and medical writer. He was one of the first to discuss feigned illness in a work published in 1595, entitled *De Lis qui Morbum Simulant Deprehendensis'.*

SILVER. A precious metal. In astrology (q.v.), metals were associated with the planets (q.v.), and silver was associated with the moon (q.v.). As the moon was believed to influence the onset of epilepsy (q.v.), it was thought that silver could be used in its treatment. Frequently it was used in the form of silver nitrate, which was first prepared by Geber, an Arab alchemist, in A.D. 800. This practice persisted until the nineteenth century.
Bibliography: Whitwell, J. R. 1936. *Historical notes on psychiatry.*

SIMEON STYLITES, SAINT (c.387– 459). A Christian ascetic (q.v.). For nine years he lived in a small cell in a Syrian monastery. He then went to Antioch and lived on a seventy-foot high pillar. He remained there for thirty years, preaching to the crowds and attracting many imitators. He is said to have died of an untreated ulcer.
Bibliography: Attwater, D. 1965. *The Penguin dictionary of saints.*

SIMMEL, ERNST (1882–1942). A German physician and pioneer of psychosomatic medicine (q.v.). He believed that repressed ideas and fantasies were responsible for hysterical (*see* HYSTERIA) states with somatic symptoms. He opened a psychoanalytic sanatorium near Berlin in the 1920s. He is remembered for his valuable studies of war neuroses (*see* NEUROSIS).
Bibliography: Alexander, F. G., and Selesnick, S. T. 1966. *The history of psychiatry.*

SIMON, HERMANN (1867–1947). A German psychiatrist and the major supporter of work therapy for the mentally ill. For many years he was superintendent of the mental hospitals of Warstein and then of Gütersloh, where he introduced his methods of active treatment. His successes generated interest in other countries, especially in the Netherlands and Switzerland.

The "Gütersloher system" was widely employed, although some believed that it led to regimentation.

Bibliography: Simon, H. 1929. *Die aktivere Krankenbehandlung in der Irrenanstalt.*

SIMON, THEODORE (1873–1961). A French psychologist and psychiatrist. After graduating from medical school he formed a lasting association with Alfred Binet (q.v.), which led to joint research in the laboratory of physiological psychology at the Sorbonne. Simon became head of the asylum of La Seine Inferieur. In 1905, in collaboration with Binet, he devised a scale for the measurement of intelligence. The project was a result of work connected with the organization of special classes for retarded children in public schools. The scale, composed of thirty items arranged in order of increasing difficulty, was later modified to correlate age and intelligence in normal children. The test, known as the Binet-Simon scale (q.v.), became widely used throughout the world.

Bibliography: Binet, A., and Simon, T. 1911. *Le mesure du dévelopment de l'intelligence chez les jeunes enfants.*

SIROCCO (*or* SCIROCCO). A dry, dusty, violent wind (q.v.) originating in Algiers. Passing over the sea, it becomes humid before reaching Southern Italy. It was believed to be one of the causes of insanity in Italians.

Bibliography: Esquirol, J. E. D. 1845. Reprint. 1965. *Mental maladies: a treatise on insanity.*

SITWELL, EDITH (1887–1964). An English poet and critic. She had an unhappy childhood: her father was difficult and eccentric, and her mother, who had little interest in her husband or her children, was given to outbursts of wild rage. Sitwell found some warmth in the company of servants and governesses, and even in the company of the peacock kept in the grounds of her parents' house. She stated: "I was unpopular with my parents from the moment of my birth and throughout my childhood and youth." Perhaps as compensation for childhood neglect, she became eccentric in her dress and attitudes and in turn was fascinated by eccentrics whom she wrote about in a book entitled *English Eccentrics* (1933). Her autobiography was published soon after her death.

Bibliography: Sitwell, E. 1965. *Taken care of.*

SIXTUS V (1521–1590). An Italian pope, the son of a washerwoman. A meek man before becoming pope, he became a thunderous ruler overnight when given the papacy. He suffered from severe headaches whenever he

was upset and was given to violent outbursts of anger. After the Spanish ambassador had delivered a provocative speech in his presence, his agitation was so great that he became delirious and died of a stroke in a few days.
Bibliography: Gontard, F. 1959. *The popes.*

SJÖBRING, HENRIK (1879–1956). A Swedish psychiatrist extremely influential in clinical teaching. The central theme of his work dealt with the problem of individual psychology in psychiatry. He emphasized the need to consider the personality as a pathogenic factor and regarded differential psychology as governed by general psychology. The study of personality, according to him, should be undertaken from the points of subjective experience and cause and effect.
Bibliography: Essen-Möller, E. 1980. The psychology and psychiatry of Henrik Sjöbring (1879-1956). *Psychol. Medicine.* 10: 201-10.

SKAE, DAVID (1814–1873). A British physician. In 1846 he became physician superintendent to the Edinburgh Lunatic Asylum (q.v.). He lectured on insanity and devised a classification of mental diseases based on the underlying physical disorders. He defined insanity as a disease of the brain affecting the mind. He believed that many mental disorders and neurotic (*see* NEUROSIS) conditions, including severe depression and suicidal (*see* SUICIDE) wishes, were due to masturbation (q.v.). He also was interested in the legal implications of insanity and wrote a book entitled *Legal Relations on Insanity* (1861).
Bibliography: Skae, D. 1863. *The classification of the various forms of insanity on a rational and practical basis.*

SKELTON, JOHN (1460–1529). An English poet, rector of Diss, Norfolk, and tutor to Henry VIII of England. His poetry was forceful, satirical, and often outrageous and improper. He hated Cardinal Wolsey (q.v.), who refused him advancement. It is said that Skelton was the first to use the word "bedlam" (q.v.) as an insult. It appeared in a venomous poem against the cardinal, whom he called the "butcher's dog." He wrote:

"Such a mad bedleme
For to rule this realm."

Bibliography: Edwards, H. L. R. 1949. *Skelton: the life and times of an early Tudor poet.*

SKETCHES IN BEDLAM. The title of an anonymous book published in London in 1823. It gave an history of Bethlem Royal Hospital (q.v.), describing contemporary conditions there and listing its rules and regulations.

The book also contained 140 case histories of named patients, including Margaret Nicholson (q.v.) and James Hadfield (q.v.). The latter had been committed to Bethlem after attempting to kill George III (q.v.).
Bibliography: Hunter, R., and Macalpine, I. 1963. *Three hundred years of psychiatry.*

SKIN DISORDERS. Jean Esquirol (q.v.) believed that the disappearance of a cutaneous affection might cause insanity. Treatment consisted in recalling the disorder.
Bibliography: Esquirol, J. E. D. 1845. Reprint. 1965. *Mental Maladies: a treatise on insanity.*

SKOPTSY. A Russian religious sect. Its followers believe that salvation is achieved through mortification of the flesh by castration. They have their reproductive organs removed, and, in addition, women often have their breasts cut off. Their appearance is one of poor general health, flabby, bloated, and slow in movement. While they await the second coming of Christ, their major occupation is limited to the trade of money changing.
Bibliography: Hinsie, L. E., and Campbell, R. J. 1960. *Psychiatric dictionary.*

SKULLCAP. *Scutellaria galericulata*, a plant usually found in damp places. It is also called "Mad-dog weed" as it was believed to be efficacious in cases of rabies. It was considered a powerful sedative as well as the supreme remedy in cases of insanity, epilepsy (q.v.), and delirium tremens (q.v.).
Bibliography: de Bairacli Levy, L. 1974. *The illustrated herbal handbook.*

SLEEP DEPRIVATION. A form of torture for people accused of criminal offences. It was introduced in the second half of the sixteenth century by the Italian criminologist Ippolito de Marsiliis. He considered it most efficacious for obstinate prisoners.
Bibliography: de Capraris, E. 1971. Considerazioni critiche su di un documento medico-legale: le perizie sulla pazzia di T. Campanella. *Minerva medica.* 62: 3200-209.

SLEEP TREATMENT. Prolonged sleep has been used as a form of therapy in certain psychiatric and physical disorders since antiquity. The Egyptians, the Greeks and the Romans practiced incubation (q.v.). During the eighteenth and nineteenth centuries, sleep was often recommended for melancholia (q.v.). Later, sleep was induced in excited patients by dosing them with bromides (q.v.). In the 1920s Jakob Klaesi (q.v.) introduced prolonged narcosis for the treatment of schizophrenia (q.v.). Under this treatment patients were kept asleep for several days by the use of drugs (q.v.). Russian workers have now developed a method to induce and maintain sleep by applying low voltage current to the sleep centers of the brain. The technique is known as "electro-narcosis."
Bibliography: Henderson, D. K., and Gillespie, R. D. 1940. *A text-book of psychiatry.*

SLOANE, SIR HANS (1660-1753). A British physician and botanist, the first in his profession to be made a baronet. He was one of the founders of the Royal Society (q.v.), and his 50,000 books, numerous manuscripts, and various collections became the basis of the British Museum. His practice in London was very fashionable and he enjoyed a high reputation. In 1721 he edited the fourth edition of the London Pharmacopoeia. Among his works, *Natural History of Jamaica* (1696) contains passages demonstrating his awareness of psychosomatic disorders. He also established the botanical garden at Chelsea.

Bibliography: de Beer, R. 1953. *Sir Hans Sloane.*

SLOUGH OF DESPOND. An expression derived from the *Pilgrim's Progress* by John Bunyan (q.v.), where it is a deep bog encountered by Christian on his way to the Wicket Gate. It has come to mean a fit or period, of deep depression.

Bibliography: 1978. *Brewer's dictionary of phrase and fable.*

SMALL, WILLIAM STANTON (1870-1943). An American psychologist and pupil of Granville Stanley Hall (q.v.). His experiments in animal psychology are remembered for his introduction of the maze as a test of performance in rats. He used as his model the diagram of the famous Maze (q.v.) at Hampton Court (q.v.).

Bibliography: Small, W. S. 1901. Experimental study of the mental processes of the rat. II. *Am. J. Psychol.* 12: 203-32.

SMALLPOX. In the nineteenth century some physicians believed that insanity could be cured by inoculating patients with smallpox. Jean Esquirol (q.v.) expressed his scepticism of this method, although suppurations in general were believed to be beneficial in cases of mental disorders.

Bibliography: Esquirol, J.E.D. 1845. Reprint. 1965. *Mental maladies: a treatise on insanity.*

SMARAGDUS. Any green stone such as the emerald (q.v.) or jasper (q.v.). They were thought by Aristotle (q.v.) and Galen (q.v.) to ward off epilepsy (q.v.) if hung round the neck or carried in the hand. In France during the Middle Ages (q.v.), an emerald ring was thought to achieve the same end, as well as fortifying the memory (q.v.) and making its wearer less prone to lust.

See also PRECIOUS STONES.

Bibliography: Whitwell, J. R. 1936. *Historical notes on psychiatry.*

SMART, CHRISTOPHER (1722-1771). An English poet best known for his *Song of David* (1763) in which he praised King David. According to tradition, the initial verses that developed into this work were first written on the walls of a cell in Bethlem Royal Hospital (q.v.), where the author was a patient. However, Edward G. O'Donoghue, the historian of Bethlem,

could find no trace of his admission and suggested that he may have been treated in a private asylum (q.v.) paid for by his friends. O'Donoghue also suggested that his writings that appear to be descriptive of Bethlem were the results of his casual visits there. Smart was morbidly religious and often composed verse on his knees. His abnormal behavior, debts, and addiction to hartshorn were a source of comment by his contemporaries. He was an alcoholic (*see* ALCOHOLISM) and in continuous conflict with his family, who probably drove him to drink. He died in a debtors' prison.
Bibliography: Devlin, C. 1967. *Poor Kit Smart.*

SMITH, SIR GRAFTON ELLIOT (1871-1937). An Australian neurologist, renowned for his studies of the evolution of the nervous system, as well as for anthropological and ethnological research undertaken in Egypt.
Bibliography: Haymaker, W., and Schiller, F. 1970. *The founders of neurology* 2d. ed.

SMITH, HELENE. The pseudonym of Catharine Müller (q.v.).

SMITH, JOSEPH (1805-1844). The American founder of the Church of Jesus Christ of the Latter-Day Saints. He believed that angels had appeared to him in a vision and had told him where to find a hidden gospel written on golden plates. He claimed the *Book of Mormon* was written with help received during these visions. Smith founded a colony, which he governed despotically. His views, especially his espousal of polygamy, incited ridicule, hostility, and, at times, violence, but the sect attracted many followers. He was arrested on charges of treason and conspiracy and was murdered by a mob that broke into Carthage jail.
Bibliography: Brodie, F. M. 1945. *No man knows my history: the life of Joseph Smith, the Mormon prophet.*

SMITH PAPYRUS. The Edwin Smith papyrus, probably written in Egypt (q.v.) in 1550 B.C., contains the first known description of the brain, and indicates that it was believed to be the center of mental functions. The papyrus was purchased in Luxor, in 1862 by the American Egyptologist, Edwin Smith (1822-1906). In 1949 it was presented to the New York Academy of Medicine.
Bibliography: Sigerist, H. E. 1951. *A history of medicine.* Vol. 1.

SMOLLET, TOBIAS (1721-1771). A Scottish physician and writer. Although he wrote a number of novels, he wrote only one book of medical interest, *An Essay on the External Use of Water* (1752). In it he asserted that the water of Bath, then a fashionable spa, had no special curative value. He also disapproved of subjecting manic patients to cold baths (q.v.), often followed by solitary confinement in a dark church in the hopes of a mirac-

ulous cure. His novel *Sir Launcelot Greaves* (1760-1762) contains passages based on *A Treatise on Madness* (q.v.) by William Battie (q.v.) and on *Remarks on Dr. Battie's Treatise on Madness* by John Monro (q.v.). Smollet had reviewed extensively both books for the *British Magazine*. He was the first to conceive of and practice the serialization of books in periodicals.
Bibliography: Brander, L.R.M. 1951. *Smollett.*

SNAKE, SYMBOL, OF. In ancient cultures the snake was worshipped as a symbol of the principle of life because its shape was associated with the male genitals. Living snakes were frequently carried in ritual processions during special festivities, and representations of them can be found in various temples.
Bibliography: Cooper, J. C. 1978. *An illustrated encyclopaedia of traditional symbols.*

SNAKEROOT. *See* RAUWOLFIA SERPENTINA.

SNEEZING. Because in medieval times mental disorders were attributed to possession (q.v.) by the devil, who could be swallowed or inhaled into the body, it was believed that he could be expelled by sneezing. Sneezing powders, therefore, were used as a form of treatment and continued to be used even in the nineteenth century. Jean Esquirol (q.v.), for example, reported using them to such a point that they caused profuse bleeding at the nose. He claimed to have treated and cured a young man by these means.
Bibliography: Esquirol, J.E.D. 1845. Reprint. 1965. *Mental Maladies: a treatise on insanity.*

SNELL, HANNAH (1723-1792). Englishwoman born in Worcester. Her father was a dyer. In order to enlist in the fleet to search for her faithless husband, she became a transvestite and assumed the name of James Gray and masculine dress. She served for nearly five years and was wounded in both legs at the battle of Pondicherry, for which she received a pension. On her return from India she resumed female dress and took to the stage, where she sang military songs in marine uniform. She married three times. She showed such signs of abnormal behavior that in her old age she was admitted to Bethlem Royal Hospital (q.v.), where she died. Her adventures were published in a book by Robert Walker entitled *The Female Soldier,* which appeared in London in 1750.
Bibliography: Acroyd, P. 1979. *Dressing up, transvestism and drag: the history of an obsession.*

SNIADECKI, JEDRZEJ (1768-1838). A Polish physician, medical writer, and social worker. He was particularly interested in the psychophysiological aspects of man. He believed that certain character disorders, for example what he called "defects of heart," were the cause of antisocial actions and

social maladaptation. According to him, they were partially hereditary and partially due to the environmental stresses brought about by civilized society. He set forth his views in a volume entitled *Theory of Organic Beings*, which was published in 1822.
Bibliography: Bilikiewicz, T., and Lyskanowski, M. 1975. Poland. *World history of psychiatry*, ed. J. G. Howells.

SNOW. Slang expression for cocaine (q.v.). It originates from the resemblance of cocaine powder to snow in its whiteness and consistency. The expression "snow bird" refers to a cocaine addict.
Bibliography: Hinsie, L. E., and Campbell, R. J. 1960. *Psychiatric dictionary*.

SOAP. The ingestion of soap was believed to be beneficial in nervous ailments. Simon A. Tissot (q.v.) was among those who prescribed it.
Bibliography: Foucault, M. 1967. *Madness and civilization*.

SOBER HOUSE. The name proposed by Benjamin Rush (q.v.) for an asylum for alcoholics (*see* ALCOHOLISM). He published plans for it in 1810, but the project was never put into practice.
Bibliography: Hunter, R., and Macalpine, I. 1963. *Three hundred years of psychiatry*.

SOCIAL BREAKDOWN SYNDROME. The expression was first used in a volume published in 1962 by the American Public Health Association. It was entitled *Mental Disorders: A Guide to Control Methods* and was produced under the leadership of Ernest Gruenberg.
Bibliography: 1966. *Milbank Memorial Fund Quarterly*. 44 (1966): No.1, pt 2.

SOCIAL PSYCHOLOGY. The study of the relationships between one individual and another, between an individual and a group, and between one group and another. The concept of social psychology originated in the middle of the nineteenth century, but the term itself, was not used until the first decade of the twentieth century. In 1908 William McDougall (q.v.) wrote a book entitled *Social Psychology*, which gave this branch of psychology the status of a separate field.
Bibliography: Watson, R.I. 1963. *The great psychologists*.

SOCIETÀ FRENIATRICA ITALIANA. A national professional psychiatric organization founded by Andrew Verga (1811-1895) in Italy in 1873.

It branched out from an older institution that had embraced all fields of science in Italy.
Bibliography: Mora, G. 1975. Italy. In *World history of psychiatry*, ed. J. G. Howells.

SOCIETÀ FRENOPATICA ITALIANA. A psychiatric organization founded in Italy in 1861 by Biagio Miraglia (q.v.).
Bibliography: Mora, G. 1975. Italy. In *World history of psychiatry*, ed. J. G. Howells.

SOCIÉTÉ DE PSYCHOLOGIE DE PARIS. An organization for French professional workers in the field of mental disorders. Founded in 1885. Jean Charcot (q.v.) was its first president.
Bibliography: Zilboorg, G. 1941. *A history of medical psychology.*

SOCIÉTÉ MÉDICO-PSYCHOLOGIQUE. The first professional body of French psychiatrists. It was founded in 1852 under the presidency of Guillaume Ferrus (q.v.).
Bibliography: Zilboorg, G. 1941. *A history of medical psychology.*

SOCIÉTÉ PHRÉNIATRIQUE BELGE. The first Belgian psychiatric association. It was founded in 1869.
Bibliography: Zilboorg, G. 1941. *A history of medical psychology.*

SOCIETIES, PSYCHIATRIC. The nineteenth century saw the creation of the first professional associations devoted to psychiatry. The first was the Association of Medical Asylums and Officers of Hospitals for the Insane (q.v.) founded in England, in 1841. It was followed in 1844 by the Association of Medical Superintendents of American Institutions for the Insane (q.v.). By the end of the century many associations were flourishing in Europe. Most of them published their own journals, providing a forum for the discussion and propagation of new ideas in psychiatry.
Bibliography: Zilboorg, G. 1941. *A history of medical psychology.*

SOCIETY FOR FREE PSYCHOANALYSIS. A society founded by Alfred Adler (q.v.) in 1911. It consisted of ten former members of the Viennese Psychoanalytic Society who had disagreed with the insular attitudes of Sigmund Freud's (q.v.) close associates. A year later it changed its name to The Society for Individual Psychology.
Bibliography: Alexander, F. G., and Selesnick, S. T. 1966. *The history of psychiatry.*

SOCIETY FOR IMPROVING THE CONDITION OF THE INSANE. An organization founded in 1842 in London by Sir Alexander Morison (q.v.) and Anthony Ashley Cooper, Earl of Shaftesbury (q.v.). One of its leaders was Dr. Daniel Hack Tuke (q.v.). The aim of the society was the propagation of knowledge into the causes and treatment of insanity. They hoped to

achieve this by encouraging research and improving the professional training of those who worked in asylums or were in direct contact with mental patients. The most distinguished psychiatrists of the time supported the organization and read papers at its meetings.
Bibliography: Leigh, D. 1961. *The historical development of British psychiatry.*

SOCIETY FOR THE PREVENTION OF CRUELTY TO CHILDREN, THE.
A body founded in New York City in 1871. Its creation followed the court case of Mary Ellen, a girl who had been maltreated by her adoptive parents. As there were no legal grounds or organizations, she was removed from their care by the intervention of the Society for the Prevention of Cruelty to Animals on the grounds that as a member of the animal kingdom her case could be dealt with by legislation referring to cruelty to animals.
Bibliography: Fontana, V. J. 1971. *The maltreated child: the maltreatment syndrome in children.*

SOCIETY FOR PSYCHICAL RESEARCH.
A society founded in England in 1882 by William Barnet, a physicist, the Reverend Stainton Moses, Frederich W. Myers (q.v.) and Henry Sidgwick (1838-1900) a philosopher. The society investigated such parapsychological phenomena as communication with spirits, clairvoyance (q.v.), and foreknowledge of future events.
Bibliography: Ellenberger, H. F. 1970. *The discovery of the unconscious.*

SOCIETY OF HARMONY.
A training school for mesmerism (q.v.) founded in the 1780s in France. It was almost a secret organization for the propagation of the teaching of Franz Mesmer (q.v.) among laymen. Branches were opened in several cities. The society published Mesmer's views in the form of aphorisms, but, despite its efforts, it failed to gain the support of the medical profession.
Bibliography: Tinterow, M. M. 1970. *Foundations of hypnosis: from Mesmer to Freud.*

SOCIETY OF NEUROPATHOLOGY AND PSYCHIATRY.
The first Russian psychiatric association. It was founded in 1892 in Kazan. Its first president was Vladimir Bekhterev (q.v.).
Bibliography: Wortis, J., and Galach'yan, A. G. 1975. Union of Soviet Socialist Republics. In *World history of psychiatry*, ed. J. G. Howells.

SOCRATES (469-399 B.C.).
A Greek philosopher, the son of a sculptor and a midwife. His untidy person was a familiar sight in the market places where he spent his time arguing, condemning, cross-questioning, and in-

structing. His philosophy was not committed to writing but was transmitted verbally. His search for truth made him unpopular, and he was often the target of vicious attacks or of ridicule, as in the "Clouds" of Aristophanes (q.v.). His pupil Plato (q.v.) illustrated his methods of teaching and his views in his dialogues. At times Socrates claimed he was inspired through what he called "voices," suggesting that he may have suffered from auditory hallucinations (q.v.). He was prone to trancelike states. He required his students to work through their problems with his guidance, believing that happiness could be obtained by correct reasoning and self-knowledge. Ancient Greek writers described him as a strong man whose devotion to duty never flinched. His outstanding intellect was matched by a keen sense of humor. Later in life he married Xanthippe (q.v.) whose bad temper, scolding, and quarreling became proverbial. He was accused of impiety and of corrupting young people and was condemned to death by a majority of six votes among about five hundred. Surrounded by his disciples, he drank hemlock in prison and died. The scene was described by Plato in his "Phaedo".
Bibliography: Taylor, A. E. 1933. *Socrates*.

SOEMMERRING, SAMUEL THOMAS VON (1755-1830). A German anatomist who devised the present classification of cranial nerves. He believed in the Aristotelian principle that the "sensorium commune" (q.v.), was to be found in the fluid of the brain ventricles. His belief was opposed by Johann Wolfgang von Goethe (q.v.) and Immanuel Kant (q.v.), who asserted that the soul cannot be localized. Soemmerring's famous treatise, *Organ of the Soul* (1796) was dedicated to Kant. His anatomical illustrations were so accurate and clear that they continued to be used for a long time after his death.
Bibliography: Clark, E., and Dewhurst, K. 1972. *Illustrated history of brain functions*.

SOFT. An expression used to refer to someone who is not intelligent. It is derived from the belief that the brains of mentally retarded individuals show signs of softening.
Bibliography: 1978. *Brewer's dictionary of phrase and fable*.

SOLANO. A moist, easterly wind prevalent in Spain that was believed to cause insanity.
Bibliography: Esquirol, J.E.D. 1845. Reprint. 1965. *Mental maladies: a treatise on insanity*.

SOLIDISM. The name given to a school of philosophy flourishing in Greece during the third century B.C. Its followers based their study of man on anatomy and carefully considered the structure of the brain, which they

related to intelligence and to certain mental disorders. Herophilus of Chalcedon (q.v.) and Erasistratus (q.v.) were prominent solidists.
Bibliography: Zilboorg, G. 1941. *A history of medical psychology.*

SOLOMON (c.1015-933 B.C.). The third king of Israel. He was credited with great wisdom and was believed to be able to communicate with the spirit world. It was said that he could cast out demons from the body of the possessed (*see* POSSESSION) through chanting incantations (q.v.) composed by him and handed down to his followers.
Bibliography: Thieberger, F. 1947. *King Solomon.*

SOMA. A powerful liquid prescribed for many illnesses. It is also a hallucinogen. According to tradition, it was the drink from which Indra, an ancient Indian divinity, derived his strength. Mentioned in the Veda (q.v.), it is believed to have been abstracted from the mushroom fly agaric (q.v.).
Bibliography: Thomson, W.R.A. 1978. *Healing plants.*

SOMDEJ CHAOPHYA HOSPITAL. A mental hospital in Thailand (q.v.). Built in 1912 near Klong Sarn, it was the first hospital in the country to provide treatment for the mentally ill in addition to custodial care. Its first chief was an Englishman, Dr. Cathew, who introduced many innovations. One of his innovations was a peaceful orchard as a rest place for the patients. It still remains a salient feature of the hospital.
Bibliography: Sangsingkeo, P. 1975. Thailand. In *World history of psychiatry,* ed.
    J. G. Howells.

SOMERS, WILLIAM. A young boy from Nottingham, England. In 1595 he was the subject of a public service of exorcism (q.v.) by John Darrell (q.v.). Somers had feigned illness to escape from the musician to whom he had been apprenticed and was believed to be possessed (*see* POSSESSION). He encouraged this belief by producing the required symptoms. He eventually was discovered and confessed his fraud.
Bibliography: Robbins, R. H. 1970. *The encyclopedia of witchcraft and demonology.*

SOMMER, ROBERT (1864-1937). A German psychiatrist. He disagreed with the premises of Emil Kraepelin (q.v.) in his study of dementia praecox (q.v.) and argued that patients who recovered could not be included in this category.
Bibliography: Zilboorg, G. 1941. *A history of medical psychology.*

SOMNAMBULISM. The term, derived from Latin, literally means "sleepwalking," but it has been used frequently to denote trance states. As a phenomenon it has been known since antiquity when it was linked to the power of divination (q.v.). In the Middle Ages (q.v.) it was regarded as a

supernatural state during which saintly people were believed to be in conversation with Christ or the angels and sinners were believed to be under the influence of the devil. "Artificial somnambulism" (induced trance, or hypnosis) [see HYPNOTISM] was discovered by Armand-Marie-Jacques Puységur (q.v.) in 1784 and became a form of therapy. It brought the study of the unconscious (q.v.) into the realm of psychology and gave rise to widespread interest in somnambulistic phenomena. Alexandre Bertrand (q.v.) wrote a *Traité du Somnambulisme* in 1823, and Aubin Gauthier, a pious Catholic, wrote *Histoire de Somnambulisme* in 1842. He concluded his work with a devout letter to Pope Gregory XVI. Somnambulism became a common theme in literature and opera (q.v.), for example *La Sonnambula* (q.v.). With the death of Jean Charcot (q.v.) studies on hypnosis declined, and "artifical somnambulism" was replaced primarily by psychoanalysis (q.v.).
Bibliography: Chertok, L., and de Saussure, R. 1979. *The therapeutic revolution: from Mesmer to Freud.*

SONNAMBULA, LA. An opera by Vincenzo Bellini (1801-1835). It revolves round the psychosomatic manifestations of somnambulism (q.v.). Amina, the heroine, walks and talks in her sleep. During one of these episodes, she walks into the bedroom of the lord of the castle and arouses the suspicious jealousy (q.v.) of her lover, who later forgives her when he, himself, sees her dangerously sleepwalking on the roof of the mill where she lives.
Bibliography: Harewood, ed. 1969. *Kobbe's complete opera book.*

SONNENSTEIN ASYLUM. A German mental hospital near Dresden. It was opened in 1811 after the building had been converted from its former function as a castle. The army of Napoleon I (q.v.) took possession of it in 1813, turned out the patients and the staff, and used it as barracks. It was later reconstructed and continued to serve as an asylum (q.v.). It was the first in Germany to practice the new ideas of humane treatment of the mentally ill. Daniel Paul Schreber (q.v.) was a patient there.
Bibliography: Macalpine, I., and Hunter, R., eds. 1955. *Schreber: memoirs of my nervous illness.*

SOPHISTS. Greek philosophers who had no fixed abode, but traveled and taught in various places. They believed that true knowledge was impossible because sensory life was subjective, and man was "the measure of all things." Nevertheless, they focused attention on man and on his faculties, rather than on material objects that were external to him.
Bibliography: Sinclair, T. A. 1952. *History of Greek political thought.*

SOPHOCLES (c.496-405 B.C.). A Greek tragic poet and dramatist. His ambition to become an actor was thwarted by his weak voice. As a compensation he wrote plays. He represented the insane as living in an unreal world, rather than a supernatural one. His drama *Ajax* contains one of the earliest descriptions of madness. His greatest masterpiece was *Oedipus Tyrannus* from which Sigmund Freud (q.v.) derived the concept and the term "Oedipus complex" (*see* OEDIPUS). Sophocles' son Iophon brought him before the phratores (a court of the person) as unable to manage his own affairs. He defended himself with the famous words "If I am Sophocles, I am not beside myself: if I am beside myself I am not Sophocles," and supported his case by reciting passages from his drama *Oedipus Colonus*. The case was dismissed.

Bibliography: Bates, W. N. 1964. *Sophocles.*

SORANUS (A.D. 93-138). A Greek physician born in Ephesus. He studied in Alexandria and Rome. His writings on medical subjects earned him a reputation of soundness and enlightenment. Although he belonged to the Methodist school of thought, Soranus did not adhere rigidly to any doctrine but followed whatever methods seemed appropriate and reliable. In the treatment of the mentally ill, he opposed harsh measures and advised kind treatment in healthy and comfortable conditions, including light, warm rooms. Mental anguish was to be relieved by conversation and the use of drugs (q.v.) was to be limited. He used psychological measures although he remained convinced that mental disorders had an organic aetiology. In his treatise *Acute Diseases*, he classified and described satyriasis, phrenitis (q.v.), and lethargy (q.v.). In another volume, entitled *Chronic Diseases*, he listed sleep disorders, chronic headaches, epilepsy (q.v.), mania (q.v.), and melancholia (q.v.). He also devoted a chapter to pathics (q.v.), or effeminate men. His works were translated into Latin by Caelius Aurelianus (q.v.).

Bibliography: Sigerist, H. E. 1933. *Great doctors.*

SORBONNE LABORATORY. The first psychology laboratory established in France in 1889. Henri Beaunis (q.v.) and Alfred Binet (q.v.) were in charge of its work on experimental and comparative psychology.

Bibliography: Flugel, J. C. 1945. *A hundred years of psychology.*

SOUL MURDER. A term first used by Johann August Strindberg (q.v.) in 1887 in an article on *Rosmersholm* by Henrik Ibsen (q.v.). Strindberg defined it as depriving a person of his basic reason to live. The term was also used by Daniel Paul Schreber (q.v.) in his *Memoirs* (1903) and by Ibsen in his play, *John Gabriel Borkman* (1896). The manipulation of Daniel Paul Schreber by his father is a classic example of the concept.

Bibliography: Shengold, L. 1974. Soul murder: a review. *Int. J. Psychoanal. Psychoth.* 3: 366-73.

SOUQUES, ACHILLE ALEXANDER (1860-1944). A French neurologist. In 1921 he presented the results of his studies which demonstrated the importance of encephalitis lethargica as an aetiological factor in Parkinsonism.
Bibliography: McHenry, L. C. 1969. *Garrison's history of neurology.*

SOURED MILK. Compresses of soured milk and clay applied to the head are used in Russian folk medicine as treatment for insomnia. In Siberia, rye bread soaked in cucumber juice is added, and the treatment is repeated three times a day.
Bibliography: Kourennoff, P. M., and St. George, G. 1970. *Russian folk medicine.*

SOURY, JULES (1842-1915). The French author of an impressive volume on the history of the theories and doctrines associated with the nervous system. The son of a glass blower and an illiterate woman whom he adored all his life, Soury reached adolescence practically uneducated. Later in life, he developed a voracious hunger for knowledge and became well versed in philosophy, comparative religion, and anthropology. He wrote expertly on all of these subjects. The work he saw at the Salpêtrière (q.v.) so inspired him that he abandoned his previous interests and, although not qualified in medicine, dedicated himself to lecturing on the nervous system at the Sorbonne. His students were many and he soon became the talk of the Parisian literary world. He had an eccentric personality: was overly attached to his mother and unable to be separated from her even for short periods; he had the same exclusive attachment to his bed and his table and could not sleep in strange beds or eat at strange tables. With the exception of his mother, he hated women and was intolerant of Jews. He is said to have been ugly, but no record of his features remains because his only portrait was buried with his mother.
Bibliography: Soury, J. 1899. *Le système nerveux central, structure et fonctions: histoire critique des théories et des doctrines.*

SOUTH CAROLINA STATE ASYLUM. An American institution opened in Columbia, South Carolina, in 1828, following the 1821 act authorizing "the erection of a suitable building for a lunatic asylum and a school for the deaf and dumb." This act followed public clamor about lack of provisions for the mentally ill and the deaf and dumb. After the project had been

studied, it became apparent that the two categories of inmates could not coexist, and the institution was devoted to "idiots, lunatics and epileptics."
Bibliography: Deutsch, A. 1949. *The mentally ill in America.*

SOUTH SEA BUBBLE. The term by which speculation involving the South Sea Company, founded in 1711, became known after its financial collapse. Richard Hale (q.v.) affirmed that many people had become insane as a result of its collapse. According to him, those who had gained large fortunes became deranged in greater number than those who were ruined.
Bibliography: Hunter, R., and Macalpine, I. 1963. *Three hundred years of psychiatry.*

SOUTHARD, ELMER ERNEST (1876-1920). An American psychiatrist, neuropathologist, and pioneer in social psychiatry. His work on shell shock (q.v.) gave prominence to military psychiatry. He was the first director of the Boston Psychopathic Hospital, where he came in contact with many sociological problems that aroused his interest in psychiatric social work. In 1922 in collaboration with Mary C. Jarrett (q.v.) he wrote a book entitled *The Kingdom of Evils* in which they presented 100 case histories. It is considered the first textbook in psychiatric social work. His other major field of study was neurosyphilis, its diagnosis and treatment.
Bibliography: Southard, E. E., and Jarrett, M. C. 1922. Reprint. 1973. *The kingdom of evils.*

SOUTHCOTT, JOANNA (1750-1814). An English domestic servant, born of farming parents. Her adherence to Methodism (q.v.) degenerated into fanaticism. She claimed supernatural gifts and believed herself to be the woman of Revelation 12, who would bring forth to the world a second Christ. Her pregnancy was a product of hysteria (q.v.) and came to nothing. She died of a brain tumor, leaving behind a large following, a number of books of prophecy and interpretation of the Bible (q.v.), and a sealed box to be opened in time of national crisis in the presence of an assembly of bishops. One bishop was present when the box was opened in 1927, and the contents declared of no interest.
Bibliography: Balleine, G. R. 1956. *Past finding out.*

SOUTHEY, ROBERT (1774-1843). An English poet and writer. After his father's death, he was brought up by an uncle. He was expelled from Westminster School for writing an essay against flogging. As he grew older, his political views became a constant source of trouble. He became a friend of Samuel Coleridge (q.v.) while they were at Oxford University and married Coleridge's wife's sister in 1795. She became insane and died in that condition in 1837. Although he remarried in 1839, her death profoundly affected him, and he tried to submerge his depression in excessive work. He died of softening of the brain. His numerous works are little read, but his story for children, *The Three Bears*, remains popular.

Bibliography: Carnall, G. 1960. *Robert Southey and his age.*

SPAIN. Because of the influence of Arab medicine, Spain had an early tradition of enlightened treatment of the insane, who were regarded as ill and in need of care, rather than possessed (*see* POSSESSION) by devils. The first psychiatric hospital in Europe was founded in 1409 at Valencia (q.v.) and was followed by others; Zaragoza in 1425, Seville and Valladolid in 1436, Palma de Mallorca in 1456, and Toledo in 1480 (qq.v.). It was through Spanish initiative that mental hospitals were built in such overseas dominions as Mexico, San Hipólito (q.v.), and Peru, Saint Andrew's Hospital.

Bibliography: Chamberlain, A. S. 1966. Early mental hospitals in Spain. *Am. J. Psychiat.* 123: 143-49.

SPALDING, DOUGLAS (c.1840-1877). A British psychologist who is regarded as the "father of ethology." He applied experimental methods to animal psychology and studied the extent to which animal behavior can be explained by instinct or experience gained from observation of other animals. In 1873 he noticed that chicks hatched in an incubator tend to follow the first moving object they see.

Bibliography: Spalding, D. A. 1873. Reprint. 1954. Instinct with original observations on young animals. *Brit. J. Animal Behav.* 2:2-11.

SPANISH FLY. *Lytta vesicatoria*, an insect, also known as a blister beetle. It gives off an evil-smelling liquid capable of producing blisters on the human skin. Dried and powdered, it was used in the treatment of mental disorders and migraine; blisters were allowed to develop and then were opened to let out the poisonous humor (q.v.). Timothy Bright (q.v.) mentioned these insects in his *Treatise of Melancholie* (q.v.). When the production of blisters was a form of treatment of the insane, Spanish flies were used to make cantharidin, an irritant. Dickens (q.v.) mentions Spanish flies in *Martin Chuzzlewit* where Mrs. Gamp, the midwife, says "Spanish flies is the only thing to draw the nonsense out of you, and if anybody wanted to do you a kindness, they'd clap a blister of 'em on y'r head. . . ."

SPATZ, HUGO (1888-1969). A German neurologist. His work in the field of neuropathology included a morphological classification of the encephalitides, investigations of cerebral atrophies, and brain trauma.

Bibliography: Haymaker, W., and Schiller, F. 1970. *The founders of neurology.* 2d.ed.

SPEARMAN, CHARLES EDWARD (1863-1945). A British psychologist. He laid the foundation of factor analysis in psychology. His early interest had been in the field of philosophy, but at the age of thirty-four he turned to psychology and studied under Wilhelm Wundt (q.v.) at Leipzig. In 1907 Spearman became chief of a small psychological department at University College in London. His lecture tours of the United States made Americans familiar with British psychology. His studies on mental abilities demonstrated that the factor of general ability, which he called the G factor (q.v.), is common to all performances. To this, he later added other special factors. His other major contribution was in the field of statistics.

See also G FACTOR, O FACTOR, P FACTOR, and W FACTOR.

Bibliography: Spearman, C. E. 1927. *The abilities of man: their nature and measurement*.

SPEEDY SYNTHETIC METHOD. A method of treating neurasthenia (q.v.) introduced in Communist China in 1958, by Li Hsin-t'ien and Li Ch'ung-p'ei, two leading psychiatrists working in Peking. It involves the combined use of physical and psychological measures, including drugs (q.v.), acupuncture, electric shock, sleep therapy, psychotherapy (q.v.), and psychosocial therapy. Patients receive lectures on the nature of the treatment and are urged to feel optimistic about recovery, which is regarded as an accomplishment contributing to politically desirable qualities. A powerful element in the treatment program is the psychiatrist's confidence that a cure can result from his and his patients' efforts. A patient, rather than a psychiatrist, leads the group activities.

Bibliography: Chin, R., and Chin, A. S. 1969. *Psychological research in Communist China: 1949-1966*.

SPENCER, HERBERT (1820-1903). An English philosopher. He had originally trained to be a railway engineer, but turned to journalism and for a time was editor of *The Economist*. He was the founder of evolutionary philosophy in which evolution is regarded as the all-pervading principle. He claimed to have anticipated the doctrines of Charles Darwin (q.v.), and Darwin, in turn, claimed that he could not understand Spencer's philosophy. Spencer's emphasis on heredity and racial factors was exaggerated at the expense of social and environmental factors. In 1855 he wrote *Principles of Psychology* in which he discussed evolutionary doctrines applied to human development. In the 1860s he wrote several volumes that formed what he called a *System of Synthetic Philosophy*, covering metaphysics, biology, psychology, sociology and ethics. He also wrote on education and the functions of government. His works greatly influenced contemporary philosophy and psychology not only in Europe and the United States but also in Japan and India.

Bibliography: Spencer, H. 1904. *Autobiography*.

SPENCER, STANLEY (1891-1959). An English painter. His attitudes to marriage, love and sexuality were unconventional, and he depicted them in his work, often mixing sexuality with religious themes. After divorcing his first wife, Hilda Carline, he married Patricia Preece, but boasted that a few days after the marriage he was sleeping with both women because he felt that absolute sexual freedom was necessary to his art. As the three of them lived in the same village, their interactions never failed to amaze the local inhabitants. Spencer was given to writing extravagant poems on lavatory paper on the themes of sex and religion and to spreading vicious tales about his women. Patricia retaliated and then lived in such seclusion that the neighbors believed she was a witch. At the other end of the village he spent his days painting and dramatizing his own saintliness.

Bibliography: Collis, L. 1972. *A private view of Stanley Spencer*.

SPENSER, EDMUND (c.1552-1599). An English epic poet, the son of a London gentleman tradesman. As his secretary he followed Lord Grey de Wilton (1536-1593) to Ireland in 1850 to crush a rebellion. His time there was miserable, and he was often near to despair. His allegorical "Despair" in *The Faerie Queene*, written over a number of years, offers a seductive encouragement to suicide (q.v.). In the second book of the same work he presents an allegory of the human body and mind, which he compared to a building called House of Alma. He explores the house and finds that the part corresponding to the brain is divided into three parts: the back, where an old man representing memory of the past lives, the middle part is occupied by judgment in the present, and the front houses "Phantastes," a sad figure, born under Saturn (q.v.), who represents an uncertain view of the future.

Bibliography: Judson, A. C. 1945. *The life of Edmund Spenser*.

SPIELMEYER, WALTER (1879-1935). A German neurologist. During World War I, he studied injuries to peripheral nerves and published a text-book on the histopathology of the nervous system in 1922. He also investigated cerebral disorders linked to vascular disturbances. In collaboration with Oskar Vogt (q.v.), he described a type of amaurotic familial idiocy (q.v.) now known as Spielmeyer-Vogt's disease.

Bibliography: Haymaker, W., and Schiller, F. 1970. *The founders of neurology*. 2d. ed.

SPILLER, WILLIAM GIBSON (1863-1940). An American neurologist and pioneer in the field of vascular occlusions of the brain stem. He introduced cordotomy in the treatment of persistent pain. It is said that he carried specimens in his pockets and would produce a spinal cord from their depths

to underline a point or start a discussion. The works of William Shakespeare (q.v.) were the favorite source of quotations for his lectures.
Bibliography: Haymaker, W., and Schiller, F. 1970. *The founders of neurology.* 2d.ed.

SPINAL PUNCTURE. A diagnostic technique devised by Heinrich Quincke (q.v.) in 1891. He first used it as a therapeutic measure in children with hydrocephalus but quickly realized its diagnostic possibilities.
Bibliography: Haymaker, W., and Schiller, F. 1970. *The founders of neurology.* 2d. ed.

SPINNING CHAIR. During the eighteenth and nineteenth centuries a number of machines were devised to produce some form of shock to the nervous system of mental patients. The spinning chair, in various forms, was introduced to subject the patient to rapid gyration. Violent patients were calmed down to the point of collapse by its motion. Among those who designed spinning chairs were Hermann Boerhaave (q.v.) and Benjamin Rush (q.v.). The unpleasant and often dangerous effects of this form of treatment were finally realized, and spinning chairs were relegated to psychiatric museums.
Bibliography: Roback, A. A. and Kierman, T. 1969. *Pictorial history of psychology and psychiatry.*

SPINOZA, BARUCH (BENEDICT) DE (1632-1677). A Dutch philosopher and theologian. His Jewish family had left Portugal because of religious persecution, but his views were no more acceptable to Jews than they were to Christians. At the age of twenty-four he was excommunicated by the synagogue. For a time he earned a living by grinding and polishing lenses. He was influenced by René Descartes (q.v.), but, unlike him, Spinoza believed that mind and body had a psychophysiolcgial parallelism and were not two radically separate entities. The body, according to him, experienced thoughts and desires through the mind. Man has no free will because he is limited by his passions. Spinoza believed that behavior was determined by the urge for self-preservation. His work *Ethica*, posthumously published in 1677, contains many discussions on psychological matters. He gave great importance to deductive and analytical reasoning. He died a victim of an occupational disease: glass dust, inhaled in his youth, destroyed his lungs.
Bibliography: Hampshire, S. 1951. *Spinoza.*

SPIRA, FRANCESCO (fl.1540). An Italian lawyer from Padua. He converted from Catholicism to Lutheranism, but in 1548 pressure from the pope broke his resolution, and he recanted. His feelings of guilt, heightened by the terrifying prospect that his soul was damned forever, precipitated a state of deep depression and suicidal impulses. His story was told in Italy as

testimony of God's displeasure with Protestant sects. In England it was used to demonstrate the treachery of the papists. Its true interpretation should be as the case history of an individual suffering from religious mania (q.v.).
Bibliography: O'Donoghue, E. G. 1914. *The story of Bethlehem Hospital.*

SPIRIT OF SKULL. A preparation made from wine and the moss from the skulls of unburied men who had died violent deaths. In the eighteenth century it was believed to be a potent remedy for convulsions, epilepsy (q.v.), vapors (q.v.) , and pains in the head. King Charles II of England was dosed with spirit of skull during his last illness. Paracelsus (q.v.) originated the compound, which, in his formula, required three human skulls that were then pulverized and mixed with a number of liquids.
Bibliography: Thompson, C.J.S. 1929. *Mystery and art of the apothecary.*

SPIRITUALISM. When used in philosophy, the term denotes a doctrine that affirms the spirit exists as distinct from the matter. In a different sense, the term is applied to a movement that originated in the United States in the mid-nineteenth century. Its interests are centered in psychical phenomena (q.v.), are nonreligious, and call for scientific investigation. Its advocates claim communication between the living and the spirits of the dead can be achieved through mediums (q.v.) or persons with special powers. Automatic writing, table rapping, and table turning are some of the manifestations purported to denote that contact with the spirit world has been achieved. Margaret Fox (q.v.) and her sisters are believed to be the originators of the movement, which, after sweeping America, spread to Europe.
Bibliography: Nelson, G. K. 1968. *Spiritualism and society.*

SPITTING. In some ancient cultures, including Greece and Rome, it was believed that epilepsy (q.v.) was due to possession (q.v.) by evil spirits and that people in close contact with epileptics could be contaminated. Spitting was believed to prevent contagion. Theophrastus (q.v.) and Pliny the Elder (q.v.) were among those who advised this precaution.
Bibliography: Temkin, O. 1971. *The falling sickness.*

SPITZ, RENÉ A. (1887-1974). An Austrian psychoanalyst who emigrated to the United States in the early 1940s. He was a student of Sigmund Freud (q.v.) and a pioneer in the application of psychoanalytic concepts in the field of child development. *Anaclitic Depression*, written in 1946, contains his theory of depression in institutionalized young children.
Bibliography: Spitz, R. A. 1946. *Anaclitic depression.*

SPITZKA, EDWARD CHARLES (1852-1914). An American psychiatrist and neurologist. He was an expert in forensic medicine and advised at the trial of Charles J. Guiteau (q.v.), the assassin of James Garfield (1831-1881),

twentieth president of the United States. He declared the accused insane. He wrote a famous textbook on insanity in which he accepted catatonia (q.v.) as a specific disorder, as suggested by Karl Kahlbaum (q.v.). He believed that progressive and inherited neurological deterioration was responsible for mental disorders, retardation, and abnormal behavior in general. The term "paranoia" (q.v.) to describe a specific psychosis (q.v.) was first used by him in 1883.
Bibliography: Spitzka, E.C. 1887. Reprint. 1973. *Insanity: its classification, diagnosis and treatment.*

SPLEEN. When personal characteristics and certain feelings were associated with particular organs, the spleen was considered the seat of anger and aggression. Some examples are found in Shakespeare's plays. Oliver Goldsmith (q.v.) in his work *The Citizen of the World, or, Letters from a Chinese Philosopher residing in London, to his friends in the East,* wrote: "When the men of this country are once turned thirty, they regularly retire every year at proper intervals to lie of the spleen. . . .In such disposition, unhappy is the foreigner who happens to cross them. . . .If they meet no foreigner, however, to fight with, they are, in such cases, generally content with beating each other." To suffer from the spleen was synonymous with feeling depressed, as melancholia (q.v.) was often attributed to bad humors (q.v.) in the spleen. Avicenna (q.v.) was among those physicians advocating this belief. In the eighteenth century most ill-defined psychosomatic disorders were called "the spleen."
Bibliography: Zilboorg, G. 1941. *A history of medical psychology.*

SPORUS. (1st century A.D.). A Greek youth loved by Nero (q.v.) who publicly "married" him. After Nero's death, he committed suicide (q.v.) rather than endure the shame of being exhibited on the stage in the role of a ravished maiden.
Bibliography: Fedden, H. R. 1938. *Suicide.*

SPRENGER, JOHANN JACOB (c.1436-1495). A Dominican monk and professor of theology in Cologne. According to him, witches (*see* WITCHCRAFT) caused disasters, plagues, and diseases of the soul. He was a fanatic witch-hunter and, with Heinrich Kraemer (q.v.), wrote the *Malleus Maleficarum* (q.v.), a book containing a great deal of sexual psychopathology and reflecting the unhealthy psychic state of its authors. In 1481 Innocent VIII (q.v.) appointed Sprenger inquisitor of the provinces of Mainz, Trèves, and Cologne. After the publication of the *Malleus* in 1487, his power and offices increased.
Bibliography: Hughes, P., ed. 1968. *Malleus maleficarum.*

SPURZHEIM, JOHANN KASPAR (1776-1832). A German physician and phrenologist. From 1800 to 1814 he worked with Franz Gall (q.v.) and

contributed to Gall's findings on brain localizations and anatomical structure. Later, he adapted Gall's teaching. His version of the new "science of the mind," or phrenology (q.v.), received greater acceptance because of his moralizing attitude and the emphasis he placed on its importance to society in general, rather than solely to criminology. He established a detailed topography of the skull, adopted a new terminology, probed into the field of psychiatry and strenuously defended phrenology from its many detractors.
Bibliography: Spurzheim, J. K. 1832. *Phrenology, or the doctrine of the mental phenomena.*

SPURZHEIM, KARL (1809-1872). An Austrian psychiatrist and the nephew of Johann Spurzheim (q.v.). He traveled through several European countries inspecting mental hospitals. He applied what he learned to his work in the institution at Ybbs (q.v.), where he was superintendent, and in the mental hospital of Vienna, which he later directed. He promoted more accurate legal reports on mental patients. A year before his death he became president of the German Association of Psychiatry and Neurology.
Bibliography: Mora, G. 1972. Anniversaries. *Am. J. Psychiat.* 129: 657.

STAËL, GERMAINE DE (1766-1817). A French-Swiss woman of letters famous for her literary salons. She was born in Switzerland as Anne Louise Germaine Necker. Her unhappy marriage to the Swedish ambassador to France, a man much older than her, ended in legal separation, and she had several love affairs. In 1803 her political views caused her exile from Paris and she traveled widely in Europe. Her novels *Delphine* (1802) and *Corinne* (1807) are perhaps the first modern feminist novels with a psychological slant. *Delphine* ends with the suicide (q.v.) of the heroine, the first "modern woman" of French literature; *Corinne* ends with the death by grief of an equally emancipated young woman. *Reflexions sur le Suicide*, written in 1810, is a condemnation of suicide, paradoxically written whilst she was very depressed. It refuted her earlier views in support of suicide, which she expressed in 1796 in an essay entitled *De l'Influence des Passions sur le Bonheur des Individus et des Nations*. In her *Reflexions sur le Suicide*, she wrote that the English were particularly prone to suicide because of their personalities, which she regarded as impetuous, and because of their excessive fear of criticism. She thought the French committed suicide for only practical reasons and positive misfortunes.
Bibliography: Herold, J. C. 1976. *Mistress to an age: life of Madame de Stäel.*

STAFFORD, RICHARD (1663-1703). An English writer of pamphlets, educated at Oxford University and the Middle Temple. He was an ardent Jacobite and ranted against the monarchy of William and Mary. In 1691 his abnormal behavior resulted in his admission to Bethlem Royal Hospital (q.v.), where he was imprisoned in a dark and evil-smelling cell for seven weeks. He continued to write violent and seditious pamphlets against William III even while in the hospital. These were taken out by his visitors, printed, and distributed among the people of London. This activity caused him to be closely guarded, and his visitors scrutinized. When he recovered, he promised that he would desist from writing against the king and accordingly turned his pen to composing sermons.

Bibliography: O'Donoghue, E. G. 1914. *The story of Bethlehem Hospital.*

STAHL, GEORG ERNST (1660-1734). A German physician. He taught anatomy and chemistry but maintained that these two subjects were insufficient to explain the behavior of man. Stahl's interest in human nature prompted his study of temperamental types. He used the classical concept of anima (q.v.) to explain human activities and held that the soul is the vital principle on which every organic development depends. This theory was called the doctrine of animism (q.v.) and was expounded in his book *Theoria Medica Vera* (1707). He realized the part played by emotions in mental and physical illness and emphasized the importance of taking account of the emotional life of the patient in his treatment. He believed that dreams (q.v.) could reflect abnormal bodily states by a kind of unconscious perception that he called "anima sensitiva" (q.v.). He is considered the last of the animists. His objection to the indiscriminate use of drugs (q.v.) in psychiatry greatly influenced Philippe Pinel (q.v.).

Bibliography: Cope, Z. 1957. *Sidelights on the history of medicine.*

STARK, KARL WILHELM (1787-1845). A German psychiatrist. Like many physicians of his time, he attempted a classification of mental disorders by arranging them into three classes: dysthenias, dysbulias, and dysnoesias. Each class then was subdivided into hyperform, a-form, and para-form. Under his method, various combinations were possible and multiplied the number of diseases without bringing any clarity to an already confused classification.

Bibliography: Zilboorg, G. 1941. *A history of medical psychology.*

STARK, WILLIAM (?-1813). A British architect. He designed the Glasgow Asylum for Lunatics (q.v.) which opened in 1814. Many of the ideas he incorporated into it, he gathered from the York Retreat (q.v.). He was the first architect to write on the construction of mental hospitals.

Bibliography: Stark, W. 1807. *Remarks on the construction of public hospitals for the cure of mental derangement.*

STARKE, AUGUST (1880-1954). A Dutch psychiatrist. He introduced psychoanalysis (q.v.) to the Netherlands and was one of the leaders of the Dutch Psychoanalytic Society. Because he believed that insanity was a result of faulty relationship between the individual and society, he stressed the

need to identify pathogenic factors in society. He emphasized the need for the study of comparative sociology.
Bibliography: Stam, F. C. 1975. The Netherlands. In *World history of psychiatry*, ed. J. G. Howells.

STARR, MOSES ALLEN (1854-1932). An American neurologist. He is remembered for his investigations of cerebral localization and for his studies of brain tumors. He was the author of several volumes, of a textbook on brain surgery in 1895 and an atlas of nerve cells in 1897.
Bibliography: McHenry, L. C. 1969. *Garrison's history of neurology.*

STARS, INFLUENCE OF. *See* PLANETS.

STATE CARE ACT. An American statute passed in 1890, following increasing popular pressure. It divided each state into hospital districts and expected each district to contain a state mental hospital. It further directed that all mental patients in almshouses should be transferred to state hospitals, which were to be supported by the state. Under the same act the term "asylum" was replaced with the term "hospital" and chronic and acute patients were no longer sent to separate institutions.
Bibliography: Deutsch, A. 1949. *The mentally ill in America.*

STATISTICAL METHODS. The serious application of statistical methods in psychiatric studies began in the nineteenth century with Jean Esquirol (q.v.). He was one of the first physicians to tabulate the aetiological factors of mental disorders. He kept a numerical list of the male and female patients at the Salpêtrière (q.v.), showing the factors that he considered responsible for their illness.
Bibliography: Esquirol, J.E.D. 1845. Reprint. 1965. *Mental maladies: a treatise on insanity.*

STATUTE DE PREROGATIVA REGIS. A statute of English law decreed by King Edward II in 1324. It made a distinction between lunatics (q.v.) and idiots (q.v.), and their estate is protected by special provisions.

STAUB, HUGO (1886-1942). A German lawyer. In collaboration with Franz Alexander (q.v.), he undertook the study of a series of individuals whose antisocial attitudes had brought them into conflict with the law. Staub and Alexander concluded that the subjects were motivated by unconscious antisocial factors that were acquired during the process of emotional maturation.
Bibliography: Alexander, F., and Staub, H. 1931. *The criminal, the judge and the public.*

STAVROGIN, NIKOLAI VSEVOLODOVICH. One of the most tormented and disturbed fictional characters in modern literature. He is the hero of *The Possessed* by Fyodor Dostoevsky (q.v.). Debauchery, crime, revolutionary activities, a meaningless marriage to a mentally retarded cripple, unsatisfactory love affairs, and a vain search for peace in religion culminate in his confession to a monk. His guilt at having violated a young girl, and having left her, frightened and confused, to hang herself so torments him that he finally commits suicide (q.v.) by hanging.

Bibliography: Dostoevsky, F. M. 1941. *The possessed*, trans. C. Garnett.

STEDMAN, CHARLES HARRISON (1805-1866). An American psychiatrist. He was interested in phrenology (q.v.) and in 1834 edited a translation of a book on brain anatomy by Johann Spurzheim (q.v.). In 1842, after a time in private practice, he was appointed superintendent of the Boston Lunatic Hospital (q.v.). Following his resignation from that post in 1851, he became involved in politics and served in the state senate and on the governor's council. He was one of the thirteen founders of the American Psychiatric Association (q.v.). After visiting the Boston Lunatic Hospital Charles Dickens (q.v.) warmly praised him in his *American Notes*.

Bibliography: Deutsch, A. 1949. *The mentally ill in America*.

STEELE, RICHARD (1672-1729). An Irish essayist and dramatist. He tried to present virtues and vices in their true light. In 1709 he founded *The Tatler* and in it described a visit to the "Collegiates of Moorfields," that is, Bethlem Royal Hospital (q.v.). There he said he found "five duchesses, three Earls, two Heathen Gods, an Emperor, a Prophet. . . ." These would-be dignitaries so impressed him that he vowed to discipline his mind and to guard himself against "the secret swelling of resentment," a passion that makes "such havock in the brain, and produces such disorder of imagination."

Bibliography: Whitwell, J. R. 1946. *Analecta psychiatrica*.

STEINBECK, JOHN ERNST (1902-1968). An American writer. After a sketchy education he tried a number of occupations before becoming a writer. Despite the feeling of powerful energy emanating from his books, he was often very depressed and given to psychosomatic disorders, which, in *Journal of a Novel: the East of Eden Letters* (1970) he described as "physical resentments against living." In the same book he stated: "I have no will to die but I can remember no time from earliest childhood until this morning when I would not have preferred never to have existed. . . . it is no longing for death, but a kind of hunger never to have lived." Many of his novels treat social problems with compassion, sensitivity, and passionate indignation. Of particular interest is *Of Mice and Men* (1937), the story of a mental defective written almost entirely as a dialogue. Steinbeck was the

victim of an anniversary reaction (q.v.). He found he was irritable and unable to write in the month of March. His mother suffered from the same reaction.
Bibliography: Fontenrose, J., ed. 1963. *John Steinbeck*.

STEINER, RUDOLPH (1861-1925). An Austrian social philosopher and founder of a mystical doctrine known as anthroposophy. He used the arts to educate and treat the mentally retarded. In 1919 in Stuttgart, Germany he established a center for child psychiatry that inspired many similar experiments in other parts of the world.
Bibliography: Steiner, R. 1925. *Mein Lebensgang*.

STEINTHAL, HAYIM (1823-1899). A German psychologist. His large literary output included contributions to mythology (q.v.), comparative religion, ethics, and logic. With his brother-in-law Moritz Lazarus (1824-1903), he developed the concept of group mind, which they defined as the integration of individual minds into a collective psyche that, in certain circumstances, functions as a unit. He and Lazarus are considered the founders of group psychology.
Bibliography: Roback, A. A. 1962. *History of psychology and psychiatry*.

STEKEL, WILHELM (1868-1940). An Austrian psychiatrist. He was a follower of Sigmund Freud (q.v.) and prominent member of the psychoanalytic group that met each Wednesday at Freud's house, although he later left the group. He believed that treatment of neurotic (*see* NEUROSIS) patients could be shortened by the active intervention of the therapist, who should sympathetically and intuitively understand the patient's repressed complexes and lead him toward self-awareness. In his books, including *The Interpretation of Dreams* (1912), *Peculiarites of Behaviour* (1922) and *Letters to a Mother* (1927), he emphasized sexual symbolism in all forms of behavior. He died by suicide (q.v.).
Bibliography: Stekel, W. 1950. *The autobiography of Wilhelm Stekel*, ed. E. A. Gutheil.

STENDHAL (1783-1842). The pseudonym of Marie Henri Beyle, a French writer. In his youth he entered the army, although his inclination was to write. He summarized his life in his own epitaph "He lived, wrote, loved." The followers of Sigmund Freud (q.v.) found their beliefs confirmed in many of his writings, for example, in his confession of incestuous love for his mother, who died when he was seven years old. He compensated for his feelings of inferiority, by becoming an arrogant and snobbish individual, who regarded life with condescending irony. His famous work *Le Rouge et le Noir* (1831) has been considered the first true psychological novel. It

concerns a man condemned to death for the murder of his mistress and raises many points of interest in the field of forensic psychiatry.
Bibliography: Richardson, J. 1974. *Stendhal.*

STENSEN, NIELS (1638-1686). A Danish anatomist and geologist, also known as Nicolaus Steno. After the death of his father, when he was six years old, he was brought up in the house of Jorgen Carstensen, a rich officer in the government administration. Although Stensen studied in Holland, most of his life was spent abroad, especially in Italy, where in 1675 he was ordained a priest in the Roman Catholic Church. He then gave up science and dedicated himself to missionary work, converting Lutherans to the Catholic faith by the thousands. In addition to anatomical discoveries, he was the first to approach the study of the brain scientifically rather than theoretically. His famous *Dissertation on the Anatomy of the Brain* was given in Paris in 1665.
Bibliography: Belloni, L. 1968. *Steno and brain research in the seventeenth century.*

STEPHANIE INSTITUTION. An asylum in Biedermannsdorf, Austria, for the education and welfare of feebleminded children. Named after the Crown Princess Stephanie, the institution opened in 1883. Its first director was Dr. Anton Antensteiner.
Bibliography: Kanner, L. 1964. *A history of the care and study of the mentally retarded.*

STEPHEN, JAMES KENNETH (1859-1892). An English poet. He was a sadist (*see* SADISM) a hater of women, and a homosexual (*see* HOMOSEXUALITY). He was the tutor of the duke of Clarence (1864-1892) at Cambridge University and was said to have seduced him. At one time it was rumoured that he was the notorious Jack the Ripper (q.v.).
Bibliography: Stephen, J. K. 1891. *Lapsus calami.*

STERILIZATION. A surgical procedure that leaves a person incapable of reproduction. In the early part of the twentieth century great emphasis was placed on the part that eugenics (q.v.) played in reducing the number of mentally retarded people. Sterilization of defectives was one of the measures advocated. In the United States, more than elsewhere, eugenic sterilizations were performed not only on mental defectives but also on psychotics, psychopaths, and criminals, especially if they were convicted of rape. The first sterilization law was enacted in 1907 by the state of Indiana. Although various modifications followed, by 1926, twenty-three American states had enacted sterilization laws. Canada followed with similar legislation in 1928. In Europe there was religious resistance to eugenic sterilization. Denmark, Finland, and some Swiss cantons, however, introduced statutes legalizing it.

STERN, LOUIS WILLIAM (1871-1938). A German psychologist. He studied in Berlin with Hermann Ebbinghaus (q.v.) and Carl Stumpf (q.v.). His major contributions were in the fields of differential and educational psychology but he also worked in psychophysics. In 1908, in cooperation with his wife, Clara Stern, he published a detailed study of behavior based on observation of his own three children. This was followed in 1914 by his book *Psychology of Early Childhood*. He devised the concept of "intelligence quotient." Stern was president of the German Psychological Society, but political events in Germany forced him to emigrate to the United States.
Bibliography: Stern, W. 1906-1924. *Person and thing: a plan for a philosophical world view*. 3 vols.

STERNE, LAURENCE (1713-1768). An English novelist and clergyman, born in Ireland. He disliked his mother and had a difficult adolescence. He was self-conscious, insecure, and paranoid (*see* PARANOIA). He was also consumptive, and it has been suggested that his constant amorousness was psychosomatic. His lecherous attention to a number of ladies was considered the cause of his wife's insanity. Sterne's doctor diagnosed syphilis (q.v.), as well as tuberculosis (q.v.), when he was dying, even though he claimed he had led an abstemious life for fifteen years. As a clergyman, his sermons were highly regarded, but his novel *Tristam Shandy* (1760-1768) was his greatest success. This eccentric, indecent, and overly sentimental work shows his mastery in handling satire, time, and consciousness, but was condemned by many of his contemporaries on grounds of immorality.
Bibliography: Thomson, D. 1972. *Wild excursion: the life and fiction of Laurence Sterne*.

STEVENSON, ROBERT LOUIS (1850-1894). A British writer, born in Edinburgh. His mother was tuberculotic, and it is probable that he acquired tuberculosis (q.v.) from her. Her constant ill health meant that his care was undertaken by a nanny, Alison Cunningham. Although he loved her, her austere Calvinistic beliefs implanted in him "an extreme terror of hell" that so terrorized him he often could not sleep. His father and his grandfather had been lighthouse builders, but his own love for engineering was thwarted by his ill health. After qualifying in law, he began to write and travel in search of a climate that would improve his health. In Paris he met an American lady, Fanny Osbourne (1840-1914), ten years his senior, separated from her husband, addicted to reading medical books, and a passion for invalids. She married him and took on the functions of nursing him in the same way as his nanny had done. Together they travelled the world in search of the sun. Despite his love of children, he avoided fathering a child for fear of transmitting his own poor health. He died in Samoa of cerebral thrombosis. Fanny suffered from spells of madness towards the end of her life. One of

his most psychologically interesting novels is *The Strange Case of Dr. Jekyll and Mr Hyde* (q.v.).
Bibliography: Calder, J. 1980. *R.L.S.: a life study.*

STEWART, DUGALD (1753-1828). A Scottish philosopher and pupil of Thomas Reid (q.v.) whose ideas he interpreted and popularized. His doctrines dominated American psychology, or philosophy of mind as it was then called, at a time when psychology was claiming the status of a discipline in its own right. Between 1792 and 1827 he wrote *Elements of Philosophy of the Human Mind.*
Bibliography: Boring, E. G. 1950. *A history of experimental psychology.*

STEWART INSTITUTION. The first institution for the feebleminded in Ireland. It was established in 1869 at Palmerston in Dublin.
Bibliography: Barr, M. W. 1904. *Mental defectives.*

STIGMATA. The term originally referred to the brands marking slaves and criminals in ancient Greece and Rome. It later came to mean wounds resembling those on Christ's body. Mystics believe that these wounds, appearing on certain individuals, have a supernatural origin. Others regard them as hysterical phenomena capable of rational interpretation. Saint Francis of Assisi (1182-1226) is one of the first persons known to have shown stigmata. Since then about three hundred cases have been recorded, usually involving women. One of the most recent cases was that of Therese Neumann (1898-1963). During the Inquisition (q.v.), those accused of witchcraft (q.v.) were said to have "stigmata diaboli," marks left on their bodies by the devil. In the nineteenth century the term "stigmata" acquired yet another meaning as it was applied to certain anatomical and physiological abnormalities said to confirm degeneracy in psychiatric patients. For instance, Benedict A. Morel (q.v.) believed that insanity was the result of hereditary weakness and could be detected by the "stigmata of degeneration."
Bibliography: Whitlock, F. A., and Hynes, J. V. 1978. Religious stigmatization: an historical and psychophysiological enquiry. *Psychol. Medicine.* 8: 185-202.

STILLER, BERTHOLD (1837-1922). A Hungarian physician. He described the presence of a floating tenth rib as indicative of a neurasthenic (*see* NEURASTHENIA) tendency. This anomaly is now known as the costal stigma, or, Stiller's sign.

STILLING, BENEDICT (1810-1879). A German surgeon, son of a Jewish wool merchant, who adopted the name Stilling in admiration for the writer Johann Heinrich Jung-Stilling (q.v.). He spent his time not occupied by his busy clinical practice on the study of the nervous system. He became interested in neurology following observations on what then was called "spinal irritation," a disorder of psychosomatic character. His descriptions and illustrations of the anatomy of the nervous system were published in giant-sized plates, folded a dozen times, and included in an encyclopedia of medicine and surgery. He gave the first description of the nuclei of nearly all the cranial nerves.

Bibliography: Haymaker, W., and Schiller, F. 1970. *The founders of neurology.* 2d. ed.

STIMULUS. A term introduced in the mid-eighteenth century by Robert Whytt (q.v.) while repeating an experiment first conducted in 1730 by Stephen Hales (1677-1761). The experiment was designed to elucidate reflex action. It demonstrated that a decapitated frog responded to pinching by retracting its legs but ceased to do so when its spinal cord was destroyed.

Bibliography: Watson, R. I. 1963. *The great psychologists.*

STOICISM. A school of practical philosophy founded in Greece by Zeno of Citium (q.v.) in the third century B.C. Stoics believed that happiness could be achieved by obeying the will of the Divinity, freeing oneself from the ties of passions and appetites, and avoiding tension. To them suffering was a matter of indifference and apathy; peace of mind would come with acceptance of the inevitable. They believed that those who found life uncongenial should commit suicide (q.v.). Seneca (q.v.) was a Stoic.

Bibliography: Wenley, M. 1925. *Stoicism and its influence.*

STOKE PARK HOSPITAL. The first certified institution for the mentally retarded in Britain. It was founded in 1909 by the clergyman Harold N. Burden (q.v.) and his wife. The original building, a manor, is mentioned in Domesday Book and was depicted on a dinner service of Wedgwood pottery made for Catherine the Great (q.v.) of Russia in 1774. The hospital became the nucleus of a group of institutions in the Bristol region that were later known as Stoke Park Colony. Many of the other hospital buildings in the group are also historically interesting and mentioned in various medieval records. The founders emphasized the rehabilitation of patients through domestic, agricultural, and industrial training. Physical treatment was also emphasized in the form of heliotherapy. Chapels and chaplains were appointed to all the hospitals in the group to provide spiritual care for the patients.

Bibliography: Jancar, J. 1969. *Sixty years of Stoke Park Hospital.*

STOMACH. Some ancient medical writers, for example Avicenna (q.v.), believed the stomach to be a possible seat of melancholia (q.v.). In more recent times, Philippe Pinel (q.v.) and François Broussais (q.v.) carefully considered the role of the stomach as a factor in mental disorders. Contem-

porary research has established that gastric disorders often have an emotional aetiology.
Bibliography: Wolf, S. J. 1965. *The stomach.*

STONECROP. *Sexum acre,* a succulent plant grown in coastal regions. In folk medicine, it was used in the treatment of epilepsy (q.v.), convulsions, nervous disorders, and hysteria (q.v.).
Bibliography: de Baïracli Levy, J. 1974. *The illustrated herbal handbook.*

STONE HOUSE. A building near Charing Cross in London. It was originally the home of a religious community that may have cared for the mentally ill. At some time before 1403, it became the property of Bethlem Royal Hospital (q.v.) and housed insane patients. According to John Stow (q.v.), the seventeenth-century chronicler, the patients were transferred from Stone House to Bethlem Royal Hospital because the king wanted them removed from the vicinity of his residence. Although it is not known which king ordered the transfer, taking into consideration Bethlem's first recorded admission of mental patients in 1377, it might have been Edward III or Richard II. Stone House was converted into tenements, possibly housing Richard II's falconer and his birds. In 1644 the original lease expired, and the governors of Bethlem had to bring a lawsuit to recover their property as its ownership was questioned. They won the suit and the ground of the Stone House remained in their possession until 1830, when it was leased to the government in exchange for another estate in Piccadilly.
Bibliography: O'Donoghue, E. G. 1914. *The story of Bethlehem Hospital.*

STONE OF MADNESS. In medieval times it was popularly believed that a stone in the head was the cause of insanity. It was thought that if the stone could be removed, a cure was assured. Quacks and charlatans performed bogus operations on the credulous. Hieronymus Bosch (q.v.) depicted this subject in his painting *The Cure of Folly* cleverly contrasting the deceit and ignorance apparent in the human figures with a serene and orderly landscape.
Bibliography: Baldass, L. von. 1960. *Hieronymus Bosch.*

STORRING, GUSTAV (1860–1947). A German psychologist and pupil of Wilhelm Wundt (q.v.) in Leipzig. He worked primarily in the field of psychopathology, but his inclinations were for philosophical rather than practical applications.
Bibliography: Boring, E. G. 1950. *A history of experimental psychology.*

STOUT, GEORGE FREDERICK (1860–1944). An English psychologist. He was the author of a number of textbooks on psychology. He studied the nature of consciousness, especially unconscious psychical dispositions, the relation between mind and matter, and man's knowledge of the material

aspects of the world. He popularized the term "conation" to indicate the fact and experience of striving.
Bibliography: Stout, G. F. 1903. *Groundwork of psychology.*

STOW, JOHN (c.1525–1605). An English chronicler and antiquary. In his *Survey of London* (1580) he gave a detailed description of the city and the customs then prevalent. He also listed provisions for the physically and mentally ill and referred to six songs of Tom O' Bedlam" (q.v.). These songs were later preserved by Bishop Thomas Percy (1729–1811) in *Percy's Reliques of Ancient English Poetry* (q.v.) published in 1765.
Bibliography: 1965. Stow's survey of London. *Everyman's Library No.589.*

STOWE, HARRIET BEECHER (1811–1896). An American novelist. She was brought up in a strictly Congregational household and later married a clergyman. She was a whimsical, absentminded, and often preoccupied woman. Religion played an important part in her life, although at times she was repelled by it and searched for comfort in spiritualism (q.v.). Her famous antislavery novel *Uncle Tom's Cabin* (1851-1852) is said to have been inspired by a vision. She championed the cause of the wife of Lord Byron (q.v.) in a book entitled *Lady Byron Vindicated* (1870), in which she accused Byron of incestuous (*see* INCEST) relations with his sister.
Bibliography: Wilson, F. 1941. *Crusader in crinoline: the life of Harriet Beecher Stowe.*

STRAIT-WAISTCOAT. A reinforced garment designed to restrain violent mental patients. In the eighteenth and nineteenth centuries its use gave rise to the belief that pulmonary tuberculosis (q.v.) and insanity were incompatible. The misconception arose from the fact that the strait-waistcoat reduced residual lung capacity, providing an unintentional form of therapy for those insane who also suffered from pulmonary tuberculosis.
Bibliography: Clarke, E., ed. 1971. *Modern methods in the history of medicine.*

STRAMONIUM or JIMSON WEED. The dried leaves and flowering tops of a plant of the Solanaceae family, *Datura stramonium.* It contains hyoscyamine. Jean Esquirol (q.v.) quoted the case of a shepherd who nightly provided himself with a suppositorium of stramonium and on waking related that he had been to a witches' meeting.
Bibliography: Esquirol, J. E. D. 1845. Reprint. 1965. *Mental maladies: a treatise on insanity.*

STRANGE CASE OF DR. JEKYLL AND MR. HYDE, THE. A novel by Robert Louis Stevenson (q.v.). It was inspired by the idea of multiple personality, which had grasped public imagination in the wake of the information coming from hypnotism (q.v.). Stevenson wrote that many of the subjects of his novels were suggested to him by "the little people" in his dreams who indeed dictated certain details. Dr. Jekyll, a "good" physician, recognizes that he has a "bad" side to his personality and that he can create this side at will through a drug. In his second and evil role, he calls himself Mr. Hyde and commits a terrible murder. Eventually Jekyll discovers that Mr. Hyde has taken over his life even without the drug and he cannot return to his "good" self. He ends his life by suicide (q.v.). William Brodie (q.v.) was said to be a genuine Jekyll and Hyde.

Bibliography: Stevenson, R. L. 1886. *The strange case of Dr. Jekyll and Mr. Hyde.*

STRATHMARTINE HOSPITAL. An institution for the mentally retarded founded in Scotland in 1852. The original building with room for 30 children was erected by Sir John and Lady Ogilvie on their estate at Baldovan near Dundee in gratitude for the care given to their defective child at the Abendberg Institution (q.v.). Treatment and training was based on the Abendberg Institution.

Bibliography: Kanner, L. 1964. *History of the care and study of the mentally retarded.*

STRATO (?–c.270 B.C.). A Greek natural philosopher and pupil of Aristotle (q.v.). Unlike his contemporaries he emphasized the importance of the brain in the aetiology of mental disorders.

Bibliography: Rodier, G. 1890. *La physique de Straton.*

STRATTON, GEORGE MALCOLM (1865–1957). An American psychologist and pupil of Wilhelm Wundt (q.v.) in Leipzig. In 1904 Stratton became professor of experimental psychology at Johns Hopkins University. He wrote a large number of books, including works on psychology and religion, social psychology, and the perception of change.

Bibliography: Stratton, G. M. 1929. *Social psychology of international conduct.*

STRIBLING, FRANCIS T. (1810–1874). An American psychiatrist. After a short spell in private practice he became, at the age of twenty-six, physician to the Western Lunatic Asylum (q.v.) of Virginia. He advocated occupational therapy (q.v.) for the insane and prompt treatment for acute psychiatric cases. He was one of the first to campaign for training programs for psychiatric nurses. He was among the younger founders of the American Psychiatric Association (q.v.).

Bibliography: Deutsch, A. 1949. *The mentally ill in America.*

STRIGAE. The term applied by Girolamo Cardano (q.v.) to senile, women beggars living on wild herbs. They were often deformed, emaciated, and unable to communicate effectively. He thought that there was little difference between them and those accused of demoniac possession (q.v.). He described them in his treatise *De Subtilitate*, published in 1550.

Bibliography: Rosen, G. 1968. *Madness in society.*

STRINDBERG, JOHAN AUGUST (1849–1912). A Swedish dramatist and novelist. He was the son of a bankrupted shipping agent and a domestic servant. His father was rigid, tyrannical, and punitive. His mother was of limited intelligence, over-emotional, and full of religious scruples. He was so obsessed (*see* OBSESSION) by her humble origins that he entitled his biography, written in 1886, *Son of a Servant*. There were twelve children in the family, five of them died in infancy. An elder brother was a depressive, and a sister died in a mental hospital. His childhood was emotionally and materially miserable; lack of money cut short his education. He was introspective and pessimistic. His paranoia (q.v.) was strengthened further by the notoriety he attracted with his novel *The Red Room* (1879) and by the accusations of blasphemy that followed the two-volume work *Married* (1884–1885). Consumed by rage and guilt, in 1894 he suffered the first of many severe episodes of mental disorder, which took the form of deep depression, isolation, and suicidal thoughts. He became interested in occultism, alchemy (q.v.), hypnotism (q.v.), and in many other would-be scientific pursuits that were fashionable during his lifetime. Although married three times, all three marriages were unsuccessful, primarily because of his pathological jealousy (q.v.) and his disgust with the physical side of the relationship. His condition has been diagnosed as schizophrenia (q.v.) by some and as toxic alcoholic intoxication by others. His last years were spent in seclusion and torment from the stomach cancer that killed him. Using the knowledge he gained from personal experience and from the works of Henry Maudsley (q.v.) and Théodule Ribot (q.v.), he accurately described many psychiatric illnesses in his works. *Inferno* (1897) is a study of mental abnormality; *The Father* (1887) and *Miss Julia* (1888) reflect his sexual attitudes and his hatred of women. *The Ghost Sonata* (1907) has themes of hallucinations (q.v.), mental torture, and moral retribution. It was in this work that he wrote, "Life is so horribly ugly, we human beings so utterly evil, that if a writer were to portray everything he saw and heard no one could bear to read it."

Bibliography: Sprigge, E. 1949. *The strange life of August Strindberg.*

STRUCTURAL PSYCHOLOGY. An approach analogous to anatomy. It was proposed by Edward B. Titchener (q.v.) and stressed the need to study such elements as sensations, images, ideas, and feelings. The approach clashed with functional psychology, which, using a similar analogy, could be compared to physiology.

Bibliography: Watson, R. I. 1963. *The great psychologists.*

STRÜMPELL, ERNST ADOLF VON (1853–1925). A German physician. He became famous after the publication of his textbook on internal medicine in 1833. He contributed to neurology and pioneered in the study of pseudosclerosis. Using personal observation, he pointed to the psychogenic elements in many disorders that, until then, had been considered solely from the organic point of view. He described the characteristic dorsiflexion of the hand that occurs when making a fist in patients suffering from organic hemiplegia. This anomaly is now called the Strumpell sign. He was deeply interested in music, played the violin, and met many famous composers of his time, including Johannes Brahms (q.v.). His autobiography, published in 1925, was entitled *Aus dem Leben eines Deutschen Klinitiers.*

Bibliography: Haymaker, W., and Schiller, F. 1970. *The founders of neurology.* 2d. ed.

STRUTHILL WELL. A holy well (q.v.) in Stirlingshire, Scotland. Its water was famous for its miraculous power to heal the insane. It was used for this purpose until the eighteenth century.

Bibliography: Tuke, D. H. 1882. *History of the insane in the British Isles.*

STULTITIA. A Latin term for imbecility. Galen (q.v.) believed that it was caused by excessive coldness and humidity in the brain and rarefaction of animal spirits (q.v.). He discussed these ideas in *De Symptomatum Causis.*

Bibliography: Zilboorg, G. 1941. *A history of medical psychology.*

STUMPF, CARL (1848–1936). A German philosopher and psychologist. His early interest was in music; by the time he was an adolescent he could play six musical instruments and compose music. However, he turned to philosophy and studied under Rudolf Lotze (q.v.) in Göttingen. In 1873 he became professor of philosophy at Würzburg, where he met Franz Brentano (q.v.), who remained a friend for the rest of his life and influenced much of his thinking. After a number of moves, Stumpf became professor at Berlin, where he developed a laboratory of experimental psychology (q.v.). He opposed the theories of Wilhelm Wundt (q.v.) and Hermann Ebbinghaus (q.v.). He believed that the function, or psychic process, is the proper field of study in psychology, while the contents, or appearance, should be left to phenomenology. He integrated his early love of music with philosophy by working on the psychology of music and tones. In 1900 he founded an archive of records of primitive music. His major works were *Tonpsychologie*

(1875–1890) and *Appearances and Psychic Functions* (1906). The Berlin Association for Child Psychology was founded by him as a culmination of his pioneering efforts in child studies.
Bibliography: Boring, E. G. 1950. *A history of experimental psychology.*

STYLE OF LIFE. A term used by Alfred Adler (q.v.) to describe the individuality that each person shows in his environment, his way of solving problems, and such like. According to Adler, a satisfactory style of life depended on good childhood experiences.
Bibliography: Adler, A. 1929. *The science of living.*

STYX. In Greek mythology (q.v.) the river of hate in Hades. Its waters were poisonous and made those who drank them speechless for a year.
Bibliography: *Brewer's dictionary of phrase and fable.* 1978.

SUAN SARARNROM. A mental hospital built in 1937 in the Surath region of Thailand (q.v.). It is named after the hill on which it stands. The locality was once the residence of the regent of the Surath region. The king, a frequent visitor to the residence and an admirer of its pleasant location among the trees called the hill "Suan Sararnrom," or "happy garden," and the hospital adopted it as its name.
Bibliography: Sangsingkeo, P. 1975. Thailand. In *World history of psychiatry*, ed. J. G. Howells.

SUBACTI. Supernatural beings. In ancient Rome, they were believed to cause sleep disorders, including insomnia and nightmare (q.v.). Caelius Aurelianus (q.v.) wrote at length about them.
Bibliography: Drabkin, I. E., ed., and trans. 1950. *Caelius Aurelianus on acute diseases and on chronic diseases.*

SUBCONSCIOUS. A term coined by Pierre Janet (q.v.) to describe autonomous psychological manifestations.
Bibliography: Ellenberger, H. F. 1970. *The discovery of the unconscious.*

SUBCORTICAL IRRITATION. In the nineteenth century the aetiology of mental disorders was assumed to be organic, therefore, great importance was given to the brain and the spinal cord. For example, Theodor Meynert (q.v.) believed subcortical irritation was the cause of delusions (q.v.) and hallucinations (q.v.).
Bibliography: Zilboorg, G. 1941. *A history of medical psychology.*

SUCCUBUS. An evil spirit, believed to be the devil in disguise. She was said to appear especially at night to disturb the sleep of her victims. In the

fifteenth century incubi (*see* INCUBUS) and succubi were accused of seducing men and women. Because sin and mental disease were correlated, succubi and incubi were held responsible for many manifestations of abnormal behavior. Pico della Mirandola (q.v.) was among the philosophers of that time who wrote about succubi.
Bibliography: Robbins, R. H. 1970. *The encyclopedia of witchcraft and demonology.*

SUCCUS MELANCHOLICUS. Another term for melancholic humor (q.v.). Galen (q.v.) believed that it was produced in the liver (q.v.) and the spleen (q.v.) and that it indirectly affected the brain.
Bibliography: Harkins, P.W., trans. 1963. *Galen on the passions and errors of the soul.*

SUCCUS NERVEUS. A term used by Giovanni A. Borelli (q.v.) in 1680 to indicate animal spirits (q.v.) and to explain animal motion.
Bibliography: Borelli, G. A. 1680. *De motu animalium.*

SUFFOCATION. Hysterical (*see* HYSTERIA) phenomena were attributed to the uterus (q.v.), wandering upward in the body like an animal or becoming engorged. This particular belief was prevalent at the time of Galen (q.v.). The rising of the uterus was said to produce a feeling of suffocation.
Bibliography: Veith, I. 1965. *Hysteria: the history of a disease.*

SUFISM. Islamic mysticism. It created a special community relationship and allowed the emergence of religious healers as leaders. In Anatolia in the Middle Ages (q.v.), special institutions of sufitic belief cared for the mentally ill, who were expected to work as soon as they improved. These centers were called *tekkes* and provided what now would be considered a therapeutic community.
Bibliography: Trimingham, J. S. 1974. *The Sufi orders in Islam.*

SUICIDE. A historical survey of suicide reveals that there are two kinds. There is institutionalized, ritualistic, and approved suicide, such as suttee (q.v.) and hara-kiri (q.v.) (honourable suicide), or all those forms of suicide that are expected by the community for its benefit (for example, in war; when people become old, as in Greenland; as sacrifices to gods). There is also personal suicide as a protest or revolt. At this point, it becomes the most individual act available to man. This form of suicide is usually condemned by society. There are nine cases of suicide in the Old Testament in which no criticism of it is implied. The Koran (q.v.) flatly condemns it. Ancient philosophers were divided in their opinions. Pythagoras and Socrates (qq.v.) condemned it; Zeno, Plato and Cicero (qq.v.) regarded it as permissible. The Christian Church condemned it, and, therefore, it became common to refuse burial in consecrated ground to suicides. This was officially stated by the Christian Church in 1284 at the Synod of Nimes. In the

Middle Ages (q.v.), the body of a suicide would suffer degradation. It might be dragged through the streets, hanged on a gallows head down, buried under the gallows, or pinned by astake. (See Plate 14). This attitude prevailed until the eighteenth century and later. The last burial at crossroads (q.v.) in England took place in 1823. Unless there was a defense of insanity, suicide was considered a felony and punishable by law. Frequently the goods of the victim were confiscated as he was believed to have broken his oath of loyalty. Outbreaks of mass suicide have been known, for example, in ancient Greece and in France during the revolution. In Germany, after the Franco-Prussian war, suicide clubs were formed. Yet, until the seventeenth and eighteenth centuries, there was no word for the act by which man terminates his own life. The word "suicide" first appeared in England in the middle of the seventeenth century. Before this date, it was sometimes called "self-homicide." In France, the word "suicide" appeared probably a century later. According to Jean Esquirol (q.v.), it was popularized by François Sauvages (q.v.) and Philippe Pinel (q.v.).
Bibliography: Fedden, H. R. 1938. *Suicide*.

SULEIMANIE ASYLUM. A *timarahane*, or, house of correction, for the insane founded in Constantinople (q.v.) in the early sixteenth century. It employed 150 persons to look after no more than 20 patients. Treatment included vapor baths, which often were forcibly administered to patients chained to the stone pavement of the chamber. Violent patients were confined to dungeons, but the more amenable enjoyed good food, music, and entertainment by actors and jugglers. The nearby school of medicine provided medical care, and exorcism (q.v.) and prayers were offered by the ulemas from the mosque.
Bibliography: Davidson, J. H. 1875. A visit to a Turkish asylum. *J. ment. Sci.* 21: 408-15.

SULLIVAN, HARRY STACK (1892-1949). An American psychiatrist. He systematically developed the theme of interpersonal relationships, which had not been crucial in Freudian teaching. According to him, the environment and harmful interpersonal relationships are the causes of mental disorders, including schizophrenia (q.v.). His systematic approach to the study of the development of personality is often made difficult for its reader by his use of special terms. He was the founder of the William Alanson White Foundation and its president for ten years.
Bibliography: Mullahy, P. 1970. *Psychoanalysis and interpersonal psychiatry: the contributions of Harry Stack Sullivan*.

SULLY, JAMES (1842-1923). An English psychologist and philosopher. In his earlier years he wrote on sensation and intuition, pessimism, and illu-

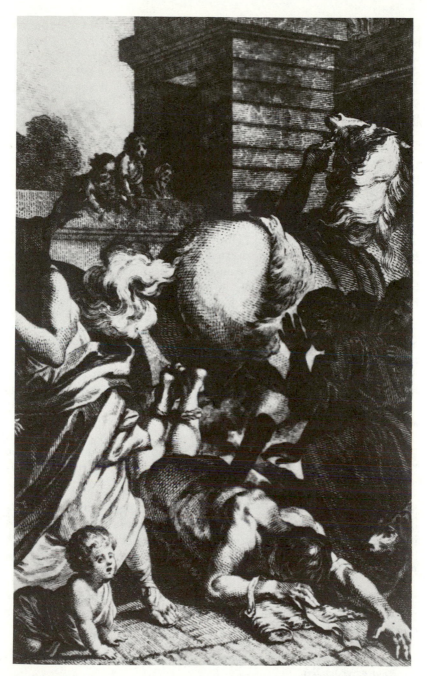

14. SUICIDE. The desecration of the corpse. This illustration from Delisle de Sales, *Philosophie de la Nature*, 1769, shows the corpse of a suicide being dragged along the streets with a stake driven through its back. By courtesy of the Department of Medical Illustration, Ipswich Hospital.

sions. He later devoted his work to child psychology (q.v.) and wrote several books in this field. In 1884 he wrote the *Teachers' Handbook of Psychology*, which was the first modern textbook written specifically for those in the educational field. His other major work, published in 1892, was entitled *The Human Mind*. In 1873 he established the British Association of Child Study.
Bibliography: Sully, J. 1918. *My life and friends*.

SUMANOVIĆ, SAVA (1896-1942). A Yugoslav painter who suffered from visual hallucinations (q.v.) and ideas of persecution. At the apex of his artistic powers, while living in France, he painted *The Drunken Boat*, which he completed in seven days and seven nights of feverish work. At the same time, his symptoms became more acute and he had to leave Paris to return home to Yugoslavia. After a brief remission, he relapsed and was admitted to Belgrade Mental Hospital. Three months later he was released and resumed painting, despite the persistence of auditory hallucinations. He successfully exhibited 410 of his paintings in Belgrade in 1939. An innocent bystander, he was killed in 1942 in a massacre of peasants.
Bibliography: Neimarevic, D., and Basicevic, D. 1971. The case of the painter Sava Sumanovic. *Proceedings of the Fifth World Congress of Psychiatry, Mexico*.

SUMMA THEOLOGICA. A work by Thomas Aquinas (q.v.). The first part of it contains the essence of Thomistic psychology. In it the nature of man is discussed, and his bodily and spiritual qualities are analyzed through his acts and habits. Man's characteristics are regarded as an integration of vegetative, sensory, and spiritual factors. The doctrines of Aristotle (q.v.) are reexamined with those of other ancient philosophers, and a new system that incorporates Greek, Arabic, and Hebrew teachings is devised. *Summa Theologica* influenced philosophers and psychologists for many generations.
Bibliography: Aquinas, T. *Summa theologica*, trans. the Fathers of the English Dominican Province. 3 vols.

SUMMERS, MONTAGUE (1880-1948). An English writer, and authority on demonology and witchcraft (q.v.) about which he wrote several books, including *History of Witchcraft and Demonology* (1926) and *The Werewolf* (1933).
Bibliography: Montague, S. 1926. *History of witchcraft and demonology*.

SUNDAY. Symptoms of emotional disorders in some patients recur at particular times. Sandor Ferenczi (q.v.) found that Sunday was the most common day of the week for these periodical returns of disturbances.
See also ANNIVERSARY REACTION.
Bibliography: Ferenczi, S. 1926. *Further contributions to the theory and technique of psychoanalysis*.

SUNDERLAND, LA ROY (1804-1885). An American supporter of Franz Mesmer (q.v.). He was a restless individual, who was easily persuaded to

join any fashionable movement. For a time, he was a supporter of antislavery and then a supporter of James Graham (q.v.). Eventually, he became disillusioned with faith healing (q.v.), another of his interests, and founded a cult that he termed "Patheism." It dealt with mental disorders and their treatment through dubious hypnotic practices.
Bibliography: Tinterow, M. M. 1970. *Foundations of hypnosis: from Mesmer to Freud.*

SUNFLOWER. *Helianthus annuus.* The seeds and leaves of the sunflower were used in Russian folk medicine to make a decoction, sweetened with honey, that was prescribed for unspecified nervous disorders.
Bibliography: Kourennoff, M. P., and St. George, G. 1970. *Russian folk medicine.*

SUPERFLUOUS MAN. The term, as originally understood, described a type of individual found in the Russian literature of the nineteenth century. He was characterized by indecision in private and public life and an inability to make meaningful relationships. These shortcomings were attributed to maladjustment in personal life and the repressive social and political practices of the time.
Bibliography: Benet, W. R. 1972. *The reader's encyclopedia.*

SUPPLICACYON FOR THE BEGGARS. A work by the English theologian Simon Fish (?-1531), circulated in London in 1529. In it he suggested that the king should take control over hospitals from the clergy and become responsible for the health, both mental and physical, and welfare of his people.
Bibliography: Rosen, G. 1968. *Madness in society.*

SUPPURATION. For centuries suppuration was believed to be beneficial in cases of mental disorders, as it was believed that the discharge provided an outlet for "bad humors." Therefore, it was artificially produced by burns, irritants, or caustic substances applied to the skin. The practice persisted until the nineteenth century and was strongly supported by such authoritative physicians as Benjamin Rush (q.v.) and Jean Esquirol (q.v.).
Bibliography: Rush, B. 1812. Reprint. 1962. *Medical inquiries and observations upon the diseases of the mind.*

SURGERY. *See* HEAD SURGERY, LOBOTOMY, and TREPANATION.

ŠURPU. An ancient Babylonian text written in cuneiform script on clay tablets. It describes phobias (q.v.), anxiety, fear, compulsions, and psychopathic (*see* PSYCHOPATHY) behavior and suggests the appropriate incantations (q.v.) to be used in therapy.

See also MAQLÛ.

Bibliography: Kinnier Wilson, J. V. 1965. *An introduction to Babylonian psychiatry.*

SURREALISM. An artistic and philosophic movement that placed the expression of subconscious thoughts and feelings above reality and logic. It originated in France around 1924, and based its tenets on concepts of the unconscious developed by Sigmund Freud (q.v.). A copy of Freud's *Introductory Lecture in Psychoanalysis* was exhibited at the Paris Office for Surrealistic Research surrounded by forks to indicate that the book was to be devoured by surrealists. Its followers sometimes went to extremes. For example, some of them regarded Jean Charcot's (q.v.) discovery of hysteria (q.v.) as "the greatest poetical discovery" of the time. Dreams (q.v.), mental illness, and abnormal psychic states were important to surrealism. The leader of the movement, André Breton (q.v.), had been a medical student who was interested in mental abnormalities and the work of Frederic Myers (q.v.), Pierre Janet (q.v.) and Freud. Surrealist writers relied on a form of automatic writing in which dictation originated from within the writer, rather than from a spirit. Frequently, this form of self-hypnosis degenerated into trances and hallucinations (q.v.). Some writers deliberately imitated the forms of expression used by psychotic (*see* PSYCHOSIS), schizophrenic (*see* SCHIZOPHRENIA), and mentally retarded patients. In the visual arts, the most characteristic surrealist painters are Salvador Dali (q.v.), Giorgio di Chirico (1888-), and Max Ernst (1891-).

Bibliography: Gaunt, W. 1973. *The Surrealists.*

SUSHRUTA. A celebrated Indian physician of the fifth century A.D.. His accounts of mental disorders and epilepsy (q.v.) are notable for their accuracy. His writings include observations on symptomatology and descriptions of states of excitement, such as, singing and crying, aimless roaming, overeating, peculiar dressing, and overtalking. He realized the importance of strong emotions in the causation of emotional disorders. He used to administer extracts of Nardus root (q.v.) to his patients in order to sedate them.

Bibliography: Whitwell, J. R. 1936. *Historical notes on psychiatry.*

SUSTO. The term applied in popular medicine in Latin America to a group of psychosomatic disorders with the common aetiology of soul loss through fright. Those afflicted believe that some evil power has deprived them of their soul. They become depressed, pale, and lethargic. They lose their appetite and interest in their persons and their surroundings. A patient,

believing that he has lost his soul, becomes extremely ill; at times his temperature rises, and he may have persistent attacks of diarrhea and vomiting.
Bibliography: Gobeil, O. 1973. El Susto: A descriptive analysis. *Internat. J. Social Psychiat.* 19: 38.

SUTHERLAND, ALEXANDER JOHN (1787-1867). An English psychiatrist. He succeeded his father as physician at Saint Luke's Hospital for Lunatics (q.v.). He was an active member of the Society for Improving the Condition of the Insane (q.v.) and was among the physicians who examined Daniel M'Naughten (q.v.). His main works include *Clinical Lectures on Insanity* (1848) and *Pathology, Morbid Anatomy and Treatment of Insanity* (1861).
Bibliography: Leigh, D. 1961. *The historical development of British psychiatry.*

SUTTEE. The term is derived from *sati*, meaning faithful wife, and is defined as "paradise." It is linked to the belief in another life in which wife and husband are reunited. Voluntary suicide (q.v.) was customary in ancient India. Hindu widows were expected to immolate themselves on their dead husbands' pyres. For a time it became a symbolic performance. The widow was required to lie on the pyre briefly and then to rise ready for a second marriage. In the sixth century, however, the Brahmins reimposed it as a physical act in order to inherit the dead couple's property. It was declared illegal in 1829 but persisted in Nepal until 1877. At least one case of suttee was reported as late as 1937. Similar customs have existed in Africa, North America, and among the Maoris, where widows were either burned alive with their husbands or strangled. In some civilizations, when a key figure died, friends and followers committed suicide to accompany him in a life beyond death.
Bibliography: Fedden, H. R. 1938. *Suicide.*

SUTTON, THOMAS (1767-1835). An English physician. He observed that heavy drinkers developed such symptoms as tremors, sweating, confusion, and agitation. He differentiated the syndrome from other forms of delirium (q.v.), related it to chronic abuse of alcohol, and termed it delirium tremens (q.v.) in a classic study of alcoholism (q.v.), which he wrote in 1813.
Bibliography: Sutton, T. 1813. *Tracts on delirium tremens.*

SUTURES. Cranial sutures were believed by the Arabs (q.v.) to represent the destiny of the individual as written by the hand of Allah. Thus, they were always carefully avoided in operations involving the skull, such as, trepanation (q.v.).
Bibliography: Brothwell, D., and Sandison, A. T. 1967. *Diseases in antiquity.*

SWEDENBORG, EMANUEL (1688-1772). A Swedish philosopher, mystic, and scientist. His father, the Lutheran bishop of Skara, was given to

seeing spirits and claimed to have brought about miraculous cures, including the cure of his girl servant, Kerstin, who tried to suffocate herself and was restored to consciousness by God's word and a good draught of Rhenish wine. Swedenborg followed his father's example, and he too deviated from orthodoxy. He was a mathematician and a scientist of genius. Among his projected inventions were mining techniques, aquatic clocks, air guns, a "flying chariot," and a method of discovering the desires and mental disorders of men by analysis. In his writings, covering physics, chemistry, anatomy, physiology, and psychology, he shifted from speculations to dogmatism and subordinated his reason to his imagination (q.v.). According to him, the soul received impressions from the senses and controlled the body, which clothed the soul and adapted itself to it in shape and form. He concluded that soul and body communicated through the brain. His remarkable scientific achievements were abandoned when, at the age of forty-six, he turned to mysticism, after having a "vision" of reptiles and toads crawling on the floor of the room in which he was having an enormous meal. The hallucination (q.v.) included the figure of God, who told him not to eat so much and that he had been chosen to interpret the true meaning of the Holy Writ. From then on, Swedenborg asserted that he experienced supernatural visions, and he dedicated his life to gloomy religious writings, which he said were dictated to him by an angel. His alleged psychical gifts made him famous. He was afraid of women and would never receive them alone. In 1744, during his stay in London, he became so excited, odd, and incoherent that he had to be lodged in a house near a doctor, who ministered to him and kept six men on guard over him. In his later years, his mind became more deranged. He lived alone on a diet of milk and bread, troubled and tempted by the bad spirits, and comforted and protected by the good ones. He accurately predicted the date of his own death. Although he did not personally originate a religious sect, his followers established one, called the New Jerusalem Church, or, New Church. William Blake (q.v.) was influenced by him. The London Swedenborg Society, founded in 1810, publishes, translates, and distributes his theological works, which include *Arcana Coelestia* (1749-1756) in eight volumes. The American Swedenborg Scientific Association is similarly concerned with his scientific works.
Bibliography: Sigstedt, C. S. 1953. *The Swedenborg epic.*

SWEET GALE. *Myrica gale*, a moorland herb used by gypsies as a remedy for many ailments, including depression, poor memory (q.v.), and insomnia. Bibliography: de Baïracli Levy, J. 1974. *Illustrated herbal handbook.*

SWEETSER, WILLIAM (1797-1875). An American psychiatrist. He believed that mind and body were one and that intellectual and emotional activities were closely linked. In 1843 he wrote a book entitled *Mental Hygiene; or an Examination of the Intellect and Passions, Designed to Il-*

lustrate their Influence on Health and Duration of Life. This was the first use of the expression "mental hygiene" (q.v.), which was later suggested by Adolf Meyer (q.v.) to describe a movement in the mental health field.
Bibliography: Deutsch, A. 1949. *The mentally ill in America.*

SWIETEN, GERARD VAN (1700-1772). A Dutch physician and pupil of Hermann Boerhaave (q.v.) whose views he helped to spread. Swieten was often quoted by medical writers such as Jean Esquirol (q.v.). He believed baths of surprise (q.v.) and bleeding (q.v.) to be the best forms of treatment in cases of insanity. He was the first to realize that, in the treatment of syphilis (q.v.), small doses of mercury (q.v.) over a long period were more efficacious than large doses over a short time. His Catholic faith caused his resignation from Leiden University, and, in 1745, he became court physician to Maria Theresa of Austria, at whose court he met Mozart. He greatly influenced medical education in Vienna. Franz Mesmer (q.v.) was among his pupils.
Bibliography: Garrison, F. H. 1929. *An introduction to the history of medicine.*

SWIFT, JONATHAN (1667-1745). A British author and clergyman, born in Dublin. He became dean of St. Patrick's in 1713. His father died before his birth, and his mother left him for three years to be brought up by a wet nurse. He had a miserable childhood and adolescence, was a poor and lazy student, associated with dissolute companions and neglected to attend lectures. His health was always poor; he often had spells of dizziness and later in life became a classic hypochondriac (*see* HYPOCHONDRIA). A confirmed pessimist, he was given to attacks of depression. His usual remark on parting from a friend was "Good night. I hope I shall not see you again." His eccentric behavior earned for him the title of "mad parson" even before he became deranged. In 1714 he was elected governor of Bethlem Royal Hospital (q.v.), and, in 1722, he used his position to ask for the admission of a man called Beaumont, who was "mad in London riding through the streets on his Irish horse with the rabble after him, and throwing his money about the street." He often referred to the hospital in his writings. In his satire *A Tale of a Tub*, written between 1689 and 1699, there is a digression in which he discusses insanity and suggests that most leaders "have generally been persons, whose reason was disturbed," therefore Bedlam should be searched for suitable candidates to command the army and to run the country. In another satire, *The Legion Club* he calls the Irish House of Commons the Bedlam of Dublin. His masterpiece *Gulliver's Travels* (1726) is a satire of mankind. His mental deterioration, which has been attributed to cerebral arteriosclerosis, began in 1736. His memory deteriorated, and eventually he was reduced to a stuporose and silent state. In 1742 the Court of Chancery, appointed guardians for him, and a commission declared him "of unsound mind and memory." In his will he provided funds for a "hospital for idiots and lunaticks," which resulted in the establishment of Saint Patrick's Hospital (q.v.) in Dublin in 1745. Swift referred to his legacy in a poem entitled 'On the Death of Dr. Swift':

> He gave what little wealth he had,
> To bukld a house for fools and mad;
> And show'd by one satiric touch,
> No nation wanted it so much.

Bibliography: Rowse, A. L. 1975. *Jonathan Swift: major prophet.*

SWINBURNE, ALGERNON CHARLES (1837-1909). An English poet and critic. He was influenced by Victor Hugo (q.v.) in Paris and the Pre-Raphaelite group in London; Dante Gabriel Rossetti (q.v.) painted a number of portraits of him. His writings were often criticized by his contemporaries because they repudiated conventional attitudes. His own life also was unconventional, especially in its sexual aspects: he enjoyed flagellation (q.v.) and visited a London brothel, where he was whipped. He had homosexual tendencies. Many of his writings are suggestive, although extremely musical; Alfred Tennyson (q.v.) called his verses "poisonus honey." Alcoholism (q.v.) eventually destroyed Swinburne's health, and his last years were spent in the house of the writer Theodore Watts-Dunton (1832-1914).
Bibliography: Thomas, D. 1979. *Swinburne: the poet in his world.*

SWINGING CHAIR. A device designed to submit mental patients to violent swinging motion. The shock to the system and the vomiting and diarrhea it produced were believed to be beneficial, especially in cases of violent behavior. Erasmus Darwin (q.v.) and Benjamin Rush (q.v.) were among the numerous enthusiastic promoters of the chair.
Bibliography: Roback, A. A., and Kierman, T. 1969. *Pictorial history of psychology and psychiatry.*

SWISS SOCIETY FOR PSYCHOANALYSIS. The first society of psychoanalysis (q.v.) in Switzerland. It was founded by Eugen Bleuler (q.v.) and Oskar Pfister (q.v.). It ceased to function in 1914 due to lack of support.

SYDENHAM, THOMAS (1624-1689). An English physician. His reliance on experience and direct observation rather than theories gained for him the title of the "English Hippocrates." He also witnessed many important events: the Great Plague, the Fire of London in 1666, the civil war, and the execution of Charles I. He was a prolific writer, best known for his *Medical Observations* (1676). He gave classic descriptions of chorea minor and "hysteric disorders," which he regarded as the most common chronic affliction. According to him, hypochondria (q.v.) was a form of hysteria (q.v.) that occurred in men. One of his favorite remedies was an alcoholic tincture of

opium (q.v.) with saffron (q.v.), which became known in the pharmacopoeia as laudanum (q.v.). He claimed that it was efficient against many disorders and insisted that he could not practice medicine without it.
Bibliography: Dewhurst, K. 1966. *Dr. Thomas Sydenham, (1624-1689): his life and original writings.*

SYLVIUS. *See* DUBOIS, JACQUES.

SYLVIUS, FRANCISCUS. *See* BOË, FRANZ DE LA.

SYM, JOHN (1581-1637). An English clergyman whose experience in the ministry prompted a remarkable treatise on counseling would-be suicides. Entitled *Life's Preservative against Self-killing* (q.v.), it outlined the signs of impending suicide (q.v.) and gave practical advice on its prevention. Sym pointed out that reasoning with depressed people is of no avail, and that it is better to attempt to find and remove the cause of their despair.
Bibliography: Rosen, J. 1971. History in the study of suicide. *Psychol. Med.* 1: 267-85.

SYMONDS, JOHN ADDINGTON (1840-1893). An English author on homosexuality (q.v.). He was a married homosexual, who found his sexual impulses nobly justified in Greek literature. He was the first to write a scholarly account on homosexuality, but the work, entitled *A Problem of Greek Ethics, an Enquiry into the Phenomenon of Sexual Inversion*, could not be published in England for moralistic reasons, hence it was published in Germany in 1873, and years later ten copies were printed in England for private circulation. In 1896 Symonds collaborated with Havelock Ellis (q.v.) in a work entitled *Sexual Inversion*, a term that Symonds preferred to homosexuality. Again, this work was first published in Germany. A year later, when it appeared in England, his family insisted that his name should be removed from the cover and tried to destroy the whole of the first edition. Efforts to suppress his homosexuality caused nervous breakdowns and despite his many achievements, including a splendid historical work, *The Renaissance in Italy* (1875-1886), Symonds felt that his output would have been greater, if "he had not been blighted by the strain of accommodating himself to conventional morality."
Bibliography: Grosskurth, P. 1964. *John Addington Symonds.*

SYMPHONIE PATHÉTIQUE. The last symphony composed by Peter Tchaikovsky (q.v.). Written just before his death, it is a remarkable human document. It voices the tragedy and pathos of his life and in its last bars anticipates his death. It is an autobiography and a requiem. He told his nephew: "Whilst working on this composition during my journey I often cried." Madame von Meck said of his music: "Your creations are an autobiography." His brother Modest also stressed the autobiographical nature of the work:

The first part represents his life, that mixture of sorrow, suffering and irresistible gleaning for the noble and good. The second movement represents the fleeting joys of his life. The third movement depicts the story of his musical development. The fourth movement represents his spiritual state during the last years of his life.

The "Lamentoso" of the last movement could be regarded as his symphonic requiem.
Bibliography: Hofmann, M. R. 1962. *Tchaikovsky*. trans. A. Heriot.

SYMPTOM COMPLEX. A term introduced by Karl Kahlbaum (q.v.) to describe a disease form that follows a definite course.
Bibliography: Kahlbaum K. L. 1973. *Catatonia*, trans. Y. Levij, and T. Pridan.

SYNAPSE. A term introduced by Charles Scott Sherrington (q.v.) in 1897 to describe those functioning connections that result from close contact between neurones.
Bibliography: Foster, M., and Sherrington, C. S. 1897. *A textbook of physiology*.

SYPHILIS. The term is derived from the poem *Syphilis sive Morbus Gallicus* written by Girolamo Fracastoro (q.v.) and published in Venice in 1530. The shepherd of the poem was named Syphilus and suffered from the disease. Until recent time, skin lesions of syphilis were confused with leprosy (q.v.) and elephantiasis, thus Manardus (1461-1536) described "leprosy" caused by sexual intercourse. Traditionally, syphilis has been said to have been introduced into Europe in epidemic form by the sailors of Christopher Columbus (1451-1506) on their return from Haiti in 1493. Not until 1913 was it demonstrated by Hideyo Noguchi (q.v.) and Joseph Moore (q.v.) that the spirocheta of syphilis is found in the brain of patients suffering from general paralysis of the insane (q.v.).
Bibliography: Pusey, W. A. 1933. *The history and epidemiology of syphilis*.

T

TABULA RASA. This term, meaning an "unmarked tablet," was used by John Locke (q.v.) to describe the state in which man is born. The experiences of life then mark the tablet.
Bibliography: Gibson, J. 1917. *Locke's theory of knowledge and its historical relation.*

TAINE, HIPPOLYTE ADOLPHE (1828-1893). A French literary critic and historian, who regarded psychology as the starting point of moral and social science. He undertook detailed research on the acquisition of language. His book *De l'intelligence*, published in 1870, is now considered the beginning of modern psychology in France. In it, he supported the views of John Stuart Mill (q.v.) and Alexander Bain (q.v.).
Bibliography: Kahn, S. J. 1953. *Science and aesthetic judgement: a study in Taine's critical method.*

TALAL I (1907-1972). A king of Jordan. He came to the throne in 1951, following the assassination of his father, Abdullah ibn Husayn (1882-1951). In less than a year he was declared insane by parliament; he was deposed and replaced by his son Hussein I (1935-).
Bibliography: Morris, J. 1959. *The Hashemite kings.*

TALION LAW. An expression referring to the primitive belief in retribution and retaliation in kind. It is summarized in the saying "an eye for an eye, a tooth for a tooth."
Bibliography: Goldenson, R. M. 1970. *The encyclopedia of human behavior.*

TALISMAN. A term derived from the Arabic and later classic Greek word meaning "mystery." Talismans, or special objects, sometimes carved with mysterious words, were believed to protect those who wore them. The

protection extended to immunity from mental disorders. A large number of talismans were believed to be efficacious against epilepsy (q.v.).
See also AMULETS.
Bibliography: Pavitt, W. T., and Pavitt, K. 1922. *Talismans, amulets and zodiacal gems.*

TALKING CURE. Talking about half-forgotten traumatic experiences was believed to have a therapeutic effect in itself. Joseph Breuer (q.v.) was among the first to enunciate this concept, which was later enlarged by Sigmund Freud (q.v.). Freud termed it "abreaction" (q.v.), or "catharsis" (q.v.).
Bibliography: Ehrenwald, J., ed. 1976. *The history of psychotherapy.*

TALMA, FRANÇOIS JOSEPH (1763-1826). A French actor, famous in France and England for his tragic roles. He was a favorite of Napoleon I (q.v.) and Louis XVIII (1755-1824). At the beginning of the French Revolution (q.v.) he suffered from unspecified mental disorders that were complicated by hallucinations (q.v.). When he was on the stage he thought that his audience was not composed of living human beings, but rather grinning skeletons. Even though this hallucination filled him with superstitious horror, he was able to continue acting without betraying any emotion.
Bibliography: Winslow, L.S.F. 1898. *Mad humanity: its forms, apparent and obscure.*

TALMUD, THE. The collection of Jewish religious books, embracing civil and ceremonial law. A part of it was codified in 200 A.D. and then expanded between 400 and 500 A.D. The Talmud considers insanity a medical condition and does not attempt to explain it in terms of demonaic or spirit possession (q.v.). Epilepsy (q.v.) is believed to be an hereditary disease that will respond to charms. Another disorder, termed *Kordiakos* (q.v.) and characterized by confusion and vertigo following contact with a vat of new wine, may be an early reference to delirium tremens (q.v.). The psychological mechanisms described anecdotally in the Talmud include the projection of guilt and the realization of unconscious wishes in dreams (q.v.). Diversion and discussion of worries are a recommended form of treatment for troubled patients.
Bibliography: Rosner, F. 1977. *Medicine in the Bible and the Talmud.*

TAMBURINI, AUGUSTO (1848-1919). An Italian psychiatrist. He promoted the welfare of the mentally ill by establishing in his hospital a training school, workshops and farms for occupational therapy (q.v.), recreational facilities, a gymnasium, and a hydrotherapy section.
Bibliography: Tamburini, A., Ferrari, G. C., and Antonini, G. 1918. *L'assistenza degli alienati in Italia e nelle varie nazioni.*

TANY (or TANNYE), THOMAS (?-? 1677). A London goldsmith known for his fanaticism and delusions (q.v.). He believed himself to be a "Jew of the tribe of Reuben" who, as the lord high priest, would rebuild the temple. He also claimed to be the earl of Essex and the king of France. In 1651, he was imprisoned in Newgate Prison (q.v.) and accused of blasphemy. As a violent man his physical assaults often led to trouble. Eventually, he was admitted to Bethlem Royal Hospital (q.v.) where he died.

Bibliography: *The dictionary of national biography.* 1900.

TARAHUMARA INDIANS. A tribe of Indians in the southwestern part of Chihuahua, Mexico. They use hallucinogenic cacti to alter their senses. They believe that plants have feelings and treat the psychotropic cacti and herbs with special respect, as they think that these plants can harm them if offended. They believe that peyote (q.v.) wards off evil forces, that some plants cause madness and death, and that others bring health and provide vision.

Bibliography: Bye, R. A., Jr. 1979. Hallucinogenic plants of the Tarahumara. *J. Ethno-pharmacology.* 1: 23-48.

TARANTISM. A form of mental disorder common in southern Italy in the seventeeth and eighteenth century. A few descriptions of it appear as early as the fifteenth century. It was attributed to the bite of the tarantula, which was believed to be poisonous. Its symptoms were deep melancholia (q.v.) with apathy and withdrawal. To combat them, those affected were kept dancing to the sound of the "tarantella," a fast dance of Neapolitan origin. (See Plate 15.) For this reason tarantism is frequently confused with dancing mania (q.v.), and frantic dancing and excitement have been listed under its symptomatology. Giorgio Baglivi (q.v.) gave a clinical description of it during the seventeenth century. Basing his facts on tradition rather than on observation, he elevated tarantism to the status of a toxic psychosis (q.v.).

Bibliography: Sigerist, H. E. 1948. The story of Tarantism. In *Music and medicine,* ed. D. Schullian and M. Schoen.

TARCHANOFF, IVAN ROMANOVICH (1848-1909). A Russian physiologist. In 1890 he described the psychogalvanic reflex, a lowering of the electrical resistance of the body, which is caused by emotional excitation. This reflex is now known as Tarchanoff's phenomenon.

Bibliography: Schmidt, J. E. 1959. *Medical discoveries: who and when.*

TARDE, GABRIEL (1843-1904). A French sociologist. He believed that social interaction included all the influences exercised between individuals. He attempted to explore and to explain logically all types of social interaction in a book entitled *Laws of Imitation* (1890). Tarde divided mental activity

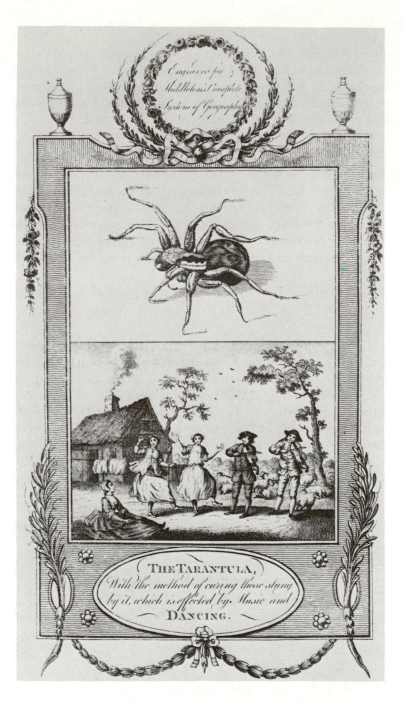

Engraved for
Middleton's Complete
System of Geography

THE TARANTULA,
With the method of curing those stung
by it, which is effected by Music and
DANCING.

15. TARANTISM. The tarantula and, below, the "tarantella" being danced to cure the victims of its sting. An eighteenth-century engraving. By courtesy of the Wellcome Trustees, Wellcome Institute for the History of Medicine, London.

into three groups: the reaction to external objects, to other minds, and to itself. He felt that belief and desire were more important than sensation.
Bibliography: Tarde, G. 1902. *Economic psychology.*

TARPEIAN ROCK. A rock on the Capitoline Hill in Rome. It was said to be guarded by the spirit of Tarpeia, who may have been a goddess of the underworld. Defective children and criminals were thrown to their death from it.

TARTARUS TARTARISATUS. A form of tartar first described by the Dutch physician Adrian Mynsicht in 1631. It was a panacea of psychiatry when all else failed.
Bibliography: Garrison, F. H. 1929. *An introduction to the history of medicine.*

TARTINI, GIUSEPPE (1692-1770). An Italian composer. Originally he was interested in the church and in law, but he gave both up in favor of music. His best known composition, *The Devil's Trill*, was said to have been played to him by the devil, who appeared to him in a dream. On waking Tartini remembered the music and wrote it down.
Bibliography: Bessy, M. 1963. *A pictorial history of magic and the supernatural.*

TARTUFFE. The hero of *Tartuffe*, a comedy by Molière (q.v.). He represents the classic psychopath, and his name has come to mean hypocrite and impostor who professes extreme piety.
Bibliography: Hall, H. G. 1970. *Molière's Tartuffe.*

TASSI, AGOSTINO (1565-1644). An Italian painter with a psychopathic (*see* PSYCHOPATHY) personality. At various times he was involved in such crimes as rape, incest (q.v.), sexual abberrations, banditry, and homicide.
Bibliography: Wittkower, R., and Wittkower, M. 1963. *Born under Saturn.*

TASSO, TORQUATO (1544-1595). An Italian poet, born in Sorrento. He suffered from auditory and visual hallucinations (q.v.). He often would converse with a spirit whom he believed to be a frequent visitor to his room. He claimed it would mix up his papers and steal his money. His nights were troubled by apparitions and mysterious lights suspended in the air. He was also a victim of persecutory delusions (q.v.) and was obsessed (*see* OBSESSION) by the fear of assassination. Tasso once described his own condition: "My mind sleeps, thinks not, my fancy is chill, and forms no image of things. I feel as if I were chained in all my operations, and as if I were overcome by an unwonted numbness and oppressive stupor." In 1579 an outburst of rage during the wedding festivities of Margherita Gonzaga caused him to be arrested, chained and imprisoned in the Ospedale di Sant'Anna, where he remained for seven years. His last years were spent in Rome and Naples. Pope Clement VIII (1536-1605) called him to Rome to be crowned poet laureate. Unfortunately, the journey proved too much for him, and he died in a monastery near Rome. Gaetano Donizetti (q.v.) composed an opera based on his life and insanity.

Bibliography: Brand, C. P. 1965. *Torquato Tasso: a study of the poet and his contribution to English literature.*

TAUSK, VICTOR (1879-1919). A Slovakian physician who became one of the most promising pupils of Sigmund Freud (q.v.). Tausk was one of nine children. His father was hypermoral and rigid in principles, although not in practice; his mother was warm and devoted to the family. Although Tausk was a handsome man and women were attracted to him, his marriage and his love affairs, including one with Lou Andreas-Salomé (q.v.), were not successful. He qualified in law. He also wrote poetry, stories, and plays, most of which were biographical. In his late twenties he suffered from a chest disease and depression that required a rest in a German sanatorium. On recovering, he decided to study medicine and to become a psychoanalyst. This was the beginning of his close contact with Freud and his dependence on him. Freud refused to analyze him, and, on his suggestion, Tausk became the first analytic patient of Helene Deutsch (q.v.), who was herself in analysis with Freud at the time. Tausk's analysis was discontinued on Freud's instructions. Some months later, faced with the unpleasantness of reversing his decision on yet another intended marriage, he committed suicide (q.v.). A gifted but difficult man, he made a particular contribution to the understanding of psychoses. Freud wrote a long and appreciative obituary for him but privately stated that he did not miss him and had considered him "a threat to the future."

Bibliography: Roazen, P. 1970. *Brother animal.*

TAVERNER, PETER. (fl. 1380-1403). Also known as Peter the porter. He was a treasurer of Bethlem Royal Hospital (q.v.) between 1388 and 1403. He was accused of embezzling funds meant for the care of the sick, stealing goods and chattels, and admitting undesirable characters, as well as unwanted children. He had used food meant for the inmates for himself and his friends, had allowed gambling and all kinds of immorality, and had extracted payment from the sick for wood and charcoal, which he bought cheaply during the summer and sold expensively in the winter. His wife sold beer at the gate of the hospital and caused such a noise that patients could not sleep. In 1403 Henry IV (q.v.) ordered an inquiry into the affairs of the hospital, and eighteen witnesses were called against Peter Taverner, who was fined and dismissed.

Bibliography: O'Donoghue, E. G. 1914. *The story of Bethlehem Hospital.*

TAVISTOCK CLINIC. A clinic established in London in 1920 with the aim of offering psychotherapy (q.v.) based on psychodynamic concepts to those patients unable to afford private treatment. Hugh Crichton-Miller was its founder and first director. The clinic was inspired by his work with army casualties during World War I. It subsequently became a pioneer in psychosomatic medicine (q.v.) and social psychiatry.

Bibliography: Dicks, H. V. 1970. *Fifty years of the Tavistock Clinic.*

TAY, WARREN (1843-1927). An English physician and ophthalmologist. In 1881 he described eye changes in a disorder due to an accumulation of fats in the cerebral cells and leading to severe mental retardation. This disorder is now known as "infantile amaurotic idiocy," or Tay-Sachs disease, as Bernard Sachs (q.v.) also studied the same disorder.

Bibliography: Tay, W. 1881. Symmetrical changes in the region of the yellow spot in each eye of an infant. *Tr. Ophth. Soc. U. K.* 1: 55-57.

TAYLOR, JEREMY (1613-1667). An English theologian and bishop of Down and Connor. In his *Ductor Dubitantium; or the Rule of Conscience* (1660), he described irrational fear, or phobia (*see* PHOBIAS), which he called "scruple." Accordingly to him, "a scruple is a great trouble of mind proceeding from a little motive, and a great indisposition, by which the conscience though sufficiently determined by proper arguments, dares not proceed to action, or if it doe, it cannot rest. . . ." He then went on to list several situations that provoke irrational fear. He also cited case histories in which he perceptively examined depression and its accompanying symptoms.

Bibliography: Hughes, H. T. 1960. *The piety of Jeremy Taylor.*

TCHAIKOVSKY, PETER ILICH (1840-1893). A Russian composer, homosexual by nature. Several individuals in his family were emotionally disturbed. His favorite brother, Modeste, and a nephew were homosexuals, an uncle was a religious fanatic, and a niece was a drug addict. His marriage was a tragic error, leading to a permanent separation after eleven weeks and to several suicide (q.v.) attempts by immersions in the icy water of the Neva river in the hope of catching pneumonia. His wife was admitted to a mental hospital. He was so obsessed with the idea that his head would fall off that he would hold it with his left hand while conducting. He formed an attachment to a wealthy widow, Nadezhda von Meck, who supported him financially and supplied him with a house. Although they corresponded for fourteen years, they never met. His fourth symphony was dedicated to her. After the break in their relationship, he composed his *Symphonie Pathétique* (q.v.), in which he expressed the tragic and melancholic aspects of his life. He regarded it as his own requiem and conducted its first performance nine

days before his death. He died of cholera, after deliberately drinking polluted water. His mother also had died of cholera.
Bibliography: Warrack, J. 1973. *Tchaikovsky.*

TEACHING OF PSYCHIATRY. In Europe the first formal teaching of psychiatry (q.v.) was untertaken by Vincenzo Chiarugi (q.v.) in the 1770s in Florence, Italy. He was followed by Philippe Pinel (1814) (q.v.) and Jean Esquirol (1817) (q.v.) in France. In Germany Ernst Horn (1806) and Johann Heinroth (1811) (q.v.) established courses in psychiatry.
Bibliography: Kraepelin, E. 1962. *One hundred years of psychiatry.*

TEDWORTH DRUMMER. The spirit of a vagrant drummer by the name of William Drury (fl. 1660). In 1662 his drum was confiscated, and he was later sentenced to transportation for some offences he had committed. From then on the house of the magistrate for Tedworth, England, John Mompesson, who had sentenced him, was haunted by drumming noises and by poltergeist (q.v.) activity. Joseph Glanvill (q.v.) investigated the phenomena and suggested that the Royal Society (q.v.) should study them. The happenings at Tedworth are probably the earliest psychical phenomena to be submitted to research by scientists.
Bibliography: Robbins, R. H. 1970. *The encyclopedia of witchcraft and demonology.*

TELEPATHY. A term coined in 1882 by Frederick W. H. Myers (q.v.) to describe "the communication of impressions of any kind from one mind to another independently of the recognized channels of sense."
See also PSYCHICAL PHENOMENA
Bibliography: Ashby, R. H. 1973. *The guidebook for the study of psychical research.*

TELESIO, BERNARDINO (1509-1588). An Italian philosopher. His system of philosophy rejected Aristotelian scholasticism (q.v.) and abstract reasoning in favor of knowledge that was based on experience and sensation from which, he believed, memory (q.v.) and reason were derived. His views on psychological matters were expressed in his book *De Natura Rerum Juxta Propria Principia* (1565-1586).
Bibliography: Van Deusen, N. C. 1932. *Telesio, the first of the moderns.*

TEMPERAMENT. The constitutional mental characteristics of man. Temperament has been of interest to both philosophers in antiquity and modern psychologists. Empedocles (q.v.) and his followers related temperament to the four bodily humors (q.v.); sanguine to blood, melancholic (*see* MELANCHOLIA) to black bile (q.v.), choleric (*see* CHOLER) to yellow bile, and phlegmatic to phlegm. Aristotle (q.v.) refined these principles and Galen (q.v.) went further by correlating disease to the temperaments. Much later, physiognomy (q.v.) linked certain facial features to personality. Typological

psychology (*see* PSYCHOLOGICAL TYPES) followed and attempted to relate physical characteristics to personality. This approach was particularly developed by Ernst Kretschmer (q.v.) and by Carl G. Jung (q.v.).
Bibliography: Jacques, D. H. 1888. *The temperaments.*

TEMPLES. Places dedicated to worship. In primitive civilizations sickness was believed to be sent by the gods, therefore, only their intercession could restore health. In time, priests transferred their activities from prayers and ceremonies to direct intervention and became physicians, but medicine remained based on temple practices. Most civilizations have practiced temple medicine, and examples can be found in Egypt (q.v.), Greece, and the Roman Empire. Perhaps the most famous temples in pre-Hippocratic times were those dedicated to Aesculapius (q.v.) in which incubation (q.v.) was the primary therapeutic approach. The separation of medicine from religion did not turn away the sick from the temples completely. Those who could not obtain a cure from science still turned for relief or comfort to the divinity. The strong suggestive influences of mystic places often succeeded when other methods failed, expecially in cases of hysterical (*see* HYSTERIA) disorders.
See also SHRINES.
Bibliography: Jayne, W. A. 1925. *The healing gods of ancient civilizations.*

TEMPLE SLEEP. *See* INCUBATION.

TEN DAYS IN A MAD-HOUSE. The title of a first-hand account of conditions in the New York Lunatic Asylum during the latter part of the nineteenth century. It was written by Nellie Bly (q.v.).
Bibliography: Bly, N. 1888. *Ten days in a mad-house.*

TENIERS, DAVID (THE YOUNGER) (1610-1690). An influential and prolific Dutch painter. His visual records of seventeenth-century rural Holland are conventional and provide an interesting contrast to the recurring themes of alchemy (q.v.), witchcraft (q.v.), the temptations of Saint Anthony, and other bizarre and suggestive motifs in his psychologically interesting pictures.
Bibliography: Davidson, J. P. 1980. *David Teniers the Younger.*

TENNESSEE LUNATIC ASYLUM. An American public institution for the mentally ill established in Nashville, Tennessee, in 1832 and opened in 1840. It was one of the state mental hospitals that were founded as a result of the curability (q.v.) cult, which changed the approach to the insane from mere custody to treatment.
Bibliography: Deutsch, A. 1949. *The mentally ill in America.*

TENNYSON, ALFRED (1809-1892). An English poet. During his lifetime he became the embodiment of Victorian sensibility and thought. His father

had been disinherited in favor of a younger brother and forced to become a clergyman; his disappointment and frustration found relief in excessive drinking and bouts of violent rage. Of the eleven children in the family, four were deeply disturbed, and one, who became insane at the age of nineteen, spent the last sixty years of his life in an asylum, the others were melancholic (see MELANCHOLIA) and eccentric. Tennyson had a lonely and miserable childhood and adolescence; he was extremely shy, untidy, and, although his writing talents were recognized, left Cambridge University without a qualification. His depression was increased by financial anxiety, the fear of becoming blind, and the worry of hereditary insanity. Instead a more tangible heredity improved his lot when his rich grandfather died leaving him a small fortune, which he later lost in an ill-fated scheme devised by Matthew Allen (q.v.), the apothecary to York Lunatic Asylum (q.v.). Tennyson changed his ways and added "d'Eyncourt" to his name, but fame still eluded him until the age of forty, when he published *In Memoriam* (1850); the poem was inspired by the death of his close friend, and prospective brother-in-law, Arthur Hallam, with whom Tennyson may have had a homosexual relationship, dating from his days at Cambridge. Marriage to Emily Sellwood had a stabilizing influence on Tennyson but his poetry changed for the worse once misery, guilt, and morbid thoughts were no longer his inspiration. In 1850, he was appointed Poet Laureate.
Bibliography: Turner, P. 1976. *Tennyson.*

TENON, JACQUES RENÉ (1724-1816). A French surgeon. In 1748 he was appointed surgeon to the Salpêtrière (q.v.). He investigated the need for mental hospitals in France and recommended several improvements, but he still advocated the use of chains to restrain the insane.
Bibliography: Zilboorg, G. 1941. *A history of medical psychology.*

TEPLOV, BORIS MIKHAILOVICH (1896-1965). A Russian neurologist remembered for his research on the typology of the nervous system and on individual differences.

TERESA (*or* THERESA), SAINT (1515-1582). A Spanish nun whose real name was Teresa de Cepeda y Ahumada. Her inclination toward mysticism was apparent even in childhood. When she was seven years old, she ran away from home hoping to be martyred among the Moors. She became a Carmelite nun before she was twenty years old and later founded numerous convents. She was given to deep melancholia (q.v.), that sometimes became so deep it extended into stupor. During ecstatic (*see* ECSTASY) states she had visions of Christ, the saints, and the devil, and she heard their voices telling

her what to do. She wrote mystical works and an autobiography entitled *Libro de su vida* (1562-1565).
Bibliography: Clissod, S. 1979. *St. Teresa of Avila.*

TERMAN, LEWIS MADISON (1877-1956). An American psychologist. He was particularly interested in intelligence tests (q.v.). His modification of the Binet scales came as the result of a series of studies published in 1916 and entitled *The Measurement of Intelligence.* He subsequently devised psychological tests for the American armed forces, for schools, and for the assessment of marital compatibility. Gifted children were the subject of one of his studies, which was published under the title of *Genetic Studies of Genius* in 1925.
Bibliography: Terman, L. M., and Merrill, M. A. 1937. *Measuring intelligence.*

TERTULLIANUS, QUINTUS SEPTIMIUS FLORENS (c. A.D. 160-230). One of the early Christian apologists, better known as Tertullian. He accepted the doctrine of the Stoics (q.v.) . He was well-versed in medicine, which he regarded as the sister of philosophy. In accordance with the beliefs of his time, he asserted that those subjected to trances and ecstatic (*see* ECSTASY) states were not in error, but divinely inspired and capable of transmitting great revelations and prophecies. Yet, he also wrote that "those who are made see one man in another, as Oreste saw his mother in his sister, Ajax beheld Ulysses in a heard of swine, Athamas and Agave wild beasts in their own children. . . ." For him the soul, which he located in the heart (q.v.), was the seat of sensation and of knowledge.
Bibliography: Barnes, T. D. 1971. *Tertullian: a historical and literary study.*

TESTA, PIETRO (1607?-1650). An Italian painter and etcher. His subjects, which were probably the cause of his lack of patrons, were strange and enigmatic and reminiscent of hallucinations (q.v.). He was a melancholic (*see* MELANCHOLIA) man, who was shy and solitary. When he drowned, it was rumored that he had committed suicide (q.v.) in a fit of depression.
Bibliography: Wittkower, R. and Wittkower, M. 1963. *Born under Saturn.*

TETANOID TYPE. A term coined by Erich R. Jaensch (q.v.) to describe an individual corresponding somewhat to the Extrovert Type (q.v.) in the typology devised by Carl G. Jung (q.v.).
See also BASEDOWOID TYPE.
Bibliography: Jaensch, E. R. 1925. *Die eidetik und die typologische Forschungsmethode.*

THAILAND. The first mental hospital in Thailand was established in 1889 at Klong Sarn, Dhonburi. A businessman by the name of Phra Bhakdi,

donated the building to King Chulalongkorn. The hospital accommodated thirty patients, and its function was mostly custodial. Treatment was primitive and included magical (*see* MAGIC) practices and herbal remedies.
Bibliography: Sangsingkeo, P. 1975. Thailand. In *World history of psychiatry*, ed. J. G. Howells.

THANATOPHOBIA. The term used by John B. Erhard (q.v.) to describe a type of depression in which the patient has a morbid fear of death.
Bibliography: Erhard, J. B. 1794. *Über die Melancholie*.

THANATOS. In Greek mythology (q.v.), the personification of death. He was believed to be the twin brother of Hypnos (q.v.). He had no father, but Night gave him birth. Sigmund Freud (q.v.) used the term to describe the death or destructive instinct.
Bibliography: Freud, S. 1920. *Beyond the pleasure principle*.

THEATER OF SPONTANEITY. A form of psychodrama (q.v.) in which the actors play unrehearsed parts. It was founded by Jacob L. Moreno (q.v.) in Vienna in 1921. From it, he developed a therapeutic approach designed to elucidate and correct faulty interpersonal relationships.
Bibliography: Moreno, J. L. 1947. *The theater of spontaneity: an introduction to psychodrama*.

THEDEN. (fl.19th century). A distinguished Prussian general. As a young man he was often in poor health. Eventually he became depressed and displayed suicidal inclinations. He was cured by drinking from twenty-four to thirty pints of cold water per day and, still on this course of water therapy (q.v.), lived to the age of eighty. His case was quoted by Jean Esquirol (q.v.).
Bibliography: Esquirol, J.E.D. 1845. Reprint. 1965. *Mental maladies: a treatise on insanity*.

THEMATIC APPERCEPTION TEST (TAT). A projection test devised in 1935 by Henry A. Murray in collaboration with Christian D. Morgan. The test involves the patient telling stories about scenes that are depicted on the cards he is shown.
Bibliography: Tomkins, S. 1947. *The thematic apperception test*.

THEMISON (c.123-43 B.C.). A Greek philosopher and physician who practiced in Rome. He was a pupil of Asclepiedes of Bithynia (q.v.). He systematized the theory of constriction and relaxation of the pores known as the *strictum and laxum* theory, and founded a school of medical thought known as "methodism." He was later criticized by Soranus (q.v.) for his cruel handling of mental patients. Among his prescriptions for them were darkness, restraint (q.v.) by chains, and deprivation of food and drink. The poet Juvenal (q.v.) satirized him and suggested that he killed more patients than he cured.

Bibliography: Zilboorg, G. 1941. *A history of medical psychology.*

THEOBROTION. A plant quoted by Pliny the Elder (q.v.) in his *Historia Naturalis.* He wrote that, according to Democritus (q.v.), it was a colorful plant with a pungent smell. It grew in Persia, where the kings used it mixed with their food or drink "for all maladies of the body and derangements of the mind."

Bibliography: Bonser, W. 1963. *The medical background of Anglo-Saxon England.*

THEODORIC (TEODORICO BORGOGNONI) (1205-1296). An Italian physician and bishop of Cervia. He was the son of Hugh of Lucca (q.v.), who taught him the art of surgery. He believed that functions could be retained even when part of the brain was removed. His name is also connected with the "soporific sponge," a sponge saturated with herbal juices that promoted drowsiness during surgical operations.

Bibliography: Garrison, F. H. 1929. *An introduction to the history of medicine.*

THEODORIC THE GREAT (c.455-526). The founder of the Ostrogothic monarchy. He was a tolerant and enlightened ruler, who brought peace and prosperity to Italy. Toward the end of his life he caused the judicial murders of Boethius (480?-?524) and of Symmachus (498-514). His guilt so disturbed him that hallucinations (q.v.) caused him to see the head of one of his victims in that of a fish he was served.

Bibliography: Hodgkin, T. 1923. *Theodoric the Goth.*

THEODOSIUS THE CENOBIARCH (c.423-529). His name means "chief of a community." He was born in Cappadocia and moved to Palestine, where he founded a monastery at Kathismus, near Bethlehem. Three hospitals were built by the side of the monastery and tended by the monks: one for the sick, one for the aged, and one for the insane. Insanity was believed to be divine punishment, and the patients were required to make penance. A special church was built for them, which they could attend while convalescing.

Bibliography: Attwater, D. 1965. *The Penguin dictionary of saints.*

THEOMANIA. A word coined by Jean Esquirol (q.v.) to indicate that class of the insane who believe they are God.

Bibliography: Esquirol, J.E.D. 1845. Reprint. 1965. *Mental maladies: a treatise on insanity.*

THEOPHRASTUS (c.372 B.C. - 287 B.C.). A Greek philosopher and botanist. He was a pupil of Plato (q.v.) and Aristotle (q.v.). Among his works are a treatise on black bile (q.v.) in which he related psychological and psychiatric observations to the humoral theory (q.v.) and a treatise on sensation, which was entitled *On Sense Perception and the Sensory Objects*. He believed that any disturbance of the brain was caused by a block in the canals carrying sensations to it. Theophrastus was among the first to recognize that opium (q.v.) relieved pain. He also is remembered for *The Characters*, a series of thirty caricatures of various human types.

Bibliography: Stratton, G. M. 1917. *Theophrastus and the Greek physiological psychology before Aristotle.*

THERAPEUTIC TRIALS. The first therapeutic trial in modern psychiatry (q.v.) was conducted on patients from Bethlem Royal Hospital (q.v.) in 1812 under the auspices of the sons of George III (q.v.), who hoped to find a cure for their father's insanity. The secret process for "Relieving and curing idiocy and lunacy and every species of insanity" was devised by Delahoyde and James Lucett (q.v.). Although for a time they managed to deceive their royal sponsors, they were eventually discredited.

Bibliography: Macalpine, I., and Hunter, R. 1969. *George III and the mad-business.*

THÉROIGNE DE MÉRICOURT (1762-1817). The pseudonym of Anne Joseph Terwagne, a famous courtesan and heroine of the French Revolution (q.v.), born in Luxembourg. In 1789 she corrupted the regiments of Flanders with money and loose women. A year later she roused the people of Liege against Versailles and haranged the mob from the terraces of the Tuileries. She set herself at the head of an army of women and was said to have decapitated a man with her sword, depite his being one of her former lovers. At the end of the revolution she became insane and was admitted to the Salpêtrière (q.v.). Jean Esquirol (q.v.) cited her case history.

Bibliography: Esquirol, J.E.D. 1845. Reprint. 1965. *Mental maladies: a treatise on insanity.*

THINKING TYPE. One of four function types classified by Carl G. Jung (q.v.). The other three are feeling, sensation and intuition types.

See also INTUITION TYPE and SENSATION TYPE.

Bibliography: Jung, C. G. 1923. *Psychological types*, trans. H. G. Baynes.

THIRUMURUGANPOONDI. An ancient Hindu shrine (q.v.) dedicated to the Lord Muruga. It was built around 100 B.C.. It is a place of pilgrimage for mental patients who gather around the temple and bathe in the three sacred wells (q.v.), under the supervision of the priests. The practice still continues, and cottages have been built to accommodate the visitors.

Bibliography: Somasundaran, O. 1973. Religious treatment of mental illness in Tamil Nadu. *Indian J. Psychiat.* 15: 38-48.

THIRUVIDAIMARUTHUR. A Hindu shrine (q.v.) in the district of Thanjavur in India. It is named after a sacred tree. It is a large and impressive temple built by the Chola King Virachola. Mental patients come to it seeking a miraculous cure.

Bibliography: Somasundaram, O. 1973. Religious treatment of mental illness in Tamil Nadu. *Indian J. Psychiat.* 15: 38-48

THISTLE. Burdock, *Arctium lappa*. In herbal folklore this plant is considered highly beneficial in a multitude of disorders. It was extensively employed in the treatment of the mentally ill. A brew made from its leaves was believed to relieve depression, dispel thoughts of suicide (q.v.), and cure loss of memory (q.v.) and insanity.

Bibliography: de Baïracli Levy, J. 1967. *Herbal handbook for everyone.*

THOMAS, DYLAN (1914–1953). A Welsh poet born in Swansea. His father, a teacher of English, was an embittered, taciturn, sarcastic man and a difficult father, who was described by Thomas's wife as "that most unhappy of all men I have ever met." His mother was unsociable and distant. A picture of his lonely childhood, estranged from his family, emerges from his autobiographical *Portrait of the Artist as a Young Dog* (1940). His disturbed young adulthood is portrayed in his *Adventures in the Skin Trade* (1955). Marriage was a strain for both partners. His irresponsibility, bizarre behavior, and alcoholism were notorious and made him, sadly, a cult figure. A book by his friend and sponsor, John Malcolm Brinnin suggests that Thomas committed suicide (q.v.) by consuming massive doses of whiskey when already dangerously ill. This theory has been strengthened by his widow, Catlin Thomas, in her book *Left Over Life to Kill* (1957): "Dylan would have made a better job of killing himself: for damnation he has done it, has he not?" His best known works are his poems, collected posthumously into one volume entitled *Collected Poems* (1953), and a play for voices, *Under Milk Wood* (1954). The latter displays great literary skill, humor, cynicism, and a forgiving, all-embracing humanity.

Bibliography: Jones, Daniel. 1977. *My friend Dylan Thomas.*

THOMISM. The ideological system of philosophy and theology of Thomas Aquinas (q.v.). It was based on the dogmatic principle of an all powerful father who is always right and controls all natural laws. Such a system discouraged investigation and change.

Bibliography: Kardiner, A. 1945. *The psychological frontiers of society.*

THOMPSON, FRANCIS (1859-1907). An English poet. He was the son of a physician and studied medicine himself but failed to qualify because of an aversion to blood and anatomical dissections. Before trying medicine, he had studied for the priesthood but had been rejected because of his unsuitable temperament. Before achieving fame, he lived a wandering life, trying to relieve his poverty by selling newspapers and matches. He became addicted

to laudanum (q.v.), possibly after reading *Confessions of an English Opium-Eater* (q.v.) by Thomas De Quincy (q.v.). The book had been given to him by his mother, shortly before her death. Treatment in a monastic hospital to relieve his addiction was only partially successful.
Bibliography: Reid, J. C. 1960. *Francis Thompson: man and poet.*

THOMPSON, GODFREY (1881-1955). A British psychologist. He continued the study of the correlation between mental traits that was begun by Francis Galton (q.v.) and further developed psychological statistics. He also was one of the psychologists who initiated the factorial analysis method of investigation. Educational psychology was another field in which he widely contributed.
Bibliography: Misiak, H., and Sexton, V. S. 1966. *History of psychology.*

THORNDIKE, EDWARD LEE (1874-1949). An American psychologist. He was a pioneer in mental testing and educational psychology. William James (q.v.) taught and inspired him, as well as offering him practical help with his animal learning experiments. When Thorndike's landlady refused to let him have chicks in his bedroom, James offered him space for them in his own house, where his children greeted the experimenter and his subjects with great delight. His experiments with a puzzle box (q.v.), which are regarded as the first laboratory studies on animal learning, proved that animals have no special insight and learn by trial and error. From animals he turned to the study of thought processes in children and to educational psychology. During World War I, he devoted much of his work to military psychology and helped to devise mental tests for the army.
Bibliography: Thorndike, E. L. 1931. *Human learning.*

THORSHAUG. The site of the first institution for the feebleminded in Christiania (now Oslo), Norway. It was opened by a Mr. Lippestad in 1871.
Bibliography: Barr, M. W. 1904. *Mental defectives.*

THRAETONA. A Persian mythological figure. He is said to have killed the serpent, or evil spirit, that caused disease. He, therefore, is regarded in Persian mythology as the first physician.
Bibliography: Elgood, C. 1951. *A medical history of Persia and the Eastern caliphate.*

THRASYLLUS. A Greek of the third century B.C. His behavior excited the curiosity of Heraclides of Pontus who recorded that the man was often seen on the Pireus, the docks of Athens, where he would note carefully the incoming and outgoing ships and their cargoes as he suffered from the delusion (q.v.) that they belonged to him. One day he recovered and became

aware that his wealth had existed only in his deranged mind. He then became sane but unhappy.
Bibliography: Rosen, G. 1968. *Madness in society.*

THREE-DIMENSIONAL THEORY. A theory developed by Wilhelm Wundt (q.v.) in 1896. According to it, it is possible to distinguish six main qualities of feeling, arranged in three pairs of opposites: pleasure — unpleasure, strain — relaxation, excitement — calm. The theory can be represented by three lines all intersecting at the zero point.
Bibliography: Wundt, W. 1896. *Grundiss der Psychologie.*

THREE KINGS. In the Middle Ages (q.v.) the names of the three wise kings, Jaspar (Casper), Melchysar (Melichior), and Baptizar (Balthazar), were engraved on cups, jewels, and other objects or charms against epilepsy (q.v.). Physicians also advised the use of such charms; for example, the French physician Bernard Gordon, who died in 1320, included it in his writings.
Bibliography: Evans, J. 1922. *Magical jewels.*

THRESHOLDS, MEASUREMENTS OF. A concept elaborated by Gustav Fechner (q.v.), who devised three independent psychophysical methods for the measurement of thresholds. He worked out that the sensation increases according to the logarithm of the stimulus (q.v.).
Bibliography: Fechner, G. T. 1860. *Elemente der psychophysic.*

THRIFT. *Ameria vluporis*, a wild plant. In herbal medicine a brew that is made from its flowers is used as a remedy for depression.
Bibliography: de Baïracli Levy, J. 1967. *Herbal handbook for everyone.*

THUDICHUM, JOHANN LUDWIG WILHELM(1829-1901). A German physician. After graduating from Giessen, he emigrated to England and settled in London, where he specialized in otolaryngology. He conducted research on the chemical identification of disease and worked on the chemical constitution of the brain. Thudichum believed that serious diseases of the brain and the spine were connected to changes in the neuroplasm and that when the chemistry of the brain was properly understood, many mental disorders could be treated. Neurochemistry was greatly advanced by his studies.
Bibliography: Drabkin, D. L. 1958. *Thudichum: chemist of the brain.*

THUGS. Originally members of the Indian religious sect that worshipped Kali (q.v.). Members propitiated the goddess by offerings of strangled victims. They became professional stranglers, who lived on the proceeds of robbery from their victims. The sect survived in India until the second half

of the nineteenth century, when British rule suppressed it. According to Meadows Taylor's investigation into the Thugs activities, at one time their victims numbered about forty thousand a year.
Bibliography: Taylor, M. 1839. *Confession of a Thug*.

THURNAM, JOHN L. (1810-1873). A British physician and medical superintendent of the York Retreat (q.v.) from 1838 to 1849. He was a great believer in the usefulness of records and statistics in psychiatry and, in 1845, he published the first book on this subject. Entitled *Observations and Essays on the Statistics of Insanity*, it examined the case histories of 244 patients treated at the York Retreat and concluded that the curability (q.v.)of insanity (q.v.) was doubtful. Another of his interests was the study of ancient skulls found in Britain.
Bibliography: Hunter, R., and Macalpine, I. 1963. *Three hundred years of psychiatry*.

THYME. *Thymus serpyllus*, a heathland plant. In addition to its oil, thymol, which is used in many preparations, a brew made from its leaves is used in herbal medicine for the treatment of nervous disorders, hysteria (q.v.), nightmares (q.v.), and psychosomatic complaints.
Bibliography: de Baïracli Levy, J. 1967. *Herbal handbook for everyone*.

THYMOS. One of the two aspects of the soul in Greek philosophy. It was that part of the soul involved in thought and emotion, and it died with the body.
Bibliography: Watson, R. I. 1963. *The great psychologists*.

TIBERINE ISLAND. An island in the Tiber River, Rome. According to legend, in 293 B.C. a group of Romans were sent to the temple of Aesculapius (q.v.) in Greece to ask the god to intercede in the plague then raging in Rome. On their return journey, they found a snake, the symbol of Aesculapius, in the boat. The snake went ashore on the Tiberine Island near Rome, and this was interpreted as a sign that a temple should be built there. The temple flourished for a long time and mental patients, treated there by incubation (q.v.) techniques, were said to be cured.
Bibliography: Mora, G. 1975. Italy. In *World history of psychiatry*, ed. J. G. Howells.

TIBERIUS, CLAUDIUS NERO (42 B.C.-A.D. 37). A Roman emperor. When he was three years old his mother, Livia Drusilla was divorced by his father, so that Augustus (63 B.C.-A.D. 14) could marry her. The same imperial power compelled him to divorce his wife and marry Augustus' notorious daughter, Julia (39 B.C.-14 A.D.), who brought him much unhappiness and shame. He succeeded Augustus as emperor, and his first years on the throne were enlightened and just. He later changed into a suspicious individual, living in continual fear of assassination. For a time he lived in

Capri and indulged in brutish sexual practices. Murders, plots, and gloom surrounded him. In his old age he became intensely superstitious and his behavior suggests that he may have been insane.
Bibliography: Seager, R. 1972. *Tiberius.*

TICEHURST ASYLUM. A private asylum (q.v.) in Sussex, England. It was opened in 1792 and run by the Newington family for over a hundred years. It was a luxury establishment for the upper classes. It possessed extensive grounds, and the patients enjoyed privacy and relative freedom. John T. Perceval (q.v.) was a patient there between 1832 and 1834. When it was damaged by fire in 1852, spacious new premises were built to replace the old house. It is still functioning as a private mental nursing home.
Bibliography: Parry-Jones, W. Ll. 1972. *The trade in lunacy: private madhouses in England in the eighteenth and nineteenth century.*

TICONAL. An Indian idol particularly honored in Bengal, India. During the feast in his honor, followers often go in trancelike states and inflict wounds upon themselves that are often serious enough to cause death.
Bibliography: Esquirol, J. E. D. 1845. Reprint. 1965. *Mental maladies: a treatise on insanity.*

TICS. The term "tique" originally was used to indicate a disorder occurring in horses. It was characterized by a sudden stop in breathing while running. In the eighteenth century, French physicians used the term to describe a number of human disorders related to the intermittent, involuntary closure of the eyes. Edouard Brissaud (q.v.) investigated patients with tics and concluded that the disorder had a psychogenic aetiology. He came to believe that those suffering from it were victims of an "abnormal psychiatric state."
Bibliography: Meige, H., and Feindel, W. 1907. *Tics and their treatment.*

TIEDEMANN, FRIEDRICH (1781-1861). A German anatomist. He conducted extensive research on the nervous system, studied the embryonic development of the brain, and determined the capacity of the skull by filling it with millet seed, which he then weighed. He also initiated the comparison of human and animal brains, thus giving impetus to comparative anatomy.
Bibliography: Clarke, E., and Dewhurst, K. 1974. *An illustrated history of brain function.*

TIMAEUS. One of the dialogues of Plato (q.v.). In it a demon is discussed in such a way that it could be linked to a spiritual guide or the superego of Sigmund Freud (q.v.).
Bibliography: Plato. *Timaeus*, trans. J. Warrington.

TIMON. A Greek misanthrope of the fifth century B.C. He was a contemporary of Socrates (q.v.). He lived in seclusion and hated all mankind, after discovering the ingratitude of his former friends. He grew a fig tree so that he could have a branch from which to hang himself. William Shakespeare (q.v.) based his tragedy *Timon of Athens* on earlier sources of the well-known story of Timon.

Bibliography: Fedden, H. R. 1938. *Suicide.*

TISSOT, CLÉMENT JOSEPH (1750-1826). A French physician. He was interested in the effects of emotion on physical diseases. In 1798, at the invitation of the Academie de Chirurgie of Paris, he wrote *On the Influence of the Passions of the Soul on Diseases, and Means of Overcoming their Ill-Effect.* According to him, cheerfulness, laughter, and music were forms of therapy that encouraged the process of recovery.

Bibliography: Zilboorg, G. 1941. *A history of medical psychology.*

TISSOT, SIMON ANDRÉ (1728-1797). A Swiss physician and the head of the College de Médecine of Lausanne. In 1761 he wrote *Avis au People sur sa Santé,* a work on public health. It became so popular that it went through ten editions and was translated into many languages. It was followed by other books on the health of scholars, whom he warned against excessive study, and the health of fashionable people, his aristocratic patients. His major work was the *Traité de l'Epilepsie* (1770) in which he isolated the clinical syndrome of epilepsy (q.v.). Although he rejected superstitions concerning the aetiology of epilepsy, he maintained that masturbation (q.v.) was an important cause and advised trephining (*see* TREPANATION) as a form of treatment. He also wrote on nervous diseases, which he believed were linked to passions and to the effect of the imagination (q.v.) on the nervous system.

Bibliography: Diethelm, O. 1975. Switzerland. In *World history of psychiatry,* ed. J. G. Howells.

TITCHENER, EDWARD BRADFORD (1867-1927). An English psychologist. His family, which on his mother's side included Thomas à Becket (1118-1170) in its ancestry, had planned for him to make a career in the church, since they thought he would make an Anglican Bishop, but changes in the family's fortunes channeled his studies in other directions. After studying at Oxford University, he became a pupil of Wilhelm Wundt (q.v.) in Leipzig, where he met many prominent psychologists. In 1895, he became professor of psychology at Cornell University in Ithaca, New York. From that date on, he lived in the United States. His main field of study was the normal adult mind, which he investigated by controlled introspective analysis. Because he believed that psychology was not firmly established in the United States, he translated books by Wundt, Oskar Külpe (q.v.), and others into English and wrote a number of textbooks as well as a four-volume treatise entitled *Experimental Psychology: A Manual of Laboratory Practice*

(1901-1905). It is now considered his most important work. For a time he was an editor of the *American Journal of Psychology* (q.v.). In 1904 he founded an informal group called the Experimental Psychologists, which after his death became the Society of Experimental Psychologists. During the last decade of his life he devoted less of his time and energy to psychology and developed other interests, including numismatics, thus his projected series of books on a system of psychology was never completed.

Bibliography: Boring, E. G. 1950. *A history of experimental psychology.*

TOAD STONE. A stone that was believed to be obtained from the head of a toad. The superstition persisted from the Middle Ages (q.v.) to the seventeenth century. Magical (*see* MAGIC) curative properties were attributed to the stone. It was believed that it was beneficial in a multitude of disorders, acted as an antidote to poison, protected its wearer from bewitchment, and cured epilepsy (q.v.) and vertigo. Albertus Magnus (q.v.) and Desiderus Erasmus (q.v.) were among those who believed in it. Queen Elizabeth I (1533-1603) had a toad stone set in gold.

Bibliography: Forbes, T. R. 1972. Lapis bufonis: the growth and decline of a medical superstition. *Yale J. Biol. Med.* 45: 139-49.

TOBACCO. Perhaps the first narcotic to be used in South America. Its consumption there was orginally restricted to ritual ceremonies. The earliest detailed description of tobacco was written in 1577 by the Spanish physician and botanist Nicholas Monardes (1493-1588). According to him, American Indians smoked the leaf of the tobacco plant to "make themselve drunke withall, and to see the visions, and things that represent unto them that wherein they do delight." He added that by smoking they were able to predict the outcome of business transactions and other ventures. A decade later Thomas Harriot (1560-1621), an English scientist, wrote that tobacco preserved the health and cured "many grievous diseases." In 1602 Sir William Vaughan (1577-1641) suggested "cane tobacco well-dried, and taken in a silver pipe" as a remedy for hysteria (q.v.). A short while later the belief in the curative properties of tobacco declined. It was said that it "bread melancholy" and "hurt the mind," as well as causing a multitude of other ills. In 1590 the Catholic Church banned tobacco smoking under threat of excommunication. In the seventeenth century, smoking was regarded as a passing fad, but some rulers prohibited it. The Emperor Jahangir of Hindustan decreed that smokers were to have their lips cut, as tobacco damaged physical and mental health; in Russia smokers had their noses slit and, if they persisted, were condemned to death. Despite these drastic measures, tobacco smoking became popular, especially after a belief in its aphrodisiac properties had been added to its other pleasant qualities. Benjamin Rush (q.v.) thought that the smoke of tobacco had sedative properties and that

it tended "not only to produce what is called a train of perception, but to hush the agitated passions into silence and order."
Bibliography: Emboden, W. 1972. *Narcotic plants.*
Rush, B. 1786. *An Inquiry into the Influence of Physical Causes upon the Moral Faculty.*

TODD, ELI (1769-1833). An American physician. He became interested in mental disorders after investigating the conditions of patients in asylums (q.v.). In 1822 he became one of the founders of the Society for Relief of the Insane, and two years later he was elected the first superintendent of the Hartford Retreat (q.v.). Under his leadership, the need for trained personnel was recognized. He was among the first to regard alcoholism (q.v.) as a clinical disorder that needed treatment rather than punishment.
Bibliography: Dain, N. 1964. *Concepts of insanity in the United States, 1789-1865.*

TOLCATZIN. A plant indigenous to South America. The ancient Aztecs believed that ingesting its leaves would cause insanity.
Bibliography: Leon, C. A., and Rosselli, H. 1975. Latin America. In *World history of psychiatry*, ed. J. G. Howells.

TOLEDO. One of the earliest mental hospitals in Spain was founded in Toledo in 1483 by the aspostolic nuncio, Francisco Ortiz. He adapted his own house to receive the insane and called it the Hospital of the Innocents, although later the asylum (q.v.) became known simply as the House of the Nuncio. New premises were built in 1793, and, soon after, the hospital became famous for its pleasant external structure, which unfortunately was not matched by its rather cramped and dark interior.
Bibliography: Chamberlain, A. S. 1966. Early mental hospitals in Spain. *Am. J. Psychiat.* 123: 143-49.

TOLLKISTE. An early German term meaning "mad cell." One such building is mentioned in the Hamburg municipal records for 1373.
See also ASYLUMS.
Bibliography: Rosen, G. 1968. *Madness in society.*

TOLLKOBEN. A German term meaning "mad hut." Small huts were used in medieval Germany to lock up the insane. When the Grosse Hospital in Erfurt (q.v.), Germany, was rebuilt in 1385, it had such a cell included in its structure.
See also ASYLUMS.
Bibliography: Rosen, G. 1968. *Madness in society.*

TOLMAN, EDWARD CHACE (1886-1959). An American psychologist. At Harvard University he studied under Edwin Holt (q.v.) and was greatly influenced by him. Following his experiments with rats in mazes (*see* MAZE),

he concluded that most learning behavior is motivated by expectancy, rather than by reward, and by the will to reach a goal through trial and error.
Bibliography: Tolman, E. C. 1932. *Purposive behavior in animals and men.*

TOLSTOY, LEO (1828-1910). A Russian writer. His mother died when he was a baby and he retained an idealized image of her, often longing for maternal love, although an affectionate aunt cared for him. He was so ugly that at times he contemplated suicide (q.v.) as he felt that no one could love him. His own shortcomings made him despair until he came to terms with human imperfections, which he was able to do after discovering the philosophy of Jean-Jacques Rousseau (q.v.). Rousseau became his hero, and he wore a medallion depicting him around his neck. He tried to put into practice idealistic theories on his estate, but the time and the people were not ready for them, and he was regarded almost as a madman. After his marriage his life and writings provide a remarkable demonstration of marital strife. His wife, Sonya, craved his attention and was delighted when she could help with his novels, but he came to despise them and preferred his religio-philosophical works. He worshipped ideas; she reality. They were happier when they were apart; this is vividly apparent from their intimate diaries, which increased marital conflict because the couple was in the habit of reading each other's entries. *The Kreutzer Sonata* (q.v.) and *The Devil* (1889) contain autobiographical passages about his marriage. Throughout his life he felt guilty about his passionate physical nature, and in his old age he became a professed misogynist. In 1910, as the strife came to its climax, his wife accused him of homosexuality and threatened suicide. The psychiatrist Gregory Rossolimo (q.v.), after an overnight stay, gave as his diagnosis "double degeneracy, paranoia and hysteria" and advocated separation. Tolstoy fled with his doctor, and some days later was joined by his daughter Sasha. After his departure, his wife attempted suicide by drowning, and another psychiatrist was called to see her. A few days later Tolstoy lay dying of pneumonia. His wife came to him with her psychiatrist and another doctor, but, for fear of upsetting him, she was not allowed to see him until he was breathing his last.
Bibliography: Troyat, H. 1967. *Tolstoy.*

TOM O'BEDLAM. A term used to describe beggars who claimed to be patients from Bethlem Royal Hospital (q.v.) to induce sympathy and gain offerings of money, food, shelter, etc. They were not real patients, as the hospital never authorized begging. In 1675 and again in 1676, the governors of the hospital issued official disclaimers of this practice.
See also BESS O'BEDLAM.
Bibliography: O'Donoghue, E. G. 1914. *The story of Bethlehem Hospital.*

TONSURE. The shaving of the head, or of a circular patch on the crown, prescribed by some religious orders. Like trepanation (q.v.), it may have originated as an early ceremony connected with the expulsion of evil spirits. It later became a hygienic measure designed to keep the head cool and prevent those mental disorders believed to be caused by heated vapors within the skull. The Dutch physician Liéven Lemnius (q.v.) wrote of the desirability of shaving the crown of the head: "For thereby grass vapours which hurt the Memory, have more scope and liberty to evaporate and fume out." He recommended tonsure "for the redresse of certayne diseases of the head, losse of right witts, feeblenes of brayne, dottrye, phrensies, Bedlem madnesse, Melancholike affections, furie and franticke fitts. . . ." From the sixteenth to the eighteenth century, the heads of the insane were shaved to facilitate the application of blistering substances, which were believed to relieve insanity by causing suppuration (q.v.).

TOPAZ. According to Girolamo Cardano (q.v.) the topaz cures madness and makes its wearer prudent and wise.
See also PRECIOUS STONES.
Bibliography: Evans, J. 1922. *Magical jewels.*

TORMENTIL. *Potentilla erecta,* a perennial herb found in the Azores, Siberia, and Europe. In Russian folk medicine it was used to make concoctions that were prescribed for nervous disorders.
Bibliography: Kourennoff, P. M., and St. George, G.1970. *Russian folk medicine.*

TORQUEMADA, TOMÁS DE (1420?-1498). A Spanish nobleman. His grandfather had married a Jew, thus, in the eyes of his family, polluting the purity of their aristocratic blood. Torquemada grew up with a fanatic hatred of Jews. He became a Dominican monk and was appointed inquisitor general for all the Spanish territories. In 1487 he became the grand inquisitor by order of Innocent VIII (q.v.). His psychopathic (*see* PSYCHOPATHY) cruelty resulted in the death of over a thousand people at the stake and the torture and imprisonment of many more.
Bibliography: Hope, T. 1939. *Torquemada: scourge of the Jews.*

TORY ROT. Benjamin Rush (q.v.) invented this term to refer to those who had no sympathy with the American Revolution. He regarded them as mentally deranged and was convinced that many died of insanity.
Bibliography: Lloyd, J. H. 1930. Benjamin Rush and his critics. *Annals of Medical History.* Vol. 2, pp. 470-75.

TOTEM. An object of veneration among primitive people. According to Sir James Frazer (q.v.), a totem was linked to the belief in an outward soul that could take refuge in it and, thus, avoid danger. Sigmund Freud (q.v.)

investigated theories on the derivation of totemism and divided them into three groups: nominalistic, sociological, and psychological.

Bibliography: Freud, S. 1913. *Totem and tabu.*
Levi-Strauss, C. 1964. *Totemism.*

TOUCHET, ELEANOR (?-1652). An English writer of prophecies. George Ballard (1706-1755) included a biography of her in his *Memoirs of Several Ladies of Great Britain*, written in 1752. According to him, she suffered from the delusion (q.v.) that she was able to predict the future. She married Sir John Davies and had two children, one of whom was an idiot (q.v.) who died in infancy. She announced to her husband that he would soon die and accordingly dressed herself in widow's weeds, which eventually proved appropriate as Sir John died within three years of her prophecy. She interpreted the book of Daniel and saw hidden meanings in the Bible (q.v.). These she published with the result that she was tried for insulting high-ranking ecclesiastical and lay people, including the king, Charles I (1600-1649). She was imprisoned in the Gatehouse at Westminister for two years, after which she was transferred to Bethlem Royal Hospital (q.v.). She remained there for seven years, but even after her discharge, she continued to produce incoherent and fanatical writings until she died.

Bibliography: O'Donoghue, E. G. 1914. *The story of Bethlehem Hospital.*

TOULOUSE-LAUTREC, HENRI DE (1864-1901). A French painter of aristocratic birth. His father's interest in horses was exceeded only by his interest in women. His mother was overly religious. Toulouse-Lautrec called her "my poor dear saint," and could not bear to be separated from her. After two accidents in childhood, his legs atrophied and remained extremely short. His facial features were ugly, and his speech, especially when excited, almost unintelligible. Despite these handicaps, Toulouse-Lautrec never indulged in self-pity, but concentrated his pride in his body on his genitalia, the only parts that were overdeveloped. He yearned for women, but only prostitutes would accept his attentions; he practically lived in brothels and contracted syphilis (q.v.) early in life. In 1899, he was admitted to an asylum (q.v.) in Neuilly near the Bois de Boulogne. The breakdown had been precipitated by his mother's departure from Paris and followed a period of confinement at home, where he was cared for by male nurses. While in the asylum, he drew a series of circus sketches known as *Le Cirque*. These so impressed the doctors that they agreed that he could not be insane and consented to his release. Toulouse-Lautrec commented "I have purchased my liberty with my drawings." But his debauchery and alcoholism (q.v.) soon returned and hastened his death.

Bibliography: Fermigier, A. 1969. *Toulouse-Lautrec*, trans. P. Stevenson.

TOWER OF SILENCE. A special laboratory erected at Koltushi in the Soviet Union in 1913, under the supervision of Ivan Pavlov (q.v.). It con-

sisted of soundproofed rooms heated to a constant uniform temperature and artificially lighted to exclude external stimuli. The building was used for Pavlov's experiments on conditioned reflexes.
Bibliography: Babkin, B. P. 1951. *Pavlov: a biography.*

TRANQUILLIZER. A special armchair designed by Benjamin Rush (q.v.) to replace the straitjacket for violent patients. The prototype of it was made by a cabinet maker called Benjamin Lindall. The advantage of the chair was that it allowed the patient lashed to it to remain in a comfortable position while being treated. Rush called it a "tranquillizer" and claimed that it had a positive therapeutic effect in that it did not restrict the circulation or impede the flow of blood to and from the brain. Many psychiatrists, including Friedrich Groos (q.v.) and Johann C. Heinroth (q.v.) considered it an indispensible aid in their practice, but others discerned the dangers of leaving patients tied to the chair for prolonged periods of time. Carl Jacobi (q.v.) cited the case of a patient who was sat in it for six months.
Bibliography: Kraepelin, E. 1962. *One hundred years of psychiatry.*

TRANSFERENCE. The term employed by Sigmund Freud (q.v.) in 1905 to describe the "new editions and facsimiles of the tendencies and fantasies which are aroused and made conscious during the process of analysis," whereby "the person involved is replaced by the physician."
Bibliography: Freud, s. 1905. "A case of hysteria."

TRANSPORT. During the nineteenth century, specially constructed horse carriages were used to transport the insane to asylums (q.v.). They were sturdy and, usually, furnished with barred windows to prevent escape. Entry was through the rear.

TRAUMATAPHOBIA. A concept formulated by Sandor Rado (q.v.), that postulates that a traumatized ego tries to avoid further traumatic experiences.
Bibliography: Rado, S. 1953. *Recent advances in psychoanalytic therapy.*

TRAVELING. Seneca (q.v.) believed that it was of little benefit in the treatment of mental disorders and quoted the reply of Socrates (q.v.) to a melancholic (*see* MELANCHOLIA) who was disappointed at having not derived any advantage from his travels, "I am not surprised; do you not travel with yourself?" Celsus (q.v.) recommended it for those who contemplated suicide (q.v.). Jean Esquirol (q.v.) thought it was good for the insane to travel as it promoted sleep, appetite, and secretions, as well as providing the patient with material for conversation, other than his illness. In the

nineteenth century, English physicians usually sent their mental patients to France, Italy, or the colonies.
Bibliography: Esquirol, J.E.D. 1845. Reprint. 1965. *Mental Maladies: a treatise on insanity.*

TREATISE OF ANGER, A. A book by John Downame (q.v.), published in 1609. It is actually a later edition of his previous work, which was entitled, *Spiritual Physicke to Cure the Diseases of the Soul.* In this work, Downame distinguished two kinds of anger and set out to describe "the lawful, laudable, and necessarie use of just and holy Anger" and the kinds, cause, effects, and treatment of "currupt and unjust Anger."
Bibliography: Hunter, R., and Macalpine, I. 1963. *Three hundred years of psychiatry.*

TREATISE OF MELANCHOLIE, A. A textbook on psychiatry by Timothy Bright (q.v.). It was the first English book devoted exclusively to psychiatry. It was printed in London by Thomas Vautrollier and published in 1586. The volume sets forth the cause of melancholia (q.v.), describes its psychological and somatic symptoms, differentiates between melancholy and "afflicted conscience," and offers spiritual advice as well as physical prescriptions. It is interspersed with "philosophical discourses" for the entertainment of the reader. William Shakespeare (q.v.) incorporated some of Bright's material into his work, and it has been speculated (e.g. by Dover Wilson in *What Happens in 'Hamlet'?*) that the poet may have read Bright's book in proof form while helping the printer. Robert Burton (q.v.), in his *Anatomy of Melancholy* (q.v.) quoted items from the work.
Bibliography: Bright, T. 1586. Reprint. 1969. *A treatise of melancholie.*

TREATISE OF THE SPLEEN AND VAPOURS, A (or, hypochondriacal and hysterical affections.) A work by Sir Richard Blackmore (q.v.) published in London in 1725. It theorized that the spleen (q.v.) was a part of the procreational system and designed for the preservation of the species. Blackmore defined "affections of the spleen" as "a distemper belonging to the whole system of animal spirits." The treatise was a progressive work in many aspects. It considered the development of mental disorder from its mild beginning to the more severe forms as a continuum. Melancholia (q.v.), a term then reserved for insanity, was used by Blackmore to mean depression. In the section on treatment, "pacifick medicines" (q.v.) are recommended, especially opium (q.v.).
Bibliography: Hunter, R., and Macalpine, I. 1963. *Three hundred years of psychiatry.*

TREATISE ON INSANITY. The title of the English translation (1806) of *Traité Médico-philosophique sur l'aliénation mentale, ou la manie* by Philippe Pinel (q.v.). First published in 1801, it quickly gained respect and popularity in the field of mental health. It was based on his experiences at

Bicêtre (q.v.) and stressed his belief in moral medicine (q.v.). It also offered practical guidance on hospital administration.
Bibliography: Pinel, P. 1801. Reprint. 1962. *A treatise on insanity*, trans. D. D. Davis.

TREATISE ON MADNESS, A. A book by Dr. William Battie (q.v.) published in 1758. It was the first English textbook of this title and the first written by a medical author who had acquired his experience through his work in a mental hospital, Saint Luke's Hospital for Lunatics (q.v.). Battie wrote the book as a guide for his students. His views were strongly challenged by Dr. John Monro (q.v.) in a volume entitled *Remarks on Dr. Battie's Treatise on Madness* (1758). The controversy that ensued reverberated throughout the medical world of the time.
Bibliography: Hunter, R., and Macalpine, I., eds. 1962. *A psychiatric controversy of the eighteenth century.*

TREDGOLD, ALFRED FRANK (1870-1952). A British physician and authority on mental deficiency. Soon after qualifying in 1899, he was offered a research scholarship in insanity and mental disorders. It enabled him to study in depth mental deficiency in all its aspects. In 1905 he was a member of the Royal Commission on the Feebleminded. The findings of the commission led to the Mental Deficiency Act of 1913. His *Textbook on Mental Deficiency*, first published in 1908, went through several editions and continues to be considered the most authoritative work in its field. In advance of his time, he recognized the importance of family relationships in the management of mental defectives. He was also the author of a work on psychological medicine.
Bibliography: Tredgold, A. F. 1943. *Manual of psychological medicine.*

TREGAGAS, RAGNHILD (fl.1320). The first individual ever to be tried for witchcraft (q.v.) in Norway. The trial, in 1325, was conducted by Bishop Andfinn. The accused was found to be insane and acquitted.
Bibliography: Retterstøl, N. 1975. Scandinavia. In *World history of psychiatry.* ed. J. G. Howells.

TRÉLAT, ULYSSES (1795-1879). A French surgeon. In 1837 he was appointed assistant physician to Salpêtrière (q.v.). His interest in mental disorders prompted him to write *Alienation Mentale* in 1827, which was reissued in 1839 under the title *Researches Historiques sur la Folie.* He argued that mental patients should be protected from legal punishment if the crimes of which they are accused are related to their conditions. He introduced the concept and term of "arson insanity."
Bibliography: Trélat, U. 1839. *Researches historiques sur la folie.*

TREPANATION. The removal of a piece of bone from the skull. The operation is one of the earliest known to man and may date back as far as

ten thousand years. Trepaned skulls, some dating from Neolithic times, have been found in Europe, Asia, Africa, North, Central, and South America, and Oceania. It originally was performed to allow evil spirits to escape from the heads of possessed (*see* POSSESSION) people. It later was used as a form of prevention therapy. From the Middle Ages (q.v.) until the nineteenth century, it was a common procedure not only in the treatment of head injuries but also in the treatment of persistent headache, epilepsy (q.v.), and mental disorders. In the early 1900s some Cornish miners still requested a "boring" after head injuries. The operation continues to be performed in primitive African tribes. Posthumous trepanations were performed in early times in Europe and, more recently, in Africa to obtain roundels of skulls which were polished, drilled, and worn as charms against evil spirits.
Bibliography: Brothwell, D., and Sandison, A. T. 1967. *Diseases in antiquity.*

TRISKAIDEKAPHOBIA. A term derived from the Greek to indicate a morbid fear of the number thirteen. The origin of the superstition has been linked with the Last Supper, when thirteen sat at the table and one later betrayed Christ. If the thirteenth day of a month falls on a Friday, it is regarded with particular horror by the superstitious, as Friday was "hangman's day," or the day when, in England, criminals were brought to the gallows. In the United States, hotels and blocks of offices avoid numbering rooms or floors with the number thirteen.
Bibliography: Hinsie, L. E., and Campbell, R. J. 1960., *Psychiatric dictionary.*

TRISTAM (or TRISTAN). The hero of a medieval legend. A part of the legend concerns the madness of Tristam, who becomes dominated by the suspicion of Isolde's (q.v.) infidelity and vainly tries to forget her. Madness is a recurring theme throughout the story: Tristam is mad with love after drinking a magic filter; he becomes insane with jealousy (q.v.), and he pretends madness, disguising himself as a beggar, to be admitted to the presence of Isolde. In some versions of the legend both lovers experience psychosomatic death as they die of despair.
Bibliography: Sutcliff, R. 1974. *Tristan and Iseult.*

TRISTIMANIA. A term proposed by Benjamin Rush (q.v.) to replace melancholia (q.v.). He argued that because the term "melancholy," was derived from the Greek and meant black bile (q.v.), it perpetuated the wrong humoral theory (q.v.). He claimed that the term he proposed described the depressive and manic phases of the disorder, which he described as "this form of madness when erroneous opinions respecting a man's person, affairs, or condition, are the subject of his distress."
Bibliography: Rush, B. 1812. Reprint. 1962. *Medical inquiries and observations upon the diseases of the mind.*

TRITHEMIUS, JOHANNES (1462-1516). The Latinized name of Johann Tritheim, whose real name was Heidenberg. He was the abbot of a German

monastery, a great scholar, and a gentle humanist. Joachim of Brandenburg (1484-1535) asked him to write a book on witches (*see* WITCHCRAFT); he produced a treatise entitled *Antipalus Maleficiorum* (q.v.) which reflects the general hysterical fear of witches prevalent during his lifetime. He also wrote two works on the art of cipher writing, *Stenographia* and *Polygraphia*. Despite the author's protestations, they were regarded as manuals of magic (q.v.).
Bibliography: Zilboorg, G. 1941. *A history of medical psychology.*

TROLL, PATRICK. The fictitious author of a collection of letters published in 1923 under the title *Book of the Id*. The letters were addressed to a woman on the subject of the influence of the unconscious (q.v.) on her conscious life. The author was Georg Groddeck (q.v.).
Bibliography: Groddeck, G. 1950. *The Book of the Id.*

TROLLOPE, ANTHONY (1815-1882). An English novelist, born in London. He felt neglected by his parents, especially his ineffectual father. As a schoolboy he was lonely and miserable. The poverty and emotional deprivation he endured in his early life left him with a sense of inferiority that often caused him to assert himself by being disagreeable, offensive, and touchy. He worked in the General Post Office. His output as an author was enormous and his novels were extremely popular. They offer a realistic picture of nineteenth-century life and reflect an uncommon psychological understanding.
Bibliography: Pope Hennessy, J. 1971. *Anthony Trollope.*

TROMBA CULT. A practice in Madagascar in which a whole tribe offer prayers to the gods until some of those present are "possessed" (*see* POSSESSION) by the spirit of a god. In a state of ecstasy (q.v.) , they prophesy and offer answers to the questions that prompted the prayers.
Bibliography: Ellenberger, H. F. 1970. *The discovery of the unconscious.*

TROPENKOHLER. A term used to describe a disorder usually found among young African males. It resembles amok (q.v.) but is less violent. Those afflicted by it become argumentative and aggressive to the point of frenzy, but, once the attack is over, they are prostrated with exhaustion.
Bibliography: Goldenson, R. M. 1970. *The encyclopedia of human behavior.*

TROPHAEUM MARIANO-CELLENSE. A seventeenth-century illustrated manuscript. It is the diary of Christoph Haizmann (q.v.), a "possessed" (*see* POSSESSION) man.
Bibliography: Macalpine, I., and Hunter, R. 1956. *Schizophrenia 1677.*

TROPISM. A theory enunciated by Jacques Loeb (q.v.) in 1890. According to it, the behavior of organisms is dependent on physical-chemical elements;

sensation or pleasure have no importance. Tropistic behavior does not consider consciousness.
Bibliography: Loeb, J. 1918. *Forced movements, tropisms, and animal conduct.*

TROTTER, THOMAS (1760-1832). A British naval surgeon. In 1807 he wrote *A View of the Nervous Temperament.* A year later, it became the first psychiatric book to be printed in the United States. The book emphasized the importance of the emotions in precipitating somatic diseases, especially if the patient had an hereditary predisposition to mental disorders. Among the causative factors he listed were "peculiar modes of living." He wrote also on alcoholism (q.v.) which he had observed closely in the navy. His campaign against it resulted in the closure of hundreds of gin (q.v.) shops.
Bibliography: Hunter, R., and Macalpine, I. 1963. *Three hundred years of psychiatry.*

TROTTER, WILFRED BATTEN LEWIS (1872-1939). A British neurosurgeon and physiologist. His work influenced social psychology and his writings on herd psychology set forth new ideas. He also wrote on cutaneous sensation in man and on the surgery of malignant tumors of the brain and the spinal cord.
Bibliography: Trotter, W. 1916. *Instincts of the herd in peace and war.*

TROTULA (c.1050 - ?). An Italian woman physician famous for her connection with the Salerno Medical School (q.v.). A medical work on the diseases of women has been attributed to her and usually is referred to as *The Trotula.* It was written in verses, probably to facilitate its memorization. Among other disorders, it mentions epilepsy (q.v.) and the black bile (q.v.) believed to cause melancholia (q.v.). The volume was popular for 500 years.
Bibliography: Harington, J. 1920. *The school of Salernum.*

TROXLER, IGNAZ PAUL VITALIS (1780-1866). A Swiss-German philosopher and physician. He was particularly interested in mental deficiency, which he regarded as a form of endemic human degeneration that could be cured. He was an admirer of the work of Jakob Guggenbühl (q.v.) and contributed a leading paper to the second issue of *Beobachtungen Über den Cretinismus* (q.v.) .
Bibliography: Kanner, L. 1964. *A history of the care and study of the mentally retarded.*

TRUTH DRUG. The popular term for scopolamine, an alkaloid. Dr. Robert E. House (1875-1930), an American obstetrician, was the first to use it as a truth drug. It causes a state of lethargy during which defences are lowered, and the patient is more likely to talk about matters that he otherwise would not reveal. It has been used to determine guilt or innocence in legal matters. Mental patients also have been given scopolamine to help in diagnosing and discovering what lies behind some states of delusion (q.v.). It is derived from *Hyoscyamus niger*, the deadly henbane (q.v.), which has been known since antiquity for its medical qualities.

TRYON, THOMAS (1634-1703). An English writer on social and philosophical subjects. He was a merchant in London but was more interested in the spiritual aspects of life. At one point he became an Anabaptist but later left the sect and lived in austerity and self-denial. He was critical of the attitudes of his contemporaries toward insanity and condemned many practices, such as bleeding (q.v.) and the prescription of drugs (q.v.) that left the patient confused and lethargic. In 1689 he wrote a book on dreams (q.v.) under the pseudonym of Philotheos Physiologus. Its title summarizes its contents: *A Treatise of Dreams and Visions, Wherein the Causes, Natures, and Uses, of Nocturnal Representations, and the Communications both of Good and Evil Angels, as also departed Souls, to Mankind are Theosophically Unfolded; that is, according to the Word of God, and the Harmony of Created Beings.* Its subtitle was *A Discourse of the Causes, Natures and Cure of Phrensie, Madness or Distraction.*
Bibliography: Hunter, R., and Macalpine, I. 1963. *Three hundred years of psychiatry.*

TSO CHUAN. A Chinese medical classic written around 100 B.C. It contains descriptions of psychopathology with references to psychosomatic disorders. The relationship between soma and psyche (q.v.) is clearly understood in it. The perfect health of the whole man is equated to the equilibrium of six natural influences; their imbalance results in physical illness or "diseases of the mind and delusions." Love, hate, pleasure, anger, sadness, and happiness are the six basic human emotions recognized in the *Tso Chuan.*
Bibliography: Chin, R., and Chin, Al-li S. 1969. *Psychological research in Communist China.*

TUBERCULOSIS. In the eighteenth and nineteenth centuries, it was believed that pulmonary tuberculosis and insanity were incompatible. It is possible that this notion arose from the fact that violent patients were restrained by the strait-waistcoat (q.v.), which acted as a form of collapse therapy, reducing the functional residual lung capacity and thus helping those insane who also suffered from tuberculosis.
Bibliography: Hunter, R. A., and Widdicombe, J. G. 1957. Tuberculosis and insanity. Historical and experimental observations on the strait-waistcoat as collapse therapy. *St. Bart's Hosp. J.* 61: 113-19.

TUBEROUS SCLEROSIS. A condition so named in 1880 by Désiré-Magloire Bourneville (q.v.). It was described in 1863 by Friedrich von Recklinghausen (q.v.). Subsequently, a case of congenital *adenoma sebaceum* (q.v.) was presented by John James Pringle (q.v.) in 1890, and in 1908, Heinrich

Vogt (1875- ?) established that the three essential elements for the condition are convulsion, sebaceous adenoma, and mental defect.

Bibliography: Kanner, L. 1964. *A history of the care and study of the mentally retarded.*

TUKE, DANIEL HACK (1827-1895). A British psychiatrist and member of a famous Yorkshire family. He was the great-grandson of William Tuke (q.v.) and the son of Samuel Tuke (q.v.). He was only twenty years old when he joined the staff of the York Retreat (q.v.) as a steward. Living among the patients, he gained first-hand knowledge of mental disorders. To this practical approach, he added the information he had gathered from literature. Although of delicate health, he decided to become a physician, the first in his family, and eventually he returned to the York Retreat in that capacity. He traveled to foreign countries to observe the management of mental patients in other hospitals. In 1880 he toured the United States and Canada and later published his observations in a volume entitled *The Insane in the United States and Canada* (1885). He was a great admirer of Philippe Pinel (q.v.), reverently visited his grave in Paris, and wrote a moving eulogy on the occasion of the unveiling of his statue at the Salpêtrière (q.v.) in 1885. Tuke was an enlightened, humane, and tolerant man, who would accept all new and useful ideas irrespective of their provenance. His *Manual of Psychological Medicine*, written in collaboration with John C. Bucknill (q.v.) in 1858, became a classic in its field. In 1892 he edited a large and encyclopedic *Dictionary of Psychological Medicine* to which he contributed many entries, including his own psychiatric classification, which was comprised of three classes with twenty-two groups. He tried to keep his nosology as simple as possible, remarking that Greek etymology had never helped the understanding of mental illness. His *Chapters in the History of the Insane in the British Isles*, originally presented in 1881 as the presidential address of the Royal Medico-Psychological Association (q.v.), is an authoritative report on the historical aspect of psychiatry in Britain.

Bibliography: Sessions, W. K., and Sessions, M. K. 1971. *The Tukes of York.*

TUKE, SIR JOHN BATTY (1835-1913). A British psychiatrist and a descendant of the Tukes of York. He was superintendent of the Fife and Kinross District Asylum in Scotland and originated an open-door system whereby the wards were no longer locked. His example was widely followed throughout the country.

Bibliography: Henderson, D. K. 1964. *The evolution of psychiatry in Scotland.*

TUKE, SAMUEL (1784-1857). A British Quaker (q.v.), the grandson of William Tuke (q.v.) and the father of Daniel H. Tuke (q.v.). He was a merchant in York, but he is remembered for his philanthropic activities and his *Description of the Retreat* in which he gave a detailed account of the history, administration, management, and methods of treatment at the famous institution founded by his grandfather. Although written by a layman, the book, first published in 1813, stimulated great interest in those concerned with mental illness. In England, the Hanwell Asylum (q.v.) was modeled on the York Retreat (q.v.), and in the United States numerous mental hospitals were founded in imitation, including the Bloomingdale Asylum, the Hartford Retreat, and the McLean Asylum (qq.v.).

Bibliography: Tuke, S. 1813. Reprint. 1964. *Description of the retreat.*

TUKE, WILLIAM (1732-1822). A British Quaker (q.v.) and a tea and coffee merchant in York, where his philanthropic work was well known. Following the mysterious circumstances in which a young Quaker woman died in York Lunatic Asylum (q.v.), he visited the institution and was appalled by what he found. He proposed to the Society of Friends that an institution of their own should be built and dedicated to the humane treatment of those Friends who became mentally ill. Respect, tolerance, kindness, and useful occupation were to replace harshness and restraint (q.v.). Accordingly, the York Retreat (q.v.) was founded. It opened in 1796 and became a model for many other mental hospitals. William Tuke supervised the institution according to his enlightened views, which, however, were greatly criticized. Even his own wife reproached him that this venture would prove to be an "idiot" child of his brain. Eventually his reforms were widely accepted and resulted in many changes for the better not only in British institutions but also throughout the world. His son, Henry Tuke (1755-1814) and his grandson, Samuel Tuke (q.v.), helped him in the humanitarian work of the York Retreat.

Bibliography: Sessions, W. K., and Sessions, E. M. 1971. *The Tukes of York.*

TURGENEV, IVAN SERGEEVICH (1818-1883). A Russian novelist. His childhood was extremely unhappy. His mother, known as "the witch," had been an abused child herself. As an adult, her marriage was unhappy, and her bitterness turned to cruelty to her own children. She beat Turgenev daily without mercy, deriving a kind of sexual satisfaction from it, which, at times, made her faint. He ran away from home but was caught and taken back to more misery. His hatred of injustice was rooted in his childhood. He was a hypochondriac (*see* HYPOCHONDRIA) all his life, and suffered from unspecific abdominal pains, like his father. He had a phobic fear of anyone touching his head because he imagined that only skin and hair covered his brain. He was a precocious child and an avid reader with a vivid curiosity for all things and a great capacity for concentration. At the age of fourteen he entered the University of Moscow and later went to Germany, where he was greatly influenced by Western culture. He became infatuated with a Spanish primadonna, Pauline Viardot-Garcia and spent the rest of his life in close contact with her and her husband. His stories, *Sportsman's Sketches* (1852) are said to have influenced the decision to abolish serfdom.

Among his many novels *A Nest of Gentlefolk* (1859) and *Fathers and Sons* (1862) are the best known. All of them show a poetic, sensitive mood, as well as progressive ideas and comments on contemporary life in Russia.
Bibliography: Schapiro, L. 1978. *Turgenev: his life and times.*

TÜRK, LUDWIG (1810-1868). An Austrian physician and neurologist. His investigation into the secondary degeneration in the central nervous system was his primary contribution to medicine. His work on the degeneration of the spinal tract was not fully recognized at the time, but it provided the basis for later neurological studies.
Bibliography: Haymaker, W., and Schiller, F. 1970. *The founders of neurology.* 2d. ed.

TURKISH BATH. Turkish baths were employed from time to time in the treatment of the insane. The annual report of the Colney Hatch Asylum (q.v.) for 1877 contains the following remarks about Turkish baths: "no asylum can lay claim to completeness which is not furnished with this apparatus for eliminating poisons and renewing life."
Bibliography: Tuke, D. H. 1892. *A dictionary of psychological medicine.*

TURLYGOOD. A fanatical sect found in Europe in the thirteenth and fourteenth centuries. Its members were thought to be insane. They sometimes were known as Turlupins. William Shakespeare (q.v.) referred to them in *King Lear.*
Bibliography: Whitwell, J. R. 1946. *Analecta psychiatrica.*

TURNER, DANIEL (1667-1741). An English physician and member of the Barber-Surgeon's Company. In 1717 he wrote *A Practical Dissertation of the Venereal Disease* in which he gave a detailed description of the obsessional (*see* OBSESSION) fears of certain patients who were convinced that they were suffering from syphilis (q.v.). He was impressed by this phobia (q.v.), which led to such demanding behavior that sometimes doctors also were drawn into their patients' false beliefs and converted the phobia into a delusion (q.v.). In 1723 Turner became the first recipient of an honorary medical degree from Yale University.
Bibliography: Hunter, R., and Macalpine, I. 1963. *Three hundred years of psychiatry.*

TURNER, JOSEPH MALLORD WILLIAM (1775-1851). An English painter, famous for his landscapes. His father, a barber, was a mean and narrowminded man. He was said to have praised his child only when the latter hoarded small coins. Turner's mother, an excitable and mentally unstable woman, was, for a time, a patient of Bethlem Royal Hospital (q.v.). She died in a private asylum (q.v.). His childhood was spent almost in poverty, in near-sordid surroundings, which he tried to avoid by isolating

himself. This was the beginning of his lifelong habit of self-imposed solitude and secretiveness. He was fond of fishing and spent whole days in this occupation, even during heavy rain. Because he was an atrocious writer and could not spell, some clauses of his will could not be implemented because they were incomprehensible. His conversation was poor, and his general knowledge was less than adequate. Alcohol had a special attraction for him, and he would paint with a dirty bottle of sherry constantly by his side and seldom went out without a flask of gin in his pocket. Meanness and munificence alternated in him. He liked to conceal his identity and often would pretend to be someone else, or would disappear for days, leaving no trace of his whereabouts. He had disappeared in this way when he was found by accident in a disreputable street on his death bed. Thomas Monro, physician to Bethlem Royal Hospital and a member of the famous Monro family (q.v.), was his protector for some time and gave him the opportunity to work in the so-called Monro Academy, an assembly of young artists under his protection.
Bibliography: Reynolds, G. 1969. *Turner*.

TURNER, WILLIAM (1510-1568). A British botanist, physician, and priest. He is considered the "father of English botany." After studying botany and medicine in Italy, he returned to England but had to take refuge abroad during the reign of Mary I (q.v.) when his books were proclaimed heretical and destroyed. Among his many books are the first essay on scientific botany and the first modern volume on ornithology. His herbal included remedies for mental disorders. In 1555, he wrote a book entitled *A New Book of Spiritual Physick for Dyverse Diseases of the Nobility and Gentlemen of Englande*. His large family and his poverty were contributing factors to his anxious and irascible personality. He did not suffer fools gladly, and he thought little of bishops. He trained his dog to snatch the hat off the head of the bishop of Bath and Wells when he visited.
Bibliography: Rohde, E. S. 1974. *The old English herbals*.

TURNER, WILLIAM (1653-1701). A British clergyman and the vicar of Walberton in Sussex. In 1697 he wrote about a case of spontaneous recovery from insanity. According to him, the man concerned, after being mentally ill for a long period, indicated one day that he had had a vision of God and wished for prayers to be said on his behalf. This was done, and he recovered. Part of the lengthy title of the work is *A Compleat History of the Most Remarkable Providences, both of Judgement and Mercy, which have Hapned in this Present Age. Extracted from the Best Writers, the Author's Own Observations, and the Numerous Relations sent Him from Divers Parts of the Three Kingdoms. . . .*
Bibliography: Hunter, R., and Macalpine, I. 1963. *Three hundred years of psychiatry*.

TUSCULANAE DISPUTATIONES. A work in five books by Cicero (q.v.). It was written between 47 and 44 B.C. and deals with the subject of happiness. In it, Cicero discussed mental diseases and stated that "disorders of the soul" were more dangerous and more numerous than those of the body. He went on to say that they should be studied and treated with diligence. Perturbations of the mind, according to him, were caused not by physical agents, but by passions, or emotions.

Bibliography: Cicero. *Tusculan disputations*, trans. J. E. King.

TUTHILL, GEORGE LEMAN (1772-1835). An English doctor, physician to Westminster, Bridewell (q.v.), and Bethlem Royal Hospital (q.v.). He was a kind, tolerant man, who was said to minister to his patients in a humane and gentlemanly fashion. He was a friend of Charles and Mary Lamb (qq.v.) and advised them during Mary's recurring periods of mental disorder.

Bibliography: Munk, W. 1878. *The roll of the Royal College of Physicians of London.*

TUTORES. A term applied in England to persons legally charged with the custody of land belonging to the mentally ill. The term was used in the statutes passed during the reign of Edward I (1272-1307).

TWELVE TABLES, THE. The earliest code of Roman law. It evolved in the fifth century B.C. and included provisions for the mentally ill, who were declared legally incompetent and deprived of freedom of action in many spheres.

Bibliography: Mora, G. 1975. Italy. In *World history of psychiatry*, ed. J. G. Howells.

TWILIGHT OF THE AMERICAN MIND. A book written in 1928 by the American physician W. B. Pitkin. It is a typical example of the unfounded panic created by the eugenic studies (*see* EUGENICS) of the time into mental deficiency, which predicted a general degeneration of the human species.

Bibliography: Pitkin, W. B. 1928. *Twilight of the American mind.*

TWIRLING STOOL. One of the many devices invented in the eighteenth century for the treatment of mental disorders. Spinning the patient was supposed to shake the contents of the skull and rearrange the brain to its normal pattern. Hermann Boerhaave (q.v.) advocated this type of treatment in his *Aphorisms: concerning the knowledge and cure of diseases*, translated into English in 1728.

Bibliography: Zilboorg, G. 1941. *A history of medical psychology.*

TYLOR, EDWARD BURNETT (1832-1917). A British anthropologist. His studies of primitive cultures, and his doctrine of animism (q.v.) contributed to the development of cultural anthropology. Many of his theories, including that of a primitive mind, were later adopted by psychoanalysis

(q.v.). He was one of the first observers to describe the custom of couvade (q.v.).
Bibliography: Tylor, E. B. 1865. *Researches into the early history of mankind and his development of civilization.*

TYSON, EDWARD (1650-1708). An English physician and Fellow of the Royal Society (q.v.). Some time after gaining his master's degree at Oxford University, he proceeded to study for a Doctorate in Physick, but when he went to present his thesis at the University of Cambridge, he was prevented from discussing it and was instead asked for the examination fee, an episode which he often wearily recounted. He was physician to Bethlem Royal Hospital (q.v.) and Bridewell (q.v.). He realized that some of the patients admitted to mental hospitals were suffering from physical ailments and proceeded to treat these before dealing with their mental disorders. He estimated that two-thirds of his patients were cured. The *Post Boy*, a news sheet of the times, published an advertisement (*see* ADVERTISING) for his services in 1699 in which he claimed that most of those in his care were cured in three months and that "several have been cured in a fortnight, and some in less time. . . ." He instituted a system of after-care for discharged patients and supplied material aid to the poorest until they could provide for themselves. He also started an outpatients department (q.v.) for former inpatients. A kind, cultured, taciturn man, he spent much time hunting for old books to add to his large collection. He was also an anatomist and published the results of his work in this field in several monographs. On his death a monument was erected to him, commemorating his devotion to the hospital he served. This monument can still be found at All Hallows Church, Twickenham, near London.
Bibliography: O'Donoghue, E. G. 1914. *The story of Bethlehem Hospital.*

TZU HSI (1835-1908). The Chinese regent and dowager empress. Although intelligent and charming, her thirst for power was insatiable and matched by a psychopathic (*see* PSYCHOPATHY) cruelty. She ruled China (q.v.) from a corrupt and feudal court, blocking reforms, hating Western countries, and listening to the malevolent whispered gossip of her 3000 eunuchs. She did not hesitate to remove those who stood in her way. Before becoming regent she was one of the concubines of the emperor Hsien Feng (1831-1861). Her future role was assured when she produced a male child, although the emperor, a sickly and debauched young man, was unlikely to have fathered the child. Her rise to absolute power began with the death of the emperor— possibly by poison administered at her instigation—and continued through more contrived deaths until she was sole regent and literally the power behind the throne, as she hid behind a yellow curtain and whispered instructions to the child emperor. He, too, soon died under suspicious circumstances. He was replaced by her nephew, who was also manoeuvred and dispatched.
Bibliography: Warner, M. 1972. *Life and times of Tz'u-hsi.*

U

UFO (UNIDENTIFIED FLYING OBJECT). Throughout history, individuals or even groups of individuals have claimed to have seen UFOs. In the Middle Ages (q.v.), fear of divine punishment was reflected in the sightings of a red cross in the sky and fiery dragons among the clouds. Because delusions (q.v.) are usually linked to the fashionable anxiety of the time, it is possible that the sighting of UFOs reflects the current interest in the possibility of life on other planets and fear that it may invade earth.
Bibliography: Chapman, R. 1969. *Unidentified flying objects.*

ULLERSPERGER, JOHANN BAPTIST (1798–1879). A German psychiatrist, particularly interested in the historical aspects of psychiatry. His short essay on the development of psychiatry in Italy, published in 1867, was followed in 1871 by a volume entitled *A History of Psychology and Psychiatry in Spain from the Oldest Times to the Present.* In it he described the Spanish theory and practice of psychiatry from the times of the Roman occupation to the nineteenth century. He included a discussion of the provisions made for the care of the mentally ill in both private and public institutions.
Bibliography: Nora G. 1971. *American Journal of Psychiatry* 128:6.

ULLOA, JOSÉ CASIMIRO (1829–1891). A Peruvian psychiatrist and the first director of the Hospital de la Misericordia, which opened in Lima, Peru, in 1859. A pioneer in humanitarian treatment, he advocated regular ward rounds, introduced a more accurate classification of patients, and promoted occupational therapy (q.v.). He was interested in psychiatric problems affecting the community and vigorously campaigned against alcoholism (q.v.).
Bibliography: Leon, C. A., and Rosselli, H. 1975. Latin America. In *World history of psychiatry*, ed. J. G. Howells.

ULPIANUS, DOMITIUS (c.A.D. 160–228). A Roman jurist and adviser to the emperor Alexander Severus (205–235). He was one of the first to

assert that an insane individual could not be held responsible for a criminal act.
Bibliography: Alexander, F. G., and Selesnick, S. T. 1966. *The history of psychiatry.*

ULYSSES (or ODYSSEUS) A legendary Greek hero. In one of the episodes of the *Odyssey* (q.v.) he feigns madness by displaying such inappropriate behavior as yoking together a horse and a bull, sowing salt instead of seeds, and ploughing sand. His behavior reflects the ancient tendency to equate mental disorders solely with irrational actions.
Bibliography: Simon, B. 1978. *Mind and madness in ancient Greece.*

UNCONSCIOUS. The idea of unconscious motivation has its roots in primitive cultures, and, at various times, early authors came near to postulating the existence of "the unconscious" as elaborated by Sigmund Freud (q.v.). The term, as it is used in psychoanalyis (q.v.), was first introduced by Pierre Janet (q.v.), before it was elaborated upon by Freud. Alfred Adler (q.v.) and Carl G. Jung (q.v.) reevaluated Freud's discoveries.
Bibliography: Ellenberger, H. F. 1970. *The discovery of the unconscious.*

UNDERSTANDING. Francis Bacon (q.v.) included understanding among the three main forces responsible for psychological reactions. The other two forces that he recognized were memory (q.v.) and imagination (q.v.).
Bibliography: Wallace, K. R. 1963. *Francis Bacon on the nature of man.*

UNFINISHED CHILDREN. A term suggested in 1866 by the English physician George E. Shuttleworth for children suffering from Down's syndrome. He hoped to abandon the term "mongolism" (q.v.), which had racial connotations.
Bibliography: Shuttleworth, G. E., and Potts, W. A. 1922. *Mentally deficient children: their treatment and training.*

UNWINS, DAVID (c.1780–1837). A British physician. He was visiting physician to a private asylum in Surrey known as Peckham House. His experiences there caused him to become particularly interested in psychiatric disorders. He did not admire those medical men who had devised classifications of mental disorders, and he placed even less trust in medico-legal opinions about insanity. He believed in early sex education as a preventive measure against later sexual problems and regarded religious practices in asylums (q.v.) as acts of benevolence irrelevant to the treatment of insanity. According to him, treatment should be planned around patient the rather than around the disease. Furthermore, he felt symptoms should be relieved by "mental medicinals," or, psychological means, rather than by drugs (q.v.).
Bibliography: Unwins, D. 1833. *A treatise on those disorders of the brain and nervous system, which are usually considered and called mental.*

UNZER, JOHANN AUGUST (1727–1799). A German physician. He believed that living organisms were organized on a purely mechanical basis

and did not need a brain or soul. He was attracted to the theories of Albrecht von Haller (q.v.) on reflexes and conducted experiments on the nerves using the spinal cord of a frog. These studies emphasized the distinction between voluntary and involuntary movements. His lucid mind was much admired by Johann Wolfgang von Goethe (q.v.).
Bibliography: Debus, A. G., ed. 1968. *World who's who in science.*

UPHAM, THOMAS (1799–1872). An American philosopher and educator. In 1827 he wrote *Elements of Intellectual Philosophy*, which was followed in 1831 by *Elements of Mental Philosophy*. The two books marked the rise of interest in psychology in the United States, although that term "psychology" was not yet used.
Bibliography: Misiak, H., and Sexton, V. S. 1966. *History of psychology.*

URANISM. A term first used in 1862 in Germany by Karl H. Ulrichs (1825–1895) to indicate homosexuality (q.v.). He derived the term from the Greek myth that claimed Aphrodite Urania inspired love between males. Karl H. Ulrichs called male homosexuals "urnings" and female homosexuals "urnides."
Bibliography: Bullough, V. L. 1976. *Sexual variance in society and history.*

URSINUS LITHUANUS. The name given by Carolus Linnaeus (q.v.) to a "wild" or "savage" child discovered in 1661 among bears in Lithuania. *See also* FERAL CHILD.
Bibliography: Barr, M. W. 1904. *Mental defectives.*

UTERUS. From ancient Egypt (q.v.) to the nineteenth century, the uterus was believed to be the cause of hysterical (*see* HYSTERIA) disorders, which, in fact, took their name from the Greek term for the uterus. The Egyptians and the Greeks thought that the uterus could move upward in the body and thus sometimes produce a feeling of suffocation (q.v.). Fumigation (q.v.) of the vagina was the treatment they recommended. The link between the uterus and hysteria continued to be asserted until the nineteenth century, and hysteria was believed to be a disease of women. Mesmerism (q.v.) and marriage (q.v.) were among the suggested therapeutic remedies.
Bibliography: Veith, I. 1965. *Hysteria: the history of a disease.*

UTICA CRIB. A contraption devised to limit a patient's freedom of movement during the night. It was a modified model of the crib-bed, which was designed in 1845 by a French physician, Dr. Aubanel. The Utica Crib consisted of a crib with a hinged lid that could be closed over the recumbent

patient. It took its name from the Utica State Hospital (q.v.), where it had been adopted on the recommendation of Dr. Amariah Brigham (q.v.).
Bibliography: Deutsch, A. 1949. *The mentally ill in America.*

UTICA STATE HOSPITAL. One of the first state lunatic asylums in the United States. It opened in 1843 in Utica, New York. Dr. Amariah Brigham (q.v.) was its first superintendent.
Bibliography: Deutsch, A. 1949. *The mentally ill in America.*

UTILITARIANISM. A school of philosophy developed in Britain during the early part of the nineteenth century. Its followers held that self-interest was all-important and that social, political, and legal activities should be directed toward providing pleasure and avoiding pain. This principle of utility, or, the greatest good for the greatest number, was advanced by Jeremy Bentham (q.v.), who originated the term in *Introduction to Principles of Morals and Legislation*, published in 1789.
Bibliography: Plamenatz, J. 1949. *The English Utilitarians.*

UTOPIA. A term derived from the Greek and meaning "nowhere land." It was used as the title of a book by Sir Thomas More (q.v.) in which he dealt with an ideal form of government.
Bibliography: *Brewer's dictionary of phrase and fable.* 1978.

UTRILLO, MAURICE (1883–1955). A French painter. He was the son of Suzanne Valadon (1867–1938), a painter who had been an acrobat before an accident forced her to leave that occupation and model for Pierre August Renoir (1841–1919) and others. He was adopted by the Spanish writer Miguel Utrillo. Utrillo became unstable and dependent upon alcohol and drugs (q.v.) early in his life. Painting was suggested to him as a form of therapy. From the age of eighteen on, he spent various periods in a number of asylums (q.v.) and nursing homes. His famous "white period" began around 1909 and lasted for five years. During it, he primarily painted views of old Montmartre. Some of these were painted on the doors of the Chateau of Saint Bernard, an asylum, and they were later removed and sold in Paris. The bleakness of his landscapes and the tiny figures dwarfed by their surroundings reflect his depression. His style later deteriorated and became more rudimentary.
Bibliography: George, W. 1967. *Utrillo.*

V

VACCINES. Preparations of microorganism used against infectious diseases. From the time of Hippocrates (q.v.), physicians have noted that physical disease sometimes alleviates the symptoms of mental disorders. This observation led to the artificial production of an infection as a form of therapy. For example, typhoid vaccines have been used to produce fever and a remission of symptoms in general paralysis of the insane (q.v.).
Bibliography: Zilboorg, G. 1941. *A history of medical psychology.*

VACHÉ, JACQUES (1895-1919). A French eccentric who influenced André Breton (q.v.). As an art student, Vaché spent his time in idleness on the fringes of the Dadaist movement (*see* DADAISM). The basic principle of his psychopathic (*see* PSYCHOPATHY) behavior was that life was futile, a kind of boring joke. He wrote that he would die when he felt like it in the company of some friends to relieve the boredom of the act. Accordingly, he took an overdose of laudanum (q.v.) after administering the same amount to two unsuspecting friends.
Bibliography: Richter, H. 1965. *Dada.*

VAGBHATTA. A famous Indian physician of the seventh century A.D. He believed that health resulted from the correct balance of air, mucus, and bile (q.v.), the three elementary substances. According to him, disease was caused by evil spirits. His clinical notes included descriptions of insanity, epilepsy (q.v.), and idiocy (*see* IDIOT). Among the causes of mental disorders, he listed strong emotions and violent passions. He advocated the sedation of violent patients through drugs obtained from the nardus root (q.v.).
Bibliography: Kutumbiah, P. 1969. *Ancient Indian medicine.*

VAGRANT ACT. The first English act of Parliament for the care and protection of the insane. It was passed in 1744, during the reign of George

II (q.v.). It dealt with those who were "furiously mad, or so far mentally afflicted as to be dangerous if left at large." Two justices of the peace were empowered to arrest the dangerously insane and have them locked up and chained in a safe place. Their possessions, if any, could be expended toward their maintenance.

See also INSANE POOR, LEGISLATION IN ENGLAND.

Bibliography: Leigh, D. 1961. *The historical development of British psychiatry.*

VAIHINGER, HANS (1852-1933). A German philosopher. He was an admirer of Immanuel Kant (q.v.) and the founder of the Kant Society, which was established in 1904. He formulated the "as if" philosophy, which was based on the conviction that many social actions were founded on beliefs that had no basis in reality, such as the unfounded statement "all men are equal." His work greatly influenced Alfred Adler (q.v.), who derived from it the conceptual framework for his own system.

Bibliography: Vaihinger, H. 1911. *Die philosophie des also ob.*

VAILALA MADNESS. Another term for cargo anxiety (q.v.).

VALDEMAR. The hero of a novel by Edgar Allan Poe (q.v.). As Valdemar is dying, a friend who practices magnetism (q.v.) prevents his spirit from leaving his body; thus, putrefaction does not occur although the body is dead. When the spirit is allowed to depart, the flesh immediately falls into decomposition. This macabre piece of fiction was used by those who wanted to discredit magnetism to demonstrate the absurd beliefs of its practitioners.

Bibliography: Poe, E. A. 1845. *The facts in the case of Mr. Valdemar.*

VALDIVIA, ANDRES DE (fl. 1570). A Spanish soldier who conquered the province of Antioquia (Nueva Granada) in South America and became its governor. In 1575 he received an anonymous letter informing him that his wife was unfaithful. He was so upset that he became deranged, and his acts against the Indians became so cruel that they murdered him.

Bibliography: Leon, C. A. and Rosselli, H. 1975. Latin America. In *World history of psychiatry*, ed. J. G. Howells.

VALDIZAN, HERMILIO (1885-1929). A Peruvian psychiatrist. His work contributed to the advancement of psychiatry in Peru. He was an outstanding lecturer, an excellent clinician, and a prolific writer, especially in the field of the history of medicine. He was also interested in mental hygiene (q.v.) and in the legal aspects of psychiatry.

Bibliography: Leon, C. A., and Rosselli, H. 1975. Latin America. In *World history of psychiatry*, ed. J. G. Howells.

VALENCIA ASYLUM. *See* SANCTA MARIA DELS INOCENTS.

VALENTINE, CHARLES W. (1879-1964). A British educational psychologist and professor of education at Birmingham University. His genetic study of young children, entitled *Psychology of Early Childhood*, was published in 1942, but he is best known for his book *Psychology and its Bearings on Education* (1950), which has become a standard textbook in the training curriculum of teachers. His last book, written when he was eighty-two years old, is entitled *The Experimental Psychology of Beauty* (1962).

Bibliography: Valentine, C. W. 1950. *Psychology and its bearings on education.*

VALERIAN. *Valeriana officinalis*, a wild plant widely used in folk medicine. The American Indians believed that it was the most efficacious remedy there was for epilepsy (q.v.), which, if it did not yield to valerian, they considered incurable. In Russian folk medicine the root of valerian was the main ingredient in an infusion that was used to treat nervous excitement, irritability, and insomnia. Taken indiscriminately, valerian causes hallucinations (q.v.) and agitation. Adolf Hitler (q.v.) is believed to have been addicted to it.

Bibliography: de Baïracli Levy, J. 1974. *The illustrated herbal handbook.*

VALLADOLID. A hospital for those "poor innocents of the city bereft of reason" in Valladolid, Spain. It was founded in 1436 by Sanche Velasque de Cuellar. On his death, he bequeathed his house and belongings to the hospital for the purpose of financing the project. Treatment in the hospital may have included valerian (q.v.) and the use of a douche (q.v.) on the patient's head, as both these measures were recommended in a book entitled *Dignotico et Cura Affectuum Melancolicorum*, which was written by Alfonso de Santa Cruz, physician to Philip II (q.v.), who also lived in Valladolid.

Bibliography: Chamberlain, A. S. 1966. Early mental hospitals in Spain. *Am. J. Psych.* 123: 143-49.

VALLAMBERT, SIMON DE (1512-1578). A French physician particularly interested in childhood diseases. He was the author of the first book on pediatrics written in French. Published in 1565 it contained observations on syphilis (q.v.) in children, a subject that no other writer had discussed before him. He suggested "la mere des enfants" as an alternative name for epilepsy (q.v.) in childhood and included in the dissertation a discussion of hydrocephalus.

Bibliography: Still, G. F. 1965. *The history of paediatrics.*

VALSAVA, ANTONIO MARIA (1666-1723). An Italian physician. He was the pupil of Marcello Malpighi (1628-1694) and the teacher of the famous Giovanni Morgagni (q.v.). In addition to his work in anatomy and surgery, he is remembered for his interest in mental disorders. He was physician at the Spedale di Sant Orsola in Bologna, which, in 1710, opened a special department for the mentally ill. Valsava introduced many innovations in

psychiatric treatment, abolished the more severe forms of restraint (q.v.), and advocated a better diet (q.v.) for the mentally ill.
Bibliography: Mora, G. 1975. Italy. In *World history of psychiatry*, ed. J. G. Howells.

VAN GOGH, VINCENT WILLEM (1853-1890). A Dutch postimpressionist painter. His father, a Lutheran pastor, was a charming and popular man, who was referred to as "the handsome parson." The first child in the family died at birth and the second, Vincent, who was born on the same date a year later, was regarded as a substitute and given the same names. Every Sunday, on his way to church, he would pass the tombstone engraved with these names. His parents idealized him and could not accept his faults. Although there were five children in the family, Van Gogh remained close only to his brother Théo and to his sister Elizabeth, who described him as "a stranger to his family." He was sent to a boarding school and many years later he wrote of his feelings of loneliness on leaving home for the first time and how sad he felt when the little yellow carriage containing his parents disappeared down the road, wet with rain and flanked by spare trees. A series of failures in various jobs culminated for him in a spell as an itinerant evangelist for a religious society, which was embarrassed by his excessive zeal and lack of dignity. He then began to study art, but this pursuit was marred by episodes of deep depression that were sometimes triggered by unsuccessful love affairs. Absinthe (q.v.) drinking, physical neglect, attacks of fever, and, possibly, epilepsy (q.v.) may have aggravated his condition. He eventually settled for a time at the Hague, where he lived with a prostitute whom he married when she was pregnant by another man. She became the subject of his drawing entitled *Sorrow*. For a time he returned to his family at Nuenen, where he painted *The Potato Eaters*, a melancholic, haunting, dark scene of poverty. A period in Paris brought him in close contact with Toulouse-Lautrec (q.v.) and Paul Gauguin (q.v.). It was after a quarrel with Gauguin that Van Gogh cut off part of his ear lobe. The episode precipitated his admission to the asylum (q.v.) at Saint-Remy, where he frantically painted portraits of the keeper and the doctor, as well as views of the grounds. In 1890 his talents were recognized in an appreciative article, but by then depression and confusion were dominating his life. He shot himself in the same field that he had depicted full of corn but darkened by a flight of black crows. Théo became ill while organizing a commemorative exhibition for his brother and died five months later in an asylum.
Bibliography: Nagera, H. 1957. *Vincent Van Gogh: a psychological study*.

VAN MEEGEREN, HENRICUS ANTHONIUS (1889-1947). A Dutch painter and forger. He is an example of pseudologia fantastica (q.v.). He was obsessed by his own sense of importance, the need for secrecy, and the fear of being deprived of what he regarded as his own. Despite his skill and craftsmanship, he preferred to produce forgeries, which were so good that

some art experts accepted them as genuine works before scientific examination detected their fraudulence. His most famous forgery was *Christ at Emmaus*, which he presented as a newly discovered Jan Vermeer (1632-1675).
Bibliography: Kilbracken, J. G. 1967. *Van Meegeren*.

VANDERBILT, ALFRED GWYNNE (1877-1915). A member of the American family of financiers. He was pathologically superstitious and was said to be so afraid of being attacked at night by evil spirits that he kept the legs of his bed immersed in dishes of salt water, which was believed to keep devils away. He lost his life in the *Lusitania* disaster.
Bibliography: Andrews, W. 1941. *The Vanderbilt legend*.

VAPORS. A term frequently used in the eighteenth and nineteenth centuries to cover a multitude of ill-defined psychosomatic or neurotic conditions in women. Unlike the aetiology of the uterine vapors of the ancients, who believed that they originated in the uterus (q.v.) and eventually reached the brain producing mental disorders, the aetiology of the "vapors" was unclear. An attack usually was triggered by anything that displeased the lady or offended her sense of propriety. The affliction was fashionable among society ladies; it was characterized by fainting and fits. Treatment consisted mostly of hydrotherapy at fashionable spas and attending "mesmerizing" (*see* MESMERISM) sessions.
Bibliography: Pomme, P. 1763. *Treatise upon vaporous affections*.

VARGAS, JOSÉ MARIA (1786-1854). A Venezuelan physician and statesman. Before becoming president of Venezuela in 1835, he practiced and taught in Caracas. Impressed by the theories of Marie François Bichat (q.v.), he introduced them in Latin America. He was also the first in Latin America to perform dissections of the nervous system. In 1853 he took up residence in the United States.
Bibliography: Leon, C. A., and Rosselli, H. 1975. Latin America. In *World history of psychiatry*, ed. J. G. Howells.

VASOMOTOR THEORY OF THE PSYCHOSES. A complex and elaborate theory that suggested psychoses (*see* PSYCHOSIS) were caused by changes in the circulatory system. It was formulated by Theodor Meynert (q.v.) and rested on a purely anatomical basis.
Bibliography: Meynert, T. 1884. *Psychiatrie*.

VASQUEZ DE ARCE Y CEBALLOS, GREGORIO (1638-1711). A Colombian painter born in Bogota. A terse inscription on his painting of *Saint Crisanto* states that he was insane at the time of his death.
Bibliography: Rosselli, H. 1968. *Historia de la psiquiatria en Colombia*.

VAUQUELIN, NICOLAS-LOUIS (1736-1829). A French chemist and physician. He was the discoverer of chromium and beryllium and investigated organic acids and alkaloids of belladonna (q.v.). His chemical analysis of brain tissue promoted subsequent research on cerebral lipids.

Bibliography: Haymaker, W., and Schiller, F. 1970. *The founders of neurology*. 2d. ed.

VEDA, THE. The sacred books of Hinduism. They contain material relevant to normal and abnormal psychology. In them, the mind is regarded as a sixth sense organ and the seat of thought. The heart is regarded as the seat of the emotions. Because demonology is the basis of the earlier writings, incantations (q.v.), amulets (q.v.), charms, and herbs are the recommended treatment for illness. Later books of the Veda distinguish between diseases produced by supernatural causes and those produced by faulty diet (q.v.); drugs (q.v.) are suggested for those caused by diet.

Bibliography: Sigerist, H. E. 1961. *A history of medicine*. Vol. 2.

VELÁSQUEZ, DIEGO RODRIGUEZ DE SILVA Y (1599-1660). A Spanish painter. Dwarfs and mental defectives, who were employed as fools (q.v.) in the court of Madrid, were frequently the subjects of his paintings. His unflattering realism in painting Philip IV (1605-1665) and his pathetic family did not prevent him receiving lifelong court patronage.

Bibliography: Horsefield, E. 1940. Mental defectives at the court of Philip IV of Spain as portrayed by the great court painter Velásquez. *Am. J. ment. Deficiency*. 45: 152-57.

VENDIDAD, THE. A volume in the Avesta, or Zoroastrian (*see* ZOROASTER) Bible, an ancient system of Persian philosophy. The term literally means "law against demons," which reflects the belief that all diseases were caused by evil spirits. The Persians had three kinds of doctors: knife doctor, herb doctor, and word doctor. The word doctor was believed to be a healer of the soul and perhaps the equivalent of a modern psychotherapist.

Bibliography: Elgood, C. 1951. *A medical history of Persia*.

VENEZUELA. The first psychiatric institution in Venezuela was opened in Caracas in 1876. It was called Asilo National de Enajenados and was poorly staffed by untrained personnel. It closed down after sixteen years and was replaced by the Hospital Psiquiatrico Caracas.

Bibliography: Graff, H., and Blanco Acosta, H. 1971. Psychiatry in Venezuela: a brief history; *Transactions and Studies of the College of Physicians of Philadelphia*. 38: 235-39.

VENTRICULAR THEORY. A theory following the Platonic (*see* PLATO) tradition but apparently specifically Christian. It postulated that the functions of the mind, but not the soul, were located in the ventricles of the brain. Both Nemesius (q.v.) and Saint Augustine (q.v.) subscribed to it, but Andreas Vesalius (q.v.) demolished it by demonstrating that many stupid animals had brains with four ventricles like man but did not possess the same high faculties.

Bibliography: Riese, W. 1959. *A history of neurology.*

VENUS. An early Italian deity of fertility. Later she was identified with the Greek Aphrodite. As goddess of love and beauty and universal mother, she was officially worshipped by the state. During the Middle Ages (q.v.), she became the symbol of the sin of luxuria, and her pagan nudity was frowned upon. According to the beliefs of the Middle Ages, young men were tempted by her to become followers of the devil. Much guilt surrounded her image; she was depicted as the personification of vice that should be overcome by chastity and virtue. Eventually the tradition of chivalry and courtly love brought back a more pleasant picture of Venus as the inspirer of noble sentiments; her imagery was restored by many Renaissance artists who depicted her as a delightful and delighted symbol of love.

VERAGUTH, OTTO (1870-1940). A German neurologist. He described a contraction of the upper eyelid (now known as the fold of Veraguth), which is said to be found in manic-depressive patients.

VERBIGERATION. A term introduced by Karl Kahlbaum (q.v.) in a monograph on mental deterioration, published in 1874. It described the obsessional (*see* OBSESSION), meaningless chatter of psychotic (*see* PSYCHOSIS) patients.

Bibliography: Kahlbaum, K. L. 1874. Reprint. 1973. *Catatonia.*

VERLAINE, PAUL (1844-1896). A French poet. Despite a very long engagement to a sixteen-year-old girl, he found married life with her unbearable and took refuge in heavy drinking and travel. He joined the boy poet Arthur Rimbaud (q.v.), who completely subjugated him, and together they traveled through Europe, until Rimbaud threatened to end their intimacy. In despair and drunk Verlaine shot his friend in the wrist. His deep regret of this act of aggression successfully patched up the relationship for a short period, but Rimbaud, wishing to break free, staged a street incident that resulted in Verlaine's arrest. Police investigations uncovered immorality and adverse political activities. Verlaine was subsequently sentenced to two years hard labor. His wife left him, and he turned to religion for comfort. He even tried to enter a monastery to expiate his guilt. For a time he taught in England and in France. In 1877 he adopted a favorite pupil, whose death he greatly mourned in 1883. Again he turned to alcohol for comfort, and again he was imprisoned, this time for attacking his mother. For a time he lived in extreme poverty. Most of his great poetic achievements reflect his bouts of debauchery followed by the need for confession and penance. In these works, moods of sensuality alternate with mysticism.

Bibliography: Adam, A. 1963. *The art of Paul Verlaine*, trans. C. Morse.

VERMONT ASYLUM. An American institution for the insane. It was founded in Brattleboro, Vermont in 1835 through the bequest of Mrs. Anna Marsh, the wife of a physician who had cared for mental patients. She became aware of the need for better treatment facilities after Richard Whitney (q.v.), a prominent resident of Vermont, died from an overly enthusiastic application of the water cure, which entailed keeping the patient under water until he became unconscious. The institution later changed its name to Brattleboro Retreat and became a state hospital.

Bibliography: Deutsch, A. 1949. *The mentally ill in America*.

VERVAIN. *Verbena officinalis*, a plant long known for its medicinal properties. Hippocrates (q.v.) often recommended it. The Druids, the Greeks, and the Romans regarded it as sacred. Nervous disorders, epilepsy (q.v.), and insomnia were among the many ills it was reputed to cure. Also known as *Herba veneris*, it was used in witchcraft (q.v.) as an aphrodisiac.

Bibliography: Rohde, E. S. 1974. The old English herbals.

VESALIUS, ANDREAS (c.1514-1564). A Belgian anatomist, professor of surgery and anatomy at the University of Padua, and physician to the court of Charles V (q.v.) and Philip II (q.v.) of Spain. His work *De Humani Corporis Fabrica* (1543) with its accurate description of bones and the nervous sytem and beautiful illustrations executed by a pupil of Titian opened the way to scientific inquiry. His departure from the teachings of Galen (q.v.) so shocked his contemporaries that they said he was mad and justified Galen's anatomical descriptions by claiming that man had changed physically from Galen's time. The Inquisition (q.v.) condemned Vesalius to death for body snatching and for dissecting the human body, but then commuted the sentence to a forced pilgrimage to Jerusalem. Vesalius reached the sacred city but died on the return journey. Unlike the Aristotelians (*see* ARISTOTLE), who believed that the heart (q.v.) was linked to personality characteristics, Vesalius believed that the brain and the nervous system were more important but did not associate the brain with mental processes.

Bibliography: Singer, C. 1957. *A short history of anatomy and physiology from the Greeks to Harvey*.

VESANIA. A Latin term from the first century B.C. meaning insanity. Cicero (q.v.) used it, and it reappeared in the classifications of mental disorders until the nineteenth century.

Bibliography: Zilboorg, G. 1941. *A history of medical psychology*.

VICARY, THOMAS (1490?-1561). An English anatomist, surgeon to Henry VIII (1491-1547), and first master of the United Barber Surgeons. In his

writings, he borrowed freely from Henry de Mandeville, a fourteenth century surgeon. Vicary located specific faculties in specific ventricles of the brain. He placed fancy and imagination (q.v.) in the foremost ventricle, thought in the second, or middle ventricle, and memory (q.v.) in the third ventricle. Like the medieval writers, he believed that the ventricles were formed by the pia mater, which was also thought to convey the spirits from the liver (q.v.) and the heart (q.v.) to the brain. William Shakespeare (q.v.) repeated this idea in *Love's Labour Lost* (act. 4. 2): "This is a gift that I have, simple, simple; a foolish extravagent spirit, full of forms, figures, shapes, objects, ideas, apprehensions, motions, revolutions; these are begot in the ventricles of memory, nourished in the womb of pia mater, and delivered upon the mellowing of the occasion."
Bibliography: Copeman, W.S.C. 1960. *Doctors and disease in Tudor times.*

VICO, GODFREY DE (fl.1240). An Italian chaplain to Pope Innocent IV (q.v.). He was elected bishop of Bethlehem. The Pope gave him an encyclical directing the clergy of Italy, England, and Scotland to offer hospitality to the brothers of Bethlem. When the circular letter was read in the churches of London, it inspired Simon Fitz-Mary (q.v.) to give land for the establishment of the priory, that eventually became Bethlem Royal Hospital (q.v.). On October 23, 1247, Godfrey de Vico traced the boundaries at the head of a procession.
Bibliography: O'Donoghue, E. G. 1914. *The story of Bethlehem Hospital.*

VICQ D'AZYR, FELIX (1748-1794). A French anatomist and physician. He made detailed studies of the cerebral structures and described the convolutions of the lobes. His anatomical drawings of the brain were remarkable for their accuracy and stimulated subsequent research. His *Traite d'anatomie* was published in 1786.
Bibliography: Clarke, E., and Dewhurst, K. 1974. *An illustrated history of the brain function.*

VICTORIANS, THE. The reign of Queen Victoria (1819-1901) of England gave a particular flavor to nineteenth-century Europe and America. Excessive prudery in sexual matters produced an equally excessive interest in the same field. A number of books on abnormal sexuality verged on the pornographic and, like the *Malleus Maleficarum* (q.v.) some centuries earlier, provided an excuse for discussing forbidden topics. Physicians too functioned on a double level: on the one they were the exponents of reason and scientific progress, on the other they were the guardians of morals. Psychiatric disorders were attributed to sexual excesses; the sexual needs of women were denied and study for the "weaker sex" was regarded as a sure road to moral and physical destruction. Nervous ailments were common, especially in the upper classes, where they were treated with such pleasant remedies as trav-

eling (q.v.) taking the waters at fashionable spas, and other distractions. Opium (q.v.) was freely prescribed and often produced addiction. Abnormal behavior in the poor was regarded sternly and was treated by imposing discipline and religious instruction. The Victorians were the manufacturers and the victims of a system that despite many irregularities, produced social stability and prosperity but failed to improve the climate for emotional health. It was against this background that psychoanalysis (q.v.) with its emphasis on sexuality was born.
Bibliography: Haller, J. S., and Haller, R. M. 1977. *The physician and sexuality in Victorian America.*

VIERORDT, KARL VON (1818-1884). A German physiologist. He performed research on vision, hearing, and the sense of time in individuals. He also investigated in depth the development of language in children.
Bibliography: Boring, E. G. 1950. *A history of experimental psychology.*

VIEUSSENS, RAYMOND (1641-1716). A French anatomist. He attempted to localize psychological faculties in various parts of the brain and believed that the *corpora striata* were the seat of imagination (q.v.).
Bibliography: Zilboorg, G. 1941. *A history of medical psychology.*

VIGNY, ALFRED VICTOR, COMTE DE (1797-1863). A French romantic (*see* ROMANTICISM) writer. His life was a series of unfortunate events. His school days were made unhappy by the persecution he suffered from all around him. Life in the army in peace time was boring. His English wife became an invalid, and her wealth proved to be nonexistent. Victor Hugo (q.v.), his close friend, became jealous of his success. His love affair with the actress Marie Dorval was stormy and unhappy. His beloved mother whom he nursed devotedly died in 1837 when he was already suffering from depression. Melancholy (*see* MELANCHOLIA), loneliness, frustration, and a sense of defeat caused him to withdraw into the seclusion of a country estate. During the days there he nursed his hypochondriac (*see* HYPOCHONDRIA) wife and at night retired into a small room in a tower, called the "ivory tower" by Charles Sainte-Beuve (1804-1869), where he wrote. His work is permeated with stoical despair and often deals with suicide (q.v.). He believed that the Christian practice of confession had provided the inspiration for the psychological novel and his own "analytical novels" are in the form of consultations between two symbolic figures, a doctor and a poet.
Bibliography: Viallaneix, P. 1964. *Vigny par lui-meme.*

VINCENT, CLOVIS (1879-1947). A French neurologist. He was a large, clumsy, colorful figure and known to be an excellent boxer. He was regarded as the best neurosurgeon in the world by such an authority as Harvey Cushing (q.v.), who had seen him operate. Vincent was assistant to Josef

Babinski (q.v.) at the Paris Pitié. The lack of nursing help in the operating theater at the Pitié was solved satisfactorily by the assistance of Vincent's wife and his housekeeper. He introduced new techniques for the total removal of certain brain tumors and provided new forms of therapy to alleviate the consequences of head injuries.
Bibliography: Haymaker, W., and Schiller, F. 1970. *The founders of neurology.* 2d. ed.

VINCENT DE PAUL, SAINT (1580?-1660). A French priest and philanthropist. He was almoner to the queen of Henry IV (1553-1610). In addition to organizing nursing orders and institutions for foundlings, he turned an old Parisian hospital for lepers (*see* LEPROSY) into an asylum (q.v.), known as Saint Lazare (q.v.). With the help of powerful patrons, he founded a general hospital that offered shelter to beggars, prostitutes, and vagabonds, as well as to the mentally ill. He believed in the kindly treatment of the insane, but his charitable views were difficult to convert into practice because of overcrowding, poverty, and ignorance.
Bibliography: Maynard, T. 1940. *Apostle of charity.*

VINEGAR. In the Middle Ages (q.v.) vinegar was used as a remedy in the treatment of insanity. It was taken internally after it was distilled, and it was used externally, often in conjunction with ground ivy, to rub the shaven head of the patient. Aromatic vinegar was long used as a reviver for ladies succumbing to an attack of the vapors (q.v.).
Bibliography: Tuke, D. H. 1882. *History of the insane in the British Isles.*

VIOLENCE. At various times throughout history violence has been employed in the management of the mentally ill. Primitive people believed that hurting the insane would force the evil spirits possessing (*see* POSSESSION) their bodies to leave. Until the nineteenth century, even in more advanced cultures, violence in the form of binding, flogging (q.v.), sudden immersion (q.v.) in water, or spinning in special contraptions was considered therapeutic by those who believed that shocks would restore the patient's mental health.

VIOLET. A perennial herb of the *Violaceae* family. An infusion of the leaves and flowers of this plant was believed to cure difficult neurotic (*see* NEUROSIS) conditions, to improve memory (q.v.), and to bring restful sleep to the anxious. The Roman treatment for epilepsy (q.v.) included wine in which violets had been infused. Bartholomaeus Anglicus (q.v.) in his *Proprietatibus Rerum* (c.1280) advised that the smell of fresh violets "abateth heate of the braine, and refresheth and comforteth the spirites of feeling and maketh sleepe, for it cooleth and tempereth and moysteneth the braine."

Charles II (1630-1685) of England made popular the use of lozenges of sugar and violets for headache and insomnia.
Bibliography: Clarkson, R. E. 1972. *The golden age of herbs and herbals.*

VIRCHOW, RUDOLF LUDWIG CARL (1821-1902). A German pathologist. He is considered the father of modern pathology. He was a quick-tempered individual, who was feared for his sarcasm and angry outbursts. At times he appeared to be unable to accept the work of others. Because he could concentrate on more than one task at the same time, he had no difficulty in delivering a speech and proofreading it simultaneously. He refuted the germ theory of Louis Pasteur (1822-1895) and asserted that all cells are generated by other cells. His work also contributed to the field of neuropathology in mental illness. He believed social and cultural maladjustments were the causes of psychic epidemic disease. He also wrote on anthropology and spent much effort and energy in improving public health. He was considered so important that he was given a state funeral when he died. His portrait has appeared on postage stamps.
Bibliography: Ackernecht, E. H. 1953. *Rudolph Virchow, doctor, statesman, anthropologist.*

VIRGIL (*or* VERGIL, VERGILIUS), PUBLIUS MARO (70 B.C.-A.D. 19). A Roman poet. He suffered from chronic indigestion and asthma, which may account for his interest in medicine. In the twelfth book of the *Aeneid* he used his own physician in the character of Iapis. It is said that the episode concerning the wounded Aeneas was introduced only for the purpose of including a physician and praising his art. In the same epic, Virgil presented a sterotype of madness. The frenzied paroxysm described there reflects the image of insanity held by the people of his time. Incubi (*see* INCUBUS) were also mentioned in his work and their connection with mental disorder was retained for several centuries.
Bibliography: Virgil. *Aeneid*, trans. H. R. Fairclough.

VISCEROTONIA. A personality type associated with endomorphy, a physical type, in the classification of W. H. Sheldon (q.v.). It denotes passivity and pleasure in sensation.
Bibliography: Sheldon, W. H. 1940. *The varieties of human physique.*

VIS VIVA. A Latin expression meaning "living force." It was used by Christian Huygens (q.v.) in 1669 in referring to animal spirits (q.v.). It also has been used to refer to what is now known as kinetic energy.
Bibliography: Boring, E. G. 1950. *A history of experimental psychology.*

VISITING. Visits by friends and relations were considered beneficial to institutionalized mental patients. One of the strongest advocates of visiting

was Richard Hale (q.v.), physician to Bethlem Royal Hospital (q.v.) in the eighteenth century. He maintained that patients were more likely to attempt suicide (q.v.) on Sundays (q.v.) because visitors were not admitted then.
Bibliography: O'Donoghue, E. G. 1914. *The story of Bethlehem Hospital.*

VISZANIK, MICHAEL VON (1792-1872). A Hungarian physician. After obtaining his medical degree in Vienna he became interested in psychiatric disorders and was appointed physician to the Narrenturm (q.v.). He visited mental institutions in France, Switzerland, and England and introduced into his own hospital any beneficial innovations he had observed during his visits. Because of visits to other mental institutions, hydrotherapy, observation wards, and the abolition of chains became a feature of the Narrenturm. Many of his progressive ideas were incorporated in the plans for a new asylum in Brünnelfeld. He was also a teacher of psychiatry and the founder of an association for discharged mental patients in need of help.
Bibliography: Berner, P., Spiel, W., Strotzka, H., and Wyklicky, H. 1983. *Psychiatry in Vienna.*

VITALISM. A medico-philosophical concept introduced in the eighteenth century. In contrast to mechanistic theories (q.v.), it postulated the existence of a "vital principle" without which there was no life. Paul Joseph Barthez (q.v.) gave particular impetus to the vitalistic point of view, but despite the momentum it gave to medico-psychological studies, it was not accepted by many biologists because it could not be validated.
Bibliography: Watson, R. I. 1963. *The great psychologists.*

VITRUVIUS, MARCUS POLLIO. A Roman architect of the first century B.C. In the course of his travels through Northern Italy he observed the prevalence of goitre among agricultural people in the Alps. He suggested that the drinking water of the mountainous regions might be responsible for it. His observations, recorded in *De Architectura*, book 8, chapter 3, are probably the earliest on goitre.
Bibliography: Vitruvius. *De Architectura*, trans. J. R. Morgan.

VITUS, SAINT (died c. 303 A.D.). The son of a pagan senator of Sicily in the second century A.D. He was converted to Christianity by his nurse and her husband who acted as his tutor. To escape the wrath of his father, he left Sicily and took refuge in Italy. He settled in Rome where he cured the son of the emperor Diocletian (245-313). According to legend, Diocletian showed little gratitude and had Vitus thrown into a cauldron of molten lead, from which he emerged none the worse. He was then exposed to the lions, who refused to eat him. Before he could be condemned to further atrocities, an angel spirited him away. During the Middle Ages (q.v.) his cult gradually expanded, and he was invoked in cases of injury from wild beasts, hydrophobia, sudden death, and chorea. Mental patients were taken on pilgrimages to various shrines (q.v.) dedicated to him. It was believed that offerings of

gifts and dancing around his image would affect a cure. The dancing led to the term "dancing mania" (q.v.) and to the expression "Saint Vitus' dance" (q.v.) but referred to the disorders rather than to their treatment.
Bibliography: Talbot, C. H. 1967. *Medicine in medieval England.*

VIVES, JUAN LUIS (1492-1540). A Spanish philosopher, and friend of Desiderius Erasmus (q.v.). His ideas were far in advance of his time, and he is considered the father of modern psychology. He rejected the idea of planetary influences on mental phenomena, believed emotions to be more important than reason, advocated compassion for the mentally ill, and refused to regard women as intellectually inferior to men. He correlated social phenomena with abnormal behavior and understood the effect of emotion on recalling past events. He also realized how long-forgotten memories could be recalled through the association of ideas. For a time Henry VIII (1491-1547) greatly admired him, and he was invited to England in 1523. There, he enjoyed the protection of his first queen, Catherine of Aragon (1485-1536) and served as tutor to their daughter Mary I (q.v.) to whom he dedicated some of his works in the form of precepts. Thomas More (q.v.) and his family were his close friends, and he sadly missed them when Henry VIII's rejection of Catherine made his position difficult and forced him to leave England. Of his many books on education and social theory, *De Anima et Vita* (q.v.) is the most important to the field of psychology. It is considered one of the first modern works on psychology.
Bibliography: Watson, F. 1922. *Luis Vives, el gran Valenciano.*

VOGT, OSKAR (1870-1959) *and* **VOGT, CÉCILE.** (1875-1962). German neurologists who were husband and wife. Their studies concentrated on the cytoarchitecture of the brain in primates and man. They suggested that the localization of certain functions in man could be determined by studying the cerebral cortex of animals. Their studies of the thalamus led to the description of a condition characterized by athetosis. They also examined the brains of many famous people, including Nikolai Lenin (q.v.). Oskar Vogt was the founder and director of the Brain Research Institute in Berlin. He supplied hypnotism (q.v.) with a scientific basis by regarding it as a form of neurodynamic inhibition.
Bibliography: Haymaker, W. 1951. Cecile and Oskar Vogt. On the occasion of her 75th and his 80th birthday. *Neurology.* 1: 179-218.

VOISIN, FELIX (1794-1872). A French physician. After studying under Jean Esquirol (q.v.), he joined Guillaume Ferrus (q.v.) at Bicêtre (q.v.) in 1831. His major achievement was in the field of mental deficiency. In collaboration with Jean Falret (q.v.), he was the founder of a private hospital at Vanves. His views on the complex psychological changes occurring at puberty became fashionable more than a century after he proposed them in

a volume entitled *Des Causes Morales et Physiques des Maladies Mentales* (1826). According to him, mental illness was an idiopathic cerebral disorder. His major work, published in 1867, consisted of a three-volume treatise on the animal, moral, and intellectual faculties of man that was entitled '*Etudes sur la Nature de l'Homme Considéré comme être Animal, Moral et Intellectual*. In it he emphasized his belief that ethics were dependent on psychology.
Bibliography: Kanner, L. 1964. *A history of the care and study of the mentally retarded.*

VOLKMANN, ALFRED WILHELM (1800-1877). A German physiologist and professor at Halle for thirty-nine years. As well as writing on the physiology of vision, he worked with Gustav Fechner (q.v.) on the method of average error and produced a book on animal magnetism (q.v.).
Bibliography: Boring, E. G. 1950. *A history of experimental psychology.*

VOLTAIRE (1694-1778). The pen name of Jean François Marie Arouet, a French philosopher, poet, and historian. The son of a notary, his wit opened many doors, and he was welcomed into the frivolous high society of his time. Under the protection of his intimate friend, Madame du Châtelet (1706-1749), an intelligent and cultured woman, he advanced socially and financially, although his views brought him official disapproval, periods of exile, and even imprisonment. He was a leading figure of the Enlightenment. His character was a strange mixture of opposites: he lacked warmth but not humor; he was generous, yet at times mean and vindictive; enlightened yet intolerant. His vanity and irritability were well known, and his quarrels with the most notable men of his time were famous. In later years his optimism was replaced by dark pessimism, bitter rejection of the church, and contempt for authority and social institutions. He approved of suicide (q.v.) and agreed with the belief that the English were particularly prone to it, killing themselves when "the fancy took them". He also believed the spleen (q.v.) caused their melancholic (*see* MELANCHOLIA) dispositions. Constipation was the other aetiology of depression he favored. On his death the Church denied him a Christian burial.
Bibliography: Wade, I. 1970. *The intellectual development of Voltaire.*

VOLUNTARY SECLUSION. In the early nineteenth century Matthew Allen (q.v.) argued that mental patients should be allowed to enter institutions "at the commencement of the malady," rather than after they had become severely ill and were admitted under an official certificate of insanity. This was the first time that a system of voluntary patients had been suggested, but the commissioners in lunacy (q.v.) seriously disapproved of these liberal

views, which were against the legislation of the time. They reported Allen for allowing uncertified patients to reside in his establishment.
Bibliography: Hunter, R., and Macalpine, I. 1963. *Three hundred years of psychiatry.*

VOODOO. A mixture of superstition, magic (q.v.) and sorcery originating in Africa and still surviving in Haiti, other parts of the West Indies, and the Americas, especially among Negroes. The cult is based on spirit worship, and its priests, or sorcerers, are believed to possess special magic gifts. Their curses (q.v.) are believed to be so powerful that they can cause death unless counteracted by an even stronger sorcerer. Death by suggestion is not unknown among believers in voodoo.
Bibliography: Deren, M. 1953. *Divine horsemen: the living gods of Haiti.*

VULPIAN, EDMÉ FÉLIX ALFRED (1826-1887). A French physician. He worked with Jean Charcot (q.v.) at Salpêtrière (q.v.) and undertook research on the degeneration of the brain, vasomotor activity, and the action of various drugs on the nervous system. Many of Charcot's achievements were inspired and supported by him.
Bibliography: Haymaker, W., and Schiller, F. 1970. *The founders of neurology.* 2d. ed.

W

WACHSMUTH, ADOLPH (1827-1865). A German physician. He tried to organize a system of psychopathology which differentiated between organic mental disorders and functional mental disorders. He believed that psychoses are not necessarily caused by brain lesions and that brain lesions could exist without giving rise to psychotic symptoms.
Bibliography: Wachsmuth, A. 1859. *Allgemeine Pathologie der Seele*.

WACINKO. A syndrome found in the Oglala Sioux Indians. The term literally means "pouting" and indicates deep disappointment at not getting what is desired. Symptoms suggest that it is a form of reactive depression. Those affected show pathological degrees of anger, psychomotor retardation, withdrawal, mutism (q.v.), and immobility. In extreme cases, the disorder leads to suicide (q.v.).
Bibliography: Lewis, T. H. 1975. Syndrome of depression and mutism in the Oglala Sioux. *Am. J. Psych.* 132: 753-55.

WAGNER, RICHARD (1813-1883). A German composer. His first success came with the performance of *Tristan* in Munich in 1865, after he had come under the protection of the unstable Ludwig II of Bavaria (q.v.). Before this event, he often had serious financial difficulties. He tried to supplement his scarce musical earnings by writings that included *Judaism and Music* (1850), an anti-Semitic work, and the autobiographical *Communication to My Friends* (1851-1852). His debts eventually caused his imprisonment. He was extravagant and emotionally irresponsible. He also meddled unwisely in politics and attracted hostility. His love affairs were notorious. When he died, he was buried in a tomb in Bayreuth, Germany, which he had himself prepared. Ludwig II rode there alone one night to pay tribute to his much admired friend. Among his dramas are *Tannhäuser* (1843-1844), *Lohengrin*

(1846-1848), *Der Ring des Nibelungen* (1853-1874), which are all based on medieval German literary themes.

Bibliography: Newman, E. 1933-1947. *The life of Richard Wagner.* 4 vols.

WAGNER VON JAUREG, JULIUS (1857-1940). An Austrian psychiatrist and neurologist. In his work he introduced the use of malaria therapy (q.v.) in the treatment of general paralysis of the insane (q.v.). He conceived the idea that fever might be of therapeutic value in 1887; in 1917 he first innoculated paretics with tertian malarial organisms. In 1927 he was awarded the Nobel Prize for his work in this field. His physical approach provided the basis for the development of shock therapy in the treatment of psychosis (q.v.). He also advocated the addition of iodine to table salt in those areas where cretinism (q.v.) associated with goiter was endemic. His work in the fields of forensic psychiatry and pharmacology also is well known. He suffered from insomnia, which he tried to alleviate by playing long chess games with imaginary opponents.

Bibliography: Haymaker, W. and Schiller, F. 1970. *The founders of neurology.*
       2d. ed.

WAIN, LOUIS WILLIAM (1860-1939). A British artist. The first of six children, he was sickly and born with a hare lip. His poor health prevented him from going to school until he was ten years old. He also suffered from unpleasant recurring dreams (q.v.). At the age of twenty-three he upset his family by falling in love with his younger brother's governess, a woman in her thirties, whom he finally married. Three years after the marriage she died of carcinoma of the breast. During her illness, a black kitten had been her pet, and it is possible that this was significant in Wain's choice of subjects. He became known as the "man who drew cats," and the progressive deterioration of his mind was matched by the increasing distortions in his cat drawings. The death of his elder sister upset him greatly. Paranoid ideas and violent behavior caused him to be certified insane and admitted to a pauper ward in an asylum. There his drawings brought him to the attention of influential people, a fund was set up for him, and he transferred to Bethlem Royal Hospital (q.v.) and then to Napsbury Hospital, near Saint Albans, where he continued to draw.

Bibliography: Dale, R. 1969. *Louis Wain—the man who drew cats.*

WAKEFIELD, EDWARD (1774-1854). An English farmer, land agent, and philanthropist. He was the son of Priscilla Wakefield (q.v.) and continued the family tradition of working for the underprivileged. As a member of the Committee on Madhouses between 1815 and 1816 he gathered evidence and reported on the conditions of mental patients in private and public

establishments. His work among the insane brought many abuses to light, including the incarceration of William Norris (q.v.).
Bibliography: Parry-Jones, W. Ll. 1972. *The trade in lunacy.*

WAKEFIELD, PRISCILLA (1751-1832). An English Quaker (q.v.), philanthropist, and writer. She instituted several charities in London. She was the aunt of Elizabeth Fry (q.v.) and spent some time as a patient in the notorious Whitmore House (q.v.). According to John Mitford, she was beaten, dragged by her hair, and flogged in front of male patients there. With her sister, Mrs. Gurney, she was the subject of a celebrated portrait by Thomas Gainsborough (1727-1788). Her work was continued by her son Edward Wakefield (q.v.).
Bibliography: Morris, A. D. 1958. *The Hoxton madhouses.*

WAKEFIELD ASYLUM. An English mental hospital in the West Riding. It was founded in 1818. Its organization was influenced by that of the York Retreat (q.v.), and Samuel Tuke (q.v.) was consulted on the way in which it should be managed. Tuke's *Practical Hints* were published as a preface to the architect's drawings. The patients were accommodated in small groups, and a central spiral staircase provided an overall observation point. The first medical director was Sir William Ellis (q.v.), and the first matron was his wife. They introduced occupational and industrial therapy, gave their patients considerable freedom of movement, and provided a rudimentary after-care service. The asylum is now known as the Stanley Royd Hospital.
Bibliography: Poynter, R.N.I. ed. 1964. *The evolution of hospitals in Britain.*

WALDEYER-HARTZ, HEINRICH WILHELM VON (1836-1921). A German anatomist. His research in neurology (q.v.) gave prominence to the neurone theory in which the nervous system is regarded as a complex of structurally independent units called neurons. The theory was first published in 1891. Waldeyer is also credited with the introduction of the term "chromosome."
Bibliography: McHenry, L. C. 1969. *Garrison's history of neurology.*

WALES. The first asylum in Wales was opened in Haverfordwest, Pembrokeshire, in 1824. It was followed by the licensing of a house in Glamorganshire for private and pauper patients in 1843. Another asylum opened at Denbigh, North Wales, in 1847.
Bibliography: Tuke, D. H. 1882. *History of the insane in the British Isles.*

WALKER, SAYER (1748-1826). An English physician and Presbyterian minister. He often combined his two careers by treating the poor parishioners under his pastoral care. Influenced by the ideals of the French Revolution (q.v.), he was passionately on the side of freedom of speech and of a more enlightened scientific approach, especially in medicine. In 1790, he preached a sermon in London praising medical progress and the treatment of the insane. After he resigned from the ministry, having cited asthma and loss of voice as his reasons, he dedicated all his energies to medicine, especially neurology, the mind-body relationship, and psychiatric disorders. In 1796 he published *A Treatise on Nervous Diseases* in which he discussed the psychological aspects of somatic diseases and their management. The volume and much of his teachings were directed to general practitioners whose practice included neurotic and psychotic patients.

Bibliography: Hunter, R., and Macalpine, I. 1963. *Three hundred years of psychiatry*.

WALLACE, ALFRED RUSSELL (1823-1913). An English naturalist. Independently of Charles Darwin (q.v.), he originated the theory of evolution without neglecting the importance of mental factors in the process. He also provides an interesting example of the influence of the emotions on the body: he reported that after catching a new and beautiful butterfly he felt faint and suffered from migraine for the remainder of the day.

Bibliography: Wallace, A. R. 1905. *My life*.

WANG K'EN-TANG. A Chinese philosopher during the Ming dynasty in the seventeenth century. He offered advice for the diagnosis and treatment of states now recognized as schizophrenia, mania, and epilepsy (qq.v.). He described patients in the first group as given to violence and inappropriate laughter or tears. According to him, they were unlikely to recover. He said those in the second group behaved in a strange, antisocial manner, unaware of danger, abusive, stubborn, and raving. The third group consisted of patients subject to convulsions, dizziness, and the inability to recognize people.

Bibliography: Kao, J. J. 1979. *Three millenia of Chinese psychiatry*.

WARD, EDWARD (1667-1731). An English writer of satirical and humorous poetry. He is better known as Ned Ward. In his *London Spy*, a work published in monthly installments from 1698 to 1709, he described a visit to Bethlem Royal Hospital (q.v.) at Moorfields. He wrote that it was "an almshouse for madmen, a showing room for harlots, a sure market for lechers, a dry walk for loiterers." He also recorded his impressions of Bridewell (q.v.) and described the men there as "a parcel of ill-looking mortals" and the women as "shut up as close as nuns."

Bibliography: Tuke, D. H. 1882. *History of the insane in the British Isles*.

WARD, JAMES (1843-1925). An English psychologist influenced by Franz Brentano (q.v.). He was the exponent of act psychology (q.v.), which emphasized unconscious activities and opposed associationism (q.v.). He became famous as a psychologist after his contribution to the ninth edition of

the *Encyclopedia Britannica* in 1886. This was the first time that psychology had been given due importance in an encyclopedia. Ward extended the article for the eleventh edition in 1911. His system of psychology, stressing the importance of biological factors, was fully developed in *Psychological Principles*, which he wrote in 1918. In spite of abstruse ideas, he greatly influenced psychological thought, especially in England.
Bibliography: Boring, E. G. 1950. *A history of experimental psychology.*

WARDELL, SAMUEL (?-1692). One of the victims of the Salem witchcraft trials (q.v.). He confessed that he had made a pact with the devil. Becoming depressed after his proposal of marriage was rejected, he claimed he had seen a cat that changed into a black man (the devil) and promised him success in life. Wardell later retracted his confession, protesting that he was not in his right mind when he made it, but nevertheless he was found guilty and hanged.
Bibliography: Deutsch, A. 1949. *The mentally ill in America.*

"WARD No. 6." A short story by Anton Chekhov (q.v.). The protagonist is the physician of a mental hospital. He neglects his patients and withdraws into his own private world of gloomy thoughts and alcoholism (q.v.). He becomes isolated and unable to communicate with others, although he holds long philosophical discourses with one patient. His assistant finds an excuse for having him certified insane, and he is submitted to the same horrible treatment that his patients received. Just before dying he realizes the part he has played in the misery of his patients' lives in the asylum.
Bibliography: Chekhov, A. 1916-1922. *The tales of Chekhov,* trans. C. Garnett.

WARE, JOHN (1795-1864). An American physician. He wrote the first full account of delirium tremens (q.v.) in a series of papers that were later published in book form.
Bibliography: Ware, J. 1831. *Remarks on the history and treatment of delirium tremens.*

WARLINGHAM PARK HOSPITAL. A psychiatric institution in Surrey, England. It was originally known as Croydon Mental Hospital. Established in 1903, it was the first to abandon the term "asylum" and to call itself a "mental hospital." It was also the first English hospital to adopt the open-door system under Dr. T. Percy Rees.
Bibliography: Stacey, M. R. 1953. *Warlingham Park Hospital.*

WARLOCK, PETER. *See* HESELTINE, PHILIP ARNOLD.

WARMTH. According to Aristotle (q.v.) warmth was important to the functioning of the soul. He believed mental disorders would develop if the

black bile (q.v.) became either too cold or too warm. If too cold, it would produce a stuporose state, but an excess of warmth would produce frenzy and suicidal impulses.
Bibliography: *Aristotle*. (Problems, XXX.) 1831-1870, ed. I. Bekker.

WARNEFORD HOSPITAL. A psychiatric hospital near Oxford, England. It was instituted in 1813 and officially opened in 1826 with the name of Radcliffe Asylum. Its patients were drawn from the middle- and upper-classes in the Oxford area. In 1843 the Reverend Samuel Wilson Warneford (1763-1855) endowed the hospital with a substantial sum. In recognition of his generous gift, the asylum changed its name to the Warneford Lunatic Asylum. In 1849 it was granted a royal charter. A few poor patients were admitted free of charge or at reduced rates. The hospital is now part of the National Health Service.
Bibliography: Anon. 1926. *Brief history of the Warneford Hospital.*

WARREN, HOWARD CROSBY (1867-1934). An American psychologist and pupil of Wilhelm Wundt (q.v.). Although sympathetic to the tenets of behaviorism (q.v.), Warren felt that observation of overt behavior was not sufficient in research. According to him introspection methods were invaluable in scientific psychology. He wrote on the history of psychology and produced a textbook on human psychology.
Bibliography: Warren, H. C. 1922. *Elements of human psychology.*

WARTS. Folklore (q.v.) and early medical writings make frequent references to warts. Most cures rely on the power of suggestion provided through a placebo (q.v.). Many Anglo-Saxon herbals contain songs that are believed to charm warts away. Sir Kenelm Digby (q.v.) believed that the best cure for warts was a piece of bacon, which after it had been rubbed on the affected part was nailed to the framework of a window facing south. Another cure he advocated was washing by the light of a full moon (q.v.) in water held in a silver basin. Among other suggested cures were rubbing them with stolen beef, or the blood of an eel or slug, the saliva of a dog, or the hand of a corpse, or wrapping them with a spider's web and then covering them with macerated herbs. Some practices involve magical (*see* MAGIC) transference to animals or certain objects, or selling them to someone else.
Bibliography: Bonser, W. 1963. *The medical background of Anglo-Saxon England.*

WASSERMANN, AUGUST VON (1866-1925). A German bacteriologist. In 1906 he developed a blood test for the diagnosis of syphilis (q.v.).
Bibliography: Dennie, C. C. 1962. *A history of syphilis.*

WASSERMANN, JAKOB (1873-1934). A German novelist whose work is full of psychological realism. In *Caspar Hauser* (1908) the central figure is based on Kaspar Hauser (q.v.).
Bibliography: Blankenage, J. N. 1942. *The writings of Wassermann.*

WATERS, CHARLES OSCAR (1816-1892). An American physician. He gave an account of a case of chronic hereditary chorea in an adult. The disease later became known as Huntington's chorea. His description occurred in a letter to Dr. Robley Dunglison (q.v.) and was recorded by him in 1842.

Bibliography: Dunglison, R. 1842. *Practice of medicine*. Vol. 2.

WATER THERAPY. In the nineteenth century, large quantities of cold drinking water frequently were prescribed in the treatment of insanity. A tumbler every hour was the recommended dosage. Melancholia (q.v.) and a disposition to suicide (q.v.) were considered particularly responsive to this form of therapy. Other earlier forms of water therapy were the bath of surprise, the douche and the practice of immersion (qq.v.). Immersion was particularly advocated by Jan Batista Van Helmont (q.v.). In Siberia psychosomatic impotence was treated by soaking the patient overnight in cool water.

Bibliography: Esquirol, J.E.D. 1845. Reprint. 1965. *Mental maladies: a treatise on insanity.*

WATSON, JOHN BROADUS (1878-1958). An American psychologist. He believed that learning theories should describe only observable behavior. He expressed this opinion in a paper published while he was a professor of experimental and comparative psychology at Johns Hopkins University. The paper, entitled *Psychology as the Behaviorist Views It* (1913), gained for him the title of "father of behaviorism." He expanded his theories in 1919 with *Psychology from the Standpoint of a Behaviorist*. His experimental research included work on the basic reactions of infants and young children and an investigation on the ability of normal, blind, and anosonic rats to solve the problems of a maze (q.v.). He contributed to the field of educational psychology and worked on the psychological aspects of military practices during World War I. In 1918 he began working at the Henry Phipps Psychiatric Clinic (q.v.) with Adolf Meyer (q.v.). Watson was always a controversial figure, especially in the field of child care. Adverse publicity, resulting from his divorce in 1920, put an end to his academic career. For a time he turned to business enterprises and wrote for the more popular press.

See also ALBERT B.

Bibliography: Cohen, D. 1979. *J. B. Watson: the founder of behaviorism.*

WATT, HENRY J. (1879-1925). A British psychologist and pupil of Oswald Külpe (q.v.). He was appointed professor of psychology to Glasgow University in 1908. His work included books on memory (q.v.), sound, and cognition. His special field of interest was the experimental study of thought.

Bibliography: Misiak, H., and Sexton, V. S. 1966. *History of psychology.*

WATTS, ISAAC (1674-1748). An English nonconformist theologian, philosopher, and hymn writer. At the age of thirty-eight he developed a disease that left him with delusions (q.v.) of vision. He later came to believe that he was a teapot and that he was so large that he could not pass through an ordinary doorway.

Bibliography: Davis, A. P. 1943. *Isaac Watts: his life and works.*

WAUGH, EVELYN ARTHUR ST. JOHN (1903-1966). An English novelist. He was selfish, inconsiderate, and cruel to the point of sadism (q.v.). His satires of social life degenerated into such sardonic bitterness that they distressed many of his friends and acquaintances whom he used as characters in his books. He was often depressed to the point of suicide and suffered from deafness, insomnia, amnesia and paranoia (q.v.). His heavy use of hypnotics and alcohol made him worse. In 1954 he sailed for Ceylon, hoping that his health would improve. While on board he suffered from an hallucinatory psychosis that caused him to hear bodiless voices repeating his name and led him to believe that he was being persecuted. He abandoned the voyage and returned home in search of a priest who would exorcise (*see* EXORCISM) the devil possessing (*see* POSSESSION) him. A psychiatrist cured him with an effective narcotic, and a physician attributed his symptoms to bromide poisoning. Waugh was extremely superstitious and paid large sums for prayers for such things as good weather when he was giving a party. His Catholicism, however, helped to keep under control the worst side of his personality. One of his books, *The Ordeal of Gilbert Pinfold* (1956) is a fictionalized account of his psychotic illness.

Bibliography: Sykes, C. 1975. *Evelyn Waugh: a biography.*

WEATHER. For centuries atmospheric conditions have been considered significant in the aetiology of behavior disorders. Winds (q.v.), for example the sirocco (q.v.), have been blamed for producing insanity; the frequent fogs of England have been linked to depression and the high rate of suicide (q.v.) among the English. In his biography, Vittorio Alfieri (q.v.) acknowledged that weather conditions affected the quality and quantity of his literary output and John Milton (q.v.) made a similar observation.

See also CLIMATE.

Bibliography: Tromp, S. W. 1963. *Medical biometeorology.*

WEBER, CARL MARIA FRIEDRICH ERNST VON (1786-1826). A German composer. His father, a violinist and a cousin of the wife of Wolfgang Amadeus Mozart (1756-1791), considered him to be a child prodigy and forced his musical education. Parental ambition caused untold misery and nervous strain throughout his childhood. Due to a hip disease, Weber could not walk until he was four years old but could play the clavier well before that age. He was only fourteen years old when his first opera (q.v.) *Des Waldmädchen* was performed in Vienna. By the time he was seventeen years old, he was conductor of the opera at Breslau. His father's dubious

speculations resulted in accusations of embezzlement, and they were banned from Württemberg.
Bibliography: Saunders, W. 1940. *Weber*.

WEBER, ERNST HEINRICH (1795-1878). A German psychophysiologist and pioneer in the field of sensory psychology. He conducted elaborate experiments on the sense of touch and kinesthesis. His findings on the relationship between stimulus and sensation resulted in the so-called Weber's law. He also wrote a treatise on the sense of touch in which he systematized his observations and discovery of tactile sensations.
Bibliography: Weber, E. H. 1912. *The sense of touch and common feeling*, trans. B. Rand.

WECHSLER, DAVID (1896-). An American psychologist born in Rumania. He specializes in measuring intelligence in relation to age. He has devised a number of well-known intelligence tests (q.v.), contributed to the development of diagnostic techniques for assessing changes of ability, and has invented a lie detector, or psychogalvanograph.
Bibliography: Wechsler, D. 1944. *The measurements of intelligence*.

WEDNESDAY PSYCHOLOGICAL SOCIETY. Those individuals interested in problems of psychoanalysis (q.v.) who met each Wednesday evening at the home of Sigmund Freud (q.v.). The group began in 1902. In 1908 they were renamed the Viennese Psychoanalytic Society. Because of the increased size, the group could no longer meet in Freud's house; congresses were organized in various cities and attracted international interest. A dissenting society was founded by Alfred Adler (q.v.) in 1911, and in 1913 the defection of Carl Jung (q.v.) from Freud's group caused the Swiss followers to break away. Psychoanalysis, however, continued to spread, especially in the United States, and the International Psychoanalytic Association (q.v.) continued to prosper, although banned by the Nazis in Austria.
Bibliography: Fine, R. 1979. *A history of psychoanalysis*.

WEIGERT, CARL (1845-1904). A German pathologist and histologist. His new methods of staining bacteria and tissues permitted detailed study of neuroglia.
Bibliography: Haymaker, W., and Schiller, F. 1970. *The founders of neurology*. 2d. ed.

WEIKARD, MELCHIOR ADAM (1742-1803). A German physician. He classified mental diseases into two groups: disorders of mood and disorders of mind. In the first group he included depression, anxiety, shame, despair,

and suicide; in the second group he placed those disorders that are accompanied by delusions.
Bibliography: Weikard, M. A. 1790. *Der philosophische Arzt.*

WEISMANN, AUGUST (1834-1914). A German biologist. He opposed the belief that acquired characteristics are inherited and devised, instead, a theory of germ plasm, a substance passed on from generation to generation. He was one of the first to suggest that hereditary material is transmitted through chromosomes. He attacked the theories of Jean Lamarck (q.v.) and sided with Charles Darwin (q.v.) in the dispute over evolution of the species.
Bibliography: Flugel, J. C. 1965. *A hundred years of psychology.*

WEISS, ALBERT P. (1879-1931). An American psychologist born in Germany. As a behaviorist, he asserted that all psychological phenomena could be reduced to biosocial terms without some concept of consciousness for their interpretation.
Bibliography: Weiss, A. P. 1925. *A theoretical basis of human behavior.*

WEIZSÄCKER, VIKTOR VON (1886-1957). A German physician and professor of medicine. He was impressed by the ideas of Sigmund Freud (q.v.) and used psychoanalytic teachings in his explanation of the aetiological factors in bodily disorders. He also discussed the effect of somatic illness on the psyche.
Bibliography: Weizsacker, V. von 1951. *Der kranke Mensch.*

WELDON, GEORGINA (1837-1914). An English eccentric involved in spiritualism (q.v.). She believed that her pet rabbit was the reincarnation of her deceased mother. Her eccentricities led to her husband's attempts to have her certified as insane and committed to a private asylum. When an alienist (q.v.) came to take her away, she barricaded herself in the house and escaped in the disguise of a nun. She then retaliated with a series of legal actions that attracted a great deal of publicity and contributed to the reform of the laws relating to insanity. In 1878 she published her experiences under the title *The History of My Orphanage or the Outpourings of an Alleged Lunatic.*
Bibliography: Parry-Jones, W. Ll. 1972. *The trade in lunacy.*

WELLS, HERBERT GEORGE (1866-1946). An English writer, known for his science-fiction stories and satirical sociological novels. He studied biology under Thomas Huxley (q.v.) and, for a time, was a teacher. As a child he was overprotected, especially by his mother, who expected the family to keep up the appearance of comfortable prosperity, although money was scarce. He was not allowed to mix with other children for fear they would discover the family secret. His aim in life seems to have been to achieve recognition of his superior and vigorous intellect, without neglecting to live to the full. He gained the reputation of being the most successful seducer of his time. Married, with two children, he made Rebecca West (1892-) his mistress and had a son by her, but his love was never free from calculation and falseness. After ten tormented years she left him. His vanity and his reputation were all important to him, yet women were not attracted by his intellect or by his personality as a whole. One of them said that what had attracted her was the honey smell of his body. He was a diabetic, and in 1934 he founded the British Diabetic Association, feeling that there would be "something psychologically and socially valuable in the latent solidarity of people subject to a distinctive disorder." In *Mind at the End of its Tether* (1945) written shortly before his death, he expressed despair for the future of mankind.

Bibliography: Dickson, L. 1969. *H. G. Wells: his turbulent life and times.*

WELLS, THOMAS SPENCER (1818-1897). An English surgeon. He is remembered for his contribution to surgical techniques for the safe removal of the ovaries. In an age when ovariotomy (q.v.) was advocated for the treatment of hysterical (*see* HYSTERIA) disorders, he firmly stated that it was "inadmissible in any case of nervous disturbance."

Bibliography: Wells, S. Oct. 1886. *American Journal of Medical Sciences.*

WELSH, JANE BAILLIE (1801-1866). The wife of Thomas Carlyle (q.v.). She was the only child of a physician of Haddington, Scotland. She compensated for her feeble health by possessing a shrewd, querulous, and neurotic disposition. After a courtship of some years, she married Thomas Carlyle. In spite of mutual affection, the marriage was marred by her jealousy (q.v.), and her morbid introspection was increased by her childlessness. She felt that her husband neglected her and wrote her complaints, often justified, in a diary. It was written in a way to cause the maximum guilt in her husband when he found the diary after her death. In the latter part of her life she was a physical and emotional invalid. She died of shock after a trivial accident.

Bibliography: Holme, T. 1965. *The Carlyles at home.*

WELSH SPRINGS. In ancient Wales many springs, wells and streams were associated with healing of the insane. Some waters were believed to be particularly efficacious in certain disorders. Ffynon Degla, for instance, was associated with epilepsy (q.v.), Ffynon Barruc, Barry Island, with alcoholism (q.v.) and St. David's Well with melancholy.

See also HOLY WELLS.

Bibliography: Clarke, B. 1975. *Mental disorders in earlier Britain.*

WEREWOLVES. *See* LYCANTHROPY.

WERFEL, FRANZ (1890-1945). An Austrian poet and novelist. He converted from Judaism to Catholicism and became eager to convert others.

His conflict with his father is reflected in many of his poems, for example *Father and Son*. The theme is repeated in *The Murdered not the Murderer is Guilty* (1920), a novel. In his writings, fathers are always cruel, and he dwells on the manner of their death, which frequently is by murder.
Bibliography: Foltin, L. B. 1961. *Franz Werfel*.

WERNICKE, CARL (1848-1905). A German neurologist and psychiatrist. He studied under Theodor Meynert (q.v.) in Vienna and was greatly influenced by him in his search for neurological explanations of mental disorders. In 1881 he began a comprehensive account of studies on cerebral localization. The three-volume work was completed in 1883 and published in Berlin as *Lehrbuch der Gehirnkrankheiten*. Wernicke advanced many new ideas, including a description of a new syndrome, now named Wernicke's encephalopathy. He also wrote extensively on aphasia. In 1894 he published a complete system of psychiatry entitled *Grundrisser der Psychiatrie*.
Bibliography: Haymaker, W., and Schiller, F. 1970. *The founders of neurology*. 2d. ed.

WERTHEIMER, MAX (1880-1943). A Czechoslovakian psychologist who became interested in philosophy and psychology after studying law. He is considered the principal founder of the Gestalt (q.v.) school of psychology. His co-workers were Wolfgang Kohler (q.v.) and Kurt Koffka (q.v.). He objected to structuralism, which explained experiences in terms of their constituents, and asserted that experiences and perceptions cannot be split into parts if they are to be understood properly. In 1933 he left Germany because of the rise of Nazism and emigrated to the United States, where he worked at the New School for Social Research in New York. His work inspired research in many aspects of the living organism.
Bibliography: Wertheimer, M. 1945. *Productive thinking*.

WERTHER. The overly sensitive hero of *The Sorrows of Young Werther* (1774), a novel by Johann Wolfgang von Goethe (q.v.). More involved in fantasy and dreams than in reality, Werther falls in love with a practical girl. His hopeless passion leads him to suicide (q.v.). The story caused an international epidemic of suicides and created a particular type of excessive sensibility. There was even a Werther fashion in dress. Napoleon I (q.v.) read the book seven times, and the Chinese reproduced the characters of the novel on their porcelain.
Bibliography: Goethe, J. W. von. 1966. *The sufferings of young Werther*, trans. B. A. Morgan.

WESLEY, JOHN (1703-1791). An English theologian and evangelist, the founder of Methodism (q.v.). He was one of two surviving sons of fifteen children. His mother, one of twenty-five children, was a disciplinarian who

believed in blind obedience and the use of the rod to subdue children's exuberance. Almost all his sisters made unhappy marriages, and his own ended when his bad-tempered wife, a widow with four children, left him. His preaching often resulted in manifestations of contagious hysteria (q.v.) among his audience. He and his followers were banned from visiting prisons and mental hospitals because they caused the prisoners and patients to become overly excited. Wesley recounted in an entry in his diary for February 22, 1750, how he had been told to leave Bethlem Royal Hospital (q.v.) during a visit and added "so we are forbidden to go to Newgate for fear of making them wicket, and to Bedlam for fear of making them mad!" William Hogarth (q.v.) satirized his sermons in an engraving that showed a thermometer marked suicide (q.v.), "madness," "despair," "ecstasy" (q.v.), "raving," taking the temperature of a brain resting on a volume of Wesley's sermons. In his *Primitive Physic, or an Easy and Natural Method of curing most Diseases* Wesley advised that excited mental patients should be subjected to cold showers, or even "a great waterfall". Other favored remedies included apples (q.v.), the internal and external use of vinegar (q.v.) for lunacy, or the application of electricity (q.v.), which he personally had tried on melancholic patients.
Bibliography: Green, V.H.H. 1964. *John Wesley.*

WEST, ELLEN. A patient of the existential psychiatrist Otto Binswanger (q.v.). She was an intelligent and gifted young woman, suffering from a phobia of becoming fat. As a last resort she was admitted to Binswanger's sanitarium in Krenzlingen, Switzerland. After two and a half months she was declared incurable. Because of her suicidal (*see* SUICIDE) tendencies, the institution declined to be responsible for her and discharged her. She returned home to her husband and celebrated by eating without restraint, writing letters, and reading poetry. That same evening she committed suicide by poison. The 1944 publication of Binswanger's case history of this patient marked the entry of existential analysis (*see* EXISTENTIALISM) into the field of psychopathology and clinical psychiatry.
Bibliography: Rollo, M., Ernst, A., and Ellenberger, H. F., eds. 1958. *Existence.*

WESTERN LUNATIC ASYLUM. An American mental hospital established in Staunton, Virginia, in 1825 and officially opened in 1828. It was the second mental hospital in Virginia, which, with the Williamsburg Eastern State Lunatic Asylum (q.v.) already in existence, caused Virginia to become the first American state with two such institutions. Pressure for admission and overcrowding was so severe that the authorities had to restrict admission to those patients "who are either dangerous to society from their violence, or who are offensive to its moral sense by their indecency, and to those cases of derangement where there is reasonable ground to hope that the afflicted may be restored." The hospital records for 1883 show that local

politics involved the asylum in some extraordinary events. A number of patients in that year were murdered by aconite, which was added to their medications. A detective was asked to investigate the mystery and, under the assumed guise of a patient, lived in the asylum for several months. Although his findings are not available in full, it appears that the murders were committed by a political group opposed to the superintendent, with the aim to discredit him and regain control of the hospital.
Bibliography: Grob, G. N. 1973. *Mental institutions in America.*

WESTPHAL, CARL FRIEDRICH OTTO (1833-1890). A German neurologist who worked at the Berlin Charité (q.v.) under Karl Ideler (q.v.) and Wilhelm Griesinger (q.v.). He became professor of psychiatry (q.v.) in Berlin, and, later, in Leipzig. His wide range of interests in academic subjects kept him in touch with many contemporary scholars. His contributions to psychiatry came from his studies of the microscopic pathology of the brain and its links with mental disorders. Westphal was also interested in neuroses (*see* NEUROSIS) and was one of the first to describe obsessional (*see* OB-SESSION) states, which he considered to be "abortive insanity" (q.v.) and called "paranoia" (q.v.). He wrote on sexual pathology and, indeed, inaugurated the scientific study of homosexuality (q.v.) whose urges he called "contrary sexual feelings". He studied fear of open spaces, which he termed "agoraphobia." He also discovered the absence of the knee-jerk reflex (Westphal's sign) in cases of tabes dorsalis.
Bibliography: Zilboorg, G. 1941. *A history of medical psychology.*

WEYER (or WIER), JOHANN (1515-1588). A Dutch physician. He studied under Cornelius Agrippa (q.v.) and obtained a medical degree in Paris when he was twenty years old. He was court physician to Duke William of Cleves. He was interested in mental disorders and opposed the superstitious beliefs fanned by the Inquisition (q.v.). In *De Praestigiis Daemonum* (q.v.), he declared himself incredulous of possessions (q.v.) by the devil and asserted that abnormal behavior was the result of mental illness, rather than witchcraft (q.v.). He pleaded for medical treatment of the mentally ill and suggested that the confessions of the so-called witches were nothing more than reports of visual and auditory hallucinations (q.v.) experienced under the influence of some drugs (q.v.). With skill and sympathy, he described the symptoms of schizophrenia (q.v.), the phenomena of mass hysteria (q.v.), the paranoia (q.v.) of homosexuals (*see* HOMOSEXUALITY), and the significance of agitation recurring yearly on the same date. He did not accept ideas of inexplicable events without personal investigation, and, on occasion, he removed patients to his own home for better observation, as he did in the case of Barbara Kremers (q.v.). His views clashed with those of his contemporaries, who accused him of witchcraft, as they had accused his teacher Agrippa. When Duke William of Cleves became mentally disturbed following a cerebral hemorrhage, his enemies claimed that the illness was due to Weyer's sorcery. The church banned his books.

Bibliography: Wier, Johannes, 1563. Reprint. 1967. *De praestigiis daemonum.*

WEYGANDT, WILHELM (1870-1939). A German psychiatrist. Noting that the literature on idiocy was scarce, in 1915 he wrote a monograph on the subject. It became a classic and helped to focus attention on the need for institutions for mentally retarded children and for research on the condition.

Bibliography: Weygandt, W. 1915. *Idiotie and Imbezillitat.*

W FACTOR. Charles E. Spearman (q.v.) labeled the W factor an independent factor in the organization of character. According to Spearman an individual with a high W factor would act more on principle than on impulse. *See also* G FACTOR, O FACTOR, and P FACTOR.

Bibliography: Spearman, C. 1927. *The abilities of man.*

"WHAT ASYLUMS WERE, ARE AND OUGHT TO BE." A series of lectures by William A. F. Browne (q.v.). They were printed as a book in Edinburgh in 1837 under the less known title of *Browne on Insanity.* The author expressed his indignation at the conditions of asylums (q.v.) in the eighteenth century and quoted extensively from the reports of the parliamentary committee that had inquired into the state of asylums in England in 1815. Browne pointed to the negative attitude, the lack of classification, and the lethargy that condemned able-bodied patients to a life of inactivity and often led to wasted limbs. In his description of an ideal asylum, he discussed the best architecture and location for an asylum and emphasized the importance of classification. He believed patients should live in airy, sunny rooms with no bars on the windows. He went on to state that they should have visitors and a choice of activities to keep them occupied. Browne's suggestions followed the lead of Philippe Pinel (q.v.) and Jean Esquirol (q.v.) as well as the ideals of his hero, Saint Vincent de Paul (q.v.), after whom he named one of his sons. Although the book was regarded as revolutionary and rather unrealistic, many were impressed, and it was influential in his appointment as resident medical officer at the newly founded Crichton Royal Hospital (q.v.).

Bibliography: Browne, W.A.F. 1837. *Browne on insanity.*

WHIPPLE, GUY MONTROSE (1876-1941). An American psychologist. His specialty was educational psychology (q.v.) about which he wrote a number of books. He also warned the American Psychological Association (q.v.) of the damage done to the profession when unqualified persons ad-

ministered mental tests. His warning led to the establishment of special certification for consultants in clinical psychology.
Bibliography: Whipple, G. M. 1910. *Manual of mental and physical tests.*

WHIRLING CHAIR. A contraption designed to subject patients seated on it to rapid gyrations. It was in use in many asylums in the nineteenth century.
See also GYRATOR, ROTATORY MACHINE SPINNING CHAIR, SWINGING CHAIR, and TWIRLING STOOL.
Bibliography: Roback, A. A., and Kiernan, T. 1969. *Pictorial history of psychology and psychiatry.*

WHISTLER, JAMES ABBOTT MCNEIL (1834-1903). An American painter and etcher. After spending a brief part of his childhood in Russia, he studied art in Paris and eventually settled in London but remained rootless throughout his life. His style did not appeal to the public, and he was too unbending to play to popular taste. Inspite of his kindness to his mother and to his wife, he was an egotist. He was extremely vain and attacked his critics viciously. His passion for self-advertisement and his extreme conceit are demonstrated by his habit of meticulously collecting all comments upon his work, reprinting them and answering each of them as he did in his *Gentle Art of Making Enemies* (1890). John Ruskin (q.v.), already insane, decried his work, and this so angered Whistler that he started a libel action, which ended in the award of a farthing damages.
Bibliography: McMullen, R. 1973. *Victorian outsider.*

WHISTLING. During therapeutic sessions employing ayhuasca (q.v.), Peruvian healers whistle incantations (q.v.) to alleviate anxiety and tranquilize their patients who are already highly suggestible from the drug.
Bibliography: Dobkin De Rios, M. 1972. *Visionary wine: psychedelic healing in the Peruvian Amazon.*

WHITE, SAMUEL (1777-1845). An American psychiatrist. He gained his professional qualifications through apprenticeship, rather than medical school, and by the age of twenty he was in practice. His reputation was so great that he was often consulted by the American government about matters of legislation in the field of mental health. In 1830 he established a private mental hospital, the Hudson Lunatic Asylum in New York State, U.S.A., where he practiced until his death. He was one of the thirteen founders of the American Psychiatric Association (q.v.).
Bibliography: Deutsch, A. 1949. *The mentally ill in America.*

WHITE, WILLIAM ALANSON (1870-1937). An American psychiatrist. After graduating in medicine, he trained in psychiatry and in 1903 he became superintendent of Saint Elizabeth's Hospital (q.v.) in Washington, D.C. He remained there for the rest of his life and introduced many innovations. He changed the hospital's functions from custodial to therapeutic, recognized the psychological needs of mental patients, and encouraged social and recreational activities for them. White pioneered teaching in mental hospitals and opened the doors of Saint Elizabeth's to trainees in psychiatry and established a scientific tradition. His vigorous and enlightened approach to forensic psychiatry led to closer cooperation with the legal profession and the courts. With Smith E. Jelliffe (q.v.) he spread the tenets of psychoanalysis (q.v.) in the United States and in 1913 founded the *Psychoanalytic Review*, which was then the first and only English journal devoted to psychoanalysis. He was a prolific writer not only of articles and monographs but also books. His *Outlines of Psychiatry* (1907) became a classic and was printed and revised in fourteen editions. His other works supported the mental hygiene movement (q.v.), forged links with forensic psychiatry, and pioneered American psychoanalysis. An institute bearing his name was inaugurated while he was still alive in 1943, the 'William Alanson White Institute', dedicated to the training of psychoanalysts.

Bibliography: White, W. A. 1938. *The autobiography of a purpose.*

WHITE WILL (fl.1839). A tomcat who was an excellent subject for hypnotism (q.v.). He was one of the animals used in experiments by the London magnetizer and physician to the Middlesex Hospital, John Wilson in 1839. The cat easily fell into a cataleptic state, and his limbs could then be held in any position.

Bibliography: Thornton, E. M. 1976. *Hypnotism, hysteria and epilepsy: an historical synthesis.*

WHITMAN, CHARLES OTIS (1842-1910). An American zoologist. His studies on animal behavior emphasized the importance of behavioral patterns in characterizing species and provided useful lessons for students of human psychology.

Bibliography: Whitman, C. O. 1899. *Animal behavior.*

WHITMORE HOUSE. A mansion in London, formerly known as Balmes House. It was rebuilt in the seventeenth century by Sir George Whitmore (?-1654) and used as a private asylum. It was one of the Hoxton madhouses (q.v.) and was better known as Warburton's madhouse, from the name of its proprietor. It catered to aristocratic and wealthy patients, who were charged high fees. It also provided "keepers" for George III (q.v.), who was so ill-treated by them that he could not bear to see them without a shudder. The "crimes and horrors" of Warburton's madhouse were the

subject of contemporary pamphlets attributed to a former patient, John Mitford (q.v.), a relation of Lord Redesdale.
Bibliography: Morris, A. D. 1958. *The Hoxton madhouses.*

WHITNEY, RICHARD (?-1815). A prominent resident of Brattleboro, Vermont, U.S.A. He became mentally deranged and died as a result of the treatment ordered for him. His death hastened the foundation of the Vermont Asylum (q.v.), whose historian recorded the events:

A council of physicians. . . . decided upon trying, for the recovery of Mr. Whitney, a temporary suspension of his consciousness by keeping him completely immersed in water three or four minutes, or until he became insensible, and then resuscitate or awaken him to a new life. Passing through this desperate ordeal, it was hoped, would divert his mind, break the chain of unhappy associations, and thus remove the cause of his disease. Upon trial, this system of regeneration proved of no avail for, with the returning consciousness of the patient, came the knell of departed hopes, as he exclaimed, "You can't drown love!"

A second immersion (q.v.) was said to have terminated the patient's life, although another version of the story attributes his death to the overly enthusiastic administration of opium (q.v.).
Bibliography: Burnham H. 1880. *Brattleboro, Windham County, Vermont.*

WHYTT, ROBERT (1714-1766). A Scottish physician, pupil of James Monro (*see* MONRO FAMILY), and student of Hermann Boerhaave (q.v.). He was interested in the symptomatology of neurotic (*see* NEUROSIS) disorders and classified them into three groups comprised of hysteria (q.v.), hypochondriasis (q.v.), and nervous exhaustion. Under "diseases commonly called nervous" he listed "flatulent, spasmodic, hypochondriac, or hysteric" disorders. As a neurologist, he believed that nervous disorders were caused by disturbed motility within the nervous system but accused his contemporaries of using the term "nervous" for "many symptoms seemingly different, and very obscure in their nature. . . . whose nature and causes they were ignorant of." He was well aware of what he called "the laws of union between the soul and the body" and remarked that "nothing makes more sudden or more surprising changes in the body, than the several passions of the mind."
Bibliography: French, R. K. 1969. *Robert Whytt, the soul, and medicine.*

WICKMAN, OTTO IVAR (1872-1914). A Swedish neurologist whose work on poliomyelitis provided the first detailed analysis of the disease in all its infectious and neurological aspects.
Bibliography: Haymaker, W., and Schiller, F. 1970. *The founders of neurology.* 2d. ed.

WIENER, NORBERT (1894-1964). An American mathematician. He compared the brain to a computer that has self-regulating and self-corrective

devices and depends on negative feedback to maintain its stability. His work on the flow of communication led the foundation of cybernetics.
Bibliography: Wiener, N. 1950. *The human use of human beings.*

WIHTIKO (*or* **WINDIGO).** A supernatural monster in the folklore (q.v.) of certain Canadian Indians and Cree Eskimos. They believe that the monster has a heart or skeleton of ice and feeds on human flesh. Those thought to be possessed (*see* POSSESSION) by it develop a similar morbid craving and believe that they have become Wihtikos. The clinical signs of the disorder are anorexia, nausea, vomiting, anxiety, and depression. Its aetiology may be based on the fear that food will become so scarce as to make survival possible only through cannibalism.
Bibliography: Margetts, E. L. 1975. Canada. In *World history of psychiatry*, ed. J. G. Howells.

WILBERFORCE, WILLIAM (1759-1833). A British philanthropist. His father died when he was nine years old, and he inherited a considerable fortune that later allowed him to enter Parliament by bribing the electorate. At the age of twenty-six he was converted to the evangelical religious movement and suffered acute pangs of guilt at his pleasure-seeking way of life. He founded the Proclamation Society, later known as the Society for the Prevention of Vice, which attempted to suppress all forms of pleasure, including Sunday newspapers and brass bands in public parks. He also championed the abolition of slavery and campaigned against cruelty to children and animals. Charm and hypocrisy were the main traits of his personality. He married a neurotic woman who did little to improve his poor health and his recurring periods of depression. He took daily doses of opium (q.v.) to relieve his symptoms. His eldest son's debts, which he paid, destroyed his considerable fortune, and he died a poor man.
Bibliography: Furnaux, R. 1974. *William Wilberforce.*

WILBUR, HERVEY BACKUS (1820-1883). An American physician, who pioneered education in the field of mental deficiency. In 1848 he began a private school for defective children in his own home at Barre, Massachusetts. It was the first institution of its kind in the United States, and his success in training mental defectives helped to convince the state legislature to pass a bill for an experimental school organized on the same lines. Wilbur was persuaded to leave his own establishment, which was bringing him considerable financial rewards and satisfaction, to become superintendent of the new school. It opened in Albany, New York State in 1851 and then moved to Syracuse in 1855. He remained in charge of the institution until his death.

Bibliography: Kanner, L. 1964. *A history of the care and study of the mentally retarded.*

WILD BEAST TEST. An eighteenth-century English definition of the degree of insanity that would absolve an individual from responsibility of his action. The definition was given by Judge Tracy (1655-1735) in 1724 during the trial of Arnold, following his shooting of Lord Onslow. Tracy's statement, later known as the "Wild beast test" was as follows:

If a man be deprived of his reason, and consequently of his intention, he cannot be guilty. . . . It is not every kind of frantic humor or something unaccountable in a man's actions, that points him out to be such a madman as is to be exempted from punishment; it must be a man that is totally deprived of his understanding and memory, and doth not know what he is doing, no more than an infant, than a brute, or a wild beast; such a one is never the object of punishment.

Bibliography: Deutsch, A. 1949. *The mentally ill in America.*

WILD BOY OF AVEYRON (?-1828). A boy, approximately ten years old, found in 1798 by a group of hunters near Aveyron in France. He had been living in the forest, roaming about naked and eating whatever fruit and roots he could find. He was captured, and, after escaping a number of times, he was taken to the Abbé Sicard Bonnaterre (q.v.), who took him to Jean Itard (q.v.). Itard rejected the theory that the boy, who was given the name of Victor, was a mental defective. Itard believed that the boy's inability to talk and his rejection of clothing and other conventionalities were due to his past social isolation. He spent five years trying to educate the boy and to improve his behavior. The boy attracted a great deal of interest because he was regarded by philosophers and naturalists as an example of the "natural man," a concept much in vogue at the time. Itard eventually was forced to agree with Philippe Pinel (q.v.) that the boy was mentally retarded and that this infirmity probably had been the cause of his abandonment. However, the careful program of training that Itard devised for him was a valuable contribution to the education of the feebleminded and as such was espoused by Edouard O. Séguin (q.v.) to whom Itard handed the results of his experiments. Victor lived in custodial care for some thirty years.

See also FERAL CHILD.

Bibliography: Shattuck, R. 1980. *The forbidden experiment. The story of the wild boy of Aveyron.*

WILD BOY OF SALVADOR. A boy, approximately five years old, found wandering wild in the jungles of the Republic of Salvador in 1932. He was captured and taken to Jorge Ramirez Chulo, a psychologist. Within three years, Chulo had managed to educate the child to a standard appropriate

for his age. The boy, named Tamasha, apparently could remember living with animals but had no recollection of human parents.
See also FERAL CHILD.
Bibliography: Goldenson, R. M. 1970. *The encyclopedia of human behavior.*

WILDE, OSCAR FINGAL O'FLAHERTIE WILLS (1854-1900). An Irish poet and dramatist. Both his parents were unusual, excitable, and unorthodox to the extreme. His mother had longed for a daughter and, perhaps to compensate for her disappointment, dressed him as a girl until the age of nine. He grew into an awkward solitary boy, more interested in clothes, flowers, and books than games, sports, and the usual pursuits of boys. His father, William Wilde (q.v.), although eminent in his profession, was a figure of ridicule to his son, who had little affection for him. He was close to his little sister, Isola, who died in 1867 at the age of ten. He wrote of her in one of his earlier poems:

> Tread lightly, she is near,
> Speak gently, she can hear
> The daisies grow.

Thirty years after her death, he wrote an impassioned and moving letter to the *London Daily Chronicle*, condemning the imprisonment of young children and pointing out the damaging psychological effects of the harsh treatment they received in prison. He became notorious for his mode of living, his flamboyance, his alcoholic excesses, and his homosexuality (q.v.). He was tried for sodomy and condemned to two years of hard labor in Reading gaol. From prison he wrote *De Profundis*, a bitter, despairing, and dreadful letter to Lord Alfred Douglas (1870-1945) with whom he had an intimate relationship. The title, meaning "from the depths", is part of the Roman Catholic burial service. After his release from prison, he wrote anonymously *The Ballad of Reading Gaol*, a poem about the execution of a soldier for the murder of his unfaithful wife. He died in voluntary exile under an assumed name in a small Parisian hotel. Just before his death, he had been received into the Roman Catholic Church.
Bibliography: Pearson, H. 1975. *The life of Oscar Wilde.*

WILDE, WILLIAM ROBERT (1815-1876). An Irish physician, archaeologist, and writer. He was the father of Oscar Wilde (q.v.). A brilliant ocular and aural surgeon, he was also an archaeologist of note and a witty speaker, but he was ruined eventually by his dissipated way of life. He drank heavily and, despite his outlandish mode of dress, puny figure, and repulsive uncleanliness, was exceptionally attractive to women. He sired so many illegitimate children that he was uncertain of their number. After his wife, a neurotic patriot and a vitriolic poet of little merit, pressed him to discard his favorite mistress, his mistress set about to destroy him through a court case that discredited him and made him appear ridiculous. Chronic asthma and alcoholism (q.v.) contributed to the deterioration of his health, and he became depressed and apathetic. The final blow came when two of his favorite illegitimate daughters died of burns, after their dresses caught fire at a ball. He became even more neglected and eccentric. He took to his bed and died, while in the rooms below Oscar and his friends noisily and uncaringly roistered.

Bibliography: Lambert, E. 1967. *Mad with much heart.*

WILL THERAPY. A form of therapy devised by Otto Rank (q.v.). It consisted of a reexperience of the birth trauma. The patient was submitted to a severe quasi-punitive discipline. The method was adopted almost exclusively by the Pennsylvania School of Social Work, which Rank founded. His last book was entitled *Will Therapy*, 1926-31.

Bibliography: Roback, A. A. 1962. *History of psychology and psychiatry.*

WILLARD ASYLUM. An American custodial institution for incurably insane patients opened at Ovid, New York, in 1869. It was named after Dr. Sylvester D. Willard, secretary of the New York Medical Society, whose report on the care of the insane in hospitals and welfare institutions led to legislation for the insane in 1865. The act then passed provided for the creation of a state asylum of 600 beds for those individuals discharged as incurable from the local poorhouses.

Bibliography: Willard, S. D. 1865. Reprint. 1973. *Report on the condition of the insane in the county poor houses of New York.*

WILLIAMSBURG EASTERN LUNATIC ASYLUM. A mental hospital founded in 1773 in Williamsburg, Virginia. Established two years before the American Revolution, it was the first hospital for the mentally ill in British Colonial America to function entirely under the auspices of the state. Its establishment followed a 1768 act that provided for "the maintenance and care of idiots, lunaticks, and other persons of unsound mind." Its objectives were to cure "those whose cases are not become quite desperate" and to restrain "others who may be dangerous to society." It was open to all economic classes except slaves. By the middle of the nineteenth century the hospital's finances were so low that economies were necessary at the expenses of the patients' diets. During the Civil War, conditions deteriorated to the point where patients were starving. From 1779 to 1866 the hospital superintendents were drawn from the Galt family (*see* JOHN MINSON GALT).

Bibliography: Dain, N. 1971. *Disordered minds.*

WILLIS, FRANCIS (1717-1807). An English clergyman and physician. While studying theology, he became interested in medicine and practiced

without a licence until 1759, when Oxford University conferred a doctorate on him. In 1769 he became physician to Lincoln Hospital. He was particularly interested in mental disorders and ran a private madhouse in his home in Dunston and, later, ran another at Greatford (q.v.). In 1788 he was called to treat George III (q.v.). His sons, John (1751-1835) and Robert Darling (1760-1821), were also involved in the management of the king. He based his system of treatment on inculcating fear into his patients. Mechanical restraint (q.v.), violent purging (q.v.), emetics, and bleeding (q.v.) were also extensively employed by him. As physician to the king, he became fashionable, and his private madhouse soon was filled with aristocratic and rich clientele. When George III had a temporary remission of symptoms, Willis lost no time in advertising his success. He had a medal struck with his own portrait on one side and the legend "Britons Rejoice, Your King's Restored" on the other. He and his son John were rewarded by Parliament with large pensions. He was less successful in treating the queen of Portugal, but his efforts were nevertheless richly rewarded.
Bibliography: Parry-Jones, W. Ll. 1972. *The trade in lunacy.*

WILLIS, THOMAS (1621-1675). An English physician. According to John Aubrey (q.v.), he experienced some difficulties in first establishing himself in clinical practice, but in 1660 he became professor of natural philosophy at Oxford University. When he was forty-six years old, he moved to London, where he became famous for his clinical skill, his theoretical knowledge, and his interest in charitable works. His name is associated with a wide range of medical topics. He was the first to describe the sweetness of urine in diabetes, and he published many original clinical observations and anatomical descriptions. His most important contribution to neurology (q.v.) was his classification of cranial nerves, which remained in use for over a hundred years. Willis correctly reported on the cerebral circulation and wrote on mental retardation, schizophrenia (q.v.), and general paralysis of the insane (q.v.). He rejected the link between the uterus (q.v.) and hysteria (q.v.), which he regarded as a nervous disorder. According to him melancholia (q.v.) was caused by "passions of the heart" and "madness" by "vice or fault of the brain." He was first to use the term "neurology" to designate knowledge relating to the nerves. His major works include *Cerebri Anatome* (q.v.), and *De Anima Brutorum* (q.v.). He became physician to Charles II (1660-1685) and achieved honors, riches, and recognition. When he died of pneumonia at age of fifty-four, his funeral was one of the most sumptuous of the time and scandalously expensive. He is one of the few physicians to be buried in Westminster Abbey.
Bibliography: Isler, H. R. 1968. *Thomas Willis, 1621-1675: doctor and scientist.*

WILSON, KINNIER (1878-1937). An American-born neurologist raised and educated in Scotland. He worked with a group of distinguished neurologists at the National Hospital for Nervous Diseases (q.v.) in London. He described a nervous disorder associated with cirrhosis of the liver and referred to it as Kinnier Wilson's disease. In subsequent works and in his several books he clarified many issues in the field of neurology, especially those syndromes resulting from lesions of the brain stem. He was a rather dogmatic person, who, at times, ignored people's feelings in the interest of science. On one occasion, for example, he somewhat prematurely asked a patient with puzzling symptoms whether he could perform an autopsy on his brain.

Bibliography: Haymaker, W., and Schiller, F. 1970. *The founders of neurology*. 2d. ed.

WINCHESTER GOOSE. An old English expression referring to the skin rash of syphilis (q.v.). It is derived from the bishop of Winchester who licensed the brothels of Southwark in London until 1547. William Shakespeare (q.v.) also used the expression in *Troilus and Cressida*: "Some galled goose of Winchester would hiss" (5.10).

Bibliography: Whitwell, J. R. 1946. *Analecta psychiatrica*.

WINDHAM, WILLIAM FREDERICK (1840-1866). The son of an English country squire. From childhood on his behavior had been unusual and eccentric, embarrassing his family and tutors. At the age of twenty-one he married a fashionable prostitute. Later in the same year, 1861, an inquiry was held in London on his state of mind. One hundred forty witnesses were called and the hearing lasted thirty-three days. His alleged lunacy was not proven, and he was declared of sound mind. The size and the expense of the trial brought this method of public inquiry into disrepute and turned the handling of psychiatric illness from legal management to medical management. The evidence was published as a book entitled *An Inquiry into the State of Mind of W. F. Windham Esq., of Filbrigg Hall, Norfolk, before Samuel Warren Esq., Q.C. and a Special Jury.*

Bibliography: Jones, K. 1971. The Windham case. *Brit. J. Psychiat.* 119: 425-33.

WINDIGO. *See* WIHTIKO.

WIND-IN-THE-MIND. A term used in the seventeenth century in China (q.v.) to denote insanity.

Bibliography: Kiev, A., ed. 1968. *Psychiatry in the Communist world*.

WINDISCHMANN, KARL JOSEPH HIRONYMUS (1775-1839). A German mystical philosopher. He endeavored to reconcile the teachings of animal magnetism (q.v.) with those of the church. He advocated what he called "Christian healing art," a mixture of magnetism and the sacraments, which was to be practiced by priests.

Bibliography: Thornton, E. M. 1976. *Hypnotism, hysteria, and epilepsy: an historical synthesis.*

WINDS. Winds were believed to influence the course of insanity. William Shakespeare (q.v.) made reference to the influence of winds in *Hamlet*:

I am but mad north-northwest;
when the wind is southerly I know a hawk from a
handsaw.

[2.2]

In the nineteenth century, Jean Esquirol (q.v.) still included them in his list of the causes of insanity and stated that "the influence of certain winds upon the inhabitants of India, the Neapolitans, and Spaniards, explains sufficiently the effect of certain atmospheric states upon the insane."

See also KAMSIM and SIROCCO.

Bibliography: Esquirol, J.E.D. 1845. Reprint. 1965. *Mental maladies: a treatise on insanity.*

WINIFRED, SAINT. A Welsh saint of the seventh century. She was beheaded by Caradoc, her rejected suitor. According to legend a spring gushed forth from where her head fell. Saint Winifred's well (q.v.) was believed to have miraculous curative properties, especially for madness. The descendants of Caradoc were cursed and condemned to bark like dogs. It was said that their condition could be cured only by immersion (q.v.) in the well's water.

Bibliography: 1973. *Reader's digest folklore, myths and legends of Britain.*

WINNICOTT, DONALD WOODS (1897-1971). A British pediatrician and Kleinian psychoanalyst. His clinical work rested on close involvement with mothers and children. To facilitate communication with children, he devised the "squiggle games," which utilize drawings and their interpretation by the therapist and patient. His numerous books clearly describe his theories and his research.

Bibliography: Winnicott, D. D. 1971. *Therapeutic consultations in child psychiatry.*

WINSLOW, FORBES BENIGNUS (1810-1874). A British psychiatrist and the owner of two private asylums (q.v.). In 1848 he established the first British psychiatric journal known as the *Journal of Psychological Medicine and Mental Pathology* (q.v.). He wrote extensively, contributed literature to the forensic field, and often figured in famous court cases. His efforts to

popularize psychological medicine and its concepts created increased interest in the field and helped to bring about its recognition as a medical specialty.
Bibliography: Winslow, F. B. 1860. *On obscure diseases of the brain, and disorders of the mind.*

WINTER CHERRY. *Withonia somnifera*, a shrub found in the drier parts of India. Its leaves and fruits are used as a sedative and hypnotic.
Bibliography: Arber, A. 1912. *Herbals, their origin and evolution.*

WIRACOCHA. A legendary Peruvian hero. His words were said to heal the sick and restore sight to the blind.
Bibliography: Leon, C. A., and Rosselli, H. 1975. Latin America. In *World history of psychiatry*, ed. J. G. Howells.

WIRTH, WILHELM (1876-1952). A German psychologist and a student of Wilhelm Wundt (q.v.). His specialties were psychological contrast phenomena, image, and feeling. His thesis on the dulling of feeling by habit, written in 1897, was so brilliant that he was given a doctorate at the age of twenty-one, before he had even completed his training. His research and teaching covered a wide area in experimental psychology (q.v.) and produced new techniques and instruments to refine methods of measurement.
Bibliography: Murchinson, C., ed. 1936. *A history of psychology in autobiography.* Vol. 3.

WISCONSIN COUNTY CARE ACT. A statute enacted in 1881 in the state of Wisconsin. It systematized the organization of care for those suffering from chronic mental illness and supplied the counties with funds proportionate to the number of hospitalized chronic patients within them. The State Board of Charities and Reform formulated rules and regulations for the proper care of the insane and, when dissatisfied with management, could transfer patients to other county institutions, charging their maintenance to the county found wanting in its efforts. The plan was extended later to safeguard curable patients from life commitment in county institutions. It was the first plan for county care of the mentally ill and became known as the "Wisconsin system."
Bibliography: Deutsch, A. 1949. *The mentally ill in America.*

WISCONSIN STATE HOSPITAL. A mental hospital founded in Madison, Wisconsin, following legislation enacted by the state in the 1850s. Building commissioners for the hospital were appointed and based their recommendations on the advice supplied by Dr. Thomas S. Kirkbride (q.v.). The first superintendent was Dr. E. Lee, a Philadelphia physician, who was appointed in 1859, before the hospital became functional. Internal politics caused his

dismissal before the completion of the project, and the hospital was opened in 1860 with a new superintendent, Dr. P. Clement.
Bibliography: Kraus, R. F. 1972. J. Edward Lee, M. D., and the founding of the Wisconsin State Hospital. *Trans. Stud. Coll. Physicians, Phila.* 40: 120-26.

WITASEK, STEPHAN (1870-1915). An Austrian psychologist. He carried forward the principles of the school of form-quality. He wrote a textbook of psychology and a handbook on visual space-perception. His psychology of perception was based on the effect of the psychical act of producing. Educational psychology, aesthetics, and ethics were his other fields of interest.
Bibliography: Boring, E. G. 1950. *A history of experimental psychology.*

WITCH OF MALLEGEM, THE. An etching by Pieter Brueghel the Elder (q.v.). It depicts a quack cutting a stone from the head of a patient suffering from insanity while others await their turn. In the sixteenth century a stone in the head was believed to be one of the causes of lunacy, but Brueghel indicates his disbelief by showing an assistant with a lock on his lips passing stones to his master from under the table.
Bibliography: Fry, C. C. 1946. The sixteenth-century cures for lunacy. *Am. J. Psychiat.* 103: 351-52.

WITCHCRAFT. Throughout history any phenomena not easily under-stood has been attributed to supernatural forces. In early times, illness, physical and psychical, and restoration to health were often inexplicable. Thus, they gave rise to the belief that some people had mysterious powers to harm or to cure. The witch doctor usually was selected after an event such as a trance or a convulsion that could be interpreted as displaying the possession of divine powers. Sometimes he was chosen because his unusual behavior set him apart from the rest. In biblical times, witches were regarded as enemies of God, and the Bible (q.v.) stated "thou shalt not suffer a witch to live" (Exod. 12: 18). This text was used by the enthusiastic witch hunters of the Renaissance, when the church, especially in Europe, encouraged severe measures against heresy. The mentally ill inevitably became a target for persecution as the symptoms of insanity, mental retardation, and severe emotional disorder were often confused with the accepted signs of demoniac possession (q.v.). The Inquisition (q.v.) guided by the *Malleus Maleficarum* (q.v.) produced witch hunters often more deranged than their victims. They were responsible for torturing and burning hundreds of sick individuals, especially women. Women were more vulnerable than men because the church was particularly preoccupied with sexual restraint, and women were regarded as the seductive instruments of the devil, who, through them, would not only cause spiritual damage and eternal perdition, but also bring about more mundane disasters ranging from the failure of crops and the death of cattle, to sterility, impotence, and infant mortality. Thus, the destruction of the witches became a social as well as a religious duty. In England witchcraft became a felony in 1542, and causing death by witchcraft was a capital offence; in Scotland it carried the death penalty. The 1600s saw many hangings for witchcraft, and the law against it was not repealed in England until 1736 in the reign of George II (q.v.). In Switzerland, the last witch was decapitated in 1782. The cruelties of this appalling record of superstition were not directly aimed at the mentally ill. They unfortunately became considered witches and heretics because the medical knowledge of the time, with exception of a few advanced physicians such an Johann Weyer (q.v.), denied them a correct diagnosis.

Bibliography: Russell, J. B. 1980. *A history of witchcraft: sorcerers, heretics and pagans*.

WITKIEWICZ, STANISLAW IGNACY(1885-1939). A Polish painter and writer. His father was a painter, and his mother was a talented musician. Their house was a meeting place for the intellectuals of the time, but the family climate was never warm. Witkiewicz was an only child; he was educated at home and had little contact with other children. He studied philosophy, problems of aesthetics, and art theory and published works in these fields. His plays are full of restless and cruel characters trapped in nightmarish situations that are never resolved or inevitably advance toward total catastrophies. His symbolic paintings reflect his earlier inner tension and his final deterioration. He was acutely obsessional and developed bizarre rituals and phobias (q.v.). For a while he experimented with drugs (q.v.) and alcohol and meticulously noted their effect on him. After 1929, his mental state deteriorated, and his mannerisms and eccentricities increased. He was afraid of contamination and would not shake hands or touch objects he considered unclean. He felt persecuted, and his writings were full of neologisms and bizarre terminology. Although insisting that he was not ill, he became interested in psychiatry and consulted a psychiatrist, Dr. Zajackowski who diagnosed a schizophrenic process. In 1939, during the invasion of Poland, he took refuge in a wood and cut his veins after giving poison to his lover, who died with him.

Bibliography: Kowalewski, I., and Kowalewski, J. 1971. Essai d'analyse psychopathologique de la peinture de Stanislas Ignace Witkiewicz. *Encephale*. 60: 74-80.

WITMER, LIGHTNER (1867-1956). An American psychologist. He was a pupil of Wilhelm Wundt (q.v.) and of James McKeen Cattell (q.v.). In 1896 in Philadelphia, Pennsylvania, he opened the first clinic for maladjusted children and advocated the use of remedial education for children with learning difficulties. He investigated the factors that prevented the use of normal intellectual ability in children and devised criteria for the differentiation of mental defect and childhood psychosis (q.v.). His work aroused interest in child guidance and promoted the opening of many child guidance clinics (q.v.). The terms "clinical psychology" and "psychological clinic" were coined by him. In 1907, he founded *Psychological Clinic*, a journal that he edited until it ceased publication in 1935.

Bibliography: Witmer, L. 1946. *Psychiatric interviews with children.*

WITTE, EMANUEL DE (1617-1692). A Dutch painter. His unstable personality is not reflected in his interiors of churches, which are sombre and well ordered, in contrast to his debauched life. He was an eccentric man who was often in debt and in trouble for his behavior. He drank and gambled heavily. Old age found him poor and friendless. He was said to have committed suicide (q.v.).

Bibliography: Wittkower, R., and Wittkower, M. 1963. *Born under Saturn.*

WITTE, KARL (1800-1883). A German philosopher, jurist, and Dante scholar. His father dedicated himself to his son's education, which he planned in more than a thousand pages of instructions. He gave up his job as a clergyman but demanded, and obtained, a salary from the city and University of Leipzig for his self-appointed task of proving that he could produce an exceptionally well educated young man. He wrote that a man should think about his child before conception and should keep the pregnant woman healthy in mind and body. His own family life was devoted to Karl's education from the moment of his birth. A kiss or a caress was given only for some achievement; food spills were punished by a diet of bread, and implicit obedience was expected. Two young friends were briefly introduced to him but quickly removed, as the parents thought that they were a bad influence. Yet, Karl found pleasure in learning. He was only thirteen years old when he obtained his doctorate, and at the age of sixteen he was appointed professor at the University of Berlin.

Bibliography: Weiner, L., trans. 1913. *Pastor Witte. The education of Karl Witte; or the training of the child.*

WITTMANN, BLANCHE. A patient of Jean Charcot (q.v.) at the Salpêtrière (q.v.). Charcot often used this young French woman to demonstrate his three stages of hypnosis (*see* HYPNOTISM). She was nicknamed "la reine des hystériqués" and was disliked by the patients and staff because of her unpleasant manners and capriciousness. From Salpêtrière she moved to Hôtel-Dieu (q.v.), where it was discovered that she had a double personality, one hysterical (*see* HYSTERIA) and the other more balanced and aware that her behavior during demonstrations was part of an act. Under the care of Jules Janet, the brother of Pierre Janet (q.v.), she recovered enough to return to the Salpêtrière as a worker in the photographic department. She later worked in the radiology laboratory and died, after several amputations, of cancer contracted from the radiation to which she was

exposed. She is the central figure in the famous painting by Brouillet that shows Charcot surrounded by his pupils during a clinical demonstration.
Bibliography: Ellenberger, H. F. 1970. *The discovery of the unconscious.*

WOD. An Anglo-Saxon word meaning "mad." Woden was the god of the frenzied.
Bibliography: Bonser, W. 1963. *The medical background of Anglo-Saxon England.*

WÖHLER, FRIEDRICH (1800-1882). A German chemist. In 1828 he synthetised urea, an organic substance, from inorganic material and disproved the theory of vitalism (q.v.) which had asserted that such substances could be created only in living tissues.
Bibliography: Galdston, I., ed. 1967. *Historic derivations of modern psychiatry.*

WOLF, HUGO PHILIPP JAKOB (1860-1903). An Austrian composer who was famous for his beautiful songs. His life was one of hardship and frustration; as a student he was dismissed from the Vienna Conservatory on a false charge and supported himself by teaching music and writing musical criticism. His output over a short period was enormous, although periods of feverish activity were interspersed with episodes of complete inability to work. He became insane and spent the last six years of his life in an asylum.
Bibliography: Walker, F. 1951. *Hugo Wolf: a biography.*

WOLFART, KARL CHRISTIAN (1778-1832). A German physician. He was a great admirer of Franz Mesmer (q.v.) whom he visited in 1812. Wolfart begged Mesmer to continue his work and writings and published Mesmer's last book in a German translation. He was entrusted with other material, but he carelessly lost most of it. He coined the word "mesmerism" (q.v.) to describe what previously had been known as animal magnetism (q.v.).
Bibliography: Ellenberger, H. F. 1970. *The discovery of the unconscious.*

WOLF CHILD OF HESSE. A four-year-old child found in a forest in Hesse, Germany in 1544. He was believed to have survived through the care of wolves, who had made a bed of leaves for him and kept him warm at night with their own bodies. Once back into society he returned to human habits, and his intelligence was not affected by his early experiences. Carolus Linnaeus (q.v.) referred to this child and called him Lupinus Essensis.
See also FERAL CHILD.
Bibliography: Maclean, C. 1977. *The wolf children.*

WOLF CHILDREN *See* FERAL CHILD.

WOLF CHILDREN OF MIDNAPORE. A remarkable case of two girls apparently brought up by wolves in the Bengal province of India. Although there have been many reports of children raised by wild animals (wolves, sheep, cattle, bears), the wolf children of India were the first to be authenticated by photographs, a day-by-day journal, and careful investigation by a recognized scientist. The following account is based on the diary kept by the Reverend A.L. Singh, a missionary, and his wife, who trained the children, kept a diary, and wrote a book entitled *Wolf Children and Feral Men* in 1942 with the anthropologist Robert M. Zingg. Several people claimed they actually saw small human beings running along on all fours with a family consisting of a mother and father wolf and two cubs. The Reverend Singh decided to investigate these "man ghosts," as the natives called them, and succeeded in capturing the two "wolf children." Both were girls, and he took them to the orphanage which he directed. Mrs. Singh estimated that the older girl, whom they later called Kamala, was about eight years of age, while the younger one, Amala, was only about a year and a half.

When the children were discovered, their heads were covered with matted hair and their hands and knees were disfigured by sores from walking on all fours. They lapped up food from a pan, bolted meat ravenously, and growled when anyone approached while they were eating. Their teeth were sharp with long pointed canines, their eyes "glared in the dark like blue lights," their hearing was remarkably acute, and their sense of smell was so highly developed that they could smell meat from a distance of seventy yards. At night they roamed around the compound howling like a wolf. The Reverend and Mrs. Singh attempted to raise the children as newly born human beings, but they encountered great difficulties. Neither child learned to run upright, but Kamala eventually managed to walk in a somewhat awkward fashion. Her younger sister, Amala, made better progress because she was not hampered by long-term habits—but unfortunately she died a year after capture.

In the course of the next eight years, before her death at seventeen, Kamala learned to wear clothes, ceased to bare her teeth in anger, gave up prowling at night, and even developed a wariness of the dark. She learned about fifty words which she used in short sentences, and seemed to enjoy attending the morning religious services. She also developed a sense of responsibility and initiative, frequently running errands and caring for the smaller children in the orphanage. In a word, she was able to throw off her wolf-like habit patterns and develop an essentially human way of life.

See also FERAL CHILD.

Bibliography: Maclean, C. 1977. *The Wolf Children.*

WOLFENDEN REPORT. The report of the English royal commission chaired by Sir John Wolfenden (1906-). The commission was appointed by the House of Lords to investigate homosexuality (q.v.) and prostitution.

Published in 1957, the report recommended that homosexual acts involving consenting adults should not constitute a crime.
Bibliography: Weeks, J. 1977. *Coming out.*

WOLFF, CASPAR FRIEDRICH (1733-1794). A German physiologist. His theory of epigenesis, which asserted that all organisms grow out of a vital substance, or protoplasm, provided the basis for vitalism (q.v.) and greatly influenced medical psychology.
Bibliography: Zilboorg, G. 1941. *A history of medical psychology.*

WOLFF, CHRISTIAN VON (1679-1754). A German philosopher and mathematician. He popularized the term "psychology" (q.v.) and divided the discipline into empirical and rational sections. He wrote a treatise on the empirical section in 1732, and one about the rational section in 1734. Psychometry (q.v.) was also promoted by him.
Bibliography: Wolff, C. von. 1734. *Rational psychology.*

WOLF-MAN, THE (1886-1979). The name used by Sigmund Freud (q.v.) for one of his patients, who became the subject of his most famous case-history "From the History of an Infantile Neurosis." The wolf-man was the son of rich Russian landowners. His early life was spent in luxury with many material advantages but few warm relationships. As an adolescent he lost his father, his sister committed suicide (q.v.), and his semi-invalid mother seems to have dominated him. He was constantly dependent on servants. In addition to psychosomatic disorders, his neurosis (q.v.) consisted of a fear of wolves, following a disturbing dream that he had at the age of four. In 1910 he started analysis with Freud, who intepreted his phobias (q.v.) and anxieties according to the tenets of psychoanalysis (q.v.) and provided him with the needed father-figure. Two world wars considerably changed his fortunes and his background. Against his mother's wishes, but with Freud's blessing, he married a young woman who had many emotional difficulties of her own. She committed suicide in 1938, after suggesting to him that they should die together.
Bibliography: Gardiner, M., ed. 1972. *The Wolf-Man and Sigmund Freud.*
Obholzer, K. 1982. *The Wolf Man. Sixty Years Later.*

WOLLSTONECRAFT, MARY (1759-1797). An Anglo-Irish feminist and writer. Her parents provided little warmth. Her mother's love was concentrated on the first-born son, and Mary was left to fend for herself. She grew up stubborn, resentful, and awkward. After a period of earning a livelihood through teaching and as a governess, she became literary adviser to Samuel Johnson (q.v.) and became involved with a group of London radical thinkers, known as the Dissenters. In 1790 she wrote *Vindication of the Rights of Man,* which she followed with *Vindication of the Rights of Woman* (1792).

In it she advocated equality of the sexes. She went to France to observe and write about the results of the French Revolution (q.v.) and fell in love with an American captain, Gilbert Imlay. Imlay deserted her after the birth of her daughter. Disillusioned with France, she returned to London, where she attempted suicide (q.v.) by throwing herself off Putney Bridge. Because of her political views, her feminism, and her illegitimate child, she found herself isolated. In 1797, she became pregnant by William Godwin (1756-1836), the political writer who had said that marriage was "the worse of all laws", but who recanted enough to marry her. She died giving birth to their daughter, Mary, who became the wife of Percy Bysshe Shelley (q.v.) and the author of *Frankenstein* (q.v.). Her first daughter, Fanny Imlay, committed suicide.
Bibliography: Tomalin, C. 1974. *The life and death of Mary Wollstonecraft.*

WOLSEY, THOMAS (c.1473-1530). An English cleric and statesman. From humble origins he rose to great power in the church and the state as Cardinal and Lord Chancellor. His magnificence was at times greater than that of the king, which caused jealousy and friction. Although he was opposed to Anne Boleyn (1507-1536), he was obliged to conduct negotiations with the pope for the annulment of the marriage of Henry VIII (1491-1547) to Catherine of Aragon (1485-1536). He was arrogant and avaricious, but even his strong personality eventually showed signs of stress. He so brooded over his fall from grace that his health was undermined. With no hope of reconciliation with the king and charged with treason, he fell sick, elected to die, and even predicted the hour of his death. Shakespeare referred to the event in 'King Henry VIII' (IV, ii).
Bibliography: Pollard, A. F. 1929. *Wolsey.*

WOODRUFF. *Asperula odorata*, a plant used by gipsies to make medical infusions. It is reputed to be beneficial in cases of depression, hysteria (q.v.) and frigidity. It is also said to improve poor memory.
Bibliography: de Baïracli Levy, J. 1974. *The illustrated herbal handbook.*

WOODWARD, SAMUEL BAYARD (1787-1850). An American psychiatrist. He was the first president of the Association of Medical Superintendents of American Institutions for the Insane, the present American Psychiatric Association (q.v.), and the first superintendent of the Hartford Retreat (q.v.), which he helped to establish and also of the Worcester State Hospital. He was an enthusiastic admirer of Philippe Pinel (q.v.) and Jean Esquirol (q.v.) and popularized their methods in the United States. His clinical reports were widely read and established a trend for more accurate statistics in asylum psychiatry. As a physician who was actively interested in the treatment of alcoholism (q.v.), he believed in specialized medical care for alcoholics. Woodward felt he should be of service to society. He attempted to improve American psychiatry by demonstrating that insanity was curable, given appropriate and humane treatment in good time.

Bibliography: Grob, G. N. 1962. Samuel B. Woodward and the practice of psychiatry in early nineteenth-century America. *Bull. Hist. Med.* 36: 420-43.

WOODWORTH, ROBERT SESSIONS (1869-1962). An American psychologist. He was associated with Columbia University and dynamic psychology. After studying general science and mathematics, he became a high school teacher. After some years of teaching, he lectured in physiology and spent a year with Sir Charles Sherrington (q.v.) in England. In 1903 he began to teach psychology at Columbia University and succeeded James McKeen Cattell (q.v.) as a professor in 1917. He is regarded as one of the greatest and most influential teachers of psychology in America. He refused to yield to the strictures of any particular system and sought to synthetize older ideas with behaviorism (q.v.). In 1956 he was awarded the gold medal of the American Psychological Foundation (q.v.). His numerous books include *Experimental Psychology* (1938), *Contemporary Schools of Psychology* (1931), and *Dynamics of Behavior* (1958).

Bibliography: Boring, E. G. 1950. *A history of experimental psychology.*

WOOLF, VIRGINIA (1882-1941). An English writer of novels, literary criticism, and essays. She was the daughter of Sir Leslie Stephen (1832-1904), a well-known and erudite man of letters and philosopher but also a guilt-ridden depressive and a stern and tyrannical father, who saw to it that she should be well versed in the classics and in mathematics. An insane stepsister lived in the same house with them until Virginia was ten years old. Although she benefitted intellectually from the varied and stimulating background of family and friends, she remained an insecure, shy, and over-sensitive individual in spite of the brilliance of her mind and her literary achievements. When she was six years old, her half brother, who was twenty years her senior, submitted her to incestuous (*see* INCEST) relations that persisted for many years, increased her sexual inhibitions and fears, and fostered an inclination toward lesbianism (q.v.). Her first mental breakdown occurred at the age of twelve, when her mother died. A more serious one occurred ten years later on the death of her father. During this illness she became paranoid, delusional, anorexic, and tried to commit suicide (q.v.) by throwing herself out of a window. In her middle twenties she was again ill and was admitted to a nursing home, which she described as "a polite madhouse for female lunatics." On recovering, she accepted, after much hesitation, a proposal of marriage from Leonard Woolf (1880-1969) who devotedly protected and comforted her throughout their marriage. What she described as "all the horrors of the dark cupboard of illness" tormented her with insomnia, depression, severe headaches, and a morbid aversion for food, as well as all bodily functions. These symptoms, which she regarded

as almost mystical, always increased when she was about to finish a book. Her love affair with Vita Sackville-West (q.v.) did little to remedy her frigidity. Her second attempt to kill herself with an overdose of veronal was unsuccessful, but her third attempt resulted in her death by drowning in the River Ouse. In the note she left behind she stated, "I feel certain I am going mad again. I feel we can't go through another of those terrible times. . . . so I am doing what seems the best thing to do . . . . "
Bibliography: Bell, Q. 1972. *Virginia Woolf.*

WORCESTER COUNTY LUNATIC ASYLUM. A mental hospital in England. It enjoyed the distinction of having Sir Edward Elgar (q.v.) as the bandmaster for its band. He was appointed to that position in 1879 and held it for five years.

WORD ASSOCIATION. The phenomenon of the emotional preoccupations associated with certain words; it has been recognized since the time of Avicenna (q.v.). Over the years, words and the responses given to them have been the basis of many studies, including those of Sir Francis Galton, James McKeen Cattell, and Wilhelm Wundt (qq.v.). The best known theories on word association are those of Carl Jung (q.v.), who investigated responses, reaction time, and other emotion-related aspects, using a specially prepared list of 100 words.
Bibliography: Watson, R. I. 1963. *The great psychologists.*

WORDSWORTH, WILLIAM (1770-1850). An English poet. His mother died when he was eight years old. The children were separated, and William was brought up at a boarding school. He rarely met his brothers and he was completely separated from his sister Dorothy (1771-1855), with whom he formed a close relationship in later life. Childhood behavior problems and stubborness gave way to agnostic and revolutionary ideas in adolescence, which caused him to refuse to take holy orders as his guardian wished. At the same time, he developed violent headaches, possibly as a guilt reaction. In 1791, after graduating, he went to study in France, where he became an ardent advocate of the French Revolution (q.v.) and had an affair with Annette Vallon, a royalist, whom he left before the birth of their daughter. Although he supported them as best he could, he did not see them again for nearly a decade and then only to be sure that the short love affair was no obstacle to his marriage. For a while, he wrote poems containing tales of desertion, remorse, and lonely women, but he was basically disillusioned with the revolution and complacent about his abandoned love affair. He set up house with his sister Dorothy, at first in Dorset and later in the Lake District. The smallness of their cottage and their poverty did not prevent them entertaining frequent guests, especially Samuel Coleridge (q.v.), whom he called the only wonderful man he knew, Charles Lamb (q.v.), and Thomas

De Quincey (q.v.). In 1802 he married his cousin, Mary Hutchinson (1770-?) who joined them at the cottage, with Dorothy helping to bring up the children. Dorothy, always intense and excitable, had a mental breakdown from which she never recovered. In his old age Wordsworth became a man of propriety, was accepted by Victorian society and was made poet laureate in 1843. His poetry became proportionately poorer. Browning remarked that "Just for a handful of silver he left us." Among his poems are some of psychiatric interest, such as *Her Eyes Are Wild* (1799) and *The Idiot Boy* (1798).
Bibliography: Davies, H. 1980. *William Wordsworth.*

WORLD NEXT DOOR, THE. A book written in 1949 by Fritz Peters, a contemporary American author. It describes life in a mental hospital for the veterans of World War II. Peters emphasizes the brutality and homosexuality (q.v.) of some of the male aides, the limited treatment, the shortage of physicians, and the struggle of the patients' families to obtain compensation for their infirmities. Peters claimed it was a true account of events in which he deliberately changed the names of people and places to respect their privacy.
Bibliography: Peters, F. 1949. *The world next door.*

WORLD PSYCHIATRIC ASSOCIATION. An association made up of national societies of psychiatrists. The association attempts to coordinate and to advance studies on the aetiology, pathology, and treatment of mental illnesses. It was founded in 1961 under the presidency of Donald Ewen Cameron (q.v.). World congresses of psychiatry are organized by the association on occasion.

WORMS. The presence of worms in the digestive tract was often considered a cause of insanity. Jean Esquirol (q.v.) recorded that in 1811 several maniacs at the Salpêtrière (q.v.) were cured by the expulsion of worms, but he added that he did not consider this as important an aetiological factor as some of his contemporaries did.
Bibliography: Esquirol, J.E.D. 1845. Reprint. 1965. *Mental maladies: a treatise on insanity.*

WORMS, COUNCIL OF. An assembly of the Holy Roman Empire held at Worms in Germany in 868. The synod resolved that penance should be imposed on insane offenders because their illness was a direct result of their sins.
Bibliography: Kinberg, O. 1935. *Basic problems of criminology.*

WOZZECK. An opera (q.v.), written in 1925 by the Austrian composer Alban Berg (1885-1935). Wozzeck, a soldier, has visual and auditory hallucinations (q.v.). He is examined by a half-crazed doctor who uses him in his experiments. In the final scene Wozzeck, having killed his faithless lover, returns to the scene of his crime and drowns himself.

Bibliography: Harewood, ed. 1969. *Kobbe's complete opera book*.

WREN, SIR CHRISTOPHER (1632-1723). An English architect. He re-built London after the Great Fire of 1666. The building for the College of Physicians was designed by him. He illustrated *Cerebri Anatome* (q.v.) by Thomas Willis (q.v.). He was a founder and president of the Royal Society (q.v.).

Bibliography: Little, B. 1975. *Sir Christopher Wren*.

WRIGHT, THOMAS (1561-1623). An English Jesuit priest. In 1604 he wrote a book entitled *The Passions of the Minde in Generall* in which he discussed the problems of the soul and the body. He argued that some of these problems concern theologians, some philosophers, and some the physicians, yet they impinge on each other. Posing questions about the effect of physical pain on the mind, the link between imagination (q.v.) and understanding, and the role of habit in learning, he explored what was then known about neurophysiology and psychology.

Bibliography: Wright, Thomas. 1604. Reprint. 1971. *The passions of the minde in generall*.

WUNDT, WILHELM MAX (1832-1920). A German physiological psychologist. He is considered the founder of experimental psychology (q.v.). He was one of four children of a Lutheran minister, but two of his siblings died young, and his only surviving brother was eight years his senior. From the age of eight he was educated by Friedrich Müller, a vicar whom he came to love so much that his parents allowed him to live in Müller's house when he was transferred to another village. Intellectual relationships with older people compensated for Wundt's lack of childhood companions. He developed into a humourless, aggressive individual with an enormous capacity for work. His numerous books demonstrate his encyclopedic erudition. After qualifying in medicine, he worked with Johannes Müller (q.v.) at Müller's institute of physiology and then came under the influence of Hermann Helmholtz (q.v.). At that point his interests shifted from physiology to experimental psychology. In 1874 he wrote *Principles of Physiological Psychology*, which is regarded as the most important work in the history of modern psychology. In 1879 he founded at Leipzig the first formal experimental psychological laboratory (q.v.) in the world. It attracted men like Emil Kraepelin, Oswald Külpe, Granville Stanley Hall, Edward Titchener, James McKeen Cattell (qq.v.), his self-appointed assistant, and many others

who contributed a great deal to the field of psychology. To make their work known, in 1881 Wundt founded the journal *Philosophische Studien* (q.v.).
Bibliography: Boring, E. G. 1950. *A history of experimental psychology.*

WÜRZBURG SCHOOL. A German school of psychology emanating from the laboratory founded in 1896 by Oswald Külpe (q.v.). The basic belief of the school was that meanings and judgments are determined by intangible mental activities and not merely by specific images. The concept came to be called "imageless thought," and the school attempted to deal with act and content in an holistic manner, rather than limiting its investigation to basic elements, as advocated by Wilhelm Wundt (q.v.).
Bibliography: Watson, R. I. 1963. *The great psychologists.*

WYNN'S ACT. Legislation passed in 1808 in England. It gave the county justices power to provide county asylums (q.v.) for the insane poor. At first the act was permissive, rather than mandatory, and by 1844 only fifteen county asylums had been built. Most of them housed 150 to 300 patients. In 1845 the act became mandatory.
See also INSANE POOR, LEGISLATION IN ENGLAND.
Bibliography: Jones, K. 1972. *A history of the mental health services.*

WYNTER, ANDREW (1819-1876). An English physician and writer. He was editor of the *Association Medical Journal* (later known as the *British Medical Journal*). He wrote on insanity and co-authored with Joseph M. Granville (q.v.) *The Borderlands of Insanity, and other Papers.*
Bibliography: 1900. *The dictionary of national biography.*

X

XANTHIPPE. The wife of Socrates (q.v.). Her bad temper, and continuous quarreling and scolding have become proverbial. Socrates is said to have been very tolerant and patient of her shortcomings, but her views of life with him have not been recorded and this early account of a marriage problem remains one sided.
Bibliography: Krous, R. 1940. *The private and public life of Socrates.*

XI-BINEL. A disease once recognized among the Mayan Indians. They believed that those affected lost their souls through fear when they witnessed a witch (*see* WITCHCRAFT) being transformed into an unusual beast.
Bibliography: Holland, W. R., and Thorp, R. G. 1964. Highland Maya psychotherapy. *Amer. Anthropologist.* 66: 41-52.

XI-BIRIL. A group of diseases similar to Susto (q.v.) recognized by the Mayan Indians. Their common aetiological factor is soul loss through fright. Xi-binel (q.v.) is a dangerous form of it.
Bibliography: Holland, W. R., and Thorp, R. G. 1964. Highland Maya psychotherapy. *Amer. Anthropologist.* 66: 41-52.

Y

YAARI, YEHUDAH (1900-   ). A Hebrew novelist and a pioneer of agricultural settlements in Israel. Among his works is *Darke Ish* (1950), a psychological study of a young man's mental illness brought about by the war.
Bibliography: Yaari, Y. 1947. *When the candle was burning*, trans. M. Hurwitz.

YANTRA. Visual hallucination usually following self-induced hypnosis (see HYPNOTISM). It consists of a geometrically shaped, colored image that is related to the mandala (q.v.).
Bibliography: West, L. J. ed. 1962. *Hallucinations*.

YARROW. *Achillea millefolium*, a herb commonly found in pastures. It is also known as milfoil. In ancient England it was believed to be an essential part of those ceremonies accompanying incantations (q.v.) and witchcraft (q.v.). It was said to prevent hallucinations (q.v.) and fearful visions. It is mentioned in the Anglo-Saxon herbals as one of the herbs commonly used in amulets (q.v.). Nicholas Culpeper (q.v.) advised making a brew from it for "inveterate headaches," and other herbalists used it for nervous and neurotic disorders.
Bibliography: Rohde, E. S. 1974. *The Old English herbals*.

YAUYOS. A tribal group under the Inca civilization in Peru. They specialized in the treatment of head injuries and were trained to anaesthetize the patient using herbal mixtures and nerve pressure. A number of skulls have been found that indicate their practice of trepanation (q.v.). Amulets (q.v.), incantations (q.v.), and the induction of trances were part of their treatment.
Bibliography: Burland, C. A. 1967. *Peru under the Incas*.

YAVOROV, PEYU (1878-1914). The pseudonym of the Bulgarian poet and playwright Peyu Kracholov. He was obsessed with tragedy. His poetry

celebrates the oppressed and the rejected. He was involved in politics and joined the Macedonian rebels against Turkey. He was highly unstable and possibly psychotic but Bulgarian poetry benefited from his exploration of the inner self. The death of a fellow poet's sister and his unhappy marriage led to his suicide (q.v.).
Bibliography: Naydenova, G. 1957. *Peyu Yavorov.*

YBBS. A town in Austria. In 1864 the first Austrian institution for idiots (*see* IDIOT) was founded there.
Bibliography: Barr, M. W. 1904. *Mental defectives.*

YEATS, WILLIAM BUTLER (1865-1939). An Irish poet, dramatist, leader of the Irish Renaissance. As a child he was timid, easily upset, and always miserable. Romantic melancholy (*see* ROMANTICISM) and a preoccupation with the "Celtic twilight" mark his work, which was often elaborated around Irish mythology (q.v.), folkloristic beliefs, and symbolism. He was intensely interested in the occult and, in his search for mystical experiences, joined such unorthodox religious sects as the Theosophists and the Rosicrucians. In 1917, he married Georgie Hyde-Lees (1893-1968), a medium (q.v.), whose attempts at automatic writing began during their honeymoon. With her help he wrote a prose work entitled *A Vision* (1937), which is a kind of plan for a universal theology that combines philosophy and magic (q.v.). In 1923 he was awarded the Nobel Prize for literature.
Bibliography: Jeffares, A. N. 1962. *W.B. Yeats, man and poet.*

YELLOW. In the humoral theory (q.v.) this color was associated with the secretation of bile (q.v.) and, thus, with such negative qualities as jealousy (q.v.), cowardice, and treachery. For this reason, in medieval paintings Judas Iscariot (q.v.) was invariably represented clothed in yellow, and during periods of persecution, Jews were ordered to wear yellow, as betrayers of Christ.

YELLOWLEES, DAVID (1836-1921). A Scottish psychiatrist. He graduated in medicine from the University of Edinburgh at the age of twenty. His contact with the asylum at Morningside in Edinburgh aroused his interest in psychiatry and, after a time in general practice, he turned entirely to psychiatry. In 1864, he became the medical superintendent of the Morgannwg Hospital (q.v.). Ten years later he took up a similar position at the Royal Glasgow Asylum, previously known as the Glasgow Asylum for Lunatics (q.v.). He was a university lecturer in psychiatry and a president of the Royal Medico-Psychological Association (q.v.). His views on diagnosis and treatment were enlightened and humanitarian, for he promoted occupational therapy (q.v.) and forbade harsh forms of restraint (q.v.).

Favoring research in sociological and physical fields, he established one of the first asylum pathology laboratories.
Bibliography: Henderson, D. K. 1964. *The evolution of psychiatry in Scotland.*

YERKES, ROBERT MEARNS (1876-1956). An American psychologist and a pupil of William James (q.v.). His interest was the evolution of behavior from the lowest forms of animal life to man. He is regarded as the leader of American comparative psychology. During World War I, he was in charge of a group of psychologists engaged in developing intelligence tests for the army. In 1924 he became a research professor at the Institute of Human Behavior at Yale University and founded the Yale Laboratories of Primate Biology in Orange Park, Florida, which were later named the Yerkes Laboratories of Primate Biology in his honor. His work proved that learning experiences influence behavior more than instinctual drives.
Bibliography: Yerkes, R. M. 1943. *Chimpanzees: a laboratory colony.*

YIN AND YANG. The female and the male forces respectively in a Chinese theory related to the workings of the universe. It was first developed around 300 B.C. and became incorporated into Confucian philosophy (*see* CONFUCIUS). Yin is the female force, which is passive and negative; yang is the male force, active and positive. Their interaction together and with the five elements (wood, metal, fire, water, and earth), which are associated with astral bodies, colors, organs of the body, and numbers among other things, influences human behavior and controls human affairs. According to this philosophy, propitious days must be carefully determined by studying these interactions. Marriage partners must be selected from those groups that are likely to produce harmonious complements.
Bibliography: Veith, I. 1970. *The yellow emperor's classic of internal medicine.*

YOGA. A Hindu system of philosophy emphasizing meditation and based on the practice of asceticism through physical and spiritual exercises. The achievement of a state of trance is interpreted as union with God. The rules for aspiring devotees were set down in detail in the *Yoga-shastras* of Patanjali, written in the first century B.C.
Bibliography: Jaggi, O. P. 1979. *Yogic and Tantric medicine.*

YOLMELAUA. A form of oral confession practiced by the pre-Columbian Nahua Indians, who entered the Valley of Mexico around 300 A.D. It was used as a form of catharsis (q.v.) by those who needed to unburden themselves of guilt feelings. Those hearing the confessions were specially trained physicians, known as the *tlamatinimes*, who were paid for their services.

Treatment varied from advice to herbal remedies and steam baths to cleanse the body.

Bibliography: Parres, R. 1980. The first American psychiatrists. *Psychiatric Annals.* 10: 225-32.

YORK LUNATIC ASYLUM. An English lunatic asylum built in the eighteenth century by the York city architect John Carr. It is now known as Bootham Park. Despite the pride of the citizens in what was called a "truly noble institution," it quickly deteriorated. The unexplained death of one of its patients, Hannah Mills (q.v.), caused the Quakers (q.v.) to establish their own asylum, known as the York Retreat (q.v.), after William Tuke (q.v.) found conditions at the York Asylum appalling. His grandson, Samuel Tuke (q.v.), wrote a description of the York Retreat that so offended the management of the York Asylum that they protested. The controversy led to a government investigation, but, before it could occur, the worst part of the York Asylum was set on fire deliberately, causing the death of four patients. These events precipitated government action on the conditions in all asylums (q.v.) and, following the discoveries of scandalous malpractices, led to reforms.

Bibliography: Gray, J. 1814. *A history of the York Lunatic Asylum.*

YORK RETREAT, THE. A private institution founded in 1792 by the Religious Society of Friends in York, England. It developed after the death of Hannah Mills (q.v.) at the York Lunatic Asylum (q.v.) in 1791. She had been denied visitors, and the mysterious circumstances of her death led the Religious Society of Friends to suspect that she had been mistreated. William Tuke (q.v.) visited the asylum and was appalled by the conditions and the way in which patients were treated. He suggested that a special Quaker (q.v.) institution should be founded "for grievous dispensation—the loss of reason." The new institution, named The Retreat to avoid stigma attached to the term asylum (q.v.), opened its doors to Quaker patients in 1796. The first physician of the Retreat was Thomas Fowler (q.v.), who was assisted by George and Katherine Jepson (q.v.). The Retreat, because of its small size and its "family" environment, was able to initiate many reforms in hospital administration and management. It became a model for other institutions and proved that good food, fresh air, humane treatment, and occupational therapy (q.v.) were more effective forms of therapy than mechanical restraint (q.v.) and a harsh regime. Samuel Tuke (q.v.), grandson of the founder, wrote a description of the Retreat in 1813. The work, entitled *Description of the Retreat*, highlighted the contrast between it and the old York Asylum and eventually led to a government investigation of all asylums (q.v.).

Bibliography: Tuke, S. 1813. Reprint. 1965. *Description of the Retreat.*

YOUNG, EDWARD (1683-1765). An English clergyman and poet. Because he had a propensity for the morbid and liked to be reminded of death, he worked in a perpetually dark room and kept a skull on his desk. His most famous and gloomy poem *The Complaint; or Night Thoughts on Life, Death, and Immortality* (1742-1745) was the product of his meditation in such surroundings. In the poem, which consists of 10,000 lines of blank verse, he contemplated the vicissitudes of life and death. Another of his favorite places was the cemetery, where he would work among the tombs of his dead relations. Yet, despite this fascination with death, he was opposed to suicide (q.v.).

Bibliography: Wicker, C. V. 1952. *Edward Young and the fear of death.*

YOUNG, THOMAS (1773-1829). An English physicist and physician. Among his many contributions to learning, which include the deciphering of ancient Egyptian inscriptions, the most important to psychiatry were his studies on sense perception, especially vision. He challenged the corpuscular theory of light developed by Isaac Newton (q.v.) and formulated a wave theory of light that was later supported by Hermann Helmholtz (q.v.).

Bibliography: Wood, A. 1954. *Thomas Young.*

YU FU. A legendary Chinese surgeon, reputed to be able to expose the brain by trepanation (q.v.).

Bibliography: Wong, K. Chi-Min and Wu, Lien-Teh. 1932. *History of Chinese Medicine.*

Z

ZABARELLA, JACOBUS (1532-1589). An Italian philosopher and astrologer (*see* ASTROLOGY). A great Aristotelian (*see* ARISTOTLE), he wrote on numerous subjects, including the soul, the mind, and the senses. In his book *De Rebus Naturalibus* he asserted that, although the brain was the instrument of cognition, the vital spirit resided in the heart (q.v.).
Bibliography: 1959. *Symposium: the history and philosophy of the brain and its functions.*

ZACCHIA, PAOLO (1584-1659). An Italian physician. He was the founder of legal medicine in Italy and an expert on the jurisprudence of insanity. He devised a classification of mental disorders consisting of three groups: "fatuitas", or the mentally subnormal, which he divided into three degrees, depending upon severity; "insania," (q.v.) which included conditions caused by witchcraft (q.v.), melancholia (q.v.), and emotional disorders; and "phrenitis" (q.v.), which he defined as mental disorders accompanied by fever. In his volume *Questiones Medico-legales* (1621), he dealt with many aspects of mental disorders, which he believed should be assessed by a physician and not by a lawyer or a theologian. He illustrated his opinions with case histories. In making a distinction between insanity and mental deficiency, he stated his belief that the mentally retarded could not be held legally responsible for their actions, that manic patients had lucid intervals during which they were aware of their actions, and that strong emotions could lead to irresponsible behavior. He advised marriage (q.v.) for some emotional disorders and thought that melancholic individuals were more likely to suffer from demonaic possession (q.v.) than others were. Zacchia also wrote on hypochondria (q.v.) in a book entitled *De Mali Hipocondriaci*, which was published in Rome in 1635. He was physician to two popes, Innocent X (1574-1655) and Alexander VII (1599-1677).

Bibliography: Cranefield, P. F., and Federn, W. 1976. *Essays and notes on the history of medicine.*

ZAMPORINION. The popular name of a mysterious fever that struck Rio de Janeiro, Brazil, in 1777. The disease attacked the brain and the spinal medulla and, when it did not cause death, left the patient paralyzed. It took its name from a much admired Venetian singer, Zamporina, who sang in Rio de Janeiro during the same period and may have helped to divert the terrified people of the city.

Bibliography: Corney, B. G. 1912-1913. Some oddities in nomenclature. *Proc. roy. Soc. Med.* 6: 48-53.

ZAR. An Arabian ceremony for the expulsion of evil spirits believed to possess (*see* POSSESSION) those showing symptoms of mental disorders. It employs incantations (q.v.), singing, dancing, and the sacrifice of a ram whose blood is drunk by the patients. The ceremony is supervised by a *sheikha*, a woman of special skills, who is said to supply the link between the spirits and the patients. The culminating state of trance or collapse provides emotional release. Those seeking treatment are usually suffering from psychosexual disorders and are predominantly women. Zar is believed to have been introduced in Sudan and then in Egypt (q.v.) from Ethiopia in the early part of the nineteenth century, but it is possible that it is derived from earlier Christian ceremonies associated with frenzied dancing, as in the dancing mania (q.v.) of the Middle Ages (q.v.).

Bibliography: Racy, J. 1970. Psychiatry in the Arab East. *Acta Psychiatrica Scandinavica.* Supplement 211.

ZARAGOZA HOSPITAL. The general hospital in Zaragoza, Spain. It was one of the first hospitals to provide special wards for the mentally ill. Built in 1425 under the auspices of Alfonso V (1385-1458) it was financed by the citizens with money raised from various activities. Men and women of all nationalities and creeds, unless considered heretics, were cared for in two wards of some 150 beds each. Both groups were kept occupied by housework and other tasks within the institution, but distinguished patients were given private rooms and leisure. Fresh bath therapy (*see* BATHS) was a treatment of choice. Philippe Pinel (q.v.) visited the hospital and was greatly impressed by the hospital and especially praised its program of agricultural work for the patients. In 1804 the French burned the hospital, but a better and larger building with a psychiatric department was erected in 1829.

Bibliography: Chamberlain, A. S. 1966. Early mental hospitals in Spain. *Am. J. Psychiat.* 123: 143-49.

ZARATHUSTRA. *See* ZOROASTER.

ZARMANOCHEGAS. A Brahmin born in Bargosa, India. The historian Strabo (c.63 B.C.-A.D. 21) recorded that he was sent by an Indian king, to

Augustus (63 B.C.-A.D. 14) as a gift to amuse the emperor by committing suicide (q.v.) in his presence. Zarmanochegas wanted to die because he was completely happy and was afraid that something would spoil his happiness. Strabo also wrote that "he leaped upon a pyre with a laugh."
Bibliography: Fedden, H. R. 1938. *Suicide.*

ZEITSCHRIFT FÜR DAS IDIOTENWESEN. A German journal dedicated to the field of mental retardation. It was founded in Berlin in 1881 by two educators, Schröter and Reichel. Most of its articles were by theologians and educators, rather than physicians; thus, prayer was regarded as the most efficacious form of help for the feebleminded. In 1885 the journal's name was changed to *Zeitschrift für die Behandlung Schwachsinniger und Epileptiker.* At the same time its coverage was enlarged to embrace childhood psychoses (*see* PSYCHOSIS) and convulsive disorders.
Bibliography: Kanner, L. 1964. *A history of the care and study of the mentally retarded.*

ZEITSCHRIFT FÜR DIE ERFORSCHUNG UND BEHANDLUNG DES JUGENDLICHEN SCHWACHSINNS. A German journal founded in 1907 by H. Vogt and Wilhelm Weygandt (q.v.). It covered the field of childhood feeblemindedness and its related aspects including anatomical features and forensic psychiatry. After producing six issues a year until World War I, it ceased publication; it was reissued for one year in 1922.
Bibliography: Kanner, L. 1964. *A history of the care and study of the mentally retarded.*

ZEITSCHRIFT FÜR PSYCHOLOGIE UND PHYSIOLOGIE DER SINNESORGANE. A German psychological journal founded in 1890 by Hermann Ebbinghaus, Arthur König, and Hermann Helmholtz (qq.v.). Many famous contemporary physiologists were enlisted to help launch the magazine, which represented a coalition of talent in the field of experimental psychology (q.v.).
Bibliography: Boring, E. G. 1950. *A history of experimental psychology.*

ZEITSCHRIFT FÜR VÖLKERPSYCHOLOGIE UND SPRACHWISSENSCHAFT. A German journal founded by Hayin Steinthal (q.v.) and Moritz Lazarus (1824-1903) in 1860, to provide a better understanding of the philological implications of psychology.
Bibliography: Flugel, J. C. 1945. *A hundred years of psychology.*

ZEN BUDDHISM. A Chinese adaptation of Indian Buddhism. It is said to be based on the teaching of Bodhi-Dharma, an Indian patriarch of the fifth century, who, after meditating for nine years with his face to a wall, summarized his doctrines as "a vast emptiness, with nothing holy in it."

Hui-neng (638-713), a Chinese patriarch is also said to be its originator. Experts on Zen assert that it cannot be described in rational language as it is a personal experience that is only attained after years of training in meditation. The individual eventually learns to achieve *satori* (q.v.), or illumination, which is an intuitive grasp of one's true nature, devoid of intellectualizations. It leads to a feeling that one's entire life has been transformed into an increasingly effective and satisfying experience dominated by humility, love, and compassion. Zen practices and aims have been described as similar to those of psychoanalysis (q.v.), and many Western psychiatrists and psychologists, Carl Jung (q.v.) among them, have been interested in Zen techniques. Both Zen and psychoanalysis attempt to reorient behavior toward greater maturity and emotional stability.
Bibliography: Suzuki, D. T. ed. 1950. *Manual of Zen Buddhism.*

ZENO OF CITIUM (c.335-263 B.C.). A Greek philosopher and founder of Stoicism (q.v.), which took its name from the stoa poikilē (meaning "painted porch") in Athens, where Zeno taught. He committed suicide (q.v.) from sheer irritation when he fell and injured a toe. He brought about his own death by holding his breath. Stoicism stressed the importance of feelings and sensations.
Bibliography: Bevan, E. R. 1913. *Stoics and Sceptics.*

ZERO FAMILY. The fictitious name given to a family of vagrants investigated in 1905 by the Swiss psychiatrist Jörger to demonstrate the genetic transmission of mental deficiency. He claimed to have found that 20 percent of its members were imbeciles (*see* IMBECILE).
See also EUGENICS.
Bibliography: Kanner, L. 1964. *A history of the care and study of the mentally retarded.*

ZEUS. The father of the gods in Greek mythology (q.v.). The Romans called him Jupiter. According to legend, his mother, Rhea, bore him in secret to save him from his father, Kronos (q.v.), who had devoured his brothers and sisters. He was brought up in a cave by a goat, Amalthea, and eventually led a revolt against his father. Although he was considered the protector of law, justice, family, and paternal authority, his own divine behavior was very human. The number of his illegitimate children far exceeded that of his legitimate offspring, and his amorous adventures with deities and mortals of both sexes were the inspiration for works in the visual and dramatic arts and provided an acceptable excuse for the representation of many sexual perversions.
Bibliography: Graves, R. 1960. *The Greek myths.*

ZIEHEN, THEODOR (1862-1950). A German philosopher, psychologist, and psychiatrist. From 1900 until 1912, he was professor of psychiatry in

a number of German universities, but eventually he devoted all his energies to philosophy. His book on physiological psychology, which was entitled *Leitfaden der Physiologischen Psychologie* and first published in 1891, was so successful that twelve editions of it had been published by 1924. Ziehen was also the author of several works in psychiatry and philosophy.
Bibliography: Boring, E. G. 1950. *A history of experimental psychology.*

ZIMMERMANN, JOHANN GEORGE VON (1728-1795). A Swiss physician. He also analyzed those emotions that affect bodily functions, especially the digestive tract. His own loneliness caused him to experience the psychological consequences of depression and provided the material for his book *Solitude*, published in 1784. In it he discussed the advantages and disadvantages of solitude. He also wrote on the treatment and prevention of depression and other psychopathological states, as well as mysticism.
Bibliography: Diethelm, O. 1975. Switzerland. In *World history of psychiatry*, ed. J. G. Howells.

ZIMRI. A biblical figure. He was the general who assassinated Elah, the king of Israel, and usurped the throne in 876 B.C. Besieged in Tirzah, which was captured by the army, he committed suicide (q.v.), "burned the King's house over him with fire, and died."
Bibliography: 1 Kings 16:18-20.

ZINN, AUGUST (1825-1897). A German psychiatrist. After leaving Germany for political reasons, he studied in Switzerland and became a physician to the psychiatric department of Zurich University Hospital. He was influenced by the work of Wilhelm Griesinger (q.v.) and, when he became director of the psychiatric hospital of Saint Pirminsberg in the Saint Gallen canton, he introduced a system of nonrestraint, kindness, and occupational therapy (q.v.), which made the hospital a model for progressive institutions throughout Switzerland.
Bibliography: Diethelm, O. 1975. Switzerland. In *World history of psychiatry*, ed. J. G. Howells.

ZNOJMO. A town in Moravia. The first autonomous Czechoslovakian asylum for the insane was established there in 1458. It could house up to fifteen patients. The funds for the asylum were provided by the public and the town authorities, rather than by any religious order.
Bibliography: Kiev, A., ed. 1968. *Psychiatry in the Communist world.*

ZOANTHROPY. A form of insanity in which the patient believes himself to have been transformed into a beast. Jean Esquirol (q.v.) called it "a deplorable aberration of the mind, which perverts the instinct even, and persuades the lypemaniac that he is changed into a brute. . . ." He described the behavior of those suffering from zoanthropy as follows: "These wretched beings fly from their fellow men, live in the woods, churchyards and ancient ruins, and wander, howling, about the country at night. . . . Impelled by necessity or a cruel ferocity, they fall upon children, tear and slay and devour them."

See also LYCANTHROPY.

Bibliography: Esquirol, J. E. D. 1845. Reprint. 1965. *Mental maladies: a treatise on insanity.*

ZODIAC. That zone of the sky in which the sun, moon (q.v.), and brighter planets (q.v.) appear to move. In astrology (q.v.) the signs of the zodiac, denoting the divisions of the zone, have been linked to personal character-istics and have been thought to influence life events. People born under a particular sign —that is, in a certain period of the year—are said to possess a particular personality type, undergo predictable experiences, and to be suitable marriage partners to persons born under other compatible signs. Those born under Cancer (June 21 to July 22) and ruled by the moon are said to be overemotional and moody; those born under Capricorn (Decem-ber 22 to January 19) and ruled by Saturn (q.v.) have among their bad traits meanness and rigidity. Until the seventeenth century, physicians considered astrology in making their diagnoses. Those too poor to afford their fees consulted almanacs that gave guidance on appropriate days for treatment, as well as advice on many matters of social, commercial, and political im-portance. Nicholas Culpepper (q.v.) was one herbalist who combined veg-etable prescriptions with astrological advice.

Bibliography: Hone, M. 1970. *Modern textbook of astrology.*

ZOIST, THE. A journal founded in 1843 by John Elliotson (q.v.). It was devoted to the "cerebral physiology and mesmerism and their application to human welfare." Discussions on new medical and social problems were also presented. The account of surgical operations performed painlessly under hypnosis (*See* HYPNOTISM) by Dr. James Esdaile (q.v.) appeared in it in 1846. The journal ceased publication in 1856.

Bibliography: Boring, E. G. 1950. *A history of experimental psychology.*

ZOLA, ÉMILE EDOUARD CHARLES ANTOINE (1840-1902). A French novelist and social philosopher. The premature death of his father left his mother, a devoted but overpowering woman, in difficult financial circumstances. Zola was humiliated by his early poverty and felt a desperate need for affection. He left school after failing final examinations and went to live in a garret in Paris. After a few minor and poor journalistic efforts, he published a successful novel in 1868 and then confidently mapped out his whole career. He planned to write a series of works to document hu-manity. With lack of taste or moderation, but with much energy he put the plan into practice. He believed that heredity and certain cerebral disorders were the major influences on human events. Although he was branded by the prudish as a reviler of mankind for his frank descriptions of sexual matters, his novels bear the mark of the objective observer of reality. His books were considered dangerous and were banned in England. In London in 1888 his English publisher was jailed. His own life was meticulously domestic and firmly regulated by his mother and his wife. The alcoholics (*see* ALCOHOLISM), prostitutes, and their customers that he wrote about were documented by visits to the underworld conducted with the zeal of a researcher. His work was essentially moral, and he recognized the destructive role that vice plays in society.

Bibliography: Hemmings, F.W.J. 1966. *Émile Zola*.

ZOROASTER. An Iranian prophet and religious teacher. He lived sometime between 1000 B.C. and 551 B.C. He founded, or reformed, the religion of ancient Persia. His teachings were based on the doctrine that although man could choose to live a good or bad life in the supreme struggle between the creator, or spirit of goodness, and the devil, or the spirit of evil, good would finally prevail. Zoroaster regarded the body as the tomb of the immortal soul. Friedrich Nietzsche (q.v.) in his book *Thus Spake Zarathustra* (1883-1891) used him as a mouthpiece for his own views.

Bibliography: Duchesne-Guillemin, J. 1973. *Religion of ancient Iran*.

ZSCHOKKE, JOHANN HEINRICH DANIEL (1771-1848). A German writer, one of the first to compose short stories. After opening a boarding school, he became interested in educational problems of the mentally retarded. He proposed to undertake a statistical study of feeblemindedness; the investigation, which was begun under his guidance, took several years and was eventually completed in 1855.

Bibliography: Kanner, L. 1964. *A history of the care and study of the mentally retarded*.

ZWAARDEMAKER, HENDRIK (1847-1930). A Dutch physiologist. His work on the sense of smell was the first scientific exposition of the subject and brought together all that was then known about smell. He published his findings in 1895 in *Die Physiologie des Geruchs* and updated them in 1925 in another volume entitled *L'odorat*. The olfactometer was invented by him.

Bibliography: Boring, E. G. 1950. *A history of experimental psychology*.

ZWEIG, STEFAN (1881-1942). An Austrian novelist, biographer, and poet, born of a well-to-do Jewish family in Vienna. Influenced by the impressionistic movement in literature and by the teachings of Sigmund Freud (q.v.), he developed a technique that enabled him to portray his characters in intuitive psychological depth. His short stories dealt with such morbid subjects as sexual aberrations and mental illness. *Amok* (1922) is an example of this aspect of his work. He wrote several psychological biographies of literary and historical figures. For political reasons he left his country in 1934. For a time he lived in England and the United States and finally moved to Brazil, where he and his second wife committed suicide (q.v.).

Bibliography: Prater, D. A.. 1972. *European of yesterday.*

Appendix:
List of Entries by Categories

Abnormal Behavior Shown by People—Psychopaths, Hysterics, Eccentrics

Abraham-men
Acid fascism
Acte gratuit
Agrippina the Younger
Aix-en-Provence nuns
Auxonne nuns

Baker, Mary
  (*See* Mary Baker Eddy)
Baker, Rachel
Balsamo, Giuseppe
Bathory, Elizabeth
Bergier, William le
  (or Pastourel)
Bibliomania
Binggeli, Johannes
Blavatsky, Helena Petrovna
Bottell, William
Bourne, Ansel
Brinvilliers, Marie
  Madaleine d'Aubray,
  Marquise de
Brodie, William
Brothers, Richard
Brownrigg, Elizabeth

Cagliostro, Alessandro di
  (*See* Giuseppe Balsamo)
Casanova de Seingalt,
  Giovanni Giacomo
Castlereagh, Robert Steward,
  Viscount
Chorea demonomania
Chorea lasciva
Choromania
Clive, Robert, Baron Clive
  of Plassey
Colburn, Zerah
Collin, Michel
Contagion of the imagination
Curzon, George Nathaniel
  (Marquis Curzon of
  Kendleston)

Damiens, Robert François
Demandolx, Madeleine de
Dugdale, Richard
Duncan, Isadora

Earthquakes of London
Eddy, Mary Baker
El Dorado
Emmelot of Chaumont
Emmerich, Anna Katharina

Duquesnoy, Francesco
Dürer, Albrecht

Eccles (or Eagles), Solomon
Elgar, Sir Edward
Elsheimer, Adam
Ensor, Baron James
Erwartung

Farinelli, Carlo
Feltrini, Andrea
Filiger, Charles
Flannagan, John Bernard
Fleury (or Robert-Fleury),
    Joseph Nicholas Robert
Fools
Francia, Francesco Raibolini
Fuseli, John Henry

Garrick, David
Gaudí y Cornet, Antonio
Gauguin, Eugène Henri Paul
Gay, John
Géricault, Jean Louis
    André Théodore
Gershwin, George
Gesualdo, Carlo, Prince of
    Venosa
Geya (or Gheyn) Jacob de
Gillray, James
Gioconda, La
Giotto (Giotto di Bondone)
Glinka, Mikhail Ivanovich
Goes, Hugo Van der
Goya y Lucientes,
    Francisco José de
Grainger, Percy Aldridge
Greco, El
Grimaldi, Joseph
Gurney, Ivor Bertie
Guttmann-Maclay collection

Haizmann, Christoph
Hals, Frans
Handel, George Frederik
Haydon, Benjamin Robert
Heemskerck, Maerten Jacobsz Van
Heseltine, Philip Arnold

Hoffmann, Ernst Theodor
    Wilhelm (or Amadeus)
Hogarth, William
Holbein, Hans, the Younger
Huygens, Christian

Janssens, Abraham
Jokes
Josephson, Ernst

Kaulbach, Wilhelm Von
Kean, Edmund
Kokoschka, Oskar
Kreutzer Sonata

Landseer, Sir Edwin Henry
Lear, Edward
Lemoyne, François
Leonardo da Vinci
L'Étoile du nord
Lievens (or Lievensz), Jan
Linda di Chamounix
Lippi, Filippo
Liszt, Franz
Lobb, Theophilus
Lowry, Lawrence Stephen
Lucia di Lammermoor
Lucius Junius Brutus

Macklin, Charles
Mahler, Gustav
Manon Lescaut
Maria Padilla
Martin, John
Mazeppa
Medium, The
Méryon, Charles
Messerschmidt, Franz Xaver
Michelangelo, Buonarroti
Mind, Gottfried
Modigliani, Amedeo
Mondrian, Piet
Monroe, Marilyn
Monrose, Claude Louis
Morland, George
Moussorgsky, Modest Petrovich
Munch, Edvard

Cannon, Walter Bradford
Carlson, Anton J.
Cloetta, Max
Copho
Cruveilhier, Jean
Cuvier, G.L.C.F.D., Baron

Dale, Sir Henry Hallett
Dalton, John
Darwin, Charles Robert
Dodoens, Rembert
Dresser, Heinrich
Dubois, Jacques
Dubois-Reymond, Emil
Dunglison, Robley
Durand de Éros, Joseph Pierre
Durkheim, Émile

Ecker, Alexander
Egger, Emile
Ehrenberg, Christian Gottfried
Ehrlich, Paul
Einstein, Albert
Erlanger, Joseph
Ewald, Julius Richard
Exner, Sigmund

Faraday, Michael
Fleischl-Marxow, Ernst von
Flourens, Marie Jean Pierre
Følling, Ivor Asbjørn
Frey, Maximilian von
Frobenius, Leo Victor

Gall, Franz Joseph
Galton, Sir Francis
Galvani, Luigi
Gaskell, Walter Holbrook
Gasser, Herbert Spencer
Gesner, Conrad
Giddings, Franklin Henry

Hering, Ewald
Hoffmann, Moritz
Hofmann, Albert

Jennings, Herbert Spencer

Kelvin, Sir William Thomson
Kepler, Johannes
Kinsey, Alfred Charles

Lamarck, Jean Baptiste de
Langley, John Newport
Lejeune, Jerome Jean
Le Play, Pierre Guillaume
Lévi-Strauss, Claude
Linton, Ralph
Littré, Maximilien Paul
    Émile
Lodge, Sir Oliver Joseph
Loewi, Otto
Lucett, James

Malinowski, Bronislaw
    Kasper
Mannheim, Karl
Martin, Everett Dean
Mead, Margaret
Mendel, Gregor Johann
Monro, Alexander
Mooney, James
Müller, Johannes Peter
Munk, Hermann

Näcke, Paul
Nagel, Wilibald A.
Neminsky, Vladimir Pravdich
Noguchi, Hideyo

Oppenheimer, Franz

Pacchioni, Antonio
Pavlov, Ivan Petrovich
Prochaska, George
Purkyně (or Purkinje) Jan

Quetelet, Lambert Adolphe
    Jacques

Ratzel, Friedrich
Ratzenhofer, Gustav
Recklinghausen, Friedrich
    Daniel von
Rivers, William Halse
Romanes, George John

Sandow, Eugene
Saussure, Horace Bénédict de
Schaudinn, Fritz Richard
Schiff, Moritz
Schleicher, August
Schleiden, Matthias Jakob
Sechenov, Ivan Mikhailovich
Sen, Ganneth
Soemmerring, Samuel Thomas von
Stensen, Niels
Sylvius (*see* Jacques Dubois)

Tarchanoff, Ivan Romanovich
Tarde, Gabriel
Tiedemann, Friedrich
Tylor, Edward

Vierordt, Karl von
Vieussens, Raymond
Virchow, Rudolf Ludwig Carl
Volkmann, Alfred Wilhelm

Wallace, Alfred Russell
Wassermann, August von
Weigert, Carl
Weismann, August
Wiener, Norbert
Wöhler, Friedrich
Wolff, Caspar Friedrich

Zwaardemaker, Hendrik

Body Components and Body Conditions

Albinos

Bile
Black Choler

Choler

Diaphragm

Humors

Inner Senses

Left-Handedness

Mortality in the Insane

Odor of the Insane

Pulse

Sleep Deprivation
Stigmata

Uterus

Worms

Caring Professions and Occupations

Abano, Pietro D'
Actuarius, Johannes
Aesculapius
Aetius of Amida
Ager (*or* Agerius), Nicholas
Agrippa
Alcorta, Diego
Aleman, Andrew
Alexander of Tralles
Alexis of Piedmont
Allen, Matthew
Allen, Thomas
Alpini, Prospero
Arbuthnot, John
Archer, John
Archigenes
Arculanus, Johannes (*or* Arcolani, Giovanni)
Aretaeus of Cappadocia
Argyll Robertson, Douglas Moray Cooper Lamb
Arlidge, John Thomas
Arndt, Rudolf Gottfried
Arnold, Thomas
Arnold of Villanova
Arundell, John
Asclepiades
Ashbourne, John
Athenaeus of Attaleia
Aubert, Hermann

Auenbrugger, von Auenbrugg,
Leopold
Aurelianus, Caelius
(*See* Caelius Aurelianus)
Autenrieth, Ferdinand
Avenzoar
Averroes
Avicenna
Awl, William M.

Backus, Frederick
Baglivi, Giorgio
Baldi, Camillo
Banting, Sir Frederick Grant
Barrough, Philip
Basket Men
Battie, William
Bayle, Antoine Laurent Jessé
Bayle, François
Beddoes, Thomas Lovell
Beecher, Henry Knowles
Belhomme, J.E.
Bell, Luther V.
Benedikt, Moritz
Benivieni, Antonio
Berengario da Carpi, Jacopo
Bergmann, Gustav von
Bernheim, Hippolyte-Marie
Bertruccio, Niccolò
Biedl, Arthur
Bienville, M.D.T. de
Birch, John
Bircher-Benner,
Maximilian Oskar
Blackburn, I.W.
Blackmore, Sir Richard
Blake, Andrew
Blandford, G. Fielding
Blocq, Paul Oscar
Boë, Franz de la
Boerhaave, Hermann
Boissier, de Sauvages,
François
Bonet, Theóphile
Boorde, Andrew
Bouchut, Jean Antoine
Eugène
Bouillaud, Jean Baptiste

Boyle, Helen
Bozzolo, Camillo
Braid, James
Bramwell, Byron
Brandin, Abel
Breuer, Joseph
Brierre de Boismont,
Alexandre
Brigham, Amariah
Bright, Timothy
Briquet, Paul
Brodie, Sir Benjamin
Collins
Brooks, Mary
Broussais, François Joseph
Victor
Brown, John
Brown, Thomas
Browne, Sir Thomas
Brown-Sequard, Charles Édouard
Brücke, Ernst Wilhelm von
Bruele (*or* Brant), Gualtherius
Buchanan, Joseph
Bucknill, Sir John Charles
Bukht, Yishu
Burrows, George Man

Cabanis, Pierre Jean George
Caelius Aurelianus
Caius, John
Calmeil, Louis Florentin
Campbell, Alfred Walter
Campbell, Clark A.
Cardano, Girolamo
Carus, Carl Gustav
Casper, Johann Ludwig
Cassiodorus, Flavius Magnus
Aurelianus
Caton, Richard
Cerise, Laurent
Charlesworth, Edward Parker
Chatin, Gaspard Adolph
Chauliac, Guy de
Cheyne, George
Chiarugi, Vincenzo
Cirillo, Domenico
Collier, James Stanfield
Colombier, Jean

Freeman, John
Friedreich, Johannes Baptista
Friedreich, Nikolaus
Frugardi, Rogerius
   (*See* Roger of Salerno)

Gale, Thomas
Galen (Galenus Claudius)
Galt, John Minson
Gariopontus
Garland, Agnes
Gaskell, Samuel
Gaub, Hieronymus David
   (Gaubius)
Gehuchten, Arthur van
Georget, Étienne
Gerard, John
Gilbert, William
Gilles de la Tourette, Georges
Gjessing, Leiv Rolvssön
Glisson, Francis
Gohl, Johann Daniel
Gooch, Robert
Good, John Mason
Gordon, Bernard de
Granville, Joseph Mortimer
Grasset, Joseph
Greatrakes, Valentine
Greding, Johann Ernst
Gregory, John
Groddeck, Georg
Guggenbühl, (Johann) Jakob
Guillotin, Joseph Ignace
Gull, Sir William Withely

Haën, Anton de
Hahnemann, Samuel
Haindorf, Alexander
Hale, Richard
Halford, Sir Henry
Hall, John (1575-1635)
Hall, John (1733-1793)
Hall, Marshall
Hallaran, William Saunders
Haller, Albrecht von
Halliday, Sir Andrew
Hansen, C.F.
Harper, Andrew

Hartley, David
Harvey, Gideon
Harvey, William
Haslam, John
Hastings, Sir Charles
Hawkes, John
Hawkins, John
Haygarth, John
Healy, William
Helmont, Franciscus
   Mercurius van
Helmont, Jan Batista van
Hensing, Johann Thomas
Herophilus of Chalcedon
Hill, Robert Gardiner
Hippocrates of Cos
Hirschfeld, Magnus
Hitch, Samuel
Hitschmann, Edward
Hoefer, Wolfgang
Hoffmann, Friedrich
Hoffmann, Heinrich
Holland, Henry
Holmes, Sir Gordon Morgan
Holst, Fredrik
Hood, Sir William Charles
Howe, Samuel Gridley
Howitz, F.
Huarte de San Juan, Juan
   (Juan de Dois)
Hua Tho
Hübertz, Jeans Rasmussen
Hufeland, Christoph Wilhelm
Hugh of Lucca (Borgognoni,
   Ugo)
Hundt, Magnus
Hunter, Alexander
Hunter, John
Huntington, George
Hutchison, Robert

Imhotep
Ireland, William Wetherspoon
Irish, David
Itard, Jean Marie Gaspard

Jacobi, Carl Wiegant
   Maximilian

Nicholls, Frank
Nostradamus
Nurses

Oliver, Charles Augustus
Oribasius
Orta, Garcia da
O'Shaugnnessy, Sir William
  Brooke
Osler, Sir William

Paracelsus, Philippus Aureolus
Parchappe, J.B.M.
Pardoux, Bartholomy
Paré, Ambroise
Pargeter, William
Parkinson, James
Paul of Aegina
Péan, Jules Émile
Perfect, William
Perkins, Elisha
Persian Galen
Petrus Hispanus
Phaire, Thomas (or Faier,
  Phaer)
Pierce, Robert
Pineless, Friedrick
Pitres, Jean Albert
Plater, Felix
Platner, Ernst
Pollich von Mellerstadt, Martin
Pompanazzi, Pietro
Poseidonius
Pownall, James
Price, William
Prichard, James Cowles
Priests
Pringle, Sir John
Pringle, John James
Psychiatric Social Work
Purcell, John
Pussin, Jean-Baptiste

Rabelais, François
Ramazzini, Bernardino
Raulin, Joseph
Rayner, Henry
Reginald of Bath

Reid, Henry
Reid, John
Remak, Robert
Rendu, Henri Jules Louis
Retzius, Gustaf
Rhazes (Abû Bakr Muhammad
  Ibn-Zakaria y Al-Rāzi)
Riedel, Joseph Gottfried von
Riggs, Austen Fox
Ringseis, Johann Nepomuk von
Riolan, Jean
Rivière, Lazare (Riverius)
Robertson, Douglas Argyll
Roger of Salerno
  (Rogerius Frugardi)
Rolando, Luigi
Rondelet, Guillaume
Rösch, Heinrich Karl
Rosenbach, Ottomar
Rowley, William
Rufus of Ephesus
Rumpf, Theodor
Rush, James

Saint-André, François
Salicetti, Guglielmo
Salmon, Thomas William
Santorio, Santorio
Saucerotte, Nicolas
Sauvages, François
  Boissier de
Savill, Thomas Dixon
Scaliger, Julius Caesar
Scarpa, Antonio
Schenk von Grafenburg,
  Johann
Schnitzler, Arthur
Schubert, Gotthilf Heinrich von
Scot (or Scott), Michael
Scotus, Michael
  (See Michael Scot)
Scribonius Largus
Scultetus, Joannis
Séguin, Edouard Onesimus
Semmelweis, Ignaz Philipp
Semon, Felix
Sennert, Daniel
Servetus, Miguel

Clinical States

Alusia
Amaurotic Familial Idiocy
Amenomania
Amnesia
Amok
Anaclitic Depression
Anemomania
Anesthesia
Anhedonia
Anniversary Reaction
Anomia
Anorexia Nervosa
Anteneasmon
Anton Syndrome
Apanthropia
Apasara
Aphelxia
Aphemia
Arctic Hysteria
Aura in Epilepsy
Autism

Basedow's Disease
Benign Stupors
Beriberi
Black Spots

Calentura
Cargo Anxiety
Catatonia
Cerebral Hyperaemia
Cerebro-Cardiac Neuropathia
Cerebropathia Psychica
   Toxemica
Cerebrotonia
Change of Sex
Comata
Compensation Neuroses
Constipation
Cretinism
Cyclothymia

Dancing Mania
Deaf-mutism
Déjà Vu
Delahara
Délire du Toucher
Delirium

Delirium Tremens
Delusions
Delusions, Persecutory
Dementia Infantilis
Dementia Praecocissima
Dementia Praecox
Dercum's Disease
Dereistic Thinking
Dermo-Optical Perception
   (DOP)
Double
Dropsy
Dysentery
Dyslexia

Ecstasy
English Malady
Enuresis
Epilepsy
Epistaxis
Ergot Poisoning
Erotographomania
Erotomania
Espinas de la Cabeza
Exhibitionism

Fatuitate Alpina
Faxensyndrom
Feigned Insanity
Folie à Deux
Folie à Double Forme
Folie Circulaire
Folie Lucide
Formication
Furor

Gargoylism
General Paralysis of the
   Insane

Hallucinations
Happy Puppet Syndrome
Hebephrenia
Heller's Disease
Hemorrhoids
Holy Disease
Hospitalism

Triskaidekaphobia
Tristimania
Tropenkohler
Tuberculosis
Tuberous Sclerosis

Vapors
Verbigeration
Vesania

Wacinko
Werewolves

Xi-Binel
Xi-Biril

Yantra

Zamporinion
Zoanthropy

Concepts and Theories

Action Theory of Consciousness
Anima. Jungian Term
Anima Sensitiva
Animal Magnetism
Animal Soul
Animal Spirits
Animism
Aphanisis
Archetype
Archeus
Associationism
Asthenic Type
Athletic Type

Basedowoid Type
Bell-Magendie Law
Birth Trauma
Black Comedy
Body Image
Boudhi
Brain, Concepts of

Clairvoyance
Climate
Cold

Complex
Conditionalism
Consensus
Curability

Death Instinct
Degeneration
Deuterophallic
Differential Diagnosis
Differential Psychology
Dipsychism
Dreams

Effect, Law of
Elation
Emotion, Theory of
Endocrinology
English Malady
Equinoxes
Eugenics
Excitability
Extra Sensory Perception (ESP)
Extrovert Type

Genius
Gestalt
G Factor

Heart
Hormic Psychology
Humoral Theory
Hysterical Conversion

Id
Imagination
Imprinting
Inferiority Complex
Insanity, Moral
Instincts, Theory of
Introvert Type
Intuition Type
Irritability

James-Lange Theory of
    Emotion (*See* Emotion, Theory
    of)

Lashley's Principle of Equipotentiality

Life Force
Life Instincts
Liver
Love

Magnetism
Mechanistic Theories
Memory
Moral Insanity
   (*See* Insanity, Moral)

Nirvana
Noegenetic Laws
Nous

Od or Odylic Force
O Factor
Organismic Theory
Organs

Personal Equation
P Factor
Phi-Phenomenon
Physiognomy
Platonic Love
Pneuma
Polypsychism
Prana
Precocity
Prepsychotic Personality
Prognosis
Psychic Energy
Psychic Pain
Psychobiology
Psychological Reality
Psychological Types
Psychopathy
Pyknic Type

Quaternity

Sensation Type
Sentient Statue
Sentiments
Sexuality
Sick Society
Spleen

Subcortical Irritation
Superfluous Man

Tabula Rasa
Temperament
Tetanoid Type
Thinking Type
Three-Dimensional Theory
Thymos
Traumataphobia
Tropism

Unconscious
Understanding

Vasomotor Theory of the Psychoses
Ventricular Theory
Viscerotonia
Vis Viva
Vitalism

Warmth
W Factor
Word Association

Yin and Yang

**Disciplines, Schools,
Branches of Learning,
Doctrines,
Psychological Approaches**

Act Psychology
Alchemy
Applied Psychology
Astrology
Austrian School

Babylonian Medicine
Behaviorism

Child Psychiatry
Child Psychology
Chiromancy
Cnidus
Comparative Psychology
Cos

Creationists
Curanderismo
Cybernetics
Cynics
Cyrenaic School

Determinism
Developmental Psychology

Eclecticism
Educational Psychology
Elementarism
Existentialism
Experimental Psychology

Factor School

Gestalt Psychology
Graphology
Gymnasium of Cynosarges

Hedonism

Individual Psychology
Interactionism
Interpersonal Theory

Limbus of Fools

Mesopotamian Psychiatry

Nancy School
Neurology
Neuropathology
Neurophysiology

Operationism

Phrenology
Positivism
Pragmatism
Psychiatry
Psychoanalysis
Psychological Medicine, Certificate in
Psychology as a Profession
Psychosomatic Medicine
Psychosurgery

Quietism

Scholasticism
Scottish School
Skeptics (*See* Pyrrho)
Social Psychology
Solidism
Sophists
Spiritualism
Statistical Methods
Stoicism
Structural Psychology

Teaching of Psychiatry
Thomism

Utilitarianism

Würzburg School

Yoga

Zen Buddhism

**Drugs, Medicaments,
Intoxicants,
Herbs**

Absinthe
Agrimony
Antimony
Anti-Psychosis
Apples
Armenian Stone
Asafoetida
Asses' Milk
Ayhuasca

Balm
Barbiturate
Barley Water
Belladonna
Betel
Betony
Bezoar Stone
Borage
Bromides
Bugloss

Passiflora
Peony
Peppermint
Periwinkle
Peyote
Plantain
Poppy (*See* Opium)
Potable Gold
Prickly Lettuce

Qat (*See* Kat)
Queen of Hungary's Water
Quietness
Qunubu (or Qunnabu)

Rauwolfia Serpentina
Red Wool
Rose
Rosemary
Rue
Rye

Saffron
Sage
St. John's-Wort
Salvarsan
San Pedro
Siberian Tonic
Skullcap
Snakeroot (*See* Rauwolfia Serpentina)
Soma
Soured Milk
Spirit of Skull
Stonecrop
Stramonium
Sunflower
Sweet Gale

Tartarus Tartarisatus
Theobrotion
Thistle
Thrift
Thyme
Tobacco
Tolcatzin
Tormentil
Truth Drug

Valerian
Vervain
Vinegar
Violet

Winter Cherry
Woodruff

Yarrow

Educators

Alcott, Amos Bronson

Barthold, F.
Bartholomäi, F.

Comenius (or Komensky),
  John Amos

Humphreys, Milton Wylie

Mann, Horace
Montessori, Maria

Neill, Alexander Sutherland

Oporinus

Péreiré, Jacob Rodrigue
Pestalozzi, Johann Heinrich
Pfister, Oskar

Sengelmann, Heinrich Matthias

Exalted People, Sovereigns, Potentates, Rulers, Royal Personages, Popes, Etc.

Alexander III (the Great)
Amasis II
Antiochus I
Artemisia

Battus
Bayezid (Bajazet) II
Boleyn, George, Viscount
  Rochford

Messalina, Valeria
Mohammed (or Mahomet)
Mohammed Tughlak

Napoleon I (Napoleon Bonaparte)
Napoleon III (Charles Louis
    Napoleon Bonaparte)
Nebuchadnezzar
Nero, Claudius Caesar

Otho, Marcus Salvius
Otto I

Paul I
Perceval, Spencer
Perdiaccas
Peter I (or Peter the Great)
Peter III
Phagyi-Dau
Philip II
Philip V
Pius IV
Policrates
Pompadour, Jeanne Antoinette Pois-
    son, Marquise de
Pontius Pilate
Psammetichos

Richard III
Richelieu, Armand Jean
    du Plessis, Duc de
Robespierre, Maximilien François
    Marie Isidore de

Sardanapalus
Saul
Sigibaldus
Sigurd I
Sixtus V
Solomon

Talal I
Theodoric the Great
Tiberius, Claudius Nero
Tzu Hsi

Wolsey, Thomas

Feral Children

Bovinus Bambergensis

Feral Child

Hauser, Kaspar

Leblanc, Marie-Angelique

Ovinus Hibernus

Peter of Hanover

Ursinus Lithuanus

Wild Boy of Aveyron
Wild Boy of Salvador
Wolf Child of Hesse
Wolf Children
Wolf Children of Midnapore

Gems and Precious Metals

Agate
Amber
Amethyst

Beryl

Crystal

Diamond

Emerald

Galactite
Garnet

Jacinth
Jasper
Jet

Lapis Armeniacum (*See* Armenian
    Stone)
Lapis Lazuli

Onyx

Precious Stones

Ruby

Sapphire
Sardonyx
Selenite
Silver
Smaragdus

Topaz

**Hypnotism, Magnetism:
Their Practitioners and
Subjects**

Azam, Etienne Eugène

Bernard, Prudence
Bernheim, Hippolyte-Marie
Braid, James
Burkmar, Lucius

Deleuze, Joseph Philip François
Despine, Antoine
Despine, Prosper
Dods, John Bovee
Donatism
Donato (*See* Alfred d'Hont)
Dupotet de Sennevoy, J.

Ecstatici
Elliotson, John
Esdaile, James

Faria, José Custodio de

Glossolalia
Grand Hypnotisme

Hall, Spencer Timothy
Hansen, Carl
Heidenhain, Rudolf
Hell, Maximilian
Home, Daniel Dunglas
Hont, Alfred d'
Hypnotism

Insanity, Artificial

Kesuruban
Kluge, Carl Alexander Ferdinand
Kuda-Kepang

Lacordaire, Jean Baptiste
    Henri
LaFontaine, Charles
Lafayette, Marie Joseph du
    Motier, Marquis de
Lassaigne, August
Lausanne, de
Lavater Johann Kaspar
Lavoisier, Antoine Laurent
Léonie

Mesmer, Franz Anton
Mesmerism
Miller, Miss Frank

Neurypnology
Noizet, F.J.
Nollet, Jean Antoine

Okey, Elizabeth and Jane

Paradis, Maria Theresa von
Perkins, Elisha
Preiswerk, Hélène
Puységur, Amand-Marie-Jacques
    de Chastenet

Quimby, Phineas Parkhurst

Race, Victor
Richet, Charles Robert
Ringseis, Johann Nepomuk von

Sarrasin de Montferrier,
    Alexandre André Victor
Society of Harmony
Sunderland, la Roy

**Institutions, Laboratories,
Organizations and
Professional Bodies**

Abendberg Institution
Aberdeen Royal Mental Hospital

Åbo (Turku)
Académie des Sciences
Academy, the
Alcoholics Anonymous (A.A.)
Alleged Lunatics' Friend
  Society
All Hallows Hospital
Al-Mansur Hospital
Alt-Scherbitz Asylum
American Association on
  Mental Deficiency
American Breeders' Association
American Neurological
  Association
American Orthopsychiatric
  Association
American Psychiatric
  Association
American Psychological
  Association
Anthropometric Laboratory
Arbeit (Work)
Argyll and Bute Hospital
Aro
Association of Medical
  Officers of American
  Institutions for Idiots
  and Feebleminded Persons
Association of Medical Officers
  of Asylums and Hospitals
  for the Insane
Association of Medical
  Superintendents of American
  Institutions for the Insane
Asylums
Asylums, One-Man
Aversa

Baghdad Asylum
  (See Dàr-Ul-Maraftan)
Barony Parochial Asylum
Bath Mental Deficiency Colony
Belle Vue Asylum
Belmont Hospital
Bethel Colony for Epileptics
Bethel Hospital
Bethlem Royal Hospital
Bethnal House

Bexley Hospital
Bicêtre
Bloomingdale Asylum
Bootham Park (See York Lunatic
  Asylum)
Borstal System
Boston Alms House
Boston Lunatic Hospital
Botanical Lunatic Asylum
Brentry Certified Inebriate
  Reformatory
Bridewell
Brislington House
Bristol Lunatic Asylum
British Psychological Society
Broadgate Hospital
Broadmoor Hospital
Brooke House
Bucharest Central Hospital
  for Mental and Nervous
  Disorders
Burghölzli Hospital

Cairo Lunatic Asylums
Cassel Hospital
Caterham Asylum
Charenton
Charité (Germany)
Charité de Château-Thierry
Cheadle Royal Hospital
  (See Manchester Lunatic Hospital)
Child Guidance Clinics
Children's Bureau
Child Study Association
Child Welfare League of
  America
Clapham Retreat
Colditz Castle
Collegium Insanorum
Colney Hatch Asylum
Commercial Hospital and
  Lunatic Asylum
Congress of Psychology
Connecticut State Hospital
  for Insane
Coton Hill
County Asylums
Crichton Royal Hospital

Valencia Asylum (*See* Sancta Maria
  Dels Inocents)
Vermont Asylum

Wakefield Asylum
Warlingham Park Hospital
Warneford Hospital
Wednesday Psychological Society
Western Lunatic Asylum
Whitmore House
Willard Asylum
Williamsburg Eastern
  Lunatic Asylum
Wisconsin State Hospital
Worcester County Lunatic
  Asylum
World Psychiatric Association

York Lunatic Asylum
York Retreat, The

Zaragoza Hospital

Instruments and Contraptions

Aesthesiometer
Amputation Doll
Armilla
Atlanta

Baquet
Bauble
Belgian Cage
Branks

Caduceus
Camisole
Chevreul-Pendulum
Church Crosses and Pillars
Churinga
Circulating Swing
Cramp Rings

Electroencephalogram

Flute
Fool's Cap

Galton Bar
Galton Whistle
Gazing Crystal
Gyrator

Handcuffs
Headdress of Pauper Lunatics
Human Skin Belts

Idiots' Cage
Inn Signs

Leather Caps
Leg-Locks

Machines
Mad-Shirt
Magnet
Metallic Tractors
Microscope
Miroir Rotatif
Modiolus
Monument of Sympathy

Ouija Board

Padded Room
Phallus
Philosopher's Stone
Planchette

Rotatory Machine

Sanbenito
Snake, Symbol of
Spinning Chair
Strait-Waistcoat
Swinging Chair

Tranquillizer
Transport
Twirling Stool

Utica Crib

Whipping Posts (*See* Flogging)
Whirling Chair

Journals

American Journal of
   Insanity
American Journal of
   Mental Deficiency
American Journal of
   Psychiatry
American Journal of
   Psychology
Annales Médico-Psychologiques
Année Psychologique, L'
Année Sociologique, L'
Archives of Neurology
Asylum Journal, The

Beobachtungen über den
   Cretinismus
Brain
British Journal of
   Psychiatry
   (See Asylum Journal)
British Journal of
   Psychology

Excelsior

Gazette de Santé

Imago

Journal de Psychologie
Journal of Applied Psychology
Journal of Genetic Psychology
Journal of Insanity
   (See American Journal of
   Psychiatry)
Journal of Psycho-Asthenics (See
   American
   Journal of Mental Deficiency)
Journal of Psychological
   Medicine and Mental
   Pathology

Journals by Patients

Magazin zur
   Erfahrungsseelenkunde

Mind
Moonbeams

New Moon, The

Opal, The

Pedagogical Seminary, The
Philosophical Transactions, The
Philosophische Studien
Phrenological Journal
Psychological Abstracts
Psychological Review
Psychologische Forschung

Retreat Gazette

Zeitschrift für das
   Idiotenwesen
Zeitschrift für die Erforschung
   und Behandlung des
   Jugendlichen Schwachsinns
Zeitschrift für Psychologie
   und Physiologie der
   Sinnesorgane
Zeitschrift für Völkerpsychologie
   und Sprachwissenschaft

Zoist, The

Legislation, Legislators, Jurists, Legal Issues

Adoptio
Aguessau, Henry François D'

Bachofen, Johann Jakob
Bailly, Jean Sylvain
Beccaria, Cesare Bonesana di
Bentham, Jeremy
Bergasse, Nicolas
Blackstone, Sir William
Bodin, Jean
Boyington, Horatio
Bracton, Henry de
Burglary

Chambre Ardente
Chancery Lunatics

Literary Characters From Mythology, The Classics, Plays, Novels, Religious Works, Etc.

Melampus
Mephistopheles
Merlin
Micawber
Mnemosyne (*See* Mnemonics)
Moirae
Molles
Moloch
Morpheus
Moses

Narcissus
Nicolette
Niobe
Nymphs

Oedipus
Oknos
Orestes
Ormuzd
Orpheus
Othello

Pan
Panacea
Pentheus
Peter Pan
Phaedra
Pierrot
Priapus
Prig, Betsey
Proetus
Pygmalion

Rigoletto
Romulus

Salmoneus
Salome
Samson
Satyrs
Schweik
Semiramis
Silvani
Stavrogin, Nikolai
    Vsevolodovich
Styx

Subacti
Succubus

Tartuffe
Thanatos
Thraetona
Three Kings
Ticonal
Tristam
Troll, Patrick

Ulysses (or Odysseus)

Valdemar
Venus

Werther
Wihtiko (or Windigo)
Windigo (*See* Wihtiko)
Wiracocha
Wod

Zeus
Zimri

**Literary Works, Including
the Scriptures, Classical
Works, Texts, Etc.**

Adolphe
Amour Médecin, L'
*Amours du Chevalier de
    Faublas, Les*
Anatomy of Melancholy, The
André Cornélis
Anglo-Saxon Herbal
Anthropologie
Antipalus Maleficiorum
Anton Reiser
Axel
Ayur-Veda

Bacchanals
Badiano's Codex
Bartleby the Scrivener
Bedlam Poems

Locations

Movements, Religious Orders and Sects

Raymond, Fulgence
Retzius, Gustaf
Romberg, Moritz Heinrich
Rossolimo, Gregory Ivanovich
Roussy, Gustave

Sachs, Bernard
Schaffer, Karoly
Schwann, Theodor
Sherrington, Sharles Scott
Smith, Sir Grafton Elliot
Souques, Achille Alexander
Spatz, Hugo
Spielmeyer, Walter
Spiller, William Gibson
Spitzka, Edward Charles
Starr, Moses Allen

Teplov, Boris Mikhailovich
Türk, Ludwig

Veraguth, Otto
Vincent, Clovis
Vogt, Oskar and Vogt, Cécile

Waldeyer-Hartz, Heinrich
  Wilhelm von
Wernicke, Carl
Westphal, Carl Friedrich Otto
Wickman, Otto Ivar
Wilson, Kinnier

Patients

Abu Bakr El Siddig
Achilles
Alexandra of Bavaria
Anna O
Aristides, Publius Aelius

Beauchamp, Christine
Beers, Clifford W.
Blofot, Richard
Boswell, John

Cann, Sir William
Carkesse, James

Chaptal
Chevigné

Dora

Elena, F.
Elizabeth von R.
Emmy von N.
Estelle

Félida, X.

Gage, Phineas P.
Graf, Herbert (See Little Hens)
Grenville, Anne

Hauffe, Friedericke
Henry of Fordwich
Hill Folk, The

Ikara
Irene
Irma

Jukes
Justine

Kallikak Family

Little Hans
Lucie

Madame D.
Madeline
Marcelle
Marie
Markus Family
Marlborough, Duke of
Matthews, James Tilley
Miles, Hannah

Nadia
Nam
Nicholson, Margaret
Norris, William

Packard, E.P.W.
Pappenheim, Berta (See Anna O)

Nightingale, Florence
Nobel, Alfred Bernhard

Owen, Robert

Pisani, Pietro

Rahere
Recke-Volmerstein, Adalbert
 von der
Reed, Andrew

Sayago, José
Shaftesbury, Anthony Ashley
 Cooper, 7th Earl of

Theodosius the Cenobiarch
Tuke, Samuel
Tuke, William

Wakefield, Edward
Wakefield, Priscilla
Wilberforce, William

Philosophers and Theologians

Abélard, Pierre
Alcmaeon of Crotona
Alexander of Aphrodisias
Alexander of Hales
Amerling, Karl
Amiel, Henri-Frédéric
Anaxagoras of Cleomenes
Apollonius of Tyana
Aquinas, Saint Thomas
Aristotle
Augustine, Saint of Hippo
Avenarius, Richard
Averröes

Bacon, Francis
Bacon, Roger
Barthez, Paul Joseph
Bartholomaeus Anglicus
Beneke, Friedrich Eduard
Bergson, Henri
Berkelev, George

Bilfinger, Georg Bernhard
Brentano, Franz
Brown, Thomas

Cabanis, Pierre Jean George
Calanus
Calvin, John
Campanella, Tommaso
Camus, Albert
Carus, Carl Gustav
Cassiodorus, Flavius Magnus
 Aurelianus
Ch'ao Iuangfang
Cicero, Marcus Tullius
Cleanthes
Comte, Auguste
Condillac, Etienne Bonnot de
Confucius or K'ung Fu-Tzu
Cooper, Thomas
Cornelius, Hans
Critias

Democritus
Demosthenes
Descartes, René
Dessoir, Max
Dewey, John
Diogenes
Driesch, Hans Adolf Eduard
Duns Scotus, John

Eckhart, Johannes
Ehrenfels, Christian von
Empedocles
Engels, Friedrich
Epictetus
Epicurus
Erasmus, Desiderius
Erastus, Thomas
Erhard, John Benjamin

Fechner, Gustav Theodor
Fichte, Johann Gottlieb
Ficino, Marsilio
Flournoy, Théodore
Fludd, Robert
Flüe, Nicholas von Der
Friers, Jakob Friedrich

Galilei, Galileo
Gerson, Jean le Charlier de
Glanvill, Joseph
Goethe, Johann Wolfgang von
Gracián, Baltasar
Grimes, James Stanley
Groos, Karl Theodor
Gymnosophists

Haberlin, Paul
Haeckel, Ernst Heinrich
Hamilton, Sir William
Harrington, James
Hartley, David
Hartmann, Karl Robert
  Eduard von
Hegel, Georg Wilhelm
  Friedrich
Heidegger, Martin
Helmont, Franciscus
  Mercurius van
Helvetius, Claude Adrien
Heraclitus
Herbart, Johann Friedrich
Herder, Johann Gottfried von
Hickok, Laurens Perseus
Hobbes, Thomas
Hobhouse, Leonard Trelawney
Holbach, Paul Henri Dietrich I,
  Baron D'
Hooke, Robert
Hume, David
Hunayn, Ibn Ishaq
Husserl, Edmund

James, William
Jaspers, Karl Theodore
Johannitius Onan (See Hunayn Ibn
  Ishaq)
John of Salisbury
Jurieu, Pierre

Kamada, Ho
Kant, Immanuel
Kierkegaard, Søren Aabye
Klages, Ludwig

La Mettrie, Julien Offray de
Lao-Tzu (or Lao-Tze)
Le Camus, Antoine

Leibniz, Gottfried Wilhelm
Locke, John
Lucretius (Titus Lucretius
  Carus)
Lullius, Raimundus

Mach, Ernst
Maimonides, Moses
Maine de Biran, François Pierre
Malebranche, Nicholas
Marbe, Karl
Marx, Karl
Meinong, Alexius
Melanchthon, Philip
Menippus
Messer, August
Mill, James
Mill, John Stuart
Montesquieu, Charles Louis
  de Secondat, Baron de la Brède
More, Sir Thomas
Müller, Georg Elias

Nemesius
Nestorians
Newton, Sir Isaac
Nietzsche, Friedrich
  Wilhelm

Oldenburg, Henry

Pascal, Blaise
Philolaos of Croton
Pico Della Mirandola
Plato
Plotinus
Plutarch
Pompanazzi, Pietro
Porta, Giovanni Battista
  Della
Protagoras of Thrace
Psellus, Michael Constantine
Pyrrho
Pythagoras

Rabelais, François
Rauch, Frederick Augustus
Reid, Thomas

Reimarus, Hermann Samuel
Rousseau, Jean-Jacques
Royce, Josiah

Samkara
Santayana, George
Sartre, Jean-Paul
Schelling, Fredrich Wilhelm
    Joseph von
Schiller, Johann Christoph
    Friedrich von
Schopenhauer, Arthur
Schryver, Konrad (or
    Scribonius or Grophaeus)
Seneca, Lucius Annaeus
Smith, Joseph
Socrates
Sophocles
Spencer, Herbert
Spinoza, Baruch (Benedict) de
Steiner, Rudolf
Stewart, Dugald
Strato
Stumpf, Carl
Swedenborg, Emanuel

Telesio, Bernardino
Tertullianus, Quintus
    Septimius Florens
Themison
Theophrastus
Trithemius, Johannes
Troxler, Ignaz Paul Vitalis

Vaihinger, Hans
Vico, Godfrey de
Vives, Juan Luis
Voltaire

Wang K'en-Tang
Watts, Isaac
Windischmann, Karl Joseph
    Hironymus
Witte, Karl
Wolff, Christian von

Zabarella, Jacobus
Zarathustra (*See* Zoroaster)

Zeno of Citium
Ziehen, Theodor
Zoroaster

Practices and Customs

Advertising
Anagogic Interpretation
Asylum Visiting
Auto-Da-Fé

Bacchanalia
Boarding-Out of Mental
    Patients
Buttercup

Cannibalism
Cottage System
Couvade

Dancing
Divination

Falconry
Family Care
Filicide
Fixing
Flagellation
Flogging

Gift Exchange
Greatford

Hiring of Lunatics
Homosexuality

Incest
Infanticide

King's Touch

Lesbianism

Mandi-Minjak-Mendidi
Masturbation
Metoposcopy

Necromancy
New England System
Night Attendant Service

Oracles

Palmistry (*See* Chiromancy)
Penny Gates
Persecutory Child Rearing
Pinning
Polygamy

Royal Touch (*See* King's Touch)

Sterilization

Tonsure
Tromba Cult

Visiting

Yellow
Yolmelaua

Psychiatrists, Psychoanalysts and Neuropsychiatrists

Abraham, Karl
Adler, Alfred
Aichhorn, August
Allen, Frederick
Alzheimer, Alois
Andreas-Salomé, Lou
Antiphon

Baillarger, Jules
Balint, Michael
Baruk, Henri Marc
Beard, George M.
Bender, Lauretta
Berger, Hans
Bermann, Gregorio
Bernfeld, Siegfried
Bianchi, Leonardo
Bielschowsky, Max
Binswanger, Otto
Bion, Wilfred Ruprecht
Bleuler, Eugen

Bonhoeffer, Karl
Bourneville, Désiré-Magloire
Briggs, L. Vernon
Brill, Abraham Arden
Broca, Paul
Brosius, C. M.
Browne, William Alexander
    Francis
Bruns, Ludwig
Buckle, Richard Maurice
Bumke, Oswald
Burrow, N. Trigant
Butler, John

Cameron, Donald Ewen
Capgras, Jean Marie Joseph
Cerletti, Ugo
Charcot, Jean-Martin
Clérambault, Gaétan de
Clouston, Sir Thomas Smith
Conolly, John
Conrad, Klaus
Cramer, August
Crichton, Sir Alexander
Crichton-Browne, Sir James
Cueva Vallejo, Agustin
Cutter, Nehemiah

Damerow, Heinrich Philipp
    August
Dana, Charles Loomis
Daquin, Joseph
De Jong, H. Holland
Delgado, Honorio
De Sanctis, Sante
Deutsch, Helene
Down, John Langdon Haydon
Dreikurs, Rudolph
Dunbar, Helen Flanders
Dupré, Ernest Pierre
Dusser de Barenne,
    Joannes Gregorius

Earle, Pliny
Eitingon, Max
Ellis, Sir William Charles
Emminghaus, Hermann

Esquirol, Jean Étienne
  Dominique

Fairbairn, W. Ronald
Falret, Jules Ph. J.
Federn, Paul
Fenichel, Otto
Ferenczi, Sandor
Feuchtersleben, Ernst von
Forel, Auguste Henri
Freeman, Walter
Freud, Anna
Freud, Sigmund
Friedländer, Kate
Fromm, Erich
Fromm-Reichmann, Frieda

Ganser, Sigbert Joseph Maria
Gaupp, Robert Eugen
Gerard, Margaret
Gillespie, Robert Dick
Goldstein, Kurt
Gonzales Henriques, Raul
Grashey, Hubert von
Gray, John Perdue
Griesinger, Wilhelm
Groos, Friedrich
Gruhle, Hans Walther
Gudden, Bernard Aloys von
Guislain, Joseph

Hagen, Friedrich Wilhelm
Hecker, Ewald
Heinroth, Johann Christian
Held, Jan Theobald
Henderson, Sir David Kennedy
Hoch, August
Hoche, Alfred
Horney, Karen

Ideler, Karl Wilhelm
Ingenieros, José

Janet, Pierre
Jarvis, Edward
Jaspers, Karl Theodore
Jelliffe, Smith Ely
Joffroy, Alexis

Jolly, Friedrich
Jones, Ernest
Jung, Carl Gustav (1875-1961)

Kahlbaum, Karl Ludwig
Kallmann, Franz J.
Kandinsky, Viktor
  Chrisanfovich
Kanner, Leo
Kirkbride, Thomas Storey
Klaesi, Jakob
Klein, Melanie
Korsakov, Sergei
  Sergeievich
Kraepelin, Emil
Kretschmer, Ernst
Kubie, Lawrence S.
Kuffner, Karel

Laehr, Hans Heinrich
Leidesdorf, Max
Leuret, François
Lewis, Aubrey
Liébeault, Ambroise-August
Liepmann, Hugo Carl
Loewenfeld, Leopold
Lombroso, Cesare

Mapother, Edward
Marc, Charles Chretien Henri
Maudsley, Henry
Meduna, Ladislas Joseph
  von
Menninger, Karl Augustus
Meyer, Adolf
Meynert, Theodor Hermann
Mitchell, Silas Weir
Moebius, Paul Julius
Moll, Albert
Moreau de Tours, Jacques
  Joseph
Morel, Benedict Augustin
Morel, Ferdinand
Moreno, Jacob Levy
Morison, Alexander
Morita, Shoma
Morselli, Enrico

**Psychological Tests,
Techniques, Experiments,
Research Subjects**

Hall, Joseph
Hawthorne Experiments

Ink Blots
Intelligence Test

Kuleshova, Rosa

Maze

Nonsense Syllable

Otis Group Intelligence
  Scale

Puzzle Box

Raven's Progressive Matrices
Reaction Experiments

Serial Groups, Method of
Stimulus

Thematic Apperception Test
Therapeutic Trials
Thresholds, Measurements of

Psychologists, Phrenologists

Ach, Narziss J.
Alexander, Franz
Allport, Gordon W.
Angell, James Rowland
Aveling, Francis Arthur
  Powell

Bain, Alexander
Baldwin, James Mark
Bartlett, Sir Frederic
  Charles
Beaunis, Henri E.
Beck, Samuel Jacob
Bekhterev, Vladimir M.
Beneke, Friedrich Eduard
Benussi, Vittorio
Bethe, Albrecht
Binet, Alfred
Boring, Edwin Garrigues

Breuer, Joseph
Buhler, Karl
Burt, Cyril Lodowic

Carr, Harvey A.
Cattell, James McKeen
Cattell, Raymond Bernard
Claparède, Édouard
Coover, John Edgar
Culpin, Millais

Decroly, Ovide
Dessoir, Max
Dewey, John
Drever, James
Ebbinghouse, Hermann
Ellis, Havelock
Erikson, Erik Homburger
Ettlinger, Max Emil

Fechner, Gustav Theodor
Flournoy, Théodore
Fludd, Robert
Fowler, Orson Squire
Friers, Jakob Friedrich
Fröbes, Joseph
Froebel, Friedrich Wilhelm
  August

Gates, Elmer
Gelb, Adhémar Maximilian Maurice
Gesell, Arnold Lucius
Goddard, Henry Herbert
Groos, Karl Theodor

Hall, Granville Stanley
Healy, William
Hebb, Donald Olding
Hellpach, Willy
Helmholtz, Hermann Ludwig Ferdi-
  nand von
Hemingway, Ernest Millar
Herbart, Johann Friedrich
Holt, Edwin Bissell
Hornbostel, Erich von
Hull, Clark L.
Hunter, Walter S.

Whipple, Guy Montrose
Wirth, Wilhelm
Witasek, Stephan
Witmer, Lightner
Woodworth, Robert Sessions
Wundt, Wilhelm Max

Yerkes, Robert Mearns

Saints

Albertus Magnus, Saint
Anthony, Saint
Aquinas, Saint Thomas
Augustine, Saint, of Hippo

Basil the Great
Benedict of Nursia, Saint
Bernadette, Saint

Catherine of Siena, Saint
Cosmas and Damian, Saints
Cyprian, Saint

Dymphna, Saint

Finan, Saint

Gregory of Nyssa, Saint
Gregory of Tours, Saint
  (Georgius Florentius)
Guthlac, Saint

Hildegard of Bingen, Saint
Hugh of Lincoln, Saint

Isidore of Seville, Saint

Jerome, Saint
Joan of Arc, Saint
João de Deus (St. John of God)
Juan de Dios (*See* João de Deus)

Kentigern, Saint

Leonard, Saint
Liguori, Alfonso Maria Di
  (Saint Alphonsus)

Loyola, Saint Ignatius of,
Luke, Saint

Mathurin de Larchant, Saint
Maya

Nicholas, Saint

Paul, Saint

Saint
Samkara
Shah Daula
Simeon Stylites, Saint

Teresa (or Theresa) Saint

Vincent de Paul, Saint
Vitus, Saint

Winifred, Saint

**Suicide: People Who
Committed Suicide; Methods
and Places of Suicide**

Agrippina the Elder
Antinous
Autochiria

Beddoes, Thomas Lovell
Breath Holding
Brutus, Marcus Junius

Canary Islands
Castlereagh, Robert
  Steward, Viscount
Chatterton, Thomas
Clarke, Jeremiah
Clérambault, Gaétan de
Clive, Robert, Baron Clive
  of Plassey
Cornelius Rufus
Creech, Thomas
Crossroads

Demosthenes

Superstitions, Folklore, Charms, Spells, Amulets, Etc.

Jack the Clipper
Jarkman
Juramentado

Kindergarten
Kordiakos
Kuda-Kepang

Lagneia Furor
Larvatus
Lazaretto or Lazar House
Libido
Like Sweet Bells Jangled,
    out of Tune and Harsh
Lilliput
Lock Hospitals
Locusta
Logos
Lolita Syndrome
Longheaded
Love-Apple
Ludibria Faunorum
Lues Divina and Lues Deifica
Lunatic
Lycanthropy
Lypemania

Mad as a Hatter or the Mad
    Hatter
Mad-Doctor
Mad Parliament
Magdalene Asylums
Magnus Morbus
Mal D'Hercule
Mal D'Orient
Mandala
Mania
Mania, Caesar
Manic-Depressive Psychoses
Mare
Masochism
Matiruku
Medici
Megrims
Melampod
Melancholia
Melancholia Anglica
Melancholy Jacques

Melun
Mental Hygiene
Metapsychology
Micronomania
Mill-Reeck
Mnemonics
Mongolism
Monkeys
Monomania
Monomanie Incendiaire
Moonrakers
Moral Insanity (*See* Insanity, Moral)
Moria
Moron
Morotrophium
Morphinism
Mother-Sick

Narcissism
Neo-Freudians
Nervous Sleep
Neurasthenia
Neurosis
Noddy
Nostalgia
Nous
Nut

Oaf
Obeah
Obliging Dreams
Oblomovshtchina
Obsession
Onanism
Orenda

Panacea
Paralytic Insanity (*See*
    Insanity, Paralytic)
Paranoia
Parapathy
Paraphrenia
Paraphronsynias
Parapraxis
Paroniria
Patch
Pathics
Pathoneuroses

Vailala Madness
Vapors
Verbigeration
Vesania
Vis Viva

Wacinko
Winchester Goose
Wind-in-the-Mind
Wod

Zamporinion

Treatment (Forms of Treatment)

Analytic Group Therapy
Aversion Therapy

Bad News
Bath of Surprise
Baths
Bibliotherapy
Bilo
Bleeding
Blood Transfusion
Bomor
Boosening
    (*See* Bowssening)
Bowssening
Brass Bands

Cantharis Vesicatoria
    (*See* Spanish Fly)
Carbon Dioxide Therapy
Carriage-Driving
Cauterization
Chess
Circulating Swing
Citerrochen
Clitoris
Clyster
Craniotomy
    (*See* Trepanation)

Diet
Douche

Drama
Ducking

Electricity
Electroichthyology
Evacuants

Faith Healing
Farming
Fever Therapy
Fire
Fumigation

Gestation
Gladiator
Goat's Milk
Group Psychotherapy

Head Surgery
Horseback Riding

Immersion
Incantations
Incubation
Isolation

Leeches
Lizard
Lobotomy

Main Puteri
Malaria Therapy
Malopterurus Electricus
Marriage
Mercury
Metrazol Therapy
Moral Medicine
Moxa
Music Therapy

Narcosynthesis
Nile Electric Catfish
    (*See* Malopterurus Electricus)
Noninjurious Torture

Oat Straw Baths
Occupational Therapy
Orgone Therapy

Harsnett, Samuel
Hopkins, Matthew
Howard, Henry, Earl of
  Northampton

Impotence
Incubus
Inquisition

Jewell, John
Johnson, Mary

Kelley, Edward
Kraemer, Heinrich

Lancre, Pierre de
Leloyer, Pierre

Magic Shot
Medium
Muller, Catharine
Mutism

Nider, Johannes

Obeah

Possession
Prickers

Salem Witchcraft Trials
Satanism
Schwagelin, Anna Maria
Scot (or Scott), Reginald
Shamans
Smith, Helene
Somers, William
Sprenger, Johann Jacob
Strigae

Tedworth Drummer
Tregagas, Ragnhild

Wardell, Samuel
Witch of Mallegem, The
Witchcraft

Zar

Writers of Medical and Allied Works

Abbott, John Stevens Cabot
Austrius, Sebastianus

Bakewell, Thomas
Burdett, Henry Charles
Burton, Robert

Cassianus, Johannes
Celsus, Aulus Cornelius
Charaka
Constantine the African
Costa Ben Luca
Cureau de la Chambre, Marin

Democritus Junior
Downame, John
Drage, William

Elyot, Sir Thomas
Ent, Sir George

Fawcett, Benjamin
Forster, Thomas Ignatius
  Maria

Garzoni, Tomaso
Gerson, Jean Le Charlier de
Gilbertus Anglicus
Guainerio, Antonio

Hall, Basil
Hervey de Saint-Denis,
  Marie Jean Léon
Houllier, Jacques (Hollerius)

Kirchhoff, Theodor

Lactantius, Lucius Caelius Firmjanus
Lepois, Charles
Linguiti, Giovanni Maria

MacDonald, Arthur
Maxwell, William
Muratori, Ludovico Antonio

Ofhuys, Gaspar

Pannenborg, H. J. and W. A.
Pliny the Elder
 (Gaius Plinius Secundus)
Podmore, Frank

Roelans, Cornelius

Sigerist, Henry Ernest
Soury, Jules
Sym, John
Symonds, John Addington

Taylor, Jeremy
Turner, William

Upham, Thomas

Wesley, John
Wright, Thomas

Writers (Poets, Novelists, Playwrights)

Alfieri, Vittorio
Andersen, Hans Christian
Andersen, Tryggve
Aristophanes
Artaud, Antonin
Artemidorus
Aubrey, John
Auzouy, M.

Balzac, Honoré de
Barba-Jacob, Porfirio
Bashkirtseff, Marie
Baudelaire, Charles Pierre
Beattie, James
Beddoes, Thomas Lovell
Behan, Brendan
Benedictsson, Victoria Maria
Berryman, John
Blake, William
Bloomfield, Robert
Bly, Nellie
Blyton, Enid
Boccaccio, Giovanni

Borrow, George
Boswell, James
Bovey, James
Brant, Sebastian
 (See Narrenschiff)
Brentano, Clemens Maria
Breton, André
Breton, Nicholas
Brontë
Browning, Elizabeth Barrett
Browning, Robert
Buck, Pearl
Budgel, Eustace
Buffon, Georges Louis Leclerc de
Bunyan, John
Burns, Robert
Butler, Samuel
Byron, George Gordon, Lord

Calonne, Ernest de
Campanella, Tommaso
Camus, Albert
Carlyle, Thomas
Carroll, Lewis
 (See Charles Dodgson)
Cervantes Saavedra, Miguel de
Chateaubriand, François
 René, Vicomte de
Chatterton, Thomas
Chaucer, Geoffrey
Chekhov, Anton Pavlovich
Clare, John
Cockton, Henry
Cocteau, Jean
Coleridge, Samuel Taylor
Collins, William
Collins, William Wilkie
Corvo, Baron
Cotton, Nathaniel
Cowley, Abraham
Cowper, William
Crabbe, George
Creech, Thomas
Crowe, Catherine
 (née Stevens)
Cruden, Alexander

Dante Alighieri
Daudet, Alphonse

Davies, William Henry
Davy, Adam
Defoe, Daniel
Dekker, Th ̲s
Denham, Sir John
De Quincey, Thomas
Deschanel, Paul Eugène Louis
Desmarets de Saint-Sorlin, Jean
Dickens, Charles
Dickinson, Emily
Digby, Kenelm, Sir
Dobrovsky, Josef
Dodgson, Charles Lutwidge
Donne, John
Dostoevsky, Fyodor
    Mikhailovich
Doyle, Arthur Conan
Dryden, John
Ducasse, Isidore-Lucien
Dumas, Alexandre
    (Dumas Père)
Dumas, Alexandre
    (Dumas Fils)

Eeden, Frederik van
Eliot, George
    (Pseudonym of Mary Ann Evans)
Eliot, Thomas Stearns
Empedocles
Esenin, Sergei
Euripides
Evelyn, John
Ewliya, Effendi

Fadeyev, Alexander Alexandrovich
Faulkner, William
Fergusson, Robert
Fitzgerald, Francis Scott Key
Flaubert, Gustave
Forcellini, Egidio
Frazer, Sir James George

Gautier, Théophile
Gay, John
Gide, André Paul Guillaume
Giraldus Cambrensis, or
    Girard de Barri
Gissing, George

Goethe, Johann Wolfgang von
Gogol, Nikolai Vasilyevich
Goldsmith, Oliver
Goncharov, Ivan Aleksandrovich
Goncourt, Jules Alfred Huot de
Gordon, Adam Lindsay
Gorky, Maxim
Gosse, Sir Edmund William
Gray, Thomas
Grillparzer, Franz
Gurney, Ivor Bertie

Haggard, Sir Henry Rider
Hall, Radclyffe
Haller, Albrecht von
Hawker, Robert Stephen
Hazlitt, William
Heine, Heinrich
Herodotus
Herrick, Robert
Hesse, Hermann
Hill, Thomas
Hoccleve, Thomas
Hoffmann, Ernst Theodor
    Wilhelm (or Amadeus)
Hoffmann, Heinrich
Hölderlin, Johann Christian
    Friedrich
Holmes, Sir Gordon Morgan
Homer
Hugo, Victor Marie
Huxley, Aldous Leonard

Ibsen, Henrik

Jacopone da Todi
James, Henry
Johnson, Samuel
Joyce, James Augustine
    Aloysius
Jung-Stilling, Johann Heinrich
Juvenal (Decimus Junius
    Juvenalis)

Kafka, Franz
Kavan, Anna
Kawabata, Yasunari
Keats, John

(*See* Baron Corvo)
Rossetti, Christina Georgina
Rossetti, Dante Gabriel
Rousseau, Jean-Jacques
Ruskin, John

Sacher-Masoch, Leopold
  Ritter von
Sackville-West, Victoria Mary (Vita)
Sade, Donatien Alphonse
  François Comte de
Sand, George
Sappho
Sartre, Jean-Paul
Sassoon, Siegfried
Savage, Richard
Schiller, Johann Christoph
  Friedrich von
Schnitzler, Arthur
Scott, Sir Walter
Seabrook, William
Seaman, Elizabeth (*see* Nellie Bly)
Sedley, Sir Charles
Serenus Sammonicus, Quintus
Shakespeare, William
Shaw, George Bernard
Shelley, Percy Bysshe
Silva, José Asunción
Sitwell, Edith
Skelton, John
Smart, Christopher
Southey, Robert
Spenser, Edmund
Staël, Germaine de
Stafford, Richard
Steele, Richard
Steinbeck, John Ernst
Stendhal
Stephen, James Kenneth
Sterne, Laurence
Stevenson, Robert Louis
Stow, John
Stowe, Harriet Beecher

Strindberg, Johan August
Summers, Montague
Swift, Jonathan
Swinburne, Algernon Charles

Taine, Hippolyte Adolphe
Tasso, Torquato
Tennyson, Alfred
Thomas, Dylan
Thompson, Francis
Tolstoy, Leo
Trollope, Anthony
Tryon, Thomas
Turgenev, Ivan Sergeevich

Verlaine, Paul
Vigny, Alfred Victor, Comte de
Virgil (or Vergil, Vergilius),
  Publius Maro
Voltaire

Ward, Edward
Wassermann, Jakob
Waugh, Evelyn Arthur St. John
Wells, Herbert George
Werfel, Franz
Wertheimer, Max
Wilde, Oscar Fingal
  O'Flahertie Wills
Witkiewicz, Stanislaw Ignacy
Wollstonecraft, Mary
Woolf, Virginia
Wordsworth, William

Yaari, Yehudah
Yavorov, Peyu
Yeats, William Butler
Young, Edward

Zola, Émile Edouard Charles Antoine
Zschokke, Johann Heinrich Daniel
Zweig, Stefan

Index

Note: Page references for main entries are in italics. Page references that are repeated, or followed by a number in parentheses, indicate that the indexed item appears in more than one main entry on the same page.

26, 26

American Journal of Psychiatry, 26-27, 26, 28, 126, 381, 421

American Journal of Psychology, 27, 28, 397, 491, 823, 925

American Neurological Association, 13, 27, 401

American Orthopsychiatric Association, 27

American Psychiatric Association, 26, 27-28, 61, 85, 126, 139, 144, 203, 222, 276, 352, 504, 510, 666, 777, 807, 864, 881, 889, 978, 995

American Psychological Association, 28, 397, 523, 531, 977

American Psychological Foundation, 995

Amerling, Karl, 28

Amethyst, 28

Amidas, 28

Amiel, Henri-Frédéric, 28-29

Amnesia, 24, 29, 259, 340, 471, 494, 576, 747

Amnon, 29

Amok, 29, 236, 494, 630, 934

Amour Médecin, L', 29

Amours du Chevalier de Faublas, Les, 29-30

Amphiaraus, 17

Amphion, 679

Amputation doll, 30

Amulets, 30, 43, 51, 171, 304, 579, 717, 864, 906, 952, 1002(2)

Amyntas III, 719

Amyotonia congenita, 694

Amythaon, 610

Anaclitic depression, 30

Anagogic interpretation, 30

Analytic group therapy, 30-31

Analyzing instrument, 31

Ananizapta, 31

Ananke, 31

Anatomy of Melancholy, The, 6, 8, 30, 31, 97, 113, 144, 206, 240, 417, 449, 481, 503, 527, 562, 748, 825, 931

Anaxagoras of Cleomenes, 31, 33

Anaxarchus, 4

Andersen, Hans Christian, 33

Andersen, Tryggve, 33

Andfinn, 932

Andreas-Salomé, Lou, 33, 910

André Cornélis, 33

Anemomania, 34

Anesthesia, 34, 128, 413, 618, 751

Anet, Claude, 801

Angell, James Rowland, 34, 248

Angelman, H., 403

Anger, A Treatise of, 262

Anglo-Saxon Herbal, 34, 717

Anhedonia, 34, 789

Anima, 34-35, 42, 61, 394, 505, 879

Animal electricity, 638

Animal magnetism, 7, 35, 69, 89, 266, 293, 340, 356, 415, 511, 580, 617, 680, 961, 992

Animals, 35; behavior of, 35, 560, 566, 807, 979; and learning, 920; psychology of, 189, 647, 783, 860, 872

Animal soul, 35

Animal spirits, 35, 112, 452, 826, 891, 893, 958

Anima sensitiva, 35-36, 879

Animism, 35–36, 879, 941

Animus, 35

Anna Bolena, 36, 693

Anna Karenina, 36

Annales Médico-Psychologiques, 36, 66, 126, 169

Anna O., 36, 125, 165, 757

Anne (Queen of England), 104, 488, 508

Année Psychologique, L', 36-37, 81, 102

Année Sociologique, L', 37

Anne of Austria, 726

Anniversary reaction, 37, 41, 608, 882, 896

Anomia, 37, 623

Anomie, 272

Anorexia nervosa, 37, 389, 661

Anouilh, Jean, 104

Anteneasmon (*sometimes called* Enthusiasmos), 37

Antensteiner, Anton, 883

Anthony *or* Antony, Saint, 37, 49

Anthropologie, 38, 450, 500

Anthropologium, 38, 450

Anthropometric Laboratory, 38, 352, 759

Anthroponomy, 451

Anticyra, 38, 417

Antimony, 38, 362, 605

Antinous, 38

Antiochus I, 38-39, 297

Antiochus III, 402

Antipalus Maleficiorum, 39, 934

Antiphon, 39

Anti-psychosis, 39

Antisthenes, 391

Anton, Gabriel, 39

Antoninus, Marcus Aurelius, 314

About The Authors

JOHN G. HOWELLS is formerly the Director of The Institute of Family
Psychiatry in Ipswich, England, and Chairman of the Section in the History
of Psychiatry of the World Psychiatric Association. He is the author of
many books on clinical psychiatry.
MARIA LIVIA OSBORN is Clinical Research Officer at The Institute of
Family Psychiatry. She is the author of numerous papers on history and
psychiatry.